ADVANCED RECONSTRUCTION

Spine

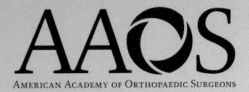

AMERICAN ACADEMY OF ORTHOPAEDIC SURGEONS

ADVANCED
RECONSTRUCTION
Spine

Edited by

Jeffrey C. Wang, MD
Chief, Orthopaedic Spine Service
Professor of Orthopaedics and Neurosurgery
Department of Orthopaedic Surgery
UCLA School of Medicine
Los Angeles, California

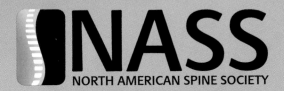

NORTH AMERICAN SPINE SOCIETY

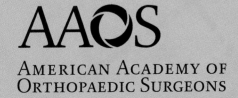

AMERICAN ACADEMY OF
ORTHOPAEDIC SURGEONS

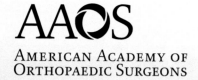

American Academy of Orthopaedic Surgeons
Board of Directors, 2011-2012

The material presented in **Advanced Reconstruction: Spine** has been made available by the American Academy of Orthopaedic Surgeons for educational purposes only. This material is not intended to present the only, or necessarily best, methods or procedures for the medical situations discussed, but rather is intended to represent an approach, view, statement, or opinion of the author(s) or producer(s), which may be helpful to others who face similar situations.

Some drugs or medical devices demonstrated in Academy courses or described in Academy print or electronic publications have not been cleared by the Food and Drug Administration (FDA) or have been cleared for specific uses only. The FDA has stated that it is the responsibility of the physician to determine the FDA clearance status of each drug or device he or she wishes to use in clinical practice.

Furthermore, any statements about commercial products are solely the opinion(s) of the author(s) and do not represent an Academy endorsement or evaluation of these products. These statements may not be used in advertising or for any commercial purpose.

CPT® is copyright 2010 American Medical Association (AMA). All rights reserved. No fee schedules, basic units, relative values, or related listings are included in CPT. The AMA assumes no liability for the data contained herein.

Published 2011 by the
American Academy of Orthopaedic Surgeons
6300 North River Road
Rosemont, IL 60018

Copyright 2011
by the American Academy of Orthopaedic Surgeons

ISBN 978-0-89203-581-6

Printed in Canada

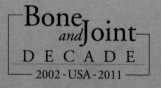

Acknowledgments

Editor, *Advanced Reconstruction: Spine*
Jeffrey C. Wang, MD

North American Spine Society
Board of Directors, 2010-2011

Gregory J. Przybylski, MD
President
Edison, NJ

Michael H. Heggeness, MD, PhD
First Vice President
Houston, TX

Charles A. Mick, MD
Second Vice President
Northampton, MA

Heidi Prather, DO
Secretary
St. Louis, MO

William C. Watters III, MD
Treasurer
Houston, TX

Ray M. Baker, MD
Past President
Bellevue, WA

Eric J. Muehlbauer, MJ, CAE
Executive Director
Burr Ridge, IL

Daniel K. Resnick, MD
Research Council Director
Madison, WI

Venu Akuthota, MD
Education Council Director
Aurora, CO

William Mitchell, MD
Health Policy Council Co-Director
Mt. Laurel, NJ

Christopher J. Standaert, MD
Health Policy Council Co-Director
Seattle, WA

Alexander J. Ghanayem, MD
Administration and Development Council Director
Maywood, IL

Charles A. Reitman, MD
Evidence Compilation and Analysis Chair
Houston, TX

Zoher Ghogawala, MD
Clinical Research Development Chair
Greenwich, CT

Jeffrey C. Wang, MD
Continuing Medical Education Chair
Los Angeles, CA

Eeric Truumees, MD
Education Publishing Chair
Austin, TX

Christopher M. Bono, MD
Professional, Economic and Regulatory Chair
Boston, MA

Raj D. Rao, MD
Advocacy Chair
Milwaukee, WI

Jerome Schofferman, MD
Section Development Chair
Daly City and San Francisco, CA

F. Todd Wetzel, MD
Governance Committee Chair
Philadelphia, PA

Marjorie Eskay-Auerbach, MD, JD
Ethics Committee Chair
Tucson, AZ

David Rothman, PhD
Ethicist
New York, NY

Contributors

Jean-Jacques Abitbol, MD, FRCSC
California Spine Group
San Diego, California

Kuniyoshi Abumi, MD
Professor
Department of Spinal Reconstruction
Hokkaido University Graduate School of Medicine
Sapporo, Japan

Todd J. Albert, MD
Chairman and Professor
Department of Orthopaedic Surgery
Thomas Jefferson University Hospital
Philadelphia, Pennsylvania

Richard Todd Allen, MD, PhD
Assistant Clinical Professor
Spine & Orthopaedic Surgery
Department of Orthopaedic Surgery
University of California, San Diego
San Diego, California

Howard S. An, MD
Department of Orthopaedic Surgery
Rush University Medical Center
Chicago, Illinois

Nomaan Ashraf, MD, MBA
Clinical Fellow, Spine Surgery
The Spine Institute of Santa Monica
Santa Monica, California

Hyun Bae, MD
Research Director
The Spine Institute of Santa Monica
Santa Monica, California

James R. Bailey, MD
Orthopaedic Surgery Resident
Department of Orthopaedic Surgery
Naval Medical Center, San Diego
San Diego, California

Hieu Ball, MD, MPH
Adult and Pediatric Spine Surgeon
California Comprehensive Spine Institute
Walnut Creek, California

Rudolf W. Beisse, MD
Head of Department
Spine Center
Orthopedic Hospital Munich
Munich, Germany

Carlo Bellabarba, MD
Associate Professor
Department of Orthopaedics and Sports Medicine – Spine
University of Washington
Harborview Medical Center
Seattle, Washington

Sigurd Berven, MD
Associate Professor in Residence
Department of Orthopaedic Surgery
University of California, San Francisco
San Francisco, California

Shay Bess, MD
Rocky Mountain Hospital for Children
Denver, Colorado

Nitin Bhatia, MD
Chief, Spine Service
Department of Orthopaedic Surgery
University of California, Irvine
Irvine, California

Henry H. Bohlman, MD
Professor of Orthopaedic Surgery
Director of University Hospitals Spine Institute
Department of Orthopaedic Surgery
University Hospitals of Cleveland Case Medical Center
Cleveland, Ohio

Richard J. Bransford, MD
Assistant Professor
Department of Orthopaedics and Sports Medicine
Harborview Medical Center
University of Washington School of Medicine
Seattle, Washington

Salvador A. Brau, MD, FACS
Visiting Assistant Clinical Professor of Surgery
Vascular Division
Keck School of Medicine
University of Southern California
Los Angeles, California

John T. Braun, MD
Associate Professor
Department of Orthopaedics and Rehabilitation
University of Vermont
Burlington, Vermont

Keith H. Bridwell, MD
Asa C. and Dorothy W. Jones Professor
  of Orthopaedic Surgery
Department of Orthopaedic Surgery
Washington University in St. Louis
St. Louis, Missouri

Darrel S. Brodke, MD
Professor and Vice Chair
Department of Orthopaedics
University of Utah
Salt Lake City, Utah

Justin Bundy, MD
Visiting Instructor
Department of Orthopaedics
University of Utah
Salt Lake City, Utah

Gregory D. Carlson, MD
Assistant Clinical Professor
Department of Orthopaedic Surgery
University of California, Irvine
Orthopaedic Specialty Institute
Orange, California

Eugene J. Carragee, MD
Department of Orthopaedic Surgery
Stanford University School of Medicine
Stanford, California

Jens R. Chapman, MD
Professor
Director of Spine Service
Hansjöerg Wyss Endowed Chair
Department of Orthopaedics and Sports Medicine
University of Washington
Seattle, Washington

Jack Chen, MD
Orthopaedic Spine Surgeon
Orthopaedic Specialty Institute
Orange, California

Woosik M. Chung, MD
Fellow in Spine Surgery
Emory Spine Center
Emory University
Atlanta, Georgia

Norman B. Chutkan, MD, FACS
Chairman
Department of Orthopaedic Surgery
Medical College of Georgia
Augusta, Georgia

John S. Clapp, MD
Orthopaedic Surgery Resident
Department of Orthopaedic Surgery
Medical College of Georgia
Augusta, Georgia

Charles H. Crawford III, MD
Spine Fellow
Department of Orthopaedic Surgery
Washington University in St. Louis
St. Louis, Missouri

Adam C. Crowl, MD
Advanced Orthopaedic Centers
Richmond, Virginia

Bradford L. Currier, MD
Professor of Orthopedics
Department of Orthopedics
Mayo Clinic
Rochester, Minnesota

Andrew Dailey, MD
Associate Professor
Department of Neurosurgery
University of Utah
Salt Lake City, Utah

Michael D. Daubs, MD
Assistant Professor
Department of Orthopaedic Surgery
University of Utah
Salt Lake City, Utah

Mark L. Dumonski, MD
Department of Orthopaedic Surgery
Rush University Medical Center
Chicago, Illinois

Jason C. Eck, DO, MS
Assistant Professor
Department of Orthopaedic Surgery
University of Massachusetts
Worcester, Massachusetts

Sanford E. Emery, MD, MBA
Professor and Chairman
Department of Orthopaedics
West Virginia University
Morgantown, West Virginia

Jason David Eubanks, MD
Fellow
Department of Orthopaedics
University of Pittsburgh Medical Center
Pittsburgh, Pennsylvania

Michael L. Fernandez, MD
Spine Fellow
Department of Orthopaedic Surgery
University of Utah
Salt Lake City, Utah

Michael Finn, MD
Fellow
Department of Orthopedics
University of Wisconsin–Madison
Madison, Wisconsin

Jeffrey S. Fischgrund, MD
Fellowship Director
Department of Orthopaedic Surgery
William Beaumont Hospital
Royal Oak, Michigan

David E. Fish, MD, MPH
Assistant Professor
Department of Orthopaedic Surgery
David Geffen School of Medicine
UCLA
Los Angeles, California

Winston Fong, MD
Spine Surgeon and Clinical Instructor
Department of Orthopaedic Surgery
UCLA Comprehensive Spine Center
Los Angeles, California

John C. France, MD
Professor of Orthopaedic and Neurosurgery
Department of Orthopaedics
West Virginia University
Morgantown, West Virginia

Christopher G. Furey, MD
Associate Professor of Orthopaedic Surgery
Department of Orthopaedic Surgery
University Hospitals of Cleveland Case Medical Center
Cleveland, Ohio

Steven R. Garfin, MD
Professor and Chair
Department of Orthopaedic Surgery
University of California, San Diego
San Diego, California

Alexander J. Ghanayem, MD
Director, Division of Spine Surgery
Professor
Department of Orthopaedic Surgery and Rehabilitation
Loyola University Medical Center
Maywood, Illinois

Anthony Gibson, MBBS
Department of Orthopaedic Surgery
University of California, San Francisco
San Francisco, California

Alex Gitelman, MD
Spine Surgery Fellow
UCLA Comprehensive Spine Center
UCLA Medical Center
Los Angeles, California

Nicolas E. Grisoni, MD
Center for Spinal Disorders
St. Anthony North Hospital
Westminster, Colorado

Eric B. Harris, MD
Director of Orthopaedic Spine Surgery
Department of Orthopaedics
Naval Medical Center
San Diego, California

Robert A. Hart, MD, MA
Associate Professor and Program Director
Department of Orthopaedics
Oregon Health and Sciences University
Portland, Oregon

John G. Heller, MD
Professor of Orthopaedic Surgery
Spine Fellowship Director
Department of Orthopaedic Surgery
The Emory Spine Center
Emory University School of Medicine
Atlanta, Georgia

Alan S. Hilibrand, MD
Professor of Orthopaedic Surgery and Neurosurgery
The Rothman Institute
Jefferson Medical College
Philadelphia, Pennsylvania

Wellington K. Hsu, MD
Assistant Professor
Department of Orthopaedic Surgery
and Department of Neurological Surgery
Northwestern University Feinberg School of Medicine
Chicago, Illinois

Serena S. Hu, MD
Professor and Vice Chair
Department of Orthopaedic Surgery
University of California, San Francisco
San Francisco, California

Manabu Ito, MD
Assistant Professor
Department of Orthopaedic Surgery
Hokkaido University Graduate School of Medicine
Sapporo, Japan

Michael E. Janssen, DO
President
Center for Spinal Disorders
St. Anthony North Hospital
Westminster, Colorado

Louis G. Jenis, MD
Clinical Associate Professor
Department of Orthopaedic Surgery
Tufts University School of Medicine
Boston Spine Group
Boston, Massachusetts

James Kang, MD
Professor
Department of Orthopaedics
University of Pittsburgh Medical Center
Pittsburgh, Pennsylvania

Geoffrey Kaung, MD, MS
Fellow, Adult Spine Surgery
Department of Orthopaedic Surgery
Oregon Health and Science University
Portland, Oregon

A. Jay Khanna, MD, MBA
Assistant Professor of Orthopaedic Surgery
and Biomedical Engineering
Department of Orthopaedic Surgery
Johns Hopkins University
Baltimore, Maryland

Choll W. Kim, MD, PhD
Associate Clinical Professor
University of California, San Diego
Spine Institute of San Diego
Center for Minimally Invasive Spine Surgery
at Alvarado Hospital
San Diego, California

Yoshihisa Kotani, MD
Assistant Professor
Department of Orthopaedic Surgery
Hokkaido University Hospital
Sapporo, Japan

Timothy R. Kuklo, MD, JD
Associate Professor
Department of Orthopaedic Surgery
Washington University in St. Louis
St. Louis, Missouri

Mark Kuper, DO
Staff Physician
Harris Methodist Hospital Fort Worth
Fort Worth, Texas

Khai S. Lam, FRCS (Orth)
Consultant Orthopaedic and Spinal Surgeon
Department of Orthopaedics
Guy's and St. Thomas' Hospitals
London, England

James Eric Lashley, MD
Associates in Orthopaedics and Sports Medicine
Dalton, Georgia

James P. Lawrence, MD, MBA
Assistant Professor
Department of Surgery
Division of Orthopaedics
Albany Medical College
Albany, New York

Charles Gerald T. Ledonio, MD
Spine Research Fellow
Department of Orthopaedic Surgery
University of Minnesota
Minneapolis, Minnesota

Steven S. Lee, MD
Orthopaedic Spine Surgery
Muir Orthopaedic Specialists
John Muir Medical Center
Walnut Creek, California

Yu-Po Lee, MD
Assistant Clinical Professor
Department of Orthopaedic Surgery
University of California, San Diego
San Diego, California

Lawrence G. Lenke, MD
The Jerome J. Gilden Professor of Orthopaedic Surgery
Professor of Neurological Surgery
Department of Orthopaedic Surgery
Washington University School of Medicine in St. Louis
St. Louis, Missouri

Isador H. Lieberman, MD, MBA, FRCSC
Professor of Surgery
Chairman
Medical Interventional and Surgical Spine Center
Cleveland Clinic Florida
Weston, Florida

Ian A. Madom, MD
Clinical Instructor
Department of Orthopaedic Surgery
Brown Alpert Medical School
Providence, Rhode Island

Kamran Majid, MD
Orthopaedic Spine Surgeon
Orthopaedic and Spine Specialists
York, Pennsylvania

Scott McGovern, MD
Fellow in Spine Surgery
Department of Orthopaedic Surgery
UCLA Comprehensive Spine Center
Santa Monica, California

Thomas Mroz, MD
Neurological Institute
Department of Orthopaedic and Neurological Surgery
Cleveland Clinic
Cleveland, Ohio

Peter O. Newton, MD
Chief of Orthopaedic Research and Scoliosis Service
Pediatric Orthopaedic and Scoliosis Center
Rady Children's Hospital
Associate Clinical Professor
Department of Orthopaedic Surgery
University of California, San Diego
San Diego, California

Joseph R. O'Brien, MD
Assistant Professor
Department of Orthopaedic Surgery
The George Washington University
Washington, D.C.

Brian A. O'Shaughnessy, MD
Fellow in Adult and Pediatric Spinal Surgery
Department of Orthopaedic Surgery
Washington University in St. Louis
Saint Louis, Missouri

Murat Pekmezci, MD
Assistant Clinical Professor
Department of Orthopedic Surgery
University of California, San Francisco
San Francisco, California

Frank M. Phillips, MD
Professor of Orthopaedic Surgery
Rush University Medical Center
Chicago, Illinois

David W. Polly, Jr, MD
Professor and Chief of Spine Service
Department of Orthopaedic Surgery
University of Minnesota
Minneapolis, Minnesota

Alexander K. Powers, MD
Fellow
Department of Neurosurgery
Washington University School of Medicine in St. Louis
St. Louis Children's Hospital
St. Louis, Missouri

A.F. Pull ter Gunne, MD
Department of Orthopaedic Surgery
Johns Hopkins Hospital
Baltimore, Maryland

Sheeraz A. Qureshi, MD, MBA
Assistant Professor of Orthopaedic Surgery
Chief of Spinal Trauma
Department of Orthopaedic Surgery
Mount Sinai Hospital
New York, New York

Ramin Raiszadeh, MD
Director of Clinical Research
Department of Orthopaedic Surgery
Spine Institute of San Diego
San Diego, California

Raj D. Rao, MD
Professor of Orthopaedic Surgery
Director of Spine Surgery
Department of Orthopaedic Surgery
Medical College of Wisconsin
Milwaukee, Wisconsin

John M. Rhee, MD
Associate Professor
Department of Orthopaedics
Emory Spine Center
Emory University School of Medicine
Atlanta, Georgia

Richard D. Rhim, MD
Department of Orthopaedic Surgery
New England Baptist Hospital
Boston, Massachusetts

K. Daniel Riew, MD
Department of Orthopaedic Surgery
Washington University in St. Louis
St. Louis, Missouri

Jeffrey A. Rihn, MD
Assistant Professor
Department of Orthopaedic Surgery
Thomas Jefferson University Hospital
The Rothman Institute
Philadelphia, Pennsylvania

Lee H. Riley III, MD
Chief of Spine Division
Associate Professor of Orthopaedic Surgery and Neurosurgery
Department of Orthopaedic Surgery
Johns Hopkins University School of Medicine
Baltimore, Maryland

Anthony Rinella, MD
Assistant Professor
Department of Orthopaedic Surgery
Loyola University Medical Center
Maywood, Illinois

M.L. Chip Routt, Jr, MD
Professor
Department of Orthopaedics and Sports Medicine – Trauma
Harborview Medical Center
Seattle, Washington

Kasra Rowshan, MD
Orthopaedic Surgeon
Department of Orthopaedic Surgery
University of California, Irvine
Orange, California

Paul T. Rubery, Jr, MD
Associate Professor of Orthopaedic Surgery and Pediatrics
Department of Orthopaedic Surgery
University of Rochester
Rochester, New York

James H. Rubright, MD
Resident Physician
Department of Orthopaedics and Rehabilitation
University of Vermont School of Medicine
  and Fletcher Allen Health Care
Burlington, Vermont

Harvinder S. Sandhu, MD
Associate Professor of Orthopaedic Surgery
Department of Orthopaedic Surgery
Hospital for Special Surgery
New York, New York

James A. Sanfilippo, MD
Spine Fellow
Clinical Instructor
Department of Orthopaedics
Emory University Spine Center
Atlanta, Georgia

Wudbhav N. Sankar, MD
Assistant Professor
Department of Orthopaedic Surgery
Children's Hospital of Philadelphia
Philadelphia, Pennsylvania

Rick C. Sasso, MD
Associate Professor of Clinical Orthopaedic Surgery
Indiana Spine Group
Indiana University School of Medicine
Indianapolis, Indiana

Thomas A. Schildhauer, MD, PhD
Professor and Chairman
Universitätsklinik für Unfallchirurgie
Medizinische Universität Graz
Graz, Austria

James Schwender, MD
Orthopaedic Spine Surgeon
Twin Cities Spine Center
Minneapolis, Minnesota

Thomas Scioscia, MD
West End Orthopaedic Clinic
Richmond, Virginia

Jonathan N. Sembrano, MD
Assistant Professor
Department of Orthopaedic Surgery
University of Minnesota
Minneapolis, Minnesota

Arya Nick Shamie, MD
Associate Professor of Orthopaedic Surgery
  and Neurosurgery
UCLA Spine Center
David Geffen School of Medicine at UCLA
Los Angeles, California

Edward D. Simmons, MD, CM, MSc, FRCSC
Clinical Professor
Department of Orthopaedic Surgery
State University of New York at Buffalo
Buffalo, New York

David L. Skaggs, MD
Endowed Chair of Pediatric Spinal Disorders
Associate Professor
Department of Orthopaedics
University of Southern California
Los Angeles, California

Michael P. Steinmetz, MD
Assistant Professor
Department of Neurosurgery
Cleveland Clinic
Cleveland, Ohio

David H. Strothman, MD
Orthopaedic Surgeon
Institute for Low Back and Neck Care
Bloomington, Minnesota

Willem S. Strydom, FCS SA (Ortho), MMED (Ortho)
Senior Clinical Fellow, Spine Surgery
Department of Orthopaedics
Guy's Hospital
London, England

Thomas Sylvester, MD
Chief Resident
Department of Orthopaedic Surgery
Loyola University Medical Center
Maywood, Illinois

Ehsan Tabaraee, MS, MD
Department of Orthopaedic Surgery
The George Washington University
Washington, D.C.

Brett A. Taylor, MD
Adult Spine Surgeon
The Orthopedic Center of St. Louis
Chesterfield, Missouri

William R. Taylor, MD
Clinical Professor of Surgery
Minimally Invasive and Complex Spine
Division of Neurosurgery
University of California, San Diego
San Diego, California

Stephen Timon, MD
Assistant Clinical Professor
Department of Orthopaedic Surgery
University of Texas Southwestern Medical Center
Dallas, Texas
North Texas Spinal Institute at All-Star Orthopaedics
Irving, Texas

Cliff Tribus, MD
Associate Professor
Department of Orthopaedics and Rehabilitative Medicine
University of Wisconsin—Madison
Madison, Wisconsin

Eeric Truumees, MD
Attending Spine Surgeon
Department of Orthopaedic Surgery
William Beaumont Hospital
Royal Oak, Michigan

Alexander Vaccaro, MD, PhD
Professor
Rothman Institute
Thomas Jefferson University
Philadelphia, Pennsylvania

Eric S. Varley, DO
Postdoctoral Research Fellow
Department of Orthopaedic Surgery
University of California, San Diego
San Diego, California

Corey J. Wallach, MD
Orthopaedic Spine Surgeon and Medical Director
The Anderson Clinic Spine Center
Arlington, Virginia

Jeffrey C. Wang, MD
Chief, Orthopaedic Spine Service
Professor of Orthopaedics and Neurosurgery
Department of Orthopaedic Surgery
UCLA School of Medicine
Los Angeles, California

Joseph K. Weistroffer, MD
Assistant Professor
Department of Orthopaedic Surgery
Northwestern University Feinberg School of Medicine
Chicago, Illinois

Christopher F. Wolf, MD
Department of Orthopaedic Surgery
UCLA
Los Angeles, California

Adam L. Wollowick, MD
Assistant Professor
Department of Orthopaedic Surgery
Albert Einstein College of Medicine
Bronx, New York

Anthony T. Yeung, MD
Associate
Desert Institute for Spine Care
Voluntary Clinical Associate Professor
Department of Orthopaedic Surgery
University of California, San Diego
San Diego, California

Christopher A. Yeung, MD
Desert Institute for Spine Care
Phoenix, Arizona

S. Tim Yoon, MD, PhD
Assistant Professor
Department of Orthopaedic Surgery
Emory University
Atlanta, Georgia

Jason P. Young, MD
Chief Resident
Department of Orthopaedic Surgery
Loyola University Medical Center
Chicago, Illinois

Paul H. Young, MD
Clinical Professor
Department of Surgery
Section of Neurosurgery
St. Louis University School of Medicine
St. Louis, Missouri

Jim A. Youssef, MD
Orthopedic Spine Surgeon
Durango Orthopedic Associates/Spine Colorado
Durango, Colorado

Warren D. Yu, MD
Associate Professor
Department of Orthopaedic Surgery
The George Washington University
Washington, D.C.

Preface

With advances in modern surgical techniques and the proliferation of new technologies, spine surgery and its indications are changing rapidly. Although several spine textbooks on focused topics are available, the need existed for a single volume that described surgical procedures in a focused, consistent, and easily accessible manner. **Advanced Reconstruction: Spine** grew out of this need.

The goal of **Advanced Reconstruction: Spine**, a combined effort of the American Academy of Orthopaedic Surgeons and the North American Spine Society, is to provide a detailed and practical guide to state-of-the-art surgical techniques. The book strives to give the reader a comprehensive understanding of the procedures used in contemporary spine surgery, including the classic procedures that are still in use. The chapters in **Advanced Reconstruction: Spine** are uniformly organized, each containing standard sections on indications, contraindications, and alternative treatments. A section on results briefly reviews the literature supporting or criticizing the procedure. The equipment and surgical preparation necessary to complete the procedure are described, as are tips for avoiding pitfalls and complications. The heart of each chapter is a step-by-step guide to the procedure as performed by the author, an expert in that particular technique. Each author was asked to include intraoperative photographs clearly illustrating the steps in the surgical technique. Although reading this book clearly is not a substitute for thorough training and supervision, I hope that **Advanced Reconstruction: Spine** will serve as a valuable and practical tool that helps spine surgeons gain an understanding of the elements of spine procedures that they may not perform on a regular basis.

I wish first to thank the authors for sharing their expertise. This group of highly skilled surgeons has generously donated their personal time in preparing the detailed chapters for this surgical textbook. I also want to thank my wife, Christina, and my family for their understanding in allowing me to devote my time to this textbook. In addition, I want to thank the Academy staff who worked long, tireless hours in developing, editing, and producing this book: Marilyn Fox, PhD, Director of Publications; Laurie Braun, Managing Editor; Michelle Bruno, Publications Assistant, Mary Steermann, Senior Manager, Production and Archives; and the production staff. This textbook would not be possible without their dedication and their passion. Finally, I would also like to thank both the American Academy of Orthopaedic Surgeons and the North American Spine Society for their support of this endeavor. I hope that you will find **Advanced Reconstruction: Spine** to be a valuable resource when preparing for spine procedures.

Jeffrey C. Wang, MD
Chief, Orthopaedic Spine Service
Professor of Orthopaedics and Neurosurgery
Department of Orthopaedic Surgery
UCLA School of Medicine
Los Angeles, California

Table of Contents

Section 1   **Cervical Spine**

1   Anterior Cervical Diskectomy and Fusion   3
     John C. France, MD

2   Cervical Arthroplasty   13
     Rick C. Sasso, MD
     James Eric Lashley, MD

3   Anterior Cervical Corpectomy and Fusion   21
     Kamran Majid, MD
     Jeffrey S. Fischgrund, MD

4   Transoral Odontoid Excision   31
     K. Daniel Riew, MD
     Adam L. Wollowick, MD
     Brett A. Taylor, MD

5   Retropharyngeal Approaches to the Upper Cervical Spine   43
     Michael Finn, MD
     Andrew Dailey, MD

6   Anterior Odontoid Screw Placement   55
     Eric B. Harris, MD
     Alexander Vaccaro, MD, PhD

7   Anterior Cervicothoracic Fusion   63
     Howard S. An, MD
     Mark L. Dumonski, MD

8   Posterior Cervical Foraminotomy and Diskectomy   71
     Jason David Eubanks, MD
     James Kang, MD

9   Minimally Invasive Posterior Laminoforaminotomy/Diskectomy   81
     Thomas Mroz, MD
     Michael P. Steinmetz, MD
     K. Daniel Riew, MD

10   Posterior Subaxial Cervical Fusion   89
     Thomas Scioscia, MD
     Adam C. Crowl, MD

11   Cervical Laminectomy and Fusion   97
     Raj D. Rao, MD
     Ian A. Madom, MD

12   Open-Door Cervical Laminaplasty   107
     Winston Fong, MD
     Scott McGovern, MD
     Jeffrey C. Wang, MD

13   Cervical Laminaplasty: French Door   115
     John G. Heller, MD
     James A. Sanfilippo, MD

14   Posterior Occipitocervical Fusion   125
     Eeric Truumees, MD

15   Posterior C2 Fixation   139
Todd J. Albert, MD
Jeffrey A. Rihn, MD

16   C1-C2 Transarticular Fixation   149
Jason C. Eck, DO, MS
Bradford L. Currier, MD

17   Fixation to C1 and C2   159
Robert A. Hart, MD, MA
Geoffrey Kaung, MD, MS

18   Posterior Cervical Wiring Technique   167
Sanford E. Emery, MD, MBA

19   Occipitocervical Fusion   175
Lee H. Riley III, MD
A.F. Pull ter Gunne, MD
A. Jay Khanna, MD, MBA

20   Posterior Cervicothoracic Fusion   183
Alexander J. Ghanayem, MD
Thomas Sylvester, MD

21   Cervical Pedicle Screw Fixation   191
Kuniyoshi Abumi, MD
Manabu Ito, MD
Yoshihisa Kotani, MD

22   Cervical Osteotomy   203
Edward D. Simmons, MD, CM, MSc, FRCSC

23   Minimally Invasive Posterior Cervical Lateral Mass Fusion   213
James P. Lawrence, MD, MBA
Alan S. Hilibrand, MD

Section 2   **Thoracic Spine**

24   Thoracic Pedicle Screw Fixation   221
Sigurd Berven, MD
Anthony Gibson, MBBS

25   Posterolateral Approaches for Thoracic Diskectomy   231
Carlo Bellabarba, MD
Richard J. Bransford, MD
Jens R. Chapman, MD

26   The Costotransversectomy Approach for Vertebrectomy   243
Michael D. Daubs, MD
Michael L. Fernandez, MD

27   Posterior Thoracic Osteotomy: Smith-Petersen Approach   253
David W. Polly, Jr, MD
Jonathan N. Sembrano, MD
Charles Gerald T. Ledonio, MD

28   Posterior Thoracic Vertebral Column Resection   265
Alexander K. Powers, MD
Brian A. O'Shaughnessy, MD
Lawrence G. Lenke, MD

29   Pedicle Subtraction Osteotomy   277
Serena S. Hu, MD
Murat Pekmezci, MD

30   Surgical Treatment of Thoracic Scoliosis   287
Brian A. O'Shaughnessy, MD
Charles H. Crawford III, MD
Keith H. Bridwell, MD

31   Transthoracic Diskectomy: Anterior Approach   303
Anthony Rinella, MD
Alex Gitelman, MD

32   Anterior Thoracoscopic Diskectomy and Anterior Release   309
Peter O. Newton, MD
Eric S. Varley, DO

33   Thoracoscopic Corpectomy and Fusion   319
Rudolf W. Beisse, MD

34   Open Transthoracic Corpectomy/Fusion   331
S. Tim Yoon, MD, PhD
James A. Sanfilippo, MD

35   Anterior Mini-Open Approach for Scoliosis Correction   339
Khai S. Lam, FRCS (Ortho)
Willem S. Strydom, FCS SA (Ortho), MMED (Ortho)

36   Fusionless Scoliosis Surgery   351
John T. Braun, MD
James Rubright, MD

37   Rib Anchors in Distraction-Based Growing Spine Implants   359
Wudbhav N. Sankar, MD
David L. Skaggs, MD

38   Posterior Fixation of Thoracolumbar Burst Fractures   371
Darrel S. Brodke, MD
Justin Bundy, MD

39   Treatment of Fractures and Dislocations at the Spinopelvic Junction   379
Thomas A. Schildhauer, MD, PhD
Carlo Bellabarba, MD
M.L. Chip Routt, Jr, MD
Jens R. Chapman, MD

Section 3   **Lumbar Spine**

40   Anterior Approaches to the Lumbar Spine   395
Salvador A. Brau, MD, FACS

41   Anterior Lumbar Interbody Fusion (With Plating)   405
Woosik M. Chung, MD
John M. Rhee, MD

42 Lumbar Arthroplasty: Anterior Approach   415
    Nicolas E. Grisoni, MD
    Michael E. Janssen, DO

43 Anterior Lumbar Corpectomy   425
    Paul T. Rubery, Jr, MD

44 Lumbar Microdiskectomy/Foraminotomy   435
    Hyun Bae, MD
    Nomaan Ashraf, MD, MBA

45 Minimally Invasive Microdiskectomy and Microforaminotomy   441
    Arya Nick Shamie, MD

46 Lumbar Laminectomy   447
    Gregory D. Carlson, MD
    Jack Chen, MD

47 Unilateral Partial Laminotomy (Laminaplasty) for Bilateral Decompression   455
    Paul H. Young, MD
    Jason P. Young, MD

48 Posterior Pedicle Screw Fixation With Posterolateral Fusion   463
    Steven S. Lee, MD

49 Percutaneous Pedicle Screw Fixation in the Lumbar Spine   471
    Yu-Po Lee, MD
    Mark Kuper, DO

50 Posterior Lumbar Interbody Fusion   477
    Hieu Ball, MD, MPH

51 Transforaminal Lumbar Interbody Fusion   485
    Stephen Timon, MD

52 Minimally Invasive Lumbar Decompression and Interbody Fusion   493
    Corey J. Wallach, MD

53 Mini-Open (Wiltse Approach) Decompression/Fusion   501
    David H. Strothman, MD
    James Schwender, MD

54 Spondylolisthesis: Decompression/Fusion and Possible Reduction   509
    Louis G. Jenis, MD
    Richard D. Rhim, MD

55 Bohlman Fibular Technique for Interbody Fusion in the Lumbosacral Spine   517
    Sheeraz A. Qureshi, MD, MBA
    Christopher G. Furey, MD
    Henry H. Bohlman, MD

56 Lateral Transpsoas Approach/Fusion   525
    Shay Bess, MD
    Jim A. Youssef, MD

57 Percutaneous Transsacral Lumbar Interbody Fusion   535
    Kasra Rowshan, MD
    Nitin Bhatia, MD

58   Pars Repair   543
      Wellington K. Hsu, MD
      Joseph K. Weistroffer, MD

59   Translaminar and Direct Facet Screw Placement   549
      Isador H. Lieberman, MD, MBA, FRCSC

60   Interspinous Spacers in the Lumbar Spine   557
      Thomas Scioscia, MD
      Adam C. Crowl, MD

61   Lumbar Osteotomy   563
      Cliff Tribus, MD

62   Treatment of Lumbar Pseudarthrosis   571
      Christopher F. Wolf, MD
      Harvinder S. Sandhu, MD
      Jeffrey C. Wang, MD

63   Sacroiliac Fixation   581
      Timothy R. Kuklo, MD, JD

64   Lumbar Scoliosis   589
      Norman B. Chutkan, MD, FACS
      John S. Clapp, MD

65   Pedicle-Based Posterior Dynamic Stabilization   599
      Warren D. Yu, MD
      Ehsan Tabaraee, MS, MD
      Joseph R. O'Brien, MD

66   Posterolateral Endoscopic Lumbar Diskectomy   611
      Anthony T. Yeung, MD
      Christopher A. Yeung, MD

Section 4   Special Topics

67   Pedicle Screw Fixation in Osteoporotic Bone   627
      James R. Bailey, MD
      Eric B. Harris, MD
      Jean-Jacques Abitbol, MD, FRCSC

68   Provocative Diskography in Spine Surgery   635
      Eugene J. Carragee, MD

69   Computer-Assisted Spine Surgery   643
      Choll W. Kim, MD, PhD
      Ramin Raiszadeh, MD
      William R. Taylor, MD
      Steven R. Garfin, MD

70   Kyphoplasty and Vertebroplasty   651
      Richard Todd Allen, MD, PhD
      Frank M. Phillips, MD

71   Spinal Epidural Injections for Lumbar Spinal Radiculopathy Pain 661
      David E. Fish, MD, MPH

      Index   669

1   Anterior Cervical Diskectomy and Fusion   3
     John C. France, MD

2   Cervical Arthroplasty   13
     Rick C. Sasso, MD
     James Eric Lashley, MD

3   Anterior Cervical Corpectomy and Fusion   21
     Kamran Majid, MD
     Jeffrey S. Fischgrund, MD

4   Transoral Odontoid Excision   31
     K. Daniel Riew, MD
     Adam L. Wollowick, MD
     Brett A. Taylor, MD

5   Retropharyngeal Approaches to the Upper Cervical Spine   43
     Michael Finn, MD
     Andrew Dailey, MD

6   Anterior Odontoid Screw Placement   55
     Eric B. Harris, MD
     Alexander Vaccaro, MD, PhD

7   Anterior Cervicothoracic Fusion   63
     Howard S. An, MD
     Mark L. Dumonski, MD

8   Posterior Cervical Foraminotomy and Diskectomy   71
     Jason David Eubanks, MD
     James Kang, MD

9   Minimally Invasive Posterior Laminoforaminotomy/Diskectomy   81
     Thomas Mroz, MD
     Michael P. Steinmetz, MD
     K. Daniel Riew, MD

10   Posterior Subaxial Cervical Fusion   89
     Thomas Scioscia, MD
     Adam C. Crowl, MD

11   Cervical Laminectomy and Fusion   97
     Raj D. Rao, MD
     Ian A. Madom, MD

12   Open-Door Cervical Laminaplasty   107
     Winston Fong, MD
     Scott McGovern, MD
     Jeffrey C. Wang, MD

13   Cervical Laminaplasty: French Door   115
     John G. Heller, MD
     James A. Sanfilippo, MD

14   Posterior Occipitocervical Fusion   125
     Eeric Truumees, MD

15 Posterior C2 Fixation   139
    Todd J. Albert, MD
    Jeffrey A. Rihn, MD

16 C1-C2 Transarticular Fixation   149
    Jason C. Eck, DO, MS
    Bradford L. Currier, MD

17 Fixation to C1 and C2   159
    Robert A. Hart, MD, MA
    Geoffrey Kaung, MD, MS

18 Posterior Cervical Wiring Technique   167
    Sanford E. Emery, MD, MBA

19 Occipitocervical Fusion   175
    Lee H. Riley III, MD
    A.F. Pull ter Gunne, MD
    A. Jay Khanna, MD, MBA

20 Posterior Cervicothoracic Fusion   183
    Alexander J. Ghanayem, MD
    Thomas Sylvester, MD

21 Cervical Pedicle Screw Fixation   191
    Kuniyoshi Abumi, MD
    Manabu Ito, MD
    Yoshihisa Kotani, MD

22 Cervical Osteotomy   203
    Edward D. Simmons, MD, CM, MSc, FRCSC

23 Minimally Invasive Posterior Cervical Lateral Mass Fusion   213
    James P. Lawrence, MD, MBA
    Alan S. Hilibrand, MD

Chapter 1

Anterior Cervical Diskectomy and Fusion

John C. France, MD

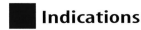

Indications

Anterior cervical diskectomy and fusion (ACDF) is a well-established technique that is used for the treatment of a variety of conditions. This chapter discusses bone graft placed at individual levels for multilevel procedures rather than a single strut extending across several levels. The latter is comparable to a corpectomy and fusion, which is discussed in another chapter.

ACDF has two components: the diskectomy and the fusion. The diskectomy can be as thorough or as limited as necessary to treat the given pathology. In most cases, the indication includes decompression of the spinal cord for myelopathy or decompression of the exiting nerve root for radiculopathy. For these indications, the fusion component simply is a means of reconstructing the defect created by the diskectomy.

In some patients, the fusion is the primary goal, and the diskectomy is done only to mobilize a segment for deformity correction or to prepare the site to accept a graft and reestablish stability, such as in the trauma setting. In the event of diskitis, the diskectomy would include a thorough dé-

bridement of the disk and possibly some of the adjacent vertebrae; then the fusion would establish stability to aid in resolving the infection.

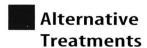

Contraindications

When considering ACDF, the surgeon must be cognizant of the pathology being treated and understand the pathomechanics involved. ACDF is not suitable for correcting certain types of pathology. For example, significant rigid kyphosis across more than one segment creating anterior cord compression that includes canal compromise at the vertebral body level would be poorly suited for a simple ACDF. Such a condition may be better treated by a corpectomy. Ossification of the posterior longitudinal ligament (OPLL) extending across multiple segments also is a contraindication to ACDF.

In trauma or other instability settings, such as inflammatory disease, the surgeon must carefully assess the degree of instability and the adequacy of the bone for reconstruction. If spinal stability is severely impaired, then an ACDF alone may be inadequate to

reestablish stability and may be contraindicated without the addition of a posterior procedure. Also, the bone quality of the vertebral body may not support the intervertebral graft or screw fixation as a stand-alone procedure. Infection is not a contraindication and may be the indication, assuming an ACDF can reestablish stability and gain adequate bony purchase as discussed previously.

Alternative Treatments

For neurocompressive pathology that is not treated adequately via ACDF, such as multilevel congenital stenosis or OPLL, a posterior procedure such as laminaplasty or laminectomy can be considered. A posterior foraminotomy also can be an alternative to ACDF for foraminal soft disk herniations causing radiculopathy. For degenerative conditions such as spondylosis or herniation causing radiculopathy, anterior diskectomy without fusion has been used to maintain motion with good initial relief of the radicular symptoms. When anterior diskectomy is performed without fusion, however, spontaneous fusion has been seen in up to 74% of patients, and distraction cannot be maintained to indirectly open the foramen and

Dr. France or an immediate family member serves as a board member, owner, officer, or committee member of AO Spine North America and has received research or institutional support from Medtronic Sofamor Danek and Synthes.

tension the ligamentum flavum. This can result in late axial pain with kyphosis. Because of these problems and the consistent success of ACDF, diskectomy without fusion has fallen out of favor. The indications for disk arthroplasty are similar to ACDF, and it has been used increasingly as an alternative procedure.

In trauma settings, the type of procedure is dictated by the morphology and neurology of the fracture, but for facet fractures or dislocations and lateral mass fractures, either a posterior fusion or ACDF can be considered. One approach may be more favorable than another, but surgeon preference often is the deciding factor. Posterior fusions have been the traditional means of treating these fractures, but ACDF has gained favor in recent years because of the ease of its patient positioning and approach and its short recovery.

For inflammatory conditions such as rheumatoid arthritis, which create a more gradual instability pattern in the subaxial cervical spine, a posterior fusion and laminectomy has been favored and has a longer track record. Patients with these conditions often have severe osteoporosis, increasing the potential for the collapse of the intervertebral strut into the bony end plate and for loss of screw fixation in the anterior vertebral body.

Results

Because ACDF is used to treat a variety of disorders, such as myelopathy, radiculopathy, fractures and dislocations, inflammatory disease, spondylosis, and infection, it is difficult to present results without a lengthy discussion of each of these conditions because the goals of treatment will vary. The one common goal for ACDF, however, is to gain a solid bony union, and many studies report on this. The number of levels treated, type of graft mate-

rial used, preparation techniques, and the use or type of hardware can vary. Numerous studies exist; only a sample of them is presented in **Table 1**. Care must be taken in evaluating these data because most are based on radiographs alone, which have not proved to be as reliable a predictor of fusion as CT. Some reasonable conclusions can be made from the literature, however, including the following observations: (1) The more levels fused, the higher the risk of nonunion; (2) plate fixation can significantly improve fusion rates for multilevel diskectomy and fusion; (3) single-level surgery has high fusion rates with both autograft and allograft (especially autograft), so it is difficult to demonstrate a clear superiority with the addition of a plate if fusion alone is the outcome measure; (4) newer polyetheretherketone (PEEK) cages perform well but have been reported only in conjunction with plating; (5) coral bone substitutes have demonstrated favorable incorporation rates, but fragmentation remains problematic; and (6) the addition of recombinant human bone morphogenetic protein 2 (rhBMP-2) improves fusion rates consistently but has unresolved issues of dysphagia, respiratory compromise, and cost. Also, the US Food and Drug Administration has not approved rhBMP-2 for use in the cervical spine.

Most of the studies in the literature are retrospective reviews, and even the few prospective studies directly comparing fusion techniques are nonrandomized. It is difficult to compare these studies because the authors' techniques vary slightly, with some burring the end plate and others leaving it intact.

Technique

Setup/Exposure
The setup for ACDF is relatively simple. The patient is supine, with a roll under the shoulders to allow gentle

neck extension to facilitate the exposure. In cases of severe stenosis with myelopathy, care should be taken to avoid excessive extension, because it might increase compression of the cord. A general-use bed in the reverse position facilitates AP and lateral fluoroscopic imaging as necessary to identify levels and assess hardware position. If autologous bone graft has been selected, then a towel bump is placed under the ipsilateral buttock for better access to the anterior pelvis. Radiographic visualization of the most caudal levels can be difficult, so the shoulders can be taped down or tied down with wrist restraints. To reduce the risk of brachial plexus palsy from continuous traction, the wrist restraints can be put on the patient and then laid at the end of the bed, where they are accessible for pulling only if it is necessary for visualization. Distracting across the disk space for graft insertion can be done internally, with posts in the vertebral bodies, or externally, with an occipitomandibular halter or Gardner-Wells tongs. I prefer to use tongs, which are placed before draping. Because the distraction force is necessary only during measurements for graft size and placement of the graft, it is not necessary to have continuous weight on the tongs. Temporary traction can be applied manually by the anesthesiologist at the appropriate times (**Figure 1**).

A transverse skin incision is made at the appropriate level based on palpable landmarks: the hyoid C3, superior border of the thyroid cartilage of C4, the inferior border of C5, and the cricoid cartilage of C6 (**Figure 2**). A transverse incision is more cosmetic than a longitudinal incision. The approach can be made along the left or right side, usually depending on the surgeon's dominant hand. Anatomically, the recurrent laryngeal nerve crosses the incision more cranially on the right side, potentially making it more vulnerable to injury when the more caudal disks are treated, but an

Table 1 Anterior Cervical Diskectomy Fusion Rates With Various Techniques

Authors (Year)	Number of Patients	Mean Patient Age in Years (Range)	Type of Study	Technique	Mean Follow-up in Months (Range)	Fusion Rate
Zdeblick and Ducker (1991)	87	Auto: 44 (24-68) Allo: 42 (28-61)	Retrospective	Smith-Robinson Freeze-dried allo vs auto No plate	28 (24-41)	1-level: auto 95%, allo 95% 2-level: allo 37%, auto 83%
Grossman et al (1992)	42	53	Retrospective	Freeze-dried fibula No plate	22.1 (9-47)	82% of levels
Brodke and Zdeblick (1992)	51	45 (19-75)	Retrospective	Smith-Robinson (burr end plates) Auto (no plate)	12 (6-25)	1-level: 97% 2-level: 94% 3-level: 87%
An et al (1995)	77	Auto: 46.1 (26-71) Allo: 48 (28-80)	Prospective	39 Smith-Robinson allo with DBM vs 38 auto No plate	Auto: 18.4 (12-33) Allo: 17.5 (12-31)	1-level: auto 73.6%, allo 52.6% 2-level: auto 76.5%, allo 62.5%
Connolly et al (1996)	43	Group 1: 52 (30-90) Group 2: 42 (22-65)	Retrospective	Smith-Robinson Auto18 no plate vs 25 plate	Plate: 16 (6-39) No plate: 17 (12-23)	All 1-level Plate 100% No plate 88%
Wang et al (2001)	59	49.3	Retrospective	Smith-Robinson Auto 40 plate vs 19 no plate	39 (2.3-7.8 yrs)	All 3-level Plate 82% No plate 63%
Baskin et al (2003)	33	Investigated group: 51.3 Controls: 47.1	Prospective RCT	18 allo/rhBMP-2 (0.6mg/level) 15 auto All plated	24	100% fusion both groups, 1-level and 2-level

Auto = autograft, allo = allograft, DMB = demineralized bone matrix, RCT = randomized controlled trial, rhBMP-2 = recombinant human bone morphogenetic protein 2.

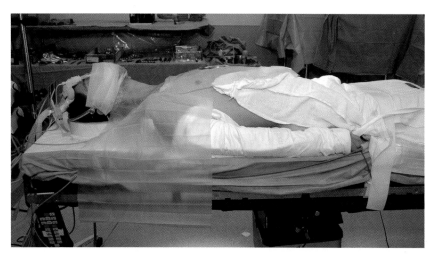

Figure 1 Clinical photograph shows the patient setup for ACDF, with a general-use bed in reverse to allow access for imaging around the head. A roll is placed under the shoulders for gentle neck extension, and Gardner-Wells tongs are in place, to be used for traction by the anesthesiologist at appropriate times during the procedure. Wrist restraints are placed for intermittent traction to assist the radiographic visualization of the lower cervical segments.

increased rate of palsy has not been well documented, so the side on which the incision is made remains surgeon preference. The platysma muscle is opened in line with the skin incision, and then a plane is developed longitudinally deep to the platysma, along the medial border of the sterno-cleidomastoid muscle (SCM). This part of the dissection can be performed as far cranial and caudal as necessary, depending on the number of levels to be included. The fascia along the medial border of the SCM is opened to the corresponding length. Next, the carotid artery is palpated with the index finger, and gentle blunt dissection is performed medial to the carotid sheath through the loose fascia

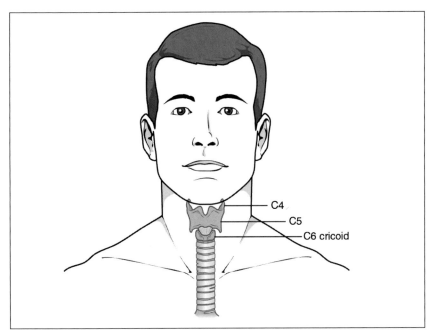

Figure 2 Illustration demonstrates the palpable external landmarks for ACDF and their corresponding disk levels: the superior border of the thyroid cartilage of C4, the inferior border of C5, and the cricoid cartilage of C6.

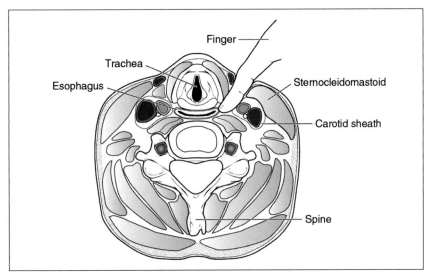

Figure 3 Illustration shows an axial view of the midcervical spine and demonstrates the interval and direction of finger dissection between the carotid sheath and the midline structures.

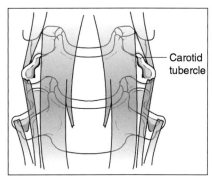

Figure 4 Illustration depicts the bony prominence called the carotid tubercle, which is palpable laterally under the longus colli muscle at C6, just below the C5-6 disk.

between the carotid sheath and trachea/esophagus (**Figure 3**). The direction is approximately toward the opposite shoulder. The vertebral bodies can now be palpated easily, and the prevertebral fascia is pushed aside with a blunt dissector.

The carotid tubercle (the most prominent anterior tubercle along the transverse process at C6 just caudal to the C5-6 disk) can be used as an internal landmark to aid in level identification (**Figure 4**). A cross-table lateral radiograph should always be used for

verification, however. An 18-gauge spinal needle with two 90° bends (with the first 1 cm from the tip) or a short blunt needle can be placed into the disk as a radiographic marker to avoid overinsertion (**Figure 5**). Once the level has been verified, electrocautery can be used to open the fascia along the medial border of the longus colli muscle on both sides. The electrocautery should be sheathed, allowing only the tip to be exposed, to minimize the risk of inadvertent damage to structures within the side walls of the exposure, such as the carotid artery (**Figure 6**). Retractor blades can be placed under the longus colli, medial to lateral, and a second set of retractors can be used longitudinally as needed (**Figure 7**).

Instruments/Equipment/ Implants Required

The equipment needed depends on the type of graft chosen and whether a plate will be used. When no additional posterior procedure is planned, a plate generally is used. Various plates are available, with no strong clinical evidence to demonstrate the superiority of any one type in a single-level ACDF. In multilevel cases and cases of significant instability, the use of dynamic plates should be cautioned. Cost, ease of application, availability, and familiarity all play a role in selection.

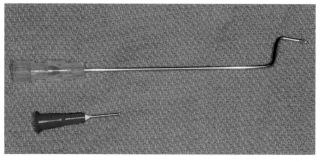

Figure 5 Photograph shows two types of needles that can be used as markers: an 18-gauge spinal needle with two 90° bends (each 1 cm in length) and a short blunt needle. Both will prevent overpenetration into the spinal canal.

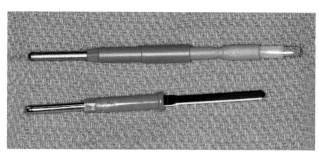

Figure 6 Photograph shows two types of electrocauteries. A sheath-protected electrocautery (top) should be used to prevent collateral side-wall damage instead of a standard cautery (bottom), which cuts and coagulates along its sides.

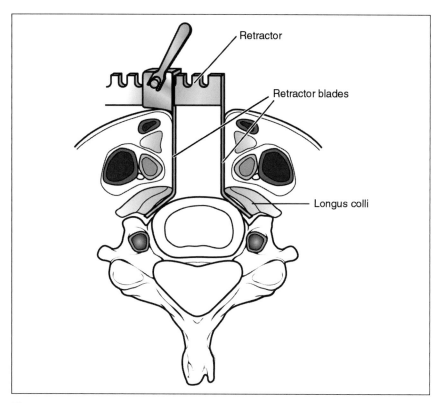

Figure 7 Illustration depicts an axial view of the spine. Retractor blades are shown placed under the longus colli muscles to prevent damage to surrounding structures.

material lacks a cancellous component. Some prefabricated allograft struts have a composition similar to that of iliac crest bone graft. Composite allografts are available that are fabricated to offer both structural cortical support and cancellous parts for rapid healing. Lastly, synthetic cages are available, made of metal or a polymer such as PEEK, and can be packed with bone.

Procedure

The anterior anulus can be excised with a No. 15 scalpel, and then the disk material is removed thoroughly with pituitary rongeurs and curets. The cartilaginous end plate should be removed without penetrating the bony cortex. The diskectomy should extend laterally out onto the uncinate processes bilaterally (**Figure 8**). The amount of decompression into the foramen depends on the pathology and indications for surgery, as does the need for osteophyte resection more centrally or removal of the posterior longitudinal ligament. Visualization into the back of the disk can be improved with focal distraction using an intervertebral spreader or vertebral body pins. The intervertebral spreader can be cumbersome and must be placed deep within the disk space to avoid iatrogenic end plate fracture. The vertebral pins must be parallel to get an even distraction. Caution must be exercised in using either technique

Various graft options are available. The graft material is chosen by surgeon preference. If autologous bone is to be used, an oscillating saw is better than osteotomes for harvesting graft to limit damage to the cortical margins. Allograft bone can be prefabricated and comes with trial sizers and kits for insertion-site preparation; it also can be sized and cut intraopera-tively by the surgeon from the fibula or tricortical iliac crest. My preference is autologous or allograft bone from the tricortical iliac crest because it has a cortical rim for immediate strength and a cancellous core for rapid incorporation. Although fibular cortical rings have a strong initial support and ultimately a good incorporation rate, the process is slower because this graft

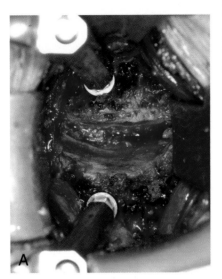

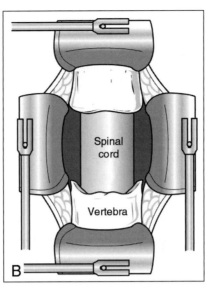

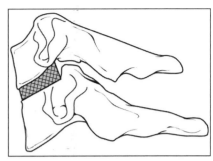

Figure 9 Illustration shows a keystone-shaped graft. This type of graft provides immediate stability. The corresponding shape is cut into the end plates to avoid a kyphosing effect.

Figure 8 Anterior cervical diskectomy **A,** In this intraoperative photograph, the uncinate processes can be seen. They can be identified deep within the disk space to define the midline and lateral margins of the decompression. **B,** Illustration of an anterior view of the spine shows the width of the diskectomy.

in osteoporotic patients, to avoid fracture that would compromise the stability of the graft/plate reconstruction. Good lighting is required, and magnification through loupes or the microscope is recommended.

After the decompression/diskectomy is complete, the site is prepared to accept the graft. With many techniques, the bony end plate is preserved to provide resistance to axial load forces. Often some perforations are made to create a bleeding surface to stimulate bone healing. Other techniques remove part of the bony end plate to accept the shape of the graft. One such technique is the keystone graft described by Simmons. This technique is simply a modification of the Smith-Robinson graft that keeps the posterior height of the graft greater than the anterior height (**Figure 9**). The Keystone technique requires some extra carpentry and distraction, but after the graft is seated fully, it has excellent intrinsic stability. This technique was developed before the use of anterior plates, when graft expulsion posed a greater problem, but it remains my preferred technique. Re-gardless of the technique used, it remains critical to use good carpentry, get a tight-fitting graft, maximize the surface area for stability and healing, and choose a material that has a track record for high union rates. The plate is no substitute for quality grafting.

The final part of the procedure is plate fixation. Bicortical fixation of the screws rarely, if ever, is necessary with modern plates. Most systems have guides and depth stops to assist with drilling and screw placement. Good initial exposure is important in helping ensure that the plate is midline and straight. If the plate is positioned close to the adjacent disk, osteophytes are more likely to develop. The clinical significance of this is not yet known, but care should be taken to maximize the distance between the end of the plate and the next disk (**Figure 10**). All traction should be released before plate fixation.

Wound Closure

Meticulous hemostasis before closure is important in minimizing hematoma formation and respiratory compromise. A drain can be inserted at this

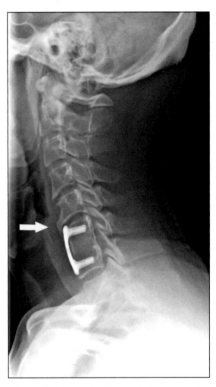

Figure 10 Lateral radiograph demonstrates an osteophyte (arrow) at the adjacent surgical level.

time to provide further security. After the retractors are removed, the fascia along the medial border of the SCM can be approximated loosely, but this is optional. The platysma must be repaired anatomically. The skin closure, using a subcutaneous suture, should be done in a fashion that provides good cosmesis. I use a running No. 2 nonabsorbable monofilament suture and elastic skin closure strips.

Postoperative Regimen

For single-level ACDF with plating, no external protection is necessary. For multiple levels or single levels above a prior fusion, the need for a hard collar depends on surgeon judgment, taking into account bone quality, screw purchase, number of fixation points, graft fit, and patient compliance. Dysphagia is common and varies in severity, so patients are begun on a soft diet, which is advanced as tolerated. They are allowed full mobility on the day of surgery unless their neurologic status is compromised. If a drain was inserted, it can be removed in the morning, and most patients can be released from the hospital on postoperative day 1. For multilevel procedures and when autologous iliac crest is used, additional hospital days may be needed. Some centers perform a single-level routine ACDF as a same-day procedure. If this is considered, great care must be taken with hemostasis because of the risk of respiratory compromise, which, although extremely rare, has the potential to be fatal if diagnosis or treatment is delayed.

Avoiding Pitfalls and Complications

The complications from this procedure can occur at the cervical or bone graft harvest site. Complications unique to the harvest site include persistent pain, fracture, and injury to the cluneal nerves or lateral femoral cutaneous nerve (LFCN). Fracture risk

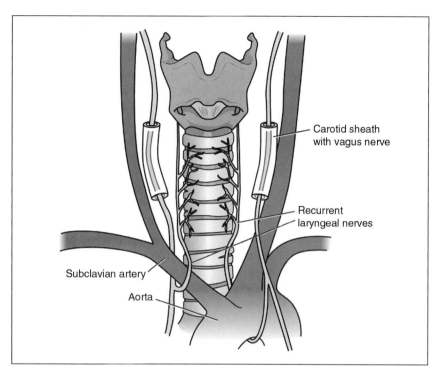

Figure 11 Illustration shows the paths of the recurrent laryngeal nerves. Note that the paths differ on the right and left sides.

can be reduced by staying two fingerbreadths posterior to the anterior superior iliac spine (ASIS) and using a saw rather than an osteotome. The surgeon must be aware of the location of the cluneal nerves and the variable location of the LFCN, which may be 1 cm anterior or up to 1 cm posterior to the ASIS. Persistent pain at the harvest site is the reason many surgeons have switched to allograft or synthetic grafts.

Several potential problems can develop at the cervical wound. Infection is relatively rare with anterior cervical surgery, but the potential exists for abscess formation posterior to the graft, which can cause spinal cord compression. The surgeon must remain vigilant and treat infections aggressively, including with surgical débridement, when identified. Injury to the structures within the walls of the exposure also can be devastating. Esophageal perforation can occur immediately or be delayed because of erosion from a retractor-related pressure necrosis or

hardware migration. If esophageal perforation is recognized intraoperatively, immediate consultation with an otolaryngologist is warranted to consider direct repair and further management. Esophageal perforation should always be considered when a postoperative infection develops. If the surgery lasts longer than 2 hours, the retractors should be released to inspect the underlying tissue for injury or pressure necrosis. At the end of every surgery, it is a good idea to inspect the esophagus before closure to assess for inadvertent injury.

Recurrent laryngeal nerve palsy is the most common neurologic injury causing unilateral vocal cord paralysis; it is often temporary, but it may be permanent. The path of the recurrent laryngeal nerves differs on the right and left sides (**Figure 11**). The surgeon should be aware of the location of the nerve during dissection and retraction. A preoperative assessment of vocal cord function is important before any revision anterior surgery, es-

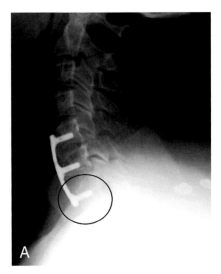 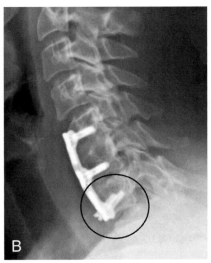

Figure 12 Lateral radiographs depict failed anterior hardware. Note the change in screw position from **A** to **B**.

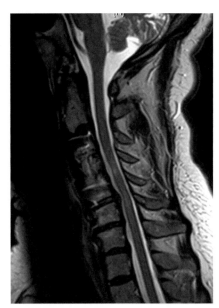

Figure 13 T2-weighted sagittal MRI demonstrates symptomatic adjacent-level disk changes caudal to the fusion at C5-6.

pecially if the surgeon plans to use the side opposite to the original incision, because bilateral paralysis can be devastating. The risk can be reduced by carefully placing retractor blades deep to the longus colli and not against the tracheoesophageal interval, and carefully retracting inferiorly. Some authors have suggested deflating the endotracheal tube balloon after the retractors are placed and then re-inflating it to allow it to adjust its position, but this has not yet been demonstrated to reduce the incidence of palsy.

Vertebral artery injury is more likely when a corpectomy is performed, but it can occur from an overly aggressive foraminotomy during simple diskectomy. The surgeon should be familiar with the location of the vertebral artery relative to the uncinate, foramen, and nerve root to reduce this risk. Spinal cord or root injury can occur, but the incidence of these complications is less than 1%. The surgeon should limit using instruments in the canal and avoid using large probes, Kerrison rongeurs, and curets. Graft retropulsion has been described as a cause of spinal cord injury. A natural lip is present on the end plates of the vertebrae posteriorly that

can aid in preventing retropulsion if left intact. Alternatively, with end plate preparation, a ridge can be created posteriorly to further minimize the risk.

Dysphagia has been identified as occurring much more frequently than originally thought and can be a persistent symptom. It is often so mild that patients will not bring it up spontaneously, but when questioned, they note its presence. Prevention may be difficult, other than standard measures such as minimizing the duration of traction that could create occult injury or scarring within the esophageal wall and avoiding hematoma.

Hardware failure and loss of fixation can occur early or late. Early failures can be related to technical errors of insertion, poor bone quality, and greater underlying instability than can be handled with an ACDF alone. Late failures more often are the result of nonunion and continued repetitive motion (**Figure 12**). **Table 1** lists some data on fusion rates with various material and levels. The environment for anterior cervical fusion is very favorable, and as a result, a variety of good graft options is available for the average patient. When the host is compromised, however, because of smoking,

prior failed fusion, irradiated bone, or multilevel fusion, then the choice of graft may play a greater role. Under such circumstances, autograft definitely should be considered. The role of recombinant human bone morphogenetic proteins (rhBMPs) is still being elucidated. They appear to enhance fusion rates but have created other issues, such as excessive soft-tissue swelling with respiratory compromise, and they remain very costly. As these issues are worked out, rhBMPs are likely to play an even greater role.

Lastly, adjacent-level degenerative changes (**Figure 13**) may occur, some from the natural history and some accelerated by the loss of motion from fusion. It is estimated that adjacent-level degenerative change with radiculopathy occurs at a rate of about 3% per year. This long-term complication has created enthusiasm for motion-sparing techniques such as disk arthroplasty.

■ Bibliography

An HS, Simpson JM, Glover JM, Stephany J: Comparison between allograft plus demineralized bone matrix versus autograft in anterior cervical fusion: A prospective multicenter study. *Spine (Phila Pa 1976)* 1995;20(20):2211-2216.

Baskin DS, Ryan P, Sonntag V, Westmark R, Widmayer MA: A prospective, randomized, controlled cervical fusion study using recombinant human bone morphogenetic protein-2 with the CORNERSTONE-SR allograft ring and the ATLANTIS anterior cervical plate. *Spine (Phila Pa 1976)* 2003;28(12):1219-1225.

Brodke DS, Zdeblick TA: Modified Smith-Robinson procedure for anterior cervical diskectomy and fusion. *Spine (Phila Pa 1976)* 1992;17(10 suppl)S427-S430.

Chau AM, Mobbs RJ: Bone graft substitutes in anterior cervical diskectomy and fusion. *Eur Spine J* 2009;18(4):449-464.

Connolly PJ, Esses SI, Kostuik JP: Anterior cervical fusion: Outcome analysis of patients fused with and without anterior cervical plates. *J Spinal Disord* 1996;9(3):202-206.

Floyd T, Ohnmeiss D: A meta-analysis of autograft versus allograft in anterior cervical fusion. *Eur Spine J* 2000;9(5): 398-403.

Fountas KN, Kapsalaki EZ, Nikolakakos LG, et al: Anterior cervical diskectomy and fusion associated complications. *Spine (Phila Pa 1976)* 2007;32(21):2310-2317.

Grossman W, Peppelman WC, Baum JA, Kraus DR: The use of freeze-dried fibular allograft in anterior cervical fusion. *Spine (Phila Pa 1976)* 1992;17(5):565-569.

Hilibrand AS, Carlson GD, Palumbo MA, Jones PK, Bohlman HH: Radiculopathy and myelopathy at segments adjacent to the site of a previous anterior cervical arthrodesis. *J Bone Joint Surg Am* 1999;81(4):519-528.

Simmons EH, Bhalla SK: Anterior cervical discectomy and fusion: A clinical and biomechanical study with eight-year follow-up. *J Bone Joint Surg Br* 1969;51(2):225-237.

Wang JC, McDonough PW, Kanim LE, Endow KK, Delamarter RB: Increased fusion rates with cervical plating for three-level anterior cervical diskectomy and fusion. *Spine (Phila Pa 1976)* 2001;26(6):643-647.

Zdeblick TA, Ducker TB: The use of freeze-dried allograft bone for anterior cervical fusions. *Spine (Phila Pa 1976)* 1991; 16(7):726-729.

Coding

CPT Codes		Corresponding ICD-9 Codes	
20930	Allograft, morselized, or placement of osteopromotive material, for spine surgery only (List separately in addition to code for primary procedure)	170.2 733.13 737.30	724.6 733.81
20931	Allograft, structural, for spine surgery only (List separately in addition to code for primary procedure)	170.2 733.13	724.6 733.81
20936	Autograft for spine surgery only (includes harvesting the graft); local (eg, ribs, spinous process, or laminar fragments) obtained from same incision (List separately in addition to code for primary procedure)	170.2 733.13	724.6 737.30
20937	Autograft for spine surgery only (includes harvesting the graft); morselized (through separate skin or fascial incision) (List separately in addition to code for primary procedure)	170.2 733.13 737.30	724.6 737.81
20938	Autograft for spine surgery only (includes harvesting the graft); structural, bicortical or tricortical (through separate skin or fascial incision) (List separately in addition to code for primary procedure)	170.2 733.13	724.6 737.81
22551	Arthrodesis, anterior interbody, including disc space preparation, discectomy, osteophytectomy and decompression of spinal cord and/or nerve roots; cervical below C2	711.01 711.03 711.05	711.02 711.04 711.06
22552	Arthrodesis, anterior interbody, including disc space preparation, discectomy, osteophytectomy and decompression of spinal cord and/or nerve roots; cervical below C2, each additional interspace (List separately in addition to code for separate procedure)	711.01 711.03 711.05	711.02 711.04 711.06
22554	Arthrodesis, anterior interbody technique, including minimal discectomy to prepare interspace (other than for decompression); cervical below C2	722.0 805.03 805.05	733.13 805.04 805.06
22845	Anterior instrumentation; 2 to 3 vertebral segments (List separately in addition to code for primary procedure)	170.2 342.9 343	342.1 342.90 343.0
22846	Anterior instrumentation; 4 to 7 vertebral segments (List separately in addition to code for primary procedure)	170.2 342.9 343	342.1 342.90 343.0

CPT copyright © 2010 by the American Medical Association. All rights reserved.

Chapter 2
Cervical Arthroplasty

Rick C. Sasso, MD
James Eric Lashley, MD

 ## Indications

In the United States, cervical arthroplasty is indicated for the treatment of cervical radiculopathy or myelopathy at a single level of the cervical spine. Preferably, the pathology results from a soft disk herniation with minimal osteophytes, minimal facet arthropathy, and obvious symptoms secondary to neural compression. Cervical arthroplasty is not indicated for the treatment of discogenic neck pain. Multilevel cervical arthroplasty has not yet been approved by the US Food and Drug Administration (FDA); however, many examples of off-label use of the procedure have been reported in the medical literature.

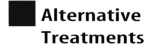

 ## Contraindications

Numerous contraindications for cervical arthroplasty have been described in different clinical studies (**Table 1**).

They generally include osteoporosis, cervical instability at the proposed level of arthroplasty, previous or active history of cervical spine infection, and moderate to severe facet arthropathy.

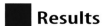

Alternative Treatments

Whether from radiculopathy or myelopathy, neural element compression in the cervical spine may be treated via an anterior or posterior approach. Anterior procedures include anterior cervical diskectomy and fusion (ACDF), usually with instrumentation. Posterior procedures include laminoforaminotomy (to decompress nerve roots) and posterior cervical laminectomy and instrumented fusion (for spinal cord compression).

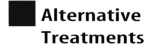

Results

Results of cervical arthroplasty can be divided into short- and long-term outcomes. Short-term results focus on how well cervical arthroplasty can treat the immediate pathology of neural compression, whereas long-term results are determined by whether arthroplasty prevents the adjacent-level degeneration associated with ACDF.

Several short-term studies have demonstrated that cervical arthroplasty is at least as effective as ACDF in reducing arm and neck pain associated with cervical radiculopathy (**Table 2**). Long-term studies are currently lacking, but midterm results show that revision rates appear to be lower after cervical arthroplasty than they are after ACDF. In addition, although pseudarthrosis is one cause of revision after ACDF, it does appear that when comparing cervical arthroplasty with ACDF, the current trend is toward fewer revisions for adjacent-level disease when arthroplasty is performed.

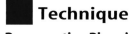

Technique
Preoperative Planning
As with any surgery, preoperative planning is essential. Preoperative radiographic studies should be

Dr. Sasso or an immediate family member serves as board member, owner, officer, or committee member of the North Meridian Surgery Center; has received royalties from Medtronic Sofamor Danek; is a member of a speakers' bureau or has made paid presentations on behalf of Ono Pharmaceutical; serves as a paid consultant to or is an employee of Medtronic Sofamor Danek; has received research or institutional support from AO North America, Cerapedics, Eli Lilly, Medtronic Sofamor Danek, and Stryker; and has stock or holds stock options in Biomet. Neither Dr. Lashley nor any immediate family member has received anything of value from or owns stock in a commercial company or institution related directly or indirectly to the subject of this chapter.

Table 1 Contraindications for Cervical Arthroplasty (Exclusion Criteria from Previous Studies)

Cervical instability at the proposed level of arthroplasty

>11° angulation

>3 mm segmental translation

"Hard disk" disease

Infection (past or present)

Inflammatory arthritides (rheumatoid arthritis, ankylosing spondylitis)

Known hypersensitivity to cobalt, chromium, molybdenum, titanium, or polyethylene

Lack of motion of target disk space evident on preoperative dynamic radiographs

Malignant disease

Metabolic bone disease

Multilevel pathology

Ossification of posterior longitudinal ligament or diffuse idiopathic skeletal hyperostosis

Osteoporosis

Postlaminectomy with kyphotic deformity

Pregnancy or possible pregnancy within 3 years of implantation

Radiographic evidence of moderate to severe osteoarthritis with loss of normal disk space height > 80%

Radiographic evidence of severe facet joint degeneration

Traumatic injury

scrutinized carefully to determine not only the level of pathology but also sources of compression, facet arthropathy, osteopenia, and sagittal alignment of the cervical spine. The surgeon also should be familiar with the specifics of each cervical device to be implanted.

Each device has unique characteristics, particular procedural steps that must be followed for implantation, and distinct implant-guided instrumentation. All of these elements must be understood and mastered to accurately and successfully implant the device. Some cervical devices require maintenance of the uncovertebral joints for joint space stability after implantation, whereas others require removal of the uncovertebral joints for appropriate placement and function. Before implanting a cervical device, the surgeon must be certain of the specifications for proper patient positioning, appropriate neural decompression, and final implantation of the

Table 2 Results of Clinical Studies on Cervical Arthroplasty

Author(s) (Year)	Number of Patients	Procedure	Mean Patient Age in Years (Range)	Mean Follow-up (Range)	Results	Success Rate
Shim et al (2006)	47	Cervical arthroplasty	45.6 (32-64)	6 months (3 to 6)	Decrease in VAS (neck and arm) Decrease in NDI	83%
Nabhan et al (*Spine*, 2007)	49	Cervical arthroplasty vs ACDF	44	(3-52 weeks)	Decrease in VAS (neck and arm) in both groups	NR
Sasso et al (2007)	115	Cervical arthroplasty vs ACDF	Arthroplasty: 42 (25-64) ACDF: 46 (29-66)	18 months (6 weeks to 24 months)	Improvement in SF-36 MCS/PCS scores Decrease in NDI, VAS (neck and arm) in both groups	94.6%
Anderson et al (2008)	463	Cervical arthroplasty vs ACDF	No difference in age reported between groups ($P > 0.05$)	(6 weeks to 24 months)	Surgically related and late medical events more common in arthroplasty group, but more severe adverse events and higher revision rate in ACDF group	NR

ACDF = anterior cervical diskectomy and fusion, NR = not reported, VAS = visual analog scale, NDI = Neck Disability Index, SF-36 = Short Form-36, MCS = mental component summary, PCS = physical component summary.

device. Meticulous technique is critical to ensure proper implantation and eventual success of the device (**Table 3**). Manufacturer-sponsored training courses, detailed surgical technique guides, and informative Web sites are available to help train surgeons to successfully implant various devices. These resources should be consulted to learn the surgical technique for each specific device.

Before surgery, a review of the indications, contraindications, risks and benefits, and prospective outcomes of the procedure should be discussed with the patient, and informed consent should be obtained. When cervical arthroplasty is planned, the patient should be informed that long-term data are not yet available. Furthermore, the patient should be informed

Table 3 Surgical Technique Pearls

1. Position the patient in a normal, lordotic position (avoid intraoperative kyphosis)
2. Fully decompress the neural structures
3. Prepare the end plates based on instrumentation/techniques of the selected cervical device (do not violate end-plate integrity)
4. Choose a correctly sized cervical device for implantation
5. Ensure correct positioning of the implanted cervical device (based on technical specifics of selected device)
6. Convert the procedure to anterior cervical diskectomy and fusion if unable to "successfully" implant the device

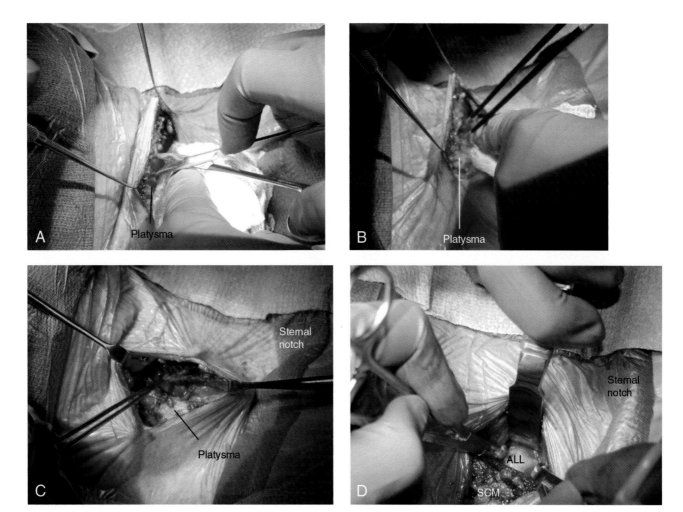

Figure 1 Intraoperative photographs showing the right-sided approach for a left C7 radiculopathy. The patient's head is to the left. **A,** The approach is started by making a transverse skin incision beginning at the midline of the neck to the medial border of the right sternocleidomastoid (SCM) muscle belly. Full-thickness skin flaps are created down to the platysma. **B,** Hemostasis is obtained, and further dissection is continued to develop full-thickness flaps, which will allow a longitudinal incision through the platysma. **C,** A longitudinal incision is made through the platysma. **D,** Blunt dissection is used to develop the plane between the sternocleidomastoid and carotid sheath (laterally) and visceral structures (medially) until the anterior aspect of the vertebral bodies is reached. ALL = anterior longitudinal ligament.

that if the surgical findings are different from those seen preoperatively, or if surgical complications arise, the arthroplasty may need to be converted to an instrumented ACDF.

Setup and Patient Positioning

The patient is first positioned supine on the surgical table and subsequently placed under general endotracheal anesthesia. The surgical incision site is then marked, based on the surgeon's preference. This can be a transverse incision in a skin crease at the proposed level of arthoplasty or a longitudinal incision (if a larger surgical field is required). The approach can be left- or right-sided; again, this is based on the surgeon's preference. Our preference is to approach on the side that is opposite the pathology. Optimal positioning of the device reproduces the natural height of the disk space to be replaced. To achieve this, the neck is gently extended by placing a soft roll (or rolled towel) underneath the neck. However, cervical myelopathy can be acutely worsened by this position. If intraoperative radiographic visualization of the cervical spine might be

blocked, the shoulders should be pulled down and held in place (generally with tape). Finally, the patient is prepared and draped in a sterile fashion.

Procedure

EXPOSURE

The skin is incised, the subcutaneous tissue plane is developed to the platysma, and the platysma is then divided in a longitudinal fashion (**Figure 1**, *A* through *C*). The interval between the sternocleidomastoid and strap muscles is developed to the anterior surface of the cervical spine (**Figure 1**, *D*). The disk space is marked with a bent needle, and an intraoperative lateral fluoroscopic image is obtained to accurately determine the appropriate level for the planned arthoplasty (**Figure 2**). Once the appropriate level is identified, blade retractors are placed under the longus colli muscles and distractor pins are placed into the vertebral bodies above and below the diseased disk (**Figure 3**). At this point, the disk is incised and the disk material is completely removed.

DECOMPRESSION

After the disk material is removed, meticulous decompression of the nerve roots and spinal cord is performed. Before removing the uncinate processes, the surgeon should know whether the implanted device requires

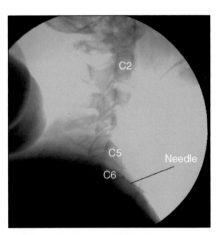

Figure 2 A bent needle is placed in the disk space as viewed through the dissection, and placement is checked with a lateral fluoroscopic radiograph. In this case, the needle was placed at the C5-C6 disk. Further dissection and disk preparation was performed accordingly at the level inferior to the placement seen here.

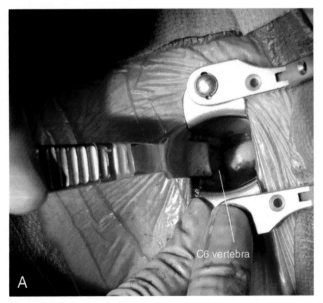
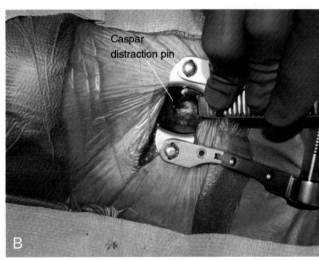

Figure 3 Placement of distraction pins. The patient's head is to the left. **A,** Blade retractors are placed beneath the longus colli muscles, and gentle retraction with a smooth handheld retractor is performed to visualize the C6 vertebral body for placement of a 12-mm Caspar distraction pin. **B,** After the superior Caspar pin has been placed, gentle retraction is performed inferiorly for placement of the C7 Caspar pin.

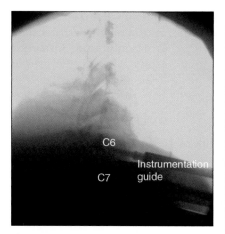

Figure 4 Lateral fluoroscopic image showing the instrumentation guide in place, which assists in preparing the disk space and vertebral bodies for the specific cervical device to be implanted.

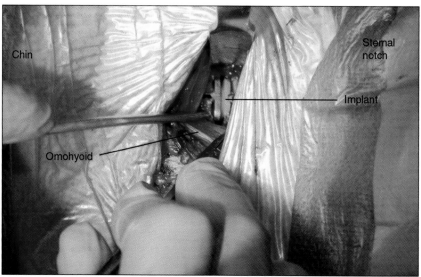

Figure 5 After the cervical device is placed, the instrumentation guide is removed, and the device is checked for positioning, stability, and mobility. The wound is irrigated, and hemostasis is obtained.

maintaining or removing the uncovertebral joints for proper implant functioning. Next, the cartilaginous portions of the end plates are completely removed.

IMPLANTATION
Before preparation of the disk space and implantation of the cervical device, the surgeon must determine the coronal center point and angle of insertion of the device. Once again, this may depend on the specifications of the particular device being implanted. The next step is preparation of the end plates (**Figure 4**) and placement of the device. After diskectomy, preparation of the disk space, and appropriate neural decompression, the instrumentation guide is placed. Mobile fluoroscopy is used to ensure that the cervical device is the appropriate height and to help position it correctly in the coronal center of the disk space. Once the device is implanted (**Figure 5**), we immediately obtain and review fluoroscopic radiographic images (**Figure 6**) to confirm placement of the device. Some surgeons also prefer to check cervical range of motion fluoroscopically at this time.

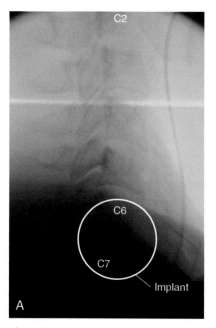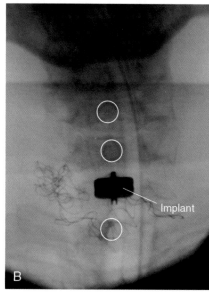

Figure 6 A, Lateral fluoroscopic image demonstrating appropriate sagittal placement and alignment of the implanted cervical device (circled in white). **B,** AP fluoroscopic image showing the superior and inferior keels of the implant in perfect alignment with the spinous process line (indicated by circles). This signifies excellent coronal alignment of the implant.

Wound Closure
When the placement and function of the cervical device is satisfactory, the wound is irrigated and hemostasis is obtained. The platysma and skin are closed in layers according to the surgeon's preference. The platysma is approximated with a running 2-0 ab-

sorbable braided suture, and the skin is closed with a running 3-0 subcuticular stitch. A topical liquid skin adhesive is then applied.

Postoperative Regimen

The cervical spine is not immobilized postoperatively. We allow patients to perform gentle range-of-motion exercises as tolerated. In addition, we prescribe nonsteroidal anti-inflammatory drugs (NSAIDs) for a short time to reduce the risk of heterotopic ossification (HO).

Avoiding Pitfalls and Complications

Complications can be easily divided into those that are common to both cervical arthroplasty and ACDF and those that are unique to cervical arthroplasty. As with ACDF, dysphagia, transient unilateral vocal cord paralysis, retropharyngeal hematoma, esophageal perforation, postoperative imaging difficulties secondary to metal artifact, and infection have all been reported following implantation of cervical arthoplasty devices. Unlike ACDF, cervical arthroplasty has both early and late complications intrinsic

to total joint arthroplasties. These include cervical device fixation issues, implant wear, and HO.

Problems with device fixation can be seen early in the postoperative period or late in postoperative follow-up. Keels, pegs, and end-plate contouring (eg, milling) are device modifications designed to achieve early stability, and titanium plasma–sprayed end plates help with bone ingrowth for late stability. Although device migration may be seen early in the postoperative period, most cervical devices achieve excellent stability by 6 months.

Implant wear always has been a concern with all types of total joint arthroplasty. Although implant wear does occur in cervical arthroplasty, it differs from that seen in large joint arthroplasties. First, the disk space is not a synovial joint. As a result, local inflammatory reaction may not be as significant as that seen in large joint arthroplasty. Second, although the same biomaterials are used in large joint and cervical arthroplasties, they may not undergo the same amount of wear. This is thought to be due to a relatively smaller biologic load at the cervical disk space, compared to a large weight-bearing joint such as the hip. To date, no long-term studies have demonstrated implant failure due to mechanical wear in cervical arthroplasty. However, a limited number of retrieval analysis studies have shown that the amount of cervical device wear seen in in vivo cases is sig-

nificantly less than that seen in simulated, in vitro mechanical models.

The purpose of cervical arthroplasty is to provide pain-free movement of the diseased disk space. One of the most difficult complications associated with any joint arthroplasty is loss of motion due to HO. HO is organized bone tissue formation in periarticular soft tissue following joint trauma or traumatic brain injury, and it has a well-known association with total joint arthroplasty. The prevalence of heterotopic bone formation in cervical arthroplasty may be greater than 60%. In spite of the presence of heterotopic bone and, in some cases, restriction of motion, improved clinical outcomes are still reported at 1-year follow-up. In one multicenter study, rates of HO were found to be lower in one center that used a routine NSAID program postoperatively.

Postoperative imaging of the cervical spine may be required for continued neurologic symptoms at the level of arthoplasty or for adjacent-level disease. Depending on the composition of the implant, varying degrees of metal artifact may occur, which may compromise appropriate visualization of the cervical spine with MRI studies, thereby affecting the appropriate diagnosis of cervical pathology. Deterioration of postoperative imaging quality is more commonly reported with cobalt-chromium implants than with titanium implants.

Bibliography

Anderson PA, Sasso RC, Riew KD: Comparison of adverse events between the Bryan artificial cervical disc and anterior cervical arthrodesis. *Spine (Phila Pa 1976)* 2008;33(12):1305-1312.

Anderson PA, Sasso RC, Riew KD: Update on cervical artificial disk replacement. *Instr Course Lect* 2007;56:237-245.

Anderson PA, Sasso RC, Rouleau JP, Carlson CS, Goffin J: The Bryan Cervical Disc: Wear properties and early clinical results. *Spine J* 2004;4(6, Suppl):303S-309S.

Chang UK, Kim DH, Lee MC, Willenberg R, Kim SH, Lim J: Changes in adjacent-level disc pressure and facet joint force after cervical arthroplasty compared with cervical discectomy and fusion. *J Neurosurg Spine* 2007;7(1):33-39.

Chang UK, Kim DH, Lee MC, Willenberg R, Kim SH, Lim J: Range of motion change after cervical arthroplasty with ProDisc-C and prestige artificial discs compared with anterior cervical discectomy and fusion. *J Neurosurg Spine* 2007;7(1):40-46.

Eck JC, Humphreys SC, Lim TH, et al: Biomechanical study on the effect of cervical spine fusion on adjacent-level intradiscal pressure and segmental motion. *Spine (Phila Pa 1976)* 2002;27(22):2431-2434.

Goffin J, Geusens E, Vantomme N, et al: Long-term follow-up after interbody fusion of the cervical spine. *J Spinal Disord Tech* 2004;17(2):79-85.

Hilibrand AS, Carlson GD, Palumbo MA, Jones PK, Bohlman HH: Radiculopathy and myelopathy at segments adjacent to the site of a previous anterior cervical arthrodesis. *J Bone Joint Surg Am* 1999;81(4):519-528.

Lind B, Zoëga B, Anderson PA: A radiostereometric analysis of the Bryan Cervical Disc prosthesis. *Spine (Phila Pa 1976)* 2007;32(8):885-891.

Mehren C, Suchomel P, Grochulla F, et al: Heterotopic ossification in total cervical artificial disc replacement. *Spine (Phila Pa 1976)* 2006;31(24):2802-2806.

Mummaneni PV, Robinson JC, Haid RW Jr: Cervical arthroplasty with the Prestige Lp cervical disc. *Neurosurgery* 2007;60(4, Suppl 2)310-315.

Nabhan A, Ahlhelm F, Pitzen T, et al: Disc replacement using Pro-Disc C versus fusion: A prospective randomised and controlled radiographic and clinical study. *Eur Spine J* 2007;16(3):423-430.

Nabhan A, Ahlhelm F, Shariat K, et al: The ProDisc-C prosthesis: Clinical and radiological experience 1 year after surgery. *Spine (Phila Pa 1976)* 2007;32(18):1935-1941.

Pickett GE, Sekhon LH, Sears WR, Duggal N: Complications with cervical arthroplasty. *J Neurosurg Spine* 2006;4(2):98-105.

Sasso RC, Smucker JD, Hacker RJ, Heller JG: Clinical outcomes of BRYAN cervical disc arthroplasty: A prospective, randomized, controlled, multicenter trial with 24-month follow-up. *J Spinal Disord Tech* 2007;20(7):481-491.

Sekhon LH, Duggal N, Lynch JJ, et al: Magnetic resonance imaging clarity of the Bryan, Prodisc-C, Prestige LP, and PCM cervical arthroplasty devices. *Spine (Phila Pa 1976)* 2007;32(6):673-680.

Shim CS, Lee SH, Park HJ, Kang HS, Hwang JH: Early clinical and radiologic outcomes of cervical arthroplasty with Bryan Cervical Disc prosthesis. *J Spinal Disord Tech* 2006;19(7):465-470.

Traynelis VC, Treharne RW: Use of Prestige LP Artificial Cervical Disc in the spine. *Expert Rev Med Devices* 2007;4(4):437-440.

Coding

CPT Codes		Corresponding ICD-9 Codes	
22554	Arthrodesis, anterior interbody technique, including minimal discectomy to prepare interspace (other than for decompression); cervical below C2	722.0 723	721
22585	Arthrodesis, anterior interbody technique, including minimal discectomy to prepare interspace (other than for decompression); each additional interspace (List separately in addition to code for primary procedure)	805 805	722.0 722.0
22845	Anterior instrumentation; 2 to 3 vertebral segments (List separately in addition to code for primary procedure)	722.52 737.30	724.6
22856	Total disc arthroplasty (artificial disc), anterior approach, including discectomy with end plate preparation (includes osteophytectomy for nerve root or spinal cord decompression and microdissection), single interspace, cervical	721.0	722.0
22861	Revision including replacement of total disc arthroplasty (artificial disc), anterior approach, single interspace; cervical	996.4	996.59
22864	Removal of total disc arthroplasty (artificial disc), anterior approach, single interspace; cervical	996.4	996.59

Chapter 3

Anterior Cervical Corpectomy and Fusion

Kamran Majid, MD
Jeffrey S. Fischgrund, MD

Indications

There are several indications for an anterior cervical corpectomy and fusion (ACCF). In burst fractures leading to neurologic deficits, the spinal canal must be decompressed (**Figure 1**). Other indications include tumor, infection, deformity, ossification of the posterior longitudinal ligament (OPLL), and spondylosis. More expeditious surgical intervention is recommended in patients with severe myelopathy, rapidly evolving deficits, multiple-level radiculopathy with persistent (3 months) disabling pain and weakness, static deficits with significant pain, and/or progressive kyphosis (**Figure 2**).

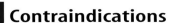

Contraindications

There are no specific contraindications to performing ACCF. However, diskectomy procedures should be considered when compression is limited to the disk level at one or two interspaces. In addition, posterior procedures should be considered in patients with predominantly posterior compression; multiple-level spondylosis or congenital stenosis; anterior bony ankylosis caused by degenerative or inflammatory disease; developmental stenosis; prior anterior neck surgery or severe anterior soft-tissue injury; continuous OPLL; and severe osteoporosis, which may increase the possibility of graft collapse.

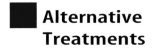

Alternative Treatments

Another way to deal with cervical pathology using an anterior approach would include performing aggressive diskectomies with specific attention to removing the compressive osteophytes from the posterior vertebral bodies. A posterior approach (laminectomy and/or fusion) may also be used in patients with pathology at multiple levels.

Results

Controversy exists as to the optimal anterior surgical treatment of patients with multiple-level spondylosis causing stenosis. Clearly, ACCF is indicated in these patients when deformity (kyphosis or spondylolisthesis) or instability is present and when compression is not limited to the disk spaces. In situations where multiple-level stenosis exists only at the disk spaces, multiple-level anterior cervical diskectomy and fusion (ACDF) may be a less technically demanding procedure, but the rate of pseudarthrosis increases as the number of levels of attempted fusion increases. Pseudarthrosis rates for one-level ACDF range from 5% to 10%. Two-level ACDF results in pseudarthrosis rates of approximately 15%. In 1998, Emery and associates reported the radiographic and clinical outcomes of patients undergoing three-level ACDF with autograft iliac crest grafting without an anterior cervical plate. Only 56% of the patients went on to solid arthrodesis at all three levels. Pseudarthrosis tended to lead to poorer clinical outcome. Emery and associates concluded that the rate of nonunion

Dr. Fischgrund or an immediate family member serves as a board member, owner, officer, or committee member of the Cervical Spine Research Society; has received royalties from DePuy; is a member of a speakers' bureau or has made paid presentations on behalf of DePuy, Smith & Nephew, and Stryker; serves as a paid consultant to or is an employee of DePuy, Smith & Nephew, Stryker, and Stout Medical; serves as an unpaid consultant to Fziomed; and has received research or institutional support from DePuy, Smith & Nephew, and Stryker. Neither Dr. Majid nor any immediate family member has received anything of value from or owns stock in a commercial company or institution related directly or indirectly to the subject of this chapter.

was unacceptable and that additional or alternative measures should be undertaken to increase the arthrodesis rate. The use of anterior instrumentation in this situation likely results in increased rates of fusion.

Anterior corpectomy with fusion relies on only two bone-healing sites but is a more technically demanding surgery. Some clinical studies involv-

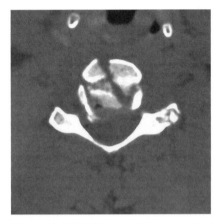

Figure 1 Axial CT scan shows a cervical burst fracture that would require a corpectomy to decompress the spinal canal.

ing ACCF procedures have reported fusion success rates > 95% (**Table 1**). Other authors have reported pseudarthrosis rates as high as 27% with autograft and 41% with allograft. In a comparison of radiographic and clinical outcomes of multiple interbody grafting and corpectomy with strut grafting, Hilibrand and associates reported a significantly higher fusion rate with strut grafting (93% versus 66%). Once again, patients with a pseudarthrosis had poorer clinical outcomes. This decrease in nonunion rates with corpectomy and strut grafting is attractive but does come with additional risks. Higher rates of graft complications and injuries to the vertebral arteries have been reported with vertebral body resections. The addition of anterior instrumentation may reduce the incidence of graft dislodgement but may adversely affect the fusion process. This idea has not been systematically studied, but some surgeons theorize that a certain amount of graft settling is necessary for bone-

graft healing/incorporation, and the addition of a static anterior cervical plate may prevent this process.

————————■

■ Technique

Setup/Exposure

ACCF is performed with the patient under general anesthesia. Positioning of the patient is of extreme importance because proper positioning will enable the surgeon to perform the surgery in a safe manner. Correct positioning of the endotracheal tube assists the surgeon, particularly in patients with herniations of upper cervical disks. If the surgeon chooses to perform the procedure on the left side of the patient's neck (**Figure 3**), the tube should be taped to the right side of the patient's mouth. A small, rolled towel is then placed between the scapulae longitudinally to allow for slight hyperextension of the neck. This will aid in exposure of the cervical spine,

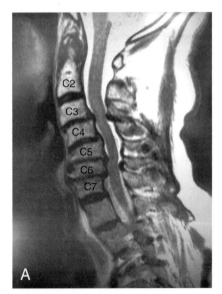

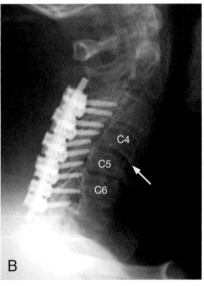

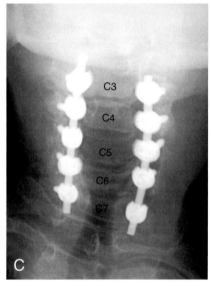

Figure 2 Images of the cervical spine of a patient obtained 1 year after the patient underwent posterior cervical laminectomy and fusion for myelopathy and radiculopathy. The myelopathy improved after the index procedure, but radiculopathy in the left arm did not remit. **A,** Midsagittal T2-weighted MRI shows severe spondylosis at multiple levels (most severe from C4 to C6) and kyphosis. **B,** Lateral radiograph also shows the spondylosis, as well as anterior subluxation of C4 on C5 (arrow). **C,** AP radiograph shows cervical spondylosis and no lateral listhesis. A decision was made to perform a corpectomy because the spine was fused posteriorly, and thus distracting the interspace to perform a diskectomy would be difficult and might not afford adequate visualization.

Table 1 Results of Anterior Cervical Corpectomy and Fusion

Authors (Year)	Number of Patients	Procedure or Approach	Mean Patient Age (Range)	Mean Follow-up (Range)	Fusion Success Rate	Results
Bernard and Whitecloud (1987)	21	ACCF	NR	32 months (12-89)	NR	16/21 with improved functional outcomes; no pseudarthroses; 1 graft dislodgement
Zdeblick and Bohlman (1989)	14	ACCF	46 years (21-73)	2.6 years (6 months-3.75 years)	NR	12/14 solid arthrodesis; 9 had complete neurologic recovery; 32° average kyphosis correction
Jamjoon et al (1991)	27	ACCF	66.9 years (39-82)	6 months (6-9)	96%	80% clinical improvements
Okada et al (1991)	37	ACCF	58 years (32-77)	49 months (28-70)	49% excellent 30% good 22% fair	29/37 satisfactory neurologic results
Swank et al (1997)	26	ACCF	51 years (30-78)	39 months (12-81)	NR	63% radiographic union; 31% symptomatic pseudarthrosis
Emery et al (1998)	55	ACCF	58 years (27-88)	(2-17 years)	NR	6 graft-related complications; 86% with preop gait disturbance improved 16 pseudarthroses 1 nonunion

ACCF = anterior cervical corpectomy and fusion; NR = not reported.

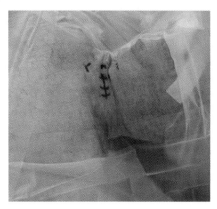

Figure 3 Intraoperative photograph shows the standard position and draping for a left-side Smith-Robinson approach to the cervical spine.

but care should be taken when performing this maneuver if patients are myelopathic. Cervical myelopathy is often worsened with neck hyperextension, and this position should be avoided during the surgical procedure. Preoperative assessment of vol-

untary neck range of motion is important in determining the amount of neck extension that can be safely used during intubation and the surgical procedure. In highly stenotic patients or in those for whom symptoms are magnified by moderate extension, fiberoptics or the use of video-guided laryngoscopic intubation is recommended. The arms should be tucked along the patient's sides, with downward traction applied to the shoulders with surgical tape. This downward traction and securing of the shoulders helps with patient positioning and is extremely useful for visualizing the lower cervical spine intraoperatively with fluoroscopy because the shoulders can often obscure the lower cervical spine when they are in the neutral position. Gardner-Wells tongs may be useful in providing intraoperative traction and are recommended when kyphosis is present.

Instruments/Equipment/Implants Required

The standard list of spine equipment found in most hospital sets should be used (**Figure 4**). This includes a full complement of Kerrison cutting tools, curets, and rongeurs. A high-speed burr with a side-cutting diamond tip is a useful and key piece of equipment for removing bone close to the dura without applying excessive pressure on the spinal cord. A hemostatic agent (a thrombin-soaked absorbable gelatin sponge, hemostatic matrix, or surgical wax) should also be available during the corpectomy. Caspar pins are especially useful to maintain distraction across the corpectomy level.

Procedure

A standard left-side anterior cervical approach is performed. Although a transverse incision may be acceptable for a one- or two-level corpectomy, a

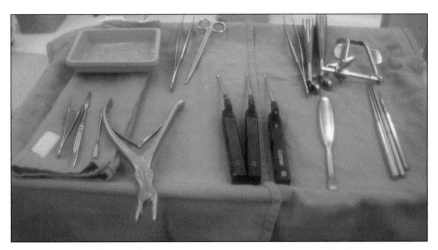

Figure 4 A representative Mayo stand with the standard instruments needed for an anterior cervical corpectomy and fusion.

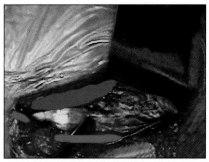

Figure 5 Intraoperative photograph shows self-retaining retractors being used during the procedure. The patient's head is to the right. Note that the longus colli muscles are dissected off the anterior vertebral body. Next, the self-retaining retractors will be placed under the longus colli muscles. Also note the relationship of the esophagus (blue area) and the carotid artery (red areas) during dissection.

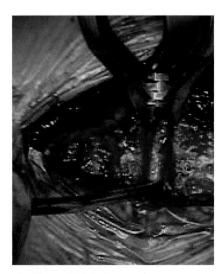

Figure 6 Intraoperative photograph of the anterior cervical spine shows a complete diskectomy of the interspace above the corpectomy level. The patient's head is to the right.

longitudinal incision should be considered for a more extensive decompression. After the exposure, the midline can be marked superior and inferior to the intended levels of decompression to help maintain orientation. Typically, the longus colli muscles are elevated 2 to 3 mm laterally to allow placement of self-retaining retractors (**Figure 5**). The uncovertebral joints provide a good landmark for defining the lateral borders. To avoid injury to the vertebral artery, dissection and decompression should not extend beyond the elevation of the longus colli.

First, diskectomies are performed at all of the involved levels. Next, a Leksell rongeur is used to create a trough in the central part of the body. The trough is widened and deepened with a 5-mm high-speed burr. A preoperative CT myelogram or MRI is useful for surgical planning and assessing the course of the vertebral arteries. At C6, a 19-mm–wide central decompression can be performed; at C3, the decompression can be only 15 mm wide.

After the posterior cortex is thinned with a high-speed burr, a small curet is used to breach the cortex along the lateral portion of the trough. This opening is then enlarged with small curets and 1- to 2-mm Kerrison rongeurs to remove any remaining bone. It is essential to elevate the bone away from the dura and the compressed spinal cord. The corpectomy trough should be at least 16 mm wide to provide adequate decompression. Routine removal of the posterior longitudinal ligament is not necessary unless ossification of the ligament or an extruded disk fragment is noted to be compressing the cord. Because of the risk of an absent dura in severe OPLL, leaving small isolated islands of OPLL has been described to avoid a large defect in the dura (**Figures 6 and 7**).

After the decompression has been completed and verified, the defect is stabilized with a structural graft (**Figures 8 and 9**).

The use of a structural autograft, such as an autologous fibula or a large iliac crest strut, is declining because of donor-site morbidity. Other options include cages packed with autologous cancellous bone graft.

The choice of graft material for strut grafting after corpectomy is controversial. Higher fusion rates with autograft are accompanied by additional risks associated with bone graft harvest. Individual patient characteristics, such as smoking history and the presence of rheumatoid arthritis, may influence the surgeon's decision to harvest the patient's iliac crest or fibula. The addition of a second surgical site for graft harvest increases the risk of infection. Specific iliac crest donor-site complications include neuroma formation, iliac crest fracture, cosmetic deformity, and persistent pain. In addition to infection, harvesting autologous fibula has been associated

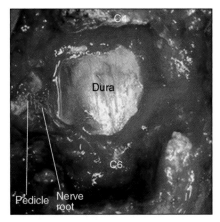

Figure 7 Intraoperative photograph taken after the corpectomy is complete. Note the wide decompression of the nerve roots above and below the corpectomy.

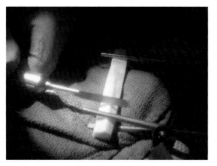

Figure 8 An allograft fibula shaft is cut with a reciprocating saw to produce the final fibula strut graft.

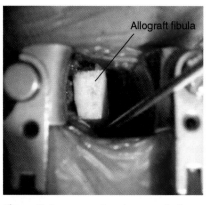

Figure 9 Intraoperative photograph shows the fibula strut graft in the space created by the corpectomy. The graft is slightly larger than the corpectomy, allowing a press fit when the graft is in place. The patient's head is at the top.

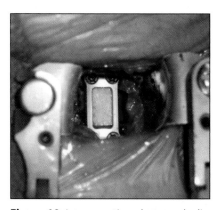

Figure 10 Intraoperative photograph displays the application of an anterior cervical plate spanning the corpectomy. The patient's head is at the top.

with injury to the peroneal nerves, contracture of the flexor hallucis longus and flexor digitorum longus tendons, the development of lower extremity deep vein thrombosis, stress fractures of the tibia, and chronic ankle pain. Thus, although the highest rates of solid fusion for ACCF have been reported for autologous grafts, the harvest of these autologous grafts is associated with significant morbidity. The use of autologous strut grafts also results in longer surgical times as well as longer hospital stays.

Alternatives to structural bone grafts have been proposed. Devices such as titanium or polyetheretherketone cages packed with autologous bone from the corpectomy site or the iliac crest have been used in combination with anterior instrumentation after decompressive corpectomy.

Acceptable rates of arthrodesis have been reported by some groups with the use of allograft fibular struts. Fusion rates for allograft bone may be enhanced by the addition of anterior instrumentation or by packing the medullary canal of the fibula with autograft bone obtained from the corpectomy. As experience with the use of osteobiologic agents increases, they may prove useful in increasing the arthrodesis rates of ACCF performed with allograft

bone. The US Food and Drug Administration (FDA) has not yet approved recombinant human bone morphogenetic protein (rhBMP-2) for use in the cervical spine. However, early experience with rhBMP-2 used in conjunction with bone allograft in ACDF has yielded excellent fusion rates. Unfortunately, multiple cases of excessive inflammatory reactions leading to airway compromise requiring reintubation have been reported in relation to this off-label procedure. These adverse reactions are postulated to be dose related, and lowering the dose of rhBMP-2 when it is used in the cervical spine may eliminate this potentially fatal event. Further research must document the safety of rhBMP-2 in the cervical spine before its widespread use can be recommended.

A cervical plate is frequently added to provide a more rigid construct in addition to providing a physical block to graft extrusion (**Figures 10** through **12**). Biomechanical studies have confirmed the increased stiffness after addition of an anterior plate to a multilevel corpectomy model. Some authors have advocated using a small inferior antikick plate, while others recommend using a dynamic plate. Currently, antikick plates are rarely used due to unacceptably high rates of pullout.

In a noninstrumented ACCF, immediate stability of the graft depends on the graft–host bone interface. An

"interference fit" is obtained by impacting the graft into place with the neck in slight extension and with traction applied to the head. The sculpting of the graft and the vertebral end plates also contributes to the initial stability. Migration most commonly occurs at the inferior end of the strut graft.

Instrumentation may be added to an ACCF to increase the immediate postoperative stability. Other potential advantages of plate osteosynthesis include reduced graft migration, reduced graft collapse, and avoidance of postoperative halo immobilization or

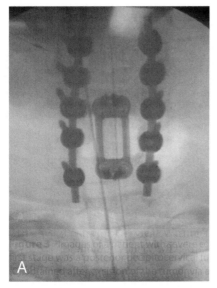 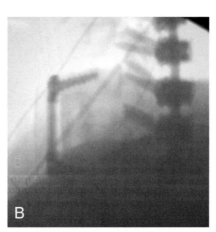

Figure 11 Postoperative AP **(A)** and lateral **(B)** cervical radiographs demonstrate proper placement of the graft and instrumentation.

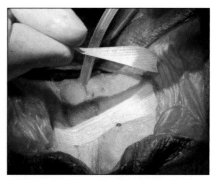

Figure 12 Intraoperative photograph shows the final closure. Note the use of a Jackson-Pratt drain, running absorbable suture, and adhesive skin-closure strips. The patient's head is to the right.

Wound Closure

Frequently, a soft drain can be placed in the wound anterior to the vertebral bodies, with the fascia over the platysma closed by simple absorbable sutures and the skin closed with a running absorbable subcuticular suture (**Figure 12**).

a secondary posterior stabilizing procedure. The plate may act as a buttress to block graft migration. Unfortunately, the use of anterior instrumentation in ACCF does not prevent graft complications.

Although compelling evidence does not exist in the current literature, most practicing spine surgeons will supplement one- and two-level corpectomies with an anterior cervical plate. The exact nature of the plate (static versus dynamic) used likely depends on the individual surgeon's training and his or her philosophy regarding whether settling of the graft must occur to obtain a solid arthrodesis. When faced with a situation in which a three-level corpectomy must be performed, many surgeons will choose to supplement the anterior procedure with posterior fixation in an attempt to reduce the likelihood of graft migration and the development of a pseudarthrosis.

During a corpectomy, the duration of soft-tissue retraction should be minimized to reduce the prevalence of dysphagia and dysphonia, which are the two most frequent symptoms after

the procedure. It may be useful to release retraction of soft tissues for a short period of time if a long retraction time is anticipated. Meticulous hemostasis should reduce the risk for a postoperative hematoma and respiratory difficulty.

When inserting a plate onto the anterior cervical spine, certain technical aspects of the procedure should be emphasized. Often, anterior osteophytes may impinge on the plate lying flush on the bone; thus, they should be removed with a rongeur or burr before placement of the plate. Unilateral screw depth should be measured before placement of the plate, with a nerve hook placed along the length of the vertebral body and measuring the length directly with a ruler. In certain trauma or tumor cases with poor bone quality, bicortical fixation is required and should be placed with fluoroscopy to determine the length of the screws. Several studies have alerted surgeons of the importance of avoiding adjacent disk degeneration by keeping the ends of the plates far away from the adjacent level.

Postoperative Regimen

With the addition of instrumentation, a firm cervical collar frequently is used postoperatively for 6 to 12 weeks. Exceptions are patients with tumors and those who have experienced trauma or who are severely osteopenic; a halo vest may be necessary for these individuals. Dislodgement of the graft or swelling usually occurs within the first week after surgery. The graft usually dislodges at the anteroinferior aspect of the lowermost vertebral body and usually is associated with a fracture of the edges of the lower vertebral body. Long-term follow-up, including periodic flexion-extension radiographs, is recommended to assess graft incorporation, particularly when allograft is used.

Avoiding Pitfalls and Complications

The most common neck problem after anterior cervical surgery is a transient sore throat or difficulty in swallowing. Many practitioners believe this complication is minor; however, most patients report significant difficulty swallowing for several weeks, along with a frequent need to fully chew their food before swallowing. The risk of injury and damage to the esophagus can be reduced by the use of dull retractors and avoiding excessive retraction. Perforation injuries to the esophagus are extremely rare but can be life threatening when they do occur. Late perforation is usually related to loosening or pullout of anterior plates or screws and is rarely due to graft extrusion. If the esophageal perforation is noted at the time of the initial surgery, all attempts should be made for an acute repair. Late perforations are technically much more difficult to repair and often require the prolonged use of nasogastric suction as well as parenteral hyperalimentation.

As with all surgical procedures, attention to detail during the approach will improve the ease of exposure and thereby allow safer decompression and reconstruction. Keeping the patient's arms at the sides improves intraoperative fluoroscopic visualization. In thick-necked patients, a longitudinal approach allows for the additional extensibility that may be needed for visualization. Loupes and a headlight or an operating microscope will further improve visualization. Undermining the platysma and a complete fascial release aids in deep dissection and manipulation. Elevation of the left and right longus colli muscles for at least one half an interspace above and below the intended diskectomies allows placement of a self-retaining retractor. This retractor may safely stay beneath these muscle bellies during the procedure and affords excellent visualization. When the extent of decompression and reconstruction is longer, a second, self-retaining retractor (with blunt blades) may be placed superiorly-inferiorly in the wound. During lengthy decompression procedures, these retractors should be removed at regular intervals to allow decompression of the soft-tissue structures. In the deep dissection, injury to the disks of adjacent levels must be avoided. Also, overstretching the longus colli muscles may result in injury to the cervical sympathetic chain and postoperative Horner syndrome.

Bibliography

Bernard TN Jr, Whitecloud TS III: Cervical spondylotic myelopathy and myeloradiculopathy: Anterior decompression and stabilization with autogenous fibula strut graft. *Clin Orthop Relat Res* 1987;221:149-160.

Breibach G, Fischgrund JS: Cervical myelopathy, in CB Bono, SR Garfin, eds: *Essentials in Orthopaedics: Spine.* Philadelphia, PA, Lippincott, Williams & Wilkins, 2004.

Emery SE, Bohlman HH, Bolesta MJ, Jones PK: Anterior cervical decompression and arthrodesis for the treatment of cervical spondylotic myelopathy: Two to seventeen-year follow-up. *J Bone Joint Surg Am* 1998;80(7):941-951.

Emery SE, Smith MD, Bohlman HH: Upper-airway obstruction after multilevel cervical corpectomy for myelopathy. *J Bone Joint Surg Am* 1991;73(4):544-551.

Fischgrund JS: Cervical radiculopathy: Part I. Anterior cervical approach, in HN Herkowitz, ed: *The Spine,* ed 5. Philadelphia, PA, Saunders Elsevier, 2006.

Fischgrund JS: Radiculopathy: Anterior discectomy with fusion, in HN Herkowitz (ed): *Cervical Spine Research Society Textbook,* ed 4. Philadelphia, PA, Lippinott-Raven, 2003.

Fujiwara K, Yonenobu K, Ebara S, Yamashita K, Ono K: The prognosis of surgery for cervical compression myelopathy: An analysis of the factors involved. *J Bone Joint Surg Br* 1989;71(3):393-398.

Hilibrand AS, Carlson GD, Palumbo MA, Jones PK, Bohlman HH: Radiculopathy and myelopathy at segments adjacent to the site of a previous anterior cervical arthrodesis. *J Bone Joint Surg Am* 1999;81(4):519-528.

Hilibrand AS, Fye MA, Emery SE, Palumbo MA, Bohlman HH: Increased rate of arthrodesis with strut grafting after multilevel anterior cervical decompression. *Spine (Phila Pa 1976)* 2002;27(2):146-151.

Jamjoom A, Williams C, Cummins B: The treatment of spondylotic cervical myelopathy by multiple subtotal vertebrectomy and fusion. *Br J Neurosurg* 1991;5(3):249-255.

Macdonald RL, Fehlings MG, Tator CH, et al: Multilevel anterior cervical corpectomy and fibular allograft fusion for cervical myelopathy. *J Neurosurg* 1997;86(6):990-997.

Okada K, Shirasaki N, Hayashi H, Oka S, Hosoya T: Treatment of cervical spondylotic myelopathy by enlargement of the spinal canal anteriorly, followed by arthrodesis. *J Bone Joint Surg Am* 1991;73(3):352-364.

Patel CK, Fischgrund JS, Herkowitz HN: Anterior cervical discectomy and fusion, in Bradford DS, Zdeblick TA, eds: *Master Techniques in Orthopaedic Surgery: The Spine*, ed 2. Philadelphia, PA, Lippincott, Williams & Wilkins, 2004.

Riew KD, Hilibrand AS, Palumbo MA, Bohlman HH: Anterior cervical corpectomy in patients previously managed with a laminectomy: Short-term complications. *J Bone Joint Surg Am* 1999;81(7):950-957.

Riew KD, Sethi NS, Devney J, Goette K, Choi K: Complications of buttress plate stabilization of cervical corpectomy. *Spine (Phila Pa 1976)* 1999;24(22):2404-2410.

Swank ML, Lowery GL, Bhat AL, McDonough RF: Anterior cervical allograft arthrodesis and instrumentation: Multilevel interbody grafting or strut graft reconstruction. *Eur Spine J* 1997;6(2):138-143.

Wada E, Suzuki S, Kanazawa A, Matsuoka T, Miyamoto S, Yonenobu K: Subtotal corpectomy versus laminoplasty for multilevel cervical spondylotic myelopathy: A long-term follow-up study over 10 years. *Spine (Phila Pa 1976)* 2001; 26(13):1443-1448.

Zdeblick TA, Bohlman HH: Cervical kyphosis and myelopathy: Treatment by anterior corpectomy and strut-grafting. *J Bone Joint Surg Am* 1989;71(2):170-182.

Coding

CPT Codes		Corresponding ICD-9 Codes	
20930	Allograft for spine surgery only; morselized (List separately in addition to code for primary procedure)	721.1 723	722 724.6
20931	Allograft for spine surgery only; structural (List separately in addition to code for primary procedure)	721.1 723.0	722 724.6
20936	Autograft for spine surgery only (includes harvesting the graft); local (eg, ribs, spinous process, or laminar fragments) obtained from same incision (List separately in addition to code for primary procedure)	724.6	722.0
20937	Autograft for spine surgery only (includes harvesting the graft); morselized (through separate skin or fascial incision) (List separately in addition to code for primary procedure)	724.6	722.0
20938	Autograft for spine surgery only (includes harvesting the graft); structural, bicortical or tricortical (through separate skin or fascial incision) (List separately in addition to code for primary procedure)	724.6 721.1	722.0
22585	Arthrodesis, anterior interbody technique, including minimal discectomy to prepare interspace (other than for decompression); each additional interspace (List separately in addition to code for primary procedure)	805	722.0
22554	Arthrodesis, anterior interbody technique, including minimal discectomy to prepare interspace (other than for decompression); cervical below C2	722.0 723	721
22845	Anterior instrumentation; 2 to 3 vertebral segments (List separately in addition to code for primary procedure)	722.52 737.30	724.6
63081	Vertebral corpectomy (vertebral body resection), partial or complete, anterior approach with decompression of spinal cord and/or nerve root(s); cervical, single segment	722.71 723	721
63082	Vertebral corpectomy (vertebral body resection), partial or complete, anterior approach with decompression of spinal cord and/or nerve root(s); cervical, each additional segment (List separately in addition to code for primary procedure)	722.71 723	721

CPT copyright © 2010 by the American Medical Association. All rights reserved.

Chapter 4
Transoral Odontoid Excision

K. Daniel Riew, MD
Adam L. Wollowick, MD
Brett A. Taylor, MD

■ Introduction

Ventral compression of the spinal cord at the craniocervical junction is an uncommon but potentially devastating situation. Certain disorders, such as rheumatoid arthritis, os odontoideum, and displaced odontoid fractures, can distort the normal anatomy of the upper cervical region and lead to severe neurologic dysfunction. To address ventral neurologic compression, resection of the odontoid process may be necessary. The most direct route to the ventral aspect of the upper cervical spine, from the clivus to the top of C3, is the transoral approach. It is nearly impossible to address pathology at these levels with a standard Smith-Robinson approach to the anterior cervical spine because the mandible blocks access to the structures above C2.

Although the upper cervical spine lies directly posterior to the oropharynx, separated from the mouth by only four thin layers of tissue, the transoral technique can be intimidating to surgeons unfamiliar with the procedure. The transoral approach has a higher rate of infection than other anterior cervical procedures; forces the surgeon to work in a narrow, deep space; and requires the use of specialized retractors. Nevertheless, with experience, careful preoperative planning and a firm understanding of the upper cervical anatomy, transoral decompression can be performed safely and result in significant neurologic improvement for the patient.

To safely perform the transoral approach to the upper cervical spine, the surgeon must fully understand the vertebral artery anatomy in this region. The midline must be correctly identified before beginning the dissection. The midline is usually defined by palpating the anterior tubercle of C1; however, pathologic conditions can severely distort the normal anatomic relationships. The longus colli muscles and anterior longitudinal ligament can help orient the surgeon once the superficial dissection is performed. At the C2-3 disk space, the vertebral arteries usually lie approximately 1 cm from the midline. The artery lies lateral to the C2 body before coursing superiorly over the transverse process. In addition, the hypoglossal nerves and eustachian tubes are typically found just lateral to the lateral masses of C1. To prevent injury to these structures, dissection should not extend beyond this point. At the base of C2 and at the level of the arch of C1, the vertebral artery is approximately 24 mm from the midline. The dissection should not be wider than 2 cm from the midline in this area. At the level of the foramen magnum, the vertebral arteries move centrally and are found about 1 cm from the midline.

———————■

■ Indications

The most general indication for a transoral approach to the upper cervical spine is extradural ventral pathology causing compression of the brainstem or upper cervical spinal cord from the clivus to the C2 vertebral body. The cause of such pathologic compression of the neurologic ele-

Dr. Riew or an immediate family member serves as a board member, owner, officer, or committee member of the Cervical Spine Research Society and the Scoliosis Research Society; has received royalties from Biomet; has received research or institutional support from Medtronic Sofamor Danek; and has stock or stock options held in Osprey. Dr. Wollowick or an immediate family member has received research or institutional support from Stryker, DePuy, and K2M. Dr. Taylor or an immediate family member serves as a board member, owner, officer, or committee member of the St. Louis Spine & Orthopaedic Surgery Center, the CT Partners of Chesterfield, and the Imaging Partners of Chesterfield.

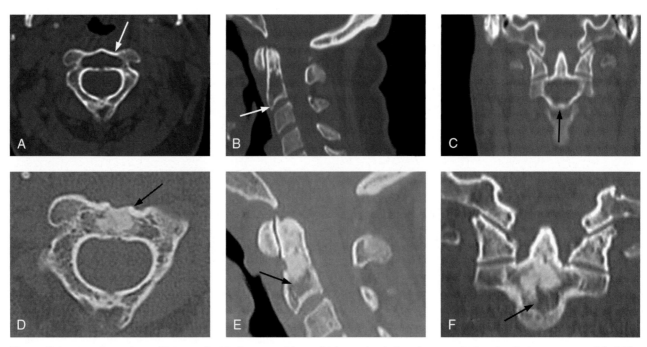

Figure 1 Images of a patient with a vertebral lesion caused by multiple myeloma, for whom medical and radiation treatment failed. The patient was treated with a transoral curettage and placement of methylmethacrylate through a small cortical window. Preoperative axial (**A**), sagittal (**B**), and coronal (**C**) CT images show an impending pathologic fracture (arrow). Axial (**D**), sagittal (**E**), and coronal (**F**) CT images at 2 years show good filling (arrow) and no recurrence of the lesion.

ments may be rheumatoid or other retro-odontoid pannus, os odontoideum and other congenital malformations, tumor, infection, or fracture. Odontoid fractures may cause upper cervical neurologic compression due to acute displacement, malunion, or nonunion of the dens. Certain tumors and infections of the upper cervical region require direct anterior exposure for removal and are best treated using the transoral approach (**Figure 1**). Additionally, rheumatoid arthritis may distort the upper cervical anatomy, leading to cranial settling, basilar invagination, and irreducible atlanto-axial subluxation. Any of these processes may result in compression of the brainstem and upper spinal cord. Other inflammatory disorders that can lead to pannus formation in the upper cervical spine include psoriasis, gout, pigmented villonodular synovitis, and os odontoideum. Occasionally, pannus formation may occur in the setting of degenerative spondylosis; this

has been referred to as "pseudotumor of the elderly."

———————————————

Contraindications

The main contraindication to the transoral approach is active infection involving the nose, mouth, and/or pharynx. In addition, dental sepsis should be fully treated before transoral surgery. The presence of vascular anomalies or vascular structures in the plane of the dissection may preclude the use of this technique, primarily because of the limited working space should it become necessary to control significant bleeding. Intradural pathology is a relative contraindication to transoral procedures because of the high risk of meningitis and encephalitis resulting from cerebrospinal fluid (CSF) contamination by oropharyngeal flora. Pathology that extends far beyond the midline or that continues

very distal or proximal to the accessible working area of the transoral route may not be amenable to isolated transoral surgery. If the ventral approach is used in these situations, an extended dissection is likely to be required, which can involve splitting the soft palate, tongue, or mandible. These extended approaches may carry a higher risk of postoperative complications than a pure transoral technique. Finally, the inability to fully open the mouth at least 25 to 30 mm may preclude a transoral approach. As a rule of thumb, to perform transoral surgery, the mouth should be able to open wide enough to allow three fingers between the upper and lower rows of teeth.

———————————————

Alternative Treatments

Many authors have demonstrated that inflammatory pannus usually sub-

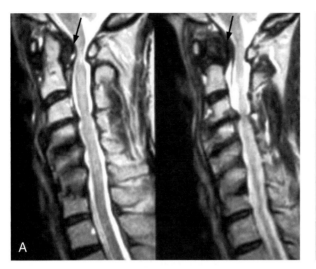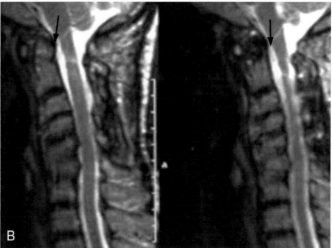

Figure 2 Images of a patient with rheumatoid arthritis who had pannus behind the dens. The patient was treated with a posterior fusion without anterior decompression. **A**, Preoperative T2-weighted sagittal MRI demonstrates the pannus (arrow) behind the dens. **B**, T2-weighted MRI obtained 6 months after surgery demonstrates resolution of the pannus (arrow).

sides following posterior fusion and stabilization of the upper cervical spine (**Figure 2**). Accordingly, we generally reserve transoral decompression and resection of the odontoid for patients with severe neurologic dysfunction that persists following posterior stabilization. Even in cases of severe basilar invagination where the dens will not resorb with time, we have found that the neurologic status improves with posterior stabilization. If there is no neurologic improvement 2 or 3 months following posterior stabilization, then we reevaluate with CT and MRI. If neural compression persists, we then proceed with anterior decompression.

Other alternative approaches include the mandible-splitting approach for a more extensile exposure, the high cervical approach, and a posterolateral approach. The mandible-splitting approach carries substantial morbidity and is not necessary to expose the atlas and axis. The high cervical approach cannot adequately visualize the anterior arch of C1 and the dens. The posterolateral approach is difficult and bloody and requires resection of the C2 nerve root. A combined approach is sometimes necessary and can avoid the morbidity associated with splitting the mandible (**Figure 3**).

Results

Several studies reporting the outcomes of transoral decompression of the craniocervical junction have been published in the literature (**Table 1**). In 1986, Crockard and associates described the outcome of 14 patients with rheumatoid arthritis who were treated with a combination of transoral resection of the odontoid and occipitocervical fusion. After an average of 18 months, nearly all patients (13 of 14) showed neurologic improvement, and all had reduced pain. There were only two minor complications of the procedure. Menezes and VanGilder described the outcome of the transoral procedure in 72 patients with a variety of upper cervical pathologies. Although only 72% required posterior stabilization, all patients showed neurologic improvement, and a wound infection occurred in only one patient. In 1989, Hadley and associates reported the results of 53 transoral pro-

cedures. After a mean follow-up of 2 years, there were no deaths attributed to the procedure, but complications occurred in three patients. All three had wound dehiscence plus additional morbidity. Neurologic improvement was found in 90% of patients at final follow-up. Grob and associates reported the results of 22 patients with rheumatoid arthritis who were treated with posterior stabilization. They specifically analyzed the status of the retrodental pannus following occipitocervical fusion. Regression of the pannus was observed in 19 of 22 patients, regardless of disease progression. They concluded that pannus is the product of instability, rather than being part of the disease process itself. This study has important implications that must be considered when deciding whether or not to proceed with a transoral decompression.

Preoperative Evaluation

The preoperative evaluation of any patient being considered for transoral

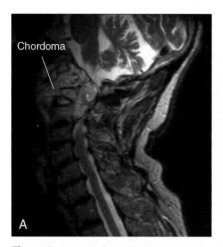
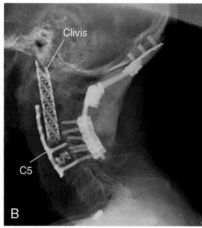
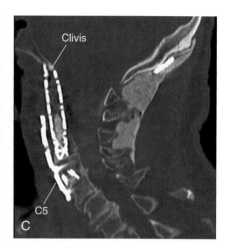

Figure 3 Images of a patient with severe cord compression from a high cervical chordoma who was treated with a two-stage procedure. The first stage was a posterior occipitocervical fusion. **A,** Preoperative T2-weighted MRI. Postoperative lateral radiograph (**B**) and sagittal CT scan (**C**) obtained after excision of the tumor via a combined transoral and high cervical approach and reconstruction from the clivus to C5.

Table 1 Results of Transoral Decompression

Author(s) (Year)	Number of Patients	Procedure or Approach	Mean Patient Age in Years (Range)	Mean Follow-up in Months (Range)	Fusion Rate	Results
Crockard et al (1986)	14	TAD + OCF	57.8 years (19-78)	17.8 (6-45)	NR	13/14 (93%) neurologic improvement 100% decreased pain No wound infections 2/14 (14%) minor complications
Menezes and VanGilder (1988)	72 (29 children)	TAD ± OCF (52/72)*	(6-82 years)	NR	NR	100% neurologic improvement 1/72 (1.4%) wound infection
Hadley et al (1989)	53	TAD ± posterior (5/53)†	54 years (2-89)	24 (6-74)	NR	3/53 (6%) morbidity 0% mortality 45/50 (90%) neurologic improvement
Grob et al (1997)	22	OCF	58.5 years (39-71)	40 (12-75)	100%	19/22 (86%) with decreased pannus, regardless of disease progression

TAD = transoral anterior decompression; OCF = occipitocervical fusion.
* Fifty-two of 72 patients required C1-2 TAD and OCF.
† Five of 53 patients had TAD and posterior fusion.

surgery begins with a thorough history and physical examination. For many patients with upper cervical pathology, stabilization of the spine is all that is necessary; however, patients with evidence of severe myelopathy or neurologic dysfunction due to ventral compression of the spinal cord or brainstem may require transoral decompression. In addition to assessing the patient's neurologic status, it is also critical to assess the overall alignment of the head and neck. Irreducible cervical kyphosis, rotatory subluxation, or fixed torticollis can distort the regional anatomy and/or preclude using the transoral approach. As previously mentioned, the mandible must be sufficiently mobile to allow adequate visualization. If there is less than 25 to 30 mm of oral clearance, it may be necessary to split the mandible to gain access to the upper cervical spine. Preoperative consultation with an otolaryngologist is helpful if there is any question about the temporomandibular joints or the amount of mandibular excursion. An ear, nose, and throat evaluation may be warranted in all patients to rule out vocal cord or pharyngeal dysfunction as well as cranial nerve abnormalities. If any problems are noted that may potentially lead to delayed postoperative extubation, a preoperative tracheostomy should be considered.

Any active dental issues such as loose teeth, untreated cavities, or other oral infections should be evaluated by a dentist or oral surgeon before undertaking the transoral approach. Furthermore, the tongue and soft palate must be sufficiently mobile to allow for retractor placement. Placement of a feeding tube or central line should be considered preoperatively, as there is sometimes a delay of several days after surgery before oral feeding is begun. In straightforward cases, such as simple decompressions of rheumatoid pannus, we rapidly advance the diet over 24 hours. However, in more complex or prolonged cases involving tumors, oral intake may be suspended for several days or more. Because of the potential for postoperative infection from oropharyngeal flora, preoperative cultures can be obtained from the mouth, nose, and throat to define an appropriate perioperative antibiotic regimen. For cases in which violation of the dura is either necessary or anticipated, preoperative placement of a lumbar drain should be considered.

All patients should have a full set of plain radiographs of the cervical spine, including open-mouth, flexion, and extension views. We obtain a CT scan with sagittal and coronal reconstructions as well as an MRI scan for all patients being considered for transoral surgery. These studies are necessary to fully assess the extent of the intraspinal pathology as well as to plan instrumentation. To define the location of the vertebral arteries and local vascular structures, a CT or magnetic resonance angiogram can be obtained as well. When possible and

practical, we prefer performing a posterior stabilization before the transoral procedure for several reasons. First, odontoid resection renders the C1-C2 articulation significantly unstable in as many as 70% of cases. The incidence of instability may approach 100% when resection of additional structures is performed. Although the risk is small, the possibility of spinal cord injury exists following odontoid resection when the patient is being turned to a prone position. Although this risk can be mitigated by halo immobilization, placement of the halo adds an unnecessary step. Second, performing the posterior approach first prevents contamination by instruments used for the transoral approach. When the anterior approach must be performed before the posterior procedure, we do both stages in the same surgical setting, but a fresh set of instruments is used for the posterior operation. We favor anterior decompression first for cases in which the cord is at risk and spinal cord monitoring is difficult to obtain, as a posterior stabilization before neural decompression might risk neurologic injury.

Techniques

Setup/Exposure

To perform the transoral procedure, we use a standard operating table and place the patient in the supine position. The head is positioned in slight extension to facilitate exposure. We have found that using oral intubation makes it easier to position the endotracheal tube away from the midline than when nasotracheal intubation is performed; however, several authors have reported using nasotracheal intubation successfully for the transoral approach. A tracheostomy is usually not necessary for transoral procedures but can improve access to the posterior pharynx and certainly provides

secure airway protection. Preoperative tracheostomy should be considered for cases that require more extensive dissection and cases in which ventilator dependence for several days is anticipated. A nasogastric tube may be placed to suction blood and secretions from the patient's stomach and to provide postoperative feeding. If necessary, the upper esophagus can be packed with gauze to prevent the ingestion of blood and other fluids.

Antibiotic prophylaxis should be given at least 30 minutes before incision. If preoperative cultures were obtained, the antibiotic regimen can be tailored to the individual patient. Otherwise, coverage with broad-spectrum antibiotics is recommended.

Instruments/Equipment/ Implants Required

We use neurophysiologic monitoring for all transoral cases. Our standard monitoring protocol includes both somatosensory-evoked potentials and transcranial motor-evoked potentials. In addition, we use the operating microscope for all transoral procedures. We have found that the microscope provides superior illumination of the surgical field and improved visualization when compared to the use of loupes and a headlamp. During the preparation, we place the bed in a 30° to 40° Trendelenburg position to prevent blood and secretions from entering the lungs. Once positioning is complete, a plastic oral drape is used to isolate the mouth. Other instruments are identified in the sections that follow.

Preparation of the Mouth

To facilitate visualization and avoid significant postoperative dysphagia and/or dysphonia, it is necessary to retract the uvula and soft palate. To retract the uvula out of the way, one can use specialized retractors from the transoral set. Sometimes these attachments are cumbersome and lose their purchase, especially if one has to reach

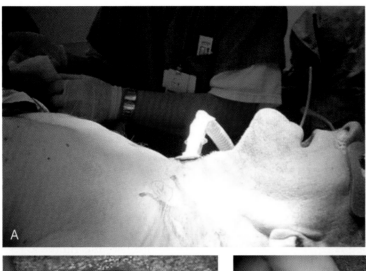

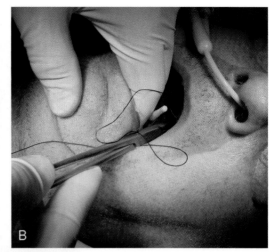

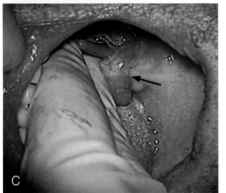

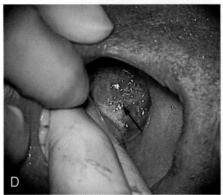

Figure 4 Clinical photographs showing the steps taken to retract the uvula. **A,** Side view shows a tube placed in the nose that exits through the mouth. Frontal views demonstrate how the uvula is sutured to the tip of the catheter (**B**), and the catheter is then pulled back through the nose (**C**) until it retracts the uvula (arrow) into the nasopharynx (**D**).

up to the clivus. In such cases, it helps to retract the uvula by suturing it to the tip of a rubber catheter inserted through the nose. To accomplish this task, a rubber catheter is passed into the pharynx through the nose. The tip of the catheter is sutured to the uvula, after which the catheter is pulled back through the nose, appropriately tensioned, and secured (**Figure 4**). If special attachments to the transoral retractors are used, the adequacy of the exposure should be assessed before the mouth is prepared. To prepare the mouth for surgery, the oral cavity is filled with povidone-iodine solution (**Figure 5,** *A*). We place the patient into a Trendelenburg position (**Figure 5,** *B*) to keep the solution from entering the lungs should the endotracheal tube cuff deflate. We generally soak the mouth for 10 minutes before re-

moving the prep solution. Finally, the field is sterilely draped according to the surgeon's typical routine and transoral retractors are placed. Several transoral retractor systems are currently available on the market. These are designed to securely hold the endotracheal tube, tongue, and posterior pharynx away from the surgical field (**Figure 6,** *A* and *B*).

Procedure: Resection of the Dens

To identify the midline for the incision, we begin by palpating the anterior tubercle of C1. In addition, the C2-3 disk space is usually prominent and defines the inferior extent of the incision. The incision is then made from the base of the clivus to the inferior aspect of the C2 vertebral body. We cut directly down to bone through

all layers of the posterior pharynx, including the pharyngeal mucosa, the superior constrictor muscles, and the anterior longitudinal ligament, using the cutting current of an electrocautery. The amount of bleeding is significantly reduced by staying in the midline, especially along the medial raphe of the pharyngeal muscles. Alternatively, the mucosa can be separated from the underlying muscles, which allows for a layered closure. Our typical incision is approximately 3 to 5 cm in length. We elevate flaps to either side of the midline but are cautious to avoid dissection beyond the lateral edge of the C2 vertebral body. If necessary, perpendicular cuts can be made to provide additional mobilization of the flaps. The soft palate can also be incised when exposure of the clivus is needed (**Figure 7,** *A* through

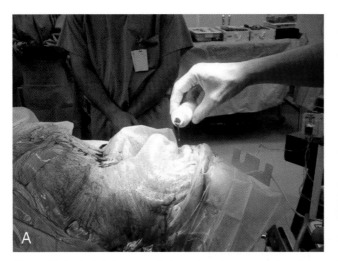
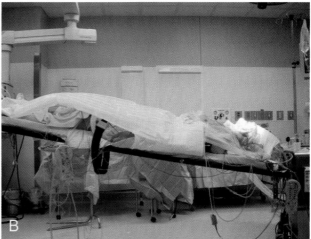

Figure 5 **A**, clinical photograph demonstrating preparation of the patient's mouth with a sterilizing solution such as a povidone-iodine. The patient is then placed into the Trendelenburg position (**B**) to keep the solution out of the lungs if the endotracheal tube deflates.

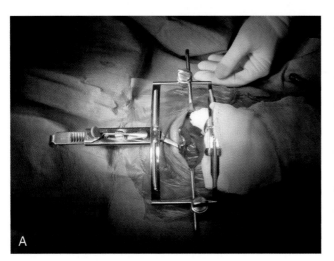
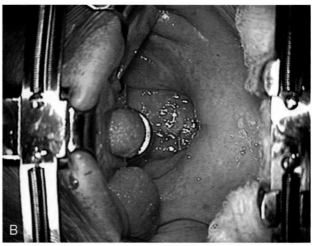

Figure 6 A transoral retractor system. The top of the patient's head is to the right. **A**, Intraoperative photograph of retractor in place. **B**, Close-up photograph of the exposure. The uvula has been retracted out of the way (right side of the photograph) and the tongue is depressed by the retractor, exposing the oropharynx.

D). However, this has been shown to lead to a high rate of postoperative dysphagia and/or dysphonia. Once the flaps are elevated, self-retaining toothed retractor blades are placed and used to retract the flaps laterally.

Once the vertebrae are fully exposed, it is necessary to resect the anterior arch of C1. We remove about 1 cm of bone in each direction from the midline, which is approximately two thirds of the entire arch. Removal of the arch can be performed with a high-speed burr or with a sharp rongeur. Enough of the anterior C1 arch must be removed to visualize the base of the odontoid and the shoulders where it joins the body of the axis. It is not uncommon to encounter pannus or granulation tissue posterior to the arch of C1 before the odontoid is visualized. Next, the odontoid must be resected, which is usually performed in one of two ways. The first method is to amputate the odontoid at its base and remove it en bloc by severing the soft-tissue connections, working in a caudal to cephalad direc-tion. We prefer to remove the dens by using a high-speed burr to resect the bone. A side-cutting matchstick burr is ideal for this purpose. It allows controlled removal of the bone while limiting the risk of tearing the underlying soft tissues. To fully remove the odontoid, it is necessary to cut the soft tissues attached to the dens, including the apical ligament, the alar ligaments, and the transverse ligament. This can be done before drilling the dens, using fine angled curet or micro-Kerrison rongeurs. A variation of removing the

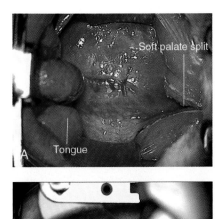

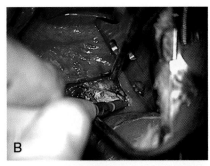

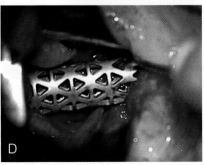

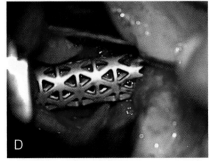

Figure 7 Exposure of the clivus. The top of the patient's head is to the right. **A**, The soft palate has been divided just lateral to the uvula to gain exposure to the clivus. **B** through **D**, Intraoperative photographs of the patient in Figure 3. **B**, Exposure through the retropharyngeal soft tissue with electrocautery. **C**, The chordoma (indicated by dashed circle) is exposed. **D**, Reconstruction using a cage that spans from the clivus to C4.

dens with the burr is to hollow out the odontoid, leaving thin lateral and posterior cortical walls of bone. The remaining bone is then removed with either fine curet or micro-Kerrison rongeurs.

The adequacy of odontoid excision is usually readily apparent by visual inspection; however, if there is any doubt, the extent of bony resection can be assessed with intraoperative imaging (radiography or fluoroscopy). As an adjunct to imaging, the cavity can be filled with radiopaque dye to improve visualization. The decompression is completed by carefully removing pannus, remaining soft tissues, and the tectorial membrane until the pulsating dura is visualized. The process of exposing the thecal sac carries a risk of CSF leakage, which places the patient at risk for meningitis and encephalitis. As the inflammatory pannus has been shown to regress following stabilization of the upper

cervical spine, it may not be necessary to expose the dura in all cases. Although resection of the soft-tissue structures around the odontoid has been shown to produce significant upper cervical instability, odontoid-sparing techniques have also been described that are thought to maintain stability. These techniques require only partial removal of the transverse ligament and the tectorial membrane, but they have been associated with instability, which can be fatal.

Wound Closure

Once the decompression is completed, it is critical to obtain meticulous hemostasis. Closure is performed using 3-0 chromic, buried sutures. We prefer to close the pharynx in a single layer, but a two-layer closure may also be performed. If the soft palate is incised, then it should be closed in two or three layers. The uvula is then separated from the previously placed

catheter, and the oropharynx is copiously irrigated. Next, the transoral retractor is removed. The tongue and posterior pharynx are visually inspected for excessive swelling. Hydrocortisone ointment can be applied to the tongue and mucosa to decrease inflammation and swelling.

Postoperative Regimen

We perform immediate posterior stabilization in all patients following odontoid resection, unless they have previous acquired or congenital fusion of the upper cervical spine. In general, we use a hard collar and manual cervical stabilization to transfer the patient from the supine to the prone position when we follow the transoral decompression with posterior fusion. If severe instability is suspected, then a halo is placed before turning the patient. As noted earlier in this chapter, whenever possible, we perform the posterior fusion before the transoral procedure. Occipitocervical stabilization is required for all patients who have complete odontoid resections because the stability of the segment depends on the ligamentous attachments to the dens. We typically use one of the commercially available occipitocervical instrumentation systems that include an occipital plate and screws connected by a rod.

For most transoral cases, we have found that immediate postoperative extubation is possible. The proximal location of the surgical field within the pharynx makes airway compromise less likely. Nevertheless, the tongue and soft tissues should be carefully inspected for severe swelling before extubating the patient. If any concern exists, the patient should remain intubated until any edema has resolved. A lateral radiograph also can be used to assist in the evaluation of local soft-tissue swelling. Oral feeding can resume immediately for most patients who have short, simple procedures; however, many require tube feeding for several days. It is best to keep the head of the bed elevated to decrease the amount of secretions pooling in the posterior pharynx. Antibiotics are continued for 24 to 48 hours after surgery. Patients who have extensive procedures are admitted to the intensive care unit until fully stabilized. Once spinal stability is ensured and the patient's respiratory status is secure, mobilization and ambulation can be initiated.

Avoiding Pitfalls and Complications

Infection has been a major concern associated with the transoral approach because dissection occurs directly through a "contaminated" field. The preponderance of oropharynGEAL flora led to early reports of infection rates that approached 60%. Currently, the incidence of postoperative infection following transoral decompression is thought to be 0% to 3%. The significant reduction in postoperative infections has been attributed to perioperative antibiotics (especially when based on preoperative cultures), meticulous hemostasis, and careful wound closure. In addition, the infection rate can be diminished by not placing bone graft or instrumentation through the transoral route. If there is any concern about infection, either in the early or late postoperative periods, then urgent imaging and/or surgical exploration should be performed. In addition, postoperative infection or retropharyngeal abscess should be considered the origins of would dehiscence until proven otherwise.

Dural tear and CSF leakage is not an infrequent occurrence with transoral decompression. Frequently, the pannus or other pathology has developed adhesions to the underlying dura that makes violation of the meninges unavoidable. As previously stated, once resection of the odontoid is completed, exposure of the dura may not be necessary because pannus typically regresses following posterior stabilization. Nevertheless, if a CSF leak occurs, it is critical to completely repair the dura whenever possible. It is necessary to completely isolate the CSF from oral flora because of the risk of meningitis and encephalitis. If a CSF leak develops, an attempt should be made to suture the dural tear. Regardless of whether closure can be performed, the repair should be supplemented with a combination of fibrin glue, tissue grafts, and dural patches. Consideration should be given to the placement of a subarachnoid lumbar drain. In addition, broad-spectrum postoperative antibiotics should be administered for at least 2 weeks because of the risk of encephalomeningitis.

Vascular injury can be a devastating complication of transoral surgery. The vertebral arteries are the vessels most at risk of injury. The importance of careful review of preoperative imaging studies to determine the location and course of the vertebral arteries cannot be overemphasized. The most likely site of vertebral artery laceration is at the lower portion of the C2 body. It is critical not to extend the dissection beyond the lateral border of the C2 body. If the vertebral artery is injured, it may be possible to repair the vessel. An attempt can also be made to simply pack the area with a hemostatic agent in an effort to control the bleeding. If the bleeding cannot be controlled, intraoperative consultation with a vascular surgeon may be required to obtain an angiogram or permanently occlude the vessel. Certainly, the latter carries a risk of stroke.

The soft tissues in the oropharynx are also at risk for injury and necrosis as a result of pressure from retractors. It is important to inspect the tongue, soft palate, and pharyngeal mucosa frequently during the procedure. While we have not found it necessary to loosen or release the retractors during most transoral procedures, it may be beneficial to do so if the surgical time exceeds 90 to 120 minutes. The use of hydrocortisone ointment on the tissues at the beginning and conclusion of the procedure may help to reduce the swelling and inflammation of the delicate soft tissues.

Spinal cord injury and worsening of neurologic function is another significant risk associated with transoral decompression. This is true for any patient undergoing surgery for severe neurologic compression and myelopathy. As noted earlier, we use spinal cord monitoring for all transoral procedures. In addition, it is important to maintain the patient's blood pressure during the operation and avoid periods of hypotension that can cause spinal cord ischemia. It is also critical to replace lost blood as needed to maintain a stable hematocrit.

Finally, transoral decompression carries a significant risk of postoperative upper cervical instability. The risk of instability is present with both resection of the dens and odontoid-sparing procedures. Our practice is to stabilize the posterior cervical spine before the transoral procedure whenever possible or to perform the posterior fusion and instrumentation immediately following the transoral approach under the same anesthetic. If neither of these options is possible, then the patient should be placed in a halo until the posterior stabilization can be performed or stability of the cranial-cervical junction is assured.

■ Bibliography

Crockard HA: Transoral surgery: Some lessons learned. *Br J Neurosurg* 1995;9(3):283-293.

Crockard HA, Pozo JL, Ransford AO, Stevens JM, Kendall BE, Essigman WK: Transoral decompression and posterior fusion for rheumatoid atlanto-axial subluxation. *J Bone Joint Surg Br* 1986;68(3):350-356.

Dickman CA, Locantro J, Fessler RG: The influence of transoral odontoid resection on stability of the craniovertebral junction. *J Neurosurg* 1992;77(4):525-530.

Di Lorenzo N: Craniocervical junction malformation treated by transoral approach: A survey of 25 cases with emphasis on postoperative instability and outcome. *Acta Neurochir (Wien)* 1992;118(3-4):112-116.

Fang HSY, Ong B: Direct anterior approach to the upper cervical spine. *J Bone Joint Surg Am* 1962;44:1588-1604.

Grob D, Würsch R, Grauer W, Sturzenegger J, Dvorak J: Atlantoaxial fusion and retrodental pannus in rheumatoid arthritis. *Spine (Phila Pa 1976)* 1997;22(14):1580-1584.

Hadley MN, Spetzler RF, Sonntag VK: The transoral approach to the superior cervical spine: A review of 53 cases of extradural cervicomedullary compression. *J Neurosurg* 1989;71(1):16-23.

Kanavel AB: Bullet located between the atlas and the base of the skull: Technique of removal through the mouth. *Surg Clin Chicago* 1917;1:361-366.

Menezes AH, VanGilder JC: Transoral-transpharyngeal approach to the anterior craniocervical junction: Ten-year experience with 72 patients. *J Neurosurg* 1988;69(6):895-903.

Young WF, Boyko O: Magnetic resonance imaging confirmation of resolution of periodontoid pannus formation following C1/C2 posterior transarticular screw fixation. *J Clin Neurosci* 2002;9(4):434-436.

Coding

CPT Codes		Corresponding ICD-9 Codes	
20930	Allograft for spine surgery only; morselized (List separately in addition to code for primary procedure)	721.1 723	722 724.6
20931	Allograft for spine surgery only; structural (List separately in addition to code for primary procedure)	721.1 723.0	722 724.6
20936	Autograft for spine surgery only (includes harvesting the graft); local (eg, ribs, spinous process, or laminar fragments) obtained from same incision (List separately in addition to code for primary procedure)	724.6	722.0
20937	Autograft for spine surgery only (includes harvesting the graft); morselized (through separate skin or fascial incision) (List separately in addition to code for primary procedure)	724.6	722.0
20938	Autograft for spine surgery only (includes harvesting the graft); structural, bicortical or tricortical (through separate skin or fascial incision) (List separately in addition to code for primary procedure)	724.6 721.1	722.0
22318	Open treatment and/or reduction of odontoid fracture(s) and or dislocation(s) (including os odontoideum), anterior approach, including placement of internal fixation; without grafting	805.01 805.11	805.02 805.12
22319	Open treatment and/or reduction of odontoid fracture(s) and or dislocation(s) (including os odontoideum), anterior approach, including placement of internal fixation; with grafting	805.01 805.11	805.02 805.12
22548	Arthrodesis, anterior transoral or extraoral technique, clivus-C1-C2 (atlas-axis), with or without excision of odontoid process	714.0 805	722.4

process to the sternoclavicular joint. Dissection is carried through the subcutaneous tissue and through the platysma in line with the skin incision. The deep cervical fascia is divided, allowing lateral retraction of the sternocleidomastoid muscle. The carotid artery can then be palpated laterally, deep to the sternocleidomastoid muscle and within the carotid sheath. The pretracheal fascia is divided sharply, while a finger is held against the carotid sheath to protect its contents. This allows lateral retraction of the carotid sheath and medial retraction of the strap muscles (sternohyoid, sternothyroid, omohyoid), trachea, and esophagus. Using the midline raphe between the longus colli muscles as a guide, the prevertebral fascia is then released, exposing the anterior longitudinal ligament and the underlying vertebral bodies and disks.

SUPRACLAVICULAR APPROACH

Although this approach can be made on either the right or the left side, the right side generally is preferred to avoid the thoracic duct on the left. A transverse incision is made parallel to and 1 cm above the clavicle, from the midline to the lateral border of the sternocleidomastoid muscle, and the platysma is divided in line with the incision. The external jugular vein and supraclavicular nerve are found within the superficial fascia just lateral to the sternocleidomastoid muscle, which should be spared if possible. The clavicular head of the sternocleidomastoid muscle is then released from its insertion. The internal jugular and subclavian veins are located just behind the sternocleidomastoid muscle and are vulnerable to injury during this release; therefore, blunt dissection should be performed between these structures and the clavicular head of the sternocleidomastoid muscle to aid in their protection. Beneath the sternocleidomastoid muscle is the omohyoid muscle, which runs obliquely across the surgical field (underlying the intermediate layer of deep fascia). At its midportion is a well-developed fascial expansion that serves as a pulley. This fascial expansion is divided transversely, permitting superior and lateral retraction of the omohyoid. The subclavian artery and its numerous branches overlying the anterior scalene muscle are next identified. The suprascapular and transverse cervical branches (running medial to lateral across the field) may be ligated if needed. The phrenic nerve is located immediately anterior to the anterior scalene muscle (crossing lateral to medial) and must be retracted medially along its entire length, along with the internal jugular vein and contents of the carotid sheath. The anterior scalene muscle is defined and divided 1 cm proximal to its insertion. The Sibson fascia (a continuation of the prevertebral fascia) is now exposed in the floor of the wound, overlying the dome of the lung. This is opened transversely, exposing the visceral pleura of the lung. The lung may be retracted inferiorly and laterally using a moist pad (taking care to not violate the pleura, as a pneumothorax would result). The trachea, the esophagus, and the recurrent laryngeal nerve are protected and retracted medially. If a left-sided approach is performed, the thoracic duct should be identified and protected. In looking downward through the thoracic inlet, structures readily identified include the sympathetic trunk (lateral to the vertebral bodies), the stellate ganglion (over the neck of the first rib), the thoracic nerve roots, and the vertebral bodies and disks. This approach can be expected to result in adequate visualization down to T1, but more distal exposure is highly dependent on various patient anatomic factors, as outlined previously in this chapter.

STERNUM-SPLITTING APPROACH

A skin incision is made longitudinally along the anterior border of the sternocleidomastoid muscle, extending inferiorly to the level of the xiphoid process. Dissection is then carried to the cervical spine as described previously in the low cervical approach. Attention is next turned to the sternum, and the aponeurosis investing both the sternal notch and the inferior xiphoid process are released sharply. All soft tissue is bluntly dissected free, both superiorly and inferiorly, in preparation for the sternotomy. A sternotomy is then performed using a saw. Once bleeding is controlled, a thoracic retractor is placed, and the strap muscles are divided. The previous cervical exposure can now be extended inferiorly by continued release of the pretracheal fascia to the level of the left brachiocephalic vein. The left brachiocephalic vein lies posterior and inferior to the undersurface of the clavicle and should be protected. (It may be ligated if necessary, but postoperative edema of the left upper extremity could be a problem.) If additional exposure is required, the inferior thyroid vein may be ligated, and the thymus may be removed. The esophagus, the trachea, and the brachiocephalic trunk are then retracted to the right, and the thoracic duct and the left common carotid artery are retracted to the left (**Figure 1**). This approach generally allows exposure from C4 to T4 (**Figure 2**).

CLAVICLE- OR MANUBRIUM-SPLITTING APPROACH

Multiple surgical approaches involve partial resection of the clavicle and/or manubrium. Among the earliest and most commonly used approaches was one described by Sundaresan and associates in 1984. A T-shaped incision is made with the horizontal limb 1 cm above the clavicles and the vertical limb in the midline, extending over the body of the sternum. The platysma is divided in line with the skin incision. Although the superficial anterior veins may be ligated, an attempt should be made to preserve the

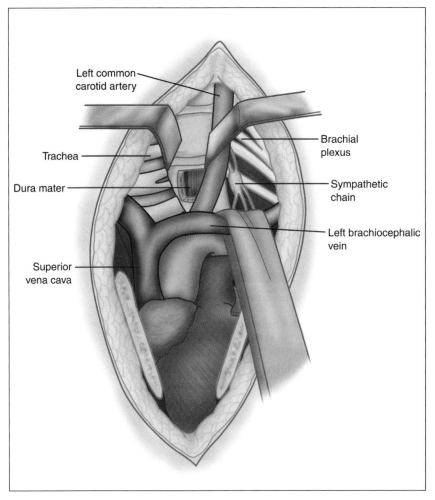

Figure 1 Illustration of the exposure provided with the sternum-spitting approach, noting the important structures encountered.

internal and external jugular veins and the supraclavicular nerve; however, they may be divided if necessary to facilitate exposure. The clavicular and sternal insertions of the sternocleidomastoid muscle are freed and reflected superiorly, as are the ipsilateral strap muscles. The sternal origin of the pectoralis major is stripped laterally as well. With the medial clavicle now exposed, it is stripped subperiosteally, and the medial third is removed through the sternoclavicular joint using a Gigli saw. A rectangular portion of the sternum is then removed using drill holes and heavy scissors (**Figure 3**). An avascular plane between

the trachea and the esophagus medially and the carotid sheath laterally is then developed to gain access to the prevertebral space. With medial retraction of the trachea and the esophagus, the right recurrent laryngeal nerve crosses the surgical field obliquely; it is vulnerable to injury and must be protected. Other variations of this approach include resecting only the medial third of the ipsilateral clavicle (leaving the manubrium intact), bilateral medial clavicle resections, and performing a midline manubriotomy (extending either into the sternum or to the manubriosternal joint), as well as a manubriectomy.

HIGH TRANSTHORACIC APPROACH

Right-sided approaches are generally preferable in gaining access to the thoracic spine, as this avoids manipulation of the aorta. However, the presenting pathology also must be taken into account, such as in scoliotic deformities (in which case the surgeon would need to approach the convexity of the curve). As mentioned previously, this is less of a concern in the upper thoracic spine (T1 through T3), as the approach is superior to the great vessels. A periscapular J-shaped incision is made beginning approximately 2.5 cm medial to the superior edge of the scapula, which is then carried down around its inferior angle to the anterior axillary line. The trapezius muscle and the latissimus dorsi are each divided as medially as possible to avoid injuring their nerve supplies, which are the spinal accessory nerves and the thoracodorsal nerves, respectively. Next, the rhomboid major is divided near its insertion into the superior scapula, followed by the serratus anterior inferiorly. The serratus anterior must be sectioned as inferiorly as possible to avoid injuring its nerve supply, the long thoracic nerve. The medial surface of the scapula is then protected with a saline-soaked sponge and is retracted superiolaterally (**Figure 4**). Next, the third rib is exposed subperiosteally along its length, and a segment spanning 1 to 2 cm from its attachment to the transverse process posteriorly to the costal cartilage anteriorly is removed. The deep periosteum is then incised in line with the rib bed.

Access to the intrapleural cavity is gained by making a transverse incision through the parietal pleura. The dome of the lung is retracted inferiorly, exposing the anterior surface of the spine. The parietal pleura overlying the upper thoracic vertebrae is incised, taking care to avoid injuring the ipsilateral superior intercostal vein and artery (running obliquely across the vertebrae T2 through T4), the

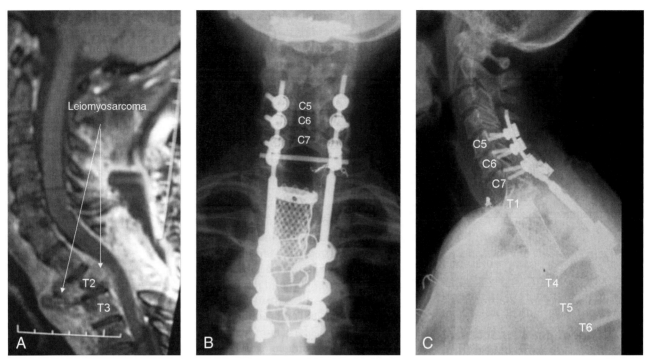

Figure 2 **A,** Sagittal T1-weighted MRI scan of a 49-year-old woman with uterine leiomyosarcoma metastatic to T2 and T3, resulting in severe myelopathy. AP (**B**) and lateral (**C**) radiographs after instrumenting the spine posteriorly from C5 to T6. A sternum-splitting approach was used, and a T2-T3 corpectomy and tumor debulking procedure was performed.

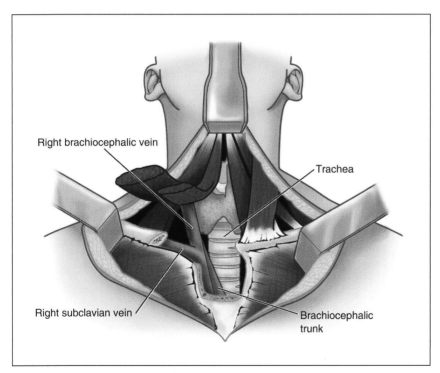

Figure 3 Illustration of the exposure following medial clavicular and partial manubrial resections, noting the relevant anatomic structures. (Adapted with permission from Sundaresan N, Shah J, Foley KM: An anterior surgical approach to the upper thoracic vertebrae. *J Neurosurg* 1984;61:686-690.)

sympathetic trunk (situated laterally), and the thoracic duct (in left-sided approaches). If visualization is required more superior to T1, the Sibson fascia is bluntly dissected above the pleural dome along the longus colli muscles. The superior intercostal artery and vein and the intercostal vessels may be ligated as needed.

COMBINED CERVICAL AND THORACIC APPROACH

Attention is first turned toward the cervical exposure. An oblique cervical incision is made parallel to the clavicle, and the platysma is incised in line with the skin incision. The fascia is then incised medial and parallel to the sternocleidomastoid muscle, which is retracted posteriorly. The carotid sheath is then identified, mobilized using blunt dissection, and retracted anteriorly. The inferior thyroid artery (at the base of the neck) is ligated and divided. The cervical vertebrae and the longus colli musculature can then

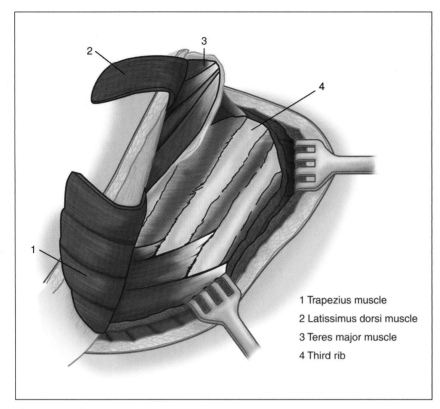

1 Trapezius muscle
2 Latissimus dorsi muscle
3 Teres major muscle
4 Third rib

Figure 4 Illustration of the exposure provided in the high transthoracic approach following superolateral retraction of the scapula and before resection of the third rib.

be identified. Dissection may then be carried down to T1. The cervical wound is packed, and attention is turned to the thoracic exposure. An incision is made along the third rib, extending from the posterior axilla to the pectoral region. Dissection is carried down to the scapula, and the inferior portion of the serratus anterior (from the medial scapula) is divided to mobilize the scapula medially and superiorly. Next, the pectoralis major, the serratus anterior, and the latissimus dorsi are divided parallel to the third rib. The scapula is then additionally mobilized by subperiosteal dissection at its inferior and lateral border and rotated superiorly. With the third rib now exposed, its periosteum is incised, and the rib is removed from the transverse process posteriorly to its sternal attachment anteriorly. The pleura is then incised (in the bed of the removed rib), and dissection is carried posteriorly to the thoracic vertebrae. The vertebrae and disks are now exposed up to the apex of the lung.

Wound Closure

If a sternotomy was performed, the split is approximated using transosseous wires. In cases of medial clavicle and manubrial resections, the bone is not reattached and is instead used as additional autograft bone. If the strap muscles were divided, they are reattached to their aponeurotic insertions at the undersurface of the sternum with interrupted, absorbable sutures, as is the sternocleidomastoid muscle. The platysma is approximated using a running absorbable suture. Suction drains are placed as needed, depending on the bleeding encountered at the conclusion of the procedure. The skin is closed either with staples or a running absorbable suture.

In the high transthoracic approach, a chest tube is placed, followed by a rib approximator. The pleura, the rib periosteum, and the intercostal musculature are closed in a running fashion using absorbable suture. Finally, the superficial musculature is closed in an interrupted fashion, and the skin is closed with staples or a running absorbable suture.

Postoperative Regimen

After cervicothoracic fusion procedures, the patient is placed in a hard collar with a thoracic extension for 6 to 8 weeks and is then weaned to a soft collar. Many cervicothoracic fusion procedures require posterior segmental fixation in addition to anterior corpectomy and strut grafting. If the posterior fixation is rigidly constructed, postoperative bracing can be done with a soft collar alone, or the overall length of bracing can be shortened. If a thoracotomy was performed, the chest tube is maintained for 2 to 3 days. Ventilator support may be needed into postoperative day 1 or longer, depending on respiratory function. Early mobilization with sitting and respiratory exercise on postoperative day 1 are important to prevent atelectasis or pneumonia.

Avoiding Pitfalls and Complications

Patient positioning should be meticulous to avoid nerve palsies in the upper extremities and to prevent malalignment of the cervical spine. If the spine cannot be placed in the optimal position initially because of deformity or neurologic compromise, the spine should be repositioned during surgery after decompression or anterior release so that the final fusion position is as normal as possible. Fusion in kyphosis will result in adjacent-segment degeneration with "adding-on" kyphotic deformity. All the vital neurovascular structures must be respected because stretching or injury to these structures may result in complications (eg, hoarseness, dysphagia, Horner syndrome, chylothorax, etc). Neuromonitoring, such as somatosensory- and motor-evoked potentials, if available, should be used to safeguard the spinal cord at the cervicothoracic junction.

Corpectomy is challenging with an anterior approach because of the increased depth of the wound and the limited exposure of the superior and inferior vertebrae. A power drill with a smooth-tipped burr may be safer than one without a smooth tip and may allow better control, with a reduced possibility of dural tears or spinal cord injury. Following corpectomy, strut grafting can be done with autograft, allograft, or cages. The vertebral end plates at the cervicothoracic junction may not be parallel, and special caution should be taken to maximize the strut–end plate contact during strut grafting. In situ distractable cages might yield an advantage in this re-gard. Anterior plating in this area is technically difficult, and it might be better to perform posterior segmental fixation to provide more biomechanically secure stabilization. Typically, fixation is done three levels above and three below the corpectomy level, using lateral mass screws in the lower cervical spine and pedicle screws in the proximal thoracic spine. Turning the patient from the supine to the prone position should be done carefully to avoid dislodgment of the graft. A turning frame may be used to help avoid complications.

 Bibliography

An HS, Vaccaro A, Cotler JM, Lin S: Spinal disorders at the cervicothoracic junction. *Spine (Phila Pa 1976)* 1994;19(22): 2557-2564.

An HS, Wise JJ, Xu R: Anatomy of the cervicothoracic junction: A study of cadaveric dissection, cryomicrotomy, and magnetic resonance imaging. *J Spinal Disord* 1999;12(6):519-525.

Boockvar JA, Philips MF, Telfeian AE, O'Rourke DM, Marcotte PJ: Results and risk factors for anterior cervicothoracic junction surgery. *J Neurosurg* 2001;94(1, suppl):12-17.

Cauchoix J, Binet JP: Anterior surgical approaches to the spine. *Ann R Coll Surg Engl* 1957;21(4):234-243.

Kurz LT, Pursel SE, Herkowitz HN: Modified anterior approach to the cervicothoracic junction. *Spine (Phila Pa 1976)* 1991;16(10, suppl):S542-S547.

Micheli LJ, Hood RW: Anterior exposure of the cervicothoracic spine using a combined cervical and thoracic approach. *J Bone Joint Surg Am* 1983;65(7):992-997.

Mihir B, Vinod L, Umesh M, Chaudhary K: Anterior instrumentation of the cervicothoracic vertebrae: Approach based on clinical and radiologic criteria. *Spine (Phila Pa 1976)* 2006;31(9):E244-E249.

Mulpuri K, LeBlanc JG, Reilly CW, et al: Sternal split approach to the cervicothoracic junction in children. *Spine (Phila Pa 1976)* 2005;30(11):E305-E310.

Pointillart V, Aurouer N, Gangnet N, Vital JM: Anterior approach to the cervicothoracic junction without sternotomy: A report of 37 cases. *Spine (Phila Pa 1976)* 2007;32(25):2875-2879.

Southwick WO, Robinson RA: Surgical approaches to the vertebral bodies in the cervical and lumbar regions. *J Bone Joint Surg Am* 1957;39(3):631-644.

Sundaresan N, Shah J, Foley KM, Rosen G: An anterior surgical approach to the upper thoracic vertebrae. *J Neurosurg* 1984;61(4):686-690.

Coding

CPT Codes		Corresponding ICD-9 Codes	
22554	Arthrodesis, anterior interbody technique, including minimal discectomy to prepare interspace (other than for decompression); cervical below C2	722.0 805.03 805.05	733.13 805.04 805.06
22845	Anterior instrumentation; 2 to 3 vertebral segments (List separately in addition to code for primary procedure)	170.2 342.9 343	342.1 342.90 343.0
20936	Autograft for spine surgery only (includes harvesting the graft); local (eg, ribs, spinous process, or laminar fragments) obtained from same incision (List separately in addition to code for primary procedure)	170.2 733.13	724.6 737.30

CPT copyright © 2010 by the American Medical Association. All rights reserved.

Chapter 8
Posterior Cervical Foraminotomy and Diskectomy

Jason David Eubanks, MD
James Kang, MD

Indications

In the treatment of nerve compression, the indications for approaching the spine anteriorly or posteriorly ultimately depend on the nature of the specific pathology. An anterior approach is favored when there is a midline or paramedian disk herniation or spur causing myelopathy or myeloradiculopathy, whereas either an anterior or a posterior approach can be used effectively to treat lateral or foraminal pathology caused by soft disk herniations (**Figure 1**) or osteophytes. Purely radicular symptoms caused by osteophytic spur compression (**Figure 2**) may be the ideal choice for a posterior cervical foraminotomy and diskectomy. Other indications for laminotomy-foraminotomy include multilevel radiculopathy secondary to spondylosis; previous anterior surgery; a patient with a short, wide neck; and stenosis at the C7-T1 junction. Finally, posterior cervical foraminotomy and diskectomy may be a useful adjunct in the prevention of C5 palsy during laminaplasty or laminectomy. A review of the literature reveals an average rate of C5 palsy of 4.6% after

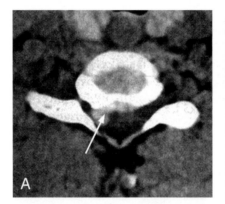
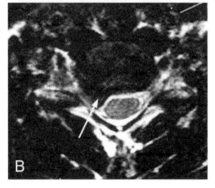
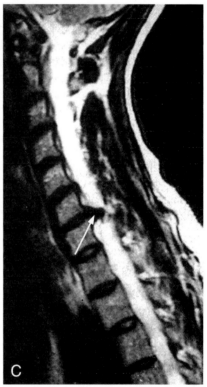

Figure 1 Axial CT (**A**), axial MRI (**B**), and sagittal MRI (**C**) images demonstrate a large, right-side soft disk herniation at the C6-C7 level (arrows). (*Adapted with permission from Korinth MC, Krüger A, Oertel M, Gilsbach JM: Posterior foraminotomy or anterior discectomy with polymethyl methacrylate interbody stabilization for cervical soft disc disease: Results in 292 patients with monoradiculopathy. Spine (Phila Pa 1976) 2006;31(11):1207-1216.*)

decompression surgery. Posterior cervical foraminotomy and diskectomy after expansive laminaplasty has been shown to decrease the incidence of C5 palsy from 4% to 0.6%.

━━━━━━■

Neither Dr. Eubanks nor any immediate family member has received anything of value from or owns stock in a commercial company or institution related directly or indirectly to the subject of this chapter. Dr. Kang or an immediate family member has received research or institutional support from Johnson & Johnson, Stryker, and Medtronic Sofamor Danek.

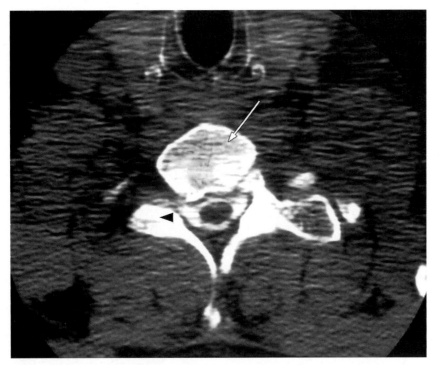

Figure 2 Axial CT myelogram at the level of a cervical disk demonstrates right-side antero-lateral spur formation (arrow) and impingement of the exiting nerve root (arrowhead). (*Adapted with permission from Epstein NE: A review of laminoforaminotomy for the management of lateral and foraminal cervical disc herniations or spurs. Surg Neurol 2002;57(4):226-234.* http://www.sciencedirect.com/science/journal/00903019.)

Contraindications

Posterior cervical foraminotomy and diskectomy is contraindicated for patients who have pure or predominant axial neck pain with few or no neurologic symptoms. For patients with a loss of cervical lordosis, posterior foraminotomy alone may not be the procedure of choice, because increased instability may result, leading to a potential kyphotic deformity. In such cases, posterior decompression may need to be supplemented with a fusion. Other contraindications to posterior cervical foraminotomy and diskectomy include a central disk herniation, gross cervical instability, or a predominance of anterior pathology (ie, large central, anterior osteophytes or ossification of the posterior longitudinal ligament) (**Figure 3**).

Alternative Treatments

Nonsurgical treatment of symptomatic cervical radiculopathy, such as bracing, therapy, traction, and medications, should be tried first. However, when these measures fail and surgical intervention is warranted, the most common alternative to posterior cervical foraminotomy and diskectomy typically entails an anterior procedure. When posterior cervical foraminotomy and diskectomy is contraindicated, the main alternatives are anterior cervical diskectomy and fusion or cervical disk replacement. When compared with anterior diskectomy and fusion, posterior cervical foraminotomy and diskectomy has the theoretical benefit of motion preservation. Although anterior diskectomy and fusion eliminates motion at the involved disk level, posterior cervical foraminotomy and diskectomy, when performed correctly, does not result in cervical instability and therefore does not require fusion. Cervical disk replacement represents another alternative, with the advantage of preserving motion at the involved disk level. As more long-term data become available on this alternative, surgeons will be better able to counsel patients on the benefits.

When compared with these alternative anterior procedures, posterior cervical foraminotomy and diskectomy also avoids some of the more salient complications associated with the anterior approach, including potential esophageal injury, major vascular injury, recurrent laryngeal paralysis, and accelerated adjacent segment degeneration. In most cases, transient postoperative dysphagia, a common complication of the anterior approach, is largely avoided with the posterior approach. Because no instability is produced and no fusion is typically required after posterior cervical foraminotomy and diskectomy, little to no postoperative bracing is required for this procedure. Finally, posterior cervical foraminotomy and diskectomy more effectively avoids the adjacent segment disease that sometimes occurs with anterior fusions. Long-term follow-up of patients who have undergone posterior cervical foraminotomy and diskectomy has demonstrated that the rate of adjacent segment degeneration is 6.7% at 10 years. This compares favorably with a reported 25.6% 10-year rate after anterior cervical arthrodesis.

Results

Posterior cervical foraminotomy (and diskectomy when indicated) has the potential to produce excellent results when used in the treatment of radiculopathy caused by lateral disk herniations or osteophytic nerve root compression. Multiple authors have documented good or excellent results (>95% efficacy) with regard to relief of radicular symptoms (**Table 1**). Randomized studies have shown that treatment of anterolateral herniations with either anterior diskectomy and fusion or posterior laminotomy–foraminotomy produces good results when compared with the alternative anterior approach for soft disk herniations. The early randomized studies tended to show slightly better outcomes for patients who underwent anterior cervical diskectomy and fusion. However, the disparity in the outcomes of these earlier studies may have resulted from the relatively new experience with the posterior approach. More recent randomized studies have shown equivalent results, corroborating the body of nonrandomized studies in the literature that supports the efficacy of posterior cervical foraminotomy and diskectomy.

—————▪

▪ Surgical Technique

Setup/Exposure

In the setup for posterior cervical foraminotomy and diskectomy, positioning of the patient in both the prone and the sitting (**Figure 4**) positions has been described in the literature. Although the prone position is more familiar to most spine surgeons, proponents of the sitting position cite reductions in surgical time, blood in the surgical field, and overall blood loss, as well as ease in obtaining lateral fluoroscopic images, as benefits of the sitting position. However, the sitting position does increase the patient's risk for developing an air embolism or intraoperative hypotension. Advantages of the prone position include lower risks of air embolism and hypotension, however, this advantage may be mitigated slightly if the bed is placed in the reverse Trendelenburg position, which raises the head.

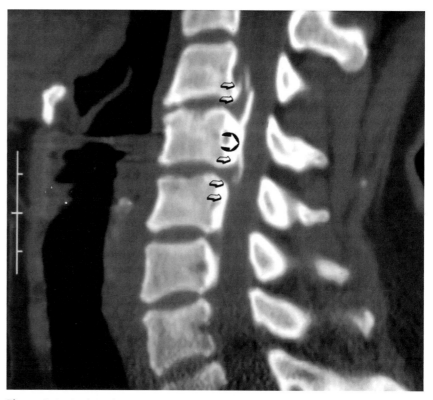

Figure 3 Sagittal CT of a patient with cervical stenosis demonstrates ossification of the posterior longitudinal ligament. The large arrow points to an area displaying the "single-layer sign," which is defined as a large focal mass of uniformly hyperdense ossification of the posterior longitudinal ligament. The small arrows point to areas displaying the "double-layer sign"; these areas are characterized by anterior and posterior rims of hyperdense ossification that are separated by a central hypodense mass, the hypertrophied but nonossified posterior longitudinal ligament. The dura often can be absent in areas of double-layer sign, and, given these CT findings, dural penetration should be suspected. (*Adapted with permission from Epstein NE: Identification of ossification of the posterior longitudinal ligament extending through the dura on preoperative computed tomographic examinations of the cervical spine. Spine (Phila Pa 1976) 2001;26(2):182-186.*)

Should a fusion be required, it can be performed more readily in the prone position as well.

In either case, general endotracheal anesthesia is administered, and the patient is prepared with the necessary arterial lines and monitoring devices, including end tidal CO_2, electrocardiogram, and pulse oximetry. Additional central venous catheters and precordial Doppler devices should be considered for patients placed in the sitting position. Intraoperative monitoring of somatosensory-evoked potentials, with or without electromyography, is certainly recommended for patients with myelopathy, although

some controversy exists as to its necessity in radiculopathy cases. Prior to final positioning, the patient is typically placed in an appropriate head holder.

Instruments/Equipment/Implants Required

Before incision, the surgeon should be equipped with either a surgical microscope or loupe magnification with sufficient lighting. Intraoperative imaging is necessary to confirm the correct level of decompression. Standard cervical spine instruments are employed (Kerrison rongeur, pituitary rongeur, nerve root retractors, nerve hook,

Table 1 Clinical Results of Posterior Cervical Foraminotomy and Diskectomy

Author(s) (Year)	Number of Patients	Procedure or Approach	Mean Patient Age (Range)	Mean Follow-up (Range)	Results
Henderson et al (1983)	736	Posterior	NR	2.8 years	Good/excellent: 91.5%
Williams (1983)	235	Posterior	NR	10 years	Relief of radicular symptoms: 96.5%
Herkowitz et al (1990)	44 (28 ACDF, 16 posterior foraminotomy)	Anterior and posterior	41 years (21-56)	4.2 years (1.6-8.2)	Anterior good/excellent: 94%; posterior good/excellent: 75%
Zeidman and Ducker (1993)	172	Posterior	48.8 years	>2 years: 77%; 1 year: 23% (mean and range NR)	Relief of radicular symptoms: 97%
Silveri et al (1997)	84 (60 at follow-up)	Posterior	44.7 years	6.1 years	Good/excellent: 98%
Kumar et al (1998)	89	Posterior	51 years (28-72)	8.6 months	Good/excellent: 95.5%
Grieve et al (2000)	77	Posterior	52 years (25-78)	40 months (17-86)	Complete or >75% resolution of pain: 70%; <75% resolution of pain: 30%
Witzmann et al (2000)	67	Posterior	43.4 years	3.1 years (1.5-7)	Relief of symptoms: 93%
Korinth et al (2006)	363 (154 anterior, 209 posterior)	ACD + PMMA and posterior	46.9 ± 10.4 years (26-76)	72.1 months	ACD Odom* grade I + II: 93.6%; posterior Odom grade I + II: 85.1%
Ruetten et al (2008)	175 (86 ACDF, 89 posterior)	ACDF and posterior	43 years (27-62)	2 years	ACDF relief of symptoms: 88%; posterior relief of symptoms: 89%

ACD = anterior cervical diskectomy, ACDF = anterior cervical diskectomy and fusion, PMMA = polymethylmethacrylate, NR = not reported.
*For explanation of the Odom scale, see Appendix.

high-speed burr, etc). In the absence of a planned fusion, no cervical hardware is required.

Procedure

The standard open technique begins with a midline incision over the area of interest, which is localized with intraoperative imaging. For unilateral pathology, the muscle is stripped in a subperiosteal fashion from the appropriate side. A burr is then taken to the posterior surface of the superior and inferior lamina, thinning it to allow

the insertion of a Kerrison rongeur into the epidural space. This laminotomy is enlarged with the Kerrison rongeur, keeping in mind that foraminal lesions typically require the resection of slightly more superior lamina than inferior lamina (**Figure 5**). Based on the surgeon's preference, either a burr and curet or a Kerrison rongeur can be used to decompress the foramen by working laterally into the medial edge of the facet. A nerve hook is inserted into the foramen to assess the sufficiency of the decompression (**Fig-

ure 6**). In most cases, a 25% to 33% facetectomy is sufficient to decompress the nerve, allowing visualization of approximately 4 mm of proximal nerve root. In some instances, however, up to 50% of the facet must be removed to appropriately decompress the exiting nerve root.

It has been suggested that a proper lateral bony resection can be determined by a change in the appearance of the compressed nerve root. This decompression will reveal an overlying vein, approximately 2 to 4 mm lateral

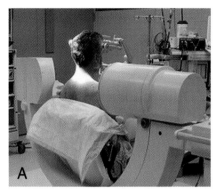
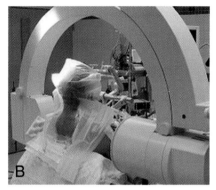
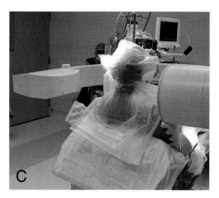

Figure 4 Photographs show a patient in the sitting position, which allows for ease of fluoroscopic imaging. The C-arm can be positioned beneath (**A**), above (**B**), or in front (**C**) of the patient. (Adapted with permission from Gala V, O'Toole J, Voyadzis J, Fessler RG: Posterior minimally invasive approaches for the cervical spine. *Orthop Clin North Am* 2007;38(3):339-349. http://www.sciencedirect.com/science/journal/00305898.)

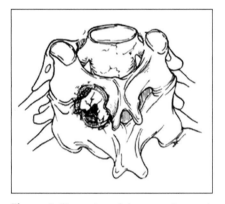

Figure 5 Illustration of the posterior cervical spine after posterior foraminotomy. The spinal cord lies centrally, with a keyhole foraminotomy allowing visualization of the exiting nerve root medial to the edge of the facet joint. (*Adapted with permission from Zeidman SM, Ducker TB: Posterior cervical laminoforaminotomy for radiculopathy: Review of 172 cases. Neurosurgery 1993;33(3): 356-362.*)

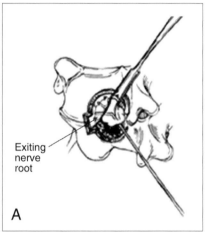
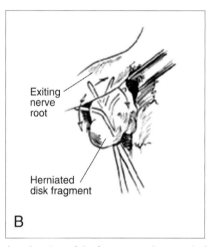

Figure 6 Illustrations show decompression and exploration of the foramen and removal of herniated disk material after posterior cervical foraminotomy. The exiting nerve root is gently retracted superiorly with a nerve root retractor (**A**), and a nerve root retractor is used to explore the foramen around the exiting nerve root for any herniated disk fragments (**B**). (*Adapted with permission from Zeidman SM, Ducker TB: Posterior cervical laminoforaminotomy for radiculopathy: Review of 172 cases. Neurosurgery 1993;33(3):356-362.*)

to the entrance of the foramen. Bleeding from this vein can be controlled via bipolar coagulation or gelatin sponge/thrombin and cottonoid packing.

A formal diskectomy is not typically necessary, because the posterior decompression sufficiently decompresses the exiting nerve root in the vast majority of cases. Disk protrusions can be described as being proximal to (**Figure 7**, *A*), anterior to (**Figure 7**, *B*), distal to (**Figure 7**, *C*), or in no contact with (**Figure 7**, *D*) the exiting nerve root. Should a diskectomy

be indicated, the exiting nerve root is usually retracted in a superior direction with a Penfield elevator or a nerve hook. This must be done with great care to avoid nerve root paralysis. A blade is used to incise the disk (**Figure 8**), and several small fragments are removed from the disk with a micropituitary rongeur or toothed forceps (**Figures 9** and **10**).

Wound Closure

As with any posterior cervical procedure, meticulous wound closure is of paramount importance. For multi-

level procedures or foraminotomies accompanying laminectomies with or without fusion, the placement of a drain deep to the fascia is often warranted. However, for single-level cases, a drain is probably unnecessary. Closure entails close approximation of the fascia, with or without reattachment to the spinous processes, as is advocated by some authors. This is then followed by separate closure of the subcutaneous and skin layers.

—■

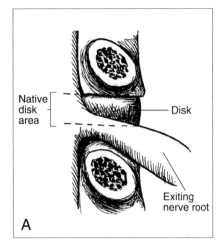

A

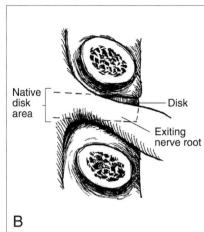

B

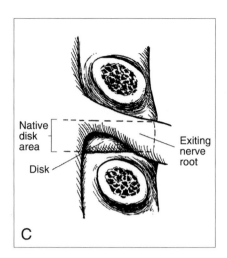

C

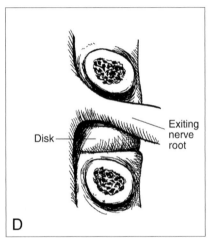

D

Figure 7 Cross-sectional illustrations show possible locations of the exiting nerve root in relation to the cervical disk and pedicles. When the exiting nerve root is distal to the disk, there is a so-called "proximal" herniation (**A**) of the disk at the shoulder of the exiting nerve root. The disk can also be anterior to (**B**), in an axillary position or distal to (**C**), or in no contact with (**D**) the exiting nerve root. (*Adapted with permission from Tanaka N, Fujimoto Y, An HS, Ikuta Y, Yasuda M: The anatomic relation among the nerve roots, intervertebral foramina, and intervertebral discs of the cervical spine. Spine (Phila Pa 1976) 2000;25(3):286-291.*)

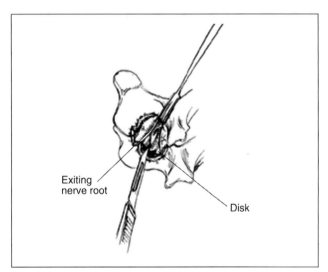

Figure 8 Illustration shows a nerve root retractor used to retract the exiting nerve root, while a blade is used to incise the disk. (*Adapted with permission from Zeidman SM, Ducker TB: Posterior cervical laminoforaminotomy for radiculopathy: Review of 172 cases. Neurosurgery 1993;33(3):356-362.*)

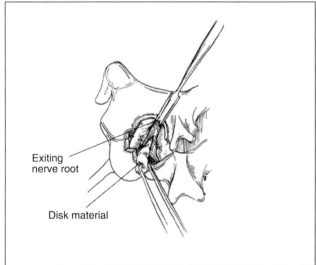

Figure 9 Illustration shows disk removal with forceps. (*Adapted with permission from Zeidman SM, Ducker TB: Posterior cervical laminoforaminotomy for radiculopathy: Review of 172 cases. Neurosurgery 1993;33(3):356-362.*)

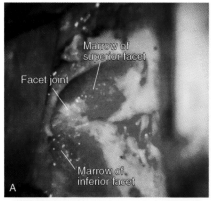
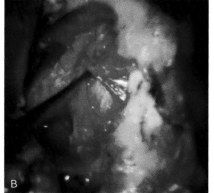
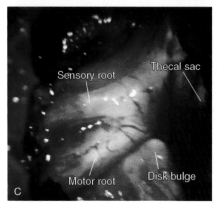
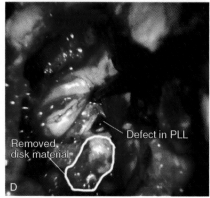

Figure 10 Intraoperative photographs of a posterior cervical foraminotomy and diskectomy. The medial portion of the facets has been removed (**A**) with exposure of the dura (**B**) and the exiting nerve root and accompanying disk bulge (**C**). With gentle retraction of the nerve root, the offending disk material is removed (**D**). PLL = posterior longitudinal ligament. (Adapted with permission from Russell S, Benjamin V: Posterior surgical approach to the cervical neural foramen for intervertebral disc disease. *Neurosurgery* 2004;54(3):662-666.)

◼ Postoperative Regimen

Patients who undergo a simple posterior cervical foraminotomy and diskectomy may be instructed to wear a soft collar postoperatively to ensure comfort. However, no collar is required, and patients are encouraged to begin moving the neck. Patients are then seen in follow-up for a wound check, subsequent serial examinations, and postoperative radiographs to ensure that no latent instability develops as a result of the decompression.

◼ Avoiding Pitfalls and Complications

Perioperative complications have been reported in up to 10% of patients undergoing posterior cervical foraminotomy and diskectomy, with intraoperative complications seen in 2.2% or more. Postoperative complications include the potential for debilitating residual neck pain, spasm, and dysfunction in anywhere from 18% to 60% of patients treated through the posterior approach. Furthermore, it is not uncommon for a patient undergoing a posterior cervical foraminotomy and diskectomy to report up to 6 weeks of postoperative radiculopathy. Appropriate counseling of patients and managing of their expectations before sur-

gery can aid in the postoperative recovery course.

Avoiding "relative hypotension," particularly when the patient is in the sitting position during the surgical procedure, can be best managed through careful intraoperative monitoring, meticulous maintenance of mean arterial pressures, and minimization of blood loss. Intraoperative monitoring of somatosensory-evoked potentials, with or without electromyography, may help minimize cord and nerve root injuries. In addition, care must be taken not to remove more than 50% of the facet joint, as it has been demonstrated that this can lead to instability that may require a secondary fusion.

Bibliography

An HS, Ahn NU: Posterior decompressive procedures for the cervical spine. *Instr Course Lect* 2003;52:471-477.

Chen BH, Natarajan RN, An HS, Andersson GB: Comparison of biomechanical response to surgical procedures used for cervical radiculopathy: Posterior keyhole foraminotomy versus anterior foraminotomy and discectomy versus anterior discectomy with fusion. *J Spinal Disord* 2001;14(1):17-20.

Clarke MJ, Ecker RD, Krauss WE, McClelland RL, Dekutoski MB: Same-segment and adjacent-segment disease following posterior cervical foraminotomy. *J Neurosurg Spine* 2007;6(1):5-9.

Epstein NE: Identification of ossification of the posterior longitudinal ligament extending through the dura on preoperative computed tomographic examinations of the cervical spine. *Spine (Phila Pa 1976)* 2001;26(2):182-186.

Epstein NE: A review of laminoforaminotomy for the management of lateral and foraminal cervical disc herniations or spurs. *Surg Neurol* 2002;57(4):226-234.

Gala VC, O'Toole JE, Voyadzis JM, Fessler RG: Posterior minimally invasive approaches for the cervical spine. *Orthop Clin North Am* 2007;38(3):339-349.

Grieve JP, Kitchen ND, Moore AJ, Marsh HT: Results of posterior cervical foraminotomy for treatment of cervical spondylitic radiculopathy. *Br J Neurosurg* 2000;14(1):40-43.

Henderson CM, Hennessy RG, Shuey HM Jr, Shackelford EG: Posterior-lateral foraminotomy as an exclusive operative technique for cervical radiculopathy: A review of 846 consecutively operated cases. *Neurosurgery* 1983;13(5):504-512.

Herkowitz HN, Kurz LT, Overholt DP: Surgical management of cervical soft disc herniation: A comparison between the anterior and posterior approach. *Spine (Phila Pa 1976)* 1990;15(10):1026-1030.

Hilibrand AS, Carlson GD, Palumbo MA, Jones PK, Bohlman HH: Radiculopathy and myelopathy at segments adjacent to the site of a previous anterior cervical arthrodesis. *J Bone Joint Surg Am* 1999;81(4):519-528.

Holly LT, Moftakhar P, Khoo LT, Wang JC, Shamie N: Minimally invasive 2-level posterior cervical foraminotomy: Preliminary clinical results. *J Spinal Disord Tech* 2007;20(1):20-24.

Komagata M, Nishiyama M, Endo K, Ikegami H, Tanaka S, Imakiire A: Prophylaxis of C5 palsy after cervical expansive laminoplasty by bilateral partial foraminotomy. *Spine J* 2004;4(6):650-655.

Korinth MC, Krüger A, Oertel MF, Gilsbach JM: Posterior foraminotomy or anterior discectomy with polymethyl methacrylate interbody stabilization for cervical soft disc disease: Results in 292 patients with monoradiculopathy. *Spine (Phila Pa 1976)* 2006;31(11):1207-1216.

Kumar GR, Maurice-Williams RS, Bradford R: Cervical foraminotomy: An effective treatment for cervical spondylotic radiculopathy. *Br J Neurosurg* 1998;12(6):563-568.

Lees F, Turner JW: Natural history and prognosis of cervical spondylosis. *Br Med J* 1963;2(5373):1607-1610.

Radhakrishnan K, Litchy WJ, O'Fallon WM, Kurland LT: Epidemiology of cervical radiculopathy: A population-based study from Rochester, Minnesota, 1976 through 1990. *Brain* 1994;117(Pt 2):325-335.

Ruetten S, Komp M, Merk H, Godolias G: Full-endoscopic cervical posterior foraminotomy for the operation of lateral disc herniations using 5.9-mm endoscopes: A prospective, randomized, controlled study. *Spine (Phila Pa 1976)* 2008; 33(9): 940-948.

Russell SM, Benjamin V: Posterior surgical approach to the cervical neural foramen for intervertebral disc disease. *Neurosurgery* 2004;54(3):662-665.

Sakaura H, Hosono N, Mukai Y, Ishii T, Yoshikawa H: C5 palsy after decompression surgery for cervical myelopathy: Review of the literature. *Spine (Phila Pa 1976)* 2003;28(21):2447-2451.

Silveri CP, Simpson JM, Simeone FA, Balderston RA: Cervical disk disease and the keyhole foraminotomy: Proven efficacy at extended long-term follow up. *Orthopedics* 1997;20(8):687-692.

Tanaka N, Fujimoto Y, An HS, Ikuta Y, Yasuda M: The anatomic relation among the nerve roots, intervertebral foramina, and intervertebral discs of the cervical spine. *Spine (Phila Pa 1976)* 2000;25(3):286-291.

Williams RW: Microcervical foraminotomy: A surgical alternative for intractable radicular pain. *Spine (Phila Pa 1976)* 1983;8(7):708-716.

Witzmann A, Hejazi N, Krasznai L: Posterior cervical foraminotomy: A follow-up study of 67 surgically treated patients with compressive radiculopathy. *Neurosurg Rev* 2000;23(4):213-217.

Zdeblick TA, Zou D, Warden KE, McCabe R, Kunz D, Vanderby R: Cervical stability after foraminotomy: A biomechanical in vitro analysis. *J Bone Joint Surg Am* 1992;74(1):22-27.

Zeidman SM, Ducker TB: Posterior cervical laminoforaminotomy for radiculopathy: Review of 172 cases. *Neurosurgery* 1993;33(3):356-362.

Coding

CPT Codes		Corresponding ICD-9 Codes	
Posterior Cervical Foraminotomy and Diskectomy			
63020	Laminotomy (hemilaminectomy), with decompression of nerve root(s), including partial facetectomy, foraminotomy and/or excision of herniated intervertebral disc, including open and endoscopically assisted approaches; 1 interspace, cervical	721.1 723.0	722
63035	Laminotomy (hemilaminectomy), with decompression of nerve root(s), including partial facetectomy, foraminotomy and/or excision of herniated intervertebral disc, including open and endoscopically-assisted approaches; each additional interspace, cervical or lumbar (List separately in addition to code for primary procedure)	721.1 723.0	722
63040	Laminotomy (hemilaminectomy), with decompression of nerve root(s), including partial facetectomy, foraminotomy and/or excision of herniated intervertebral disc, reexploration, single interspace; cervical	721.1 723.0	722
63043	Laminotomy (hemilaminectomy), with decompression of nerve root(s), including partial facetectomy, foraminotomy and/or excision of herniated intervertebral disc, reexploration, single interspace; each additional cervical interspace (List separately in addition to code for primary procedure)	721.1 723.0	722
63045	Laminectomy, facetectomy and foraminotomy (unilateral or bilateral with decompression of spinal cord, cauda equina and/or nerve root[s], [eg, spinal or lateral recess stenosis]), single vertebral segment; cervical	721.1 723.0	722
63048	Laminectomy, facetectomy and foraminotomy (unilateral or bilateral with decompression of spinal cord, cauda equina and/or nerve root[s], [eg, spinal or lateral recess stenosis]), single vertebral segment; each additional segment, cervical, thoracic, or lumbar (List separately in addition to code for primary procedure)	724.6	721.1
Additional Procedures			
22600	Arthrodesis, posterior or posterolateral technique, single level; cervical below C2 segment	723.0 721.1	722

CPT copyright © 2010 by the American Medical Association. All rights reserved.

Chapter 9

Minimally Invasive Posterior Laminoforaminotomy/Diskectomy

Thomas Mroz, MD
Michael P. Steinmetz, MD
K. Daniel Riew, MD

 ## Indications

The indications for posterior lamino-foraminotomy (PLF) in the patient with cervical radiculopathy include intractable and correlative arm pain and/or a neurologic deficit that worsens or does not improve with nonsurgical care. In the absence of neurologic demise or intractable pain, nonsurgical care generally is trialed for a minimum of 6 weeks. Posterior cervical diskectomy is indicated for patients who have soft disk herniations that are located paracentrally or intraforaminally (**Figure 1**). Therefore, this procedure typically is useful in patients in the second through fifth decades of life because of the preponderance of soft disk herniations in these populations. A PLF with or without diskectomy can be accessed via a tubular access system or through a standard midline open incision. Several reports have compared tubular access with the traditional open approach; no clear advantage of one over the other in terms of patient outcomes has been delineated in the literature. Both approaches are reasonable.

 ## Contraindications

Radiculopathy that is caused by "hard disk herniations" (disk-osteophyte complexes that occur with advanced spondylosis) are not amenable to treatment with posterior diskectomy. However, in a patient with foraminal stenosis who exhibits only radicular symptoms that are aggravated by a Spurling maneuver and are relieved by forward flexion, a PLF can be performed. Patients with centrally located disk herniations are not candidates for posterior cervical diskectomy. Other contraindications include segmental instability and severe axial neck pain. The physician should perform a careful history in patients who report "neck pain." Axial neck pain (which does not respond favorably to PLF) is different from periscapular or perimedian cervicothoracic pain, but patients often report pain in the latter two regions as "neck pain." These regional pain syndromes are often due to cervical radiculopathy, and a selective nerve root block is often helpful to differentiate them from axial neck pain. In addition, "neck pain" caused by a radiculopathy is often chronic, underscoring the importance of the history.

Alternative Treatments

Several surgical options exist for the treatment of cervical radiculopathy that is refractory to nonsurgical care. One common method is anterior cervical diskectomy and fusion (ACDF). This procedure has an established record of predictable favorable patient outcomes.

Dr. Mroz or an immediate family member serves as a board member, owner, officer, or committee member of the AO Spine North America Research Committee; is a member of a speakers' bureau or has made paid presentations on behalf of AO Spine; serves as a paid consultant to or is an employee of Globus Medical; and owns stock or stock options in Pearl Diver. Dr. Steinmetz or an immediate family member serves as a board member, owner, officer, or committee member of the Congress of Neurological Surgeons, the Council of State Neurological Societies, the American Association of Neurological Surgeons, and the CNS Joint Section on Disorders of the Spine; is a member of a speakers' bureau or has made paid presentations on behalf of Biomet; and serves as an unpaid consultant to Biomet. Dr. Riew or an immediate family member serves as a board member, owner, officer, or committee member of CSRS and KASS; has received royalties from Biomet, Medtronic Sofamor Danek, and Osprey; and owns stock or stock options in Amedica, Benvenue, Expanding Orthopaedics, Nexgen, Osprey, Paradigm Spine, PSD, Spinal Kinetics, Spineology, and Vertiflex.

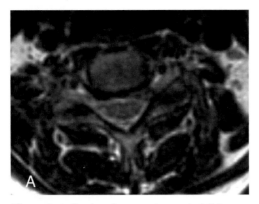 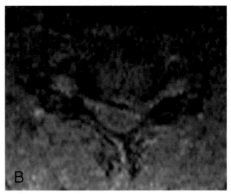 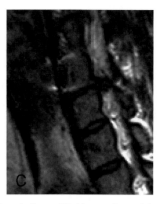

Figure 1 Indications for posterior cervical diskectomy. **A,** T2-weighted MRI shows a left intraforaminal disk herniation at C5-6 in a patient with C6 radiculopathy. This patient is a candidate for posterior diskectomy. **B,** T2-weighted MRI demonstrates a right paracentral disk herniation at C6-7 in a patient with C7 radiculopathy, indications that the patient is a candidate for posterior diskectomy. **C,** A right parasagittal T2-weighted MRI demonstrates a large right paracentral disk herniation at C6-7.

Table 1 Results of Posterior Cervical Foraminotomy

Authors (Year)	No. of Patients	Procedure	Mean Follow-up	Study Design/Level of Evidence	Results
Witzmann et al (2000)	67	Open foraminotomy	3 years	Retrospective/III	85% excellent 7% good 4% fair 3% poor
Fessler and Khoo (2002)	25 MIS 26 open	MIS vs open foraminotomy	16 months	Prospective/II	No statistically significant difference in clinical outcome between groups
Holly et al (2007)	21	2-level MIS foraminotomy	23 months	Retrospective/III	90% complete recovery 10% no improvement 1 patient required ACDF
Ruetten et al (2008)	89 MIS 86 ACDF	MIS foraminotomy vs ACDF	2 years	Randomized controlled trial/I	Operating time: MIS 28 min ACDF 68 min ($P < 0.001$) No statistically significant difference in clinical outcome of neck pain or arm as measured by NASS Instrument Scale, Hilibrand Criteria, or VAS

MIS = minimally invasive surgery; ACDF = anterior cervical diskectomy and fusion; NASS = North American Spine Society; VAS = visual analog scale.

 ## Results

Like ACDF, PLF results in acceptable outcomes in most patients. Few trials have compared PLF with and without diskectomy, but several have demonstrated both procedures to be efficacious in the treatment of cervical radiculopathy (Table 1). These studies provide level IIIb evidence, however, and involve small numbers of patients, so it is unclear whether performing a posterior diskectomy provides any actual clinical benefit compared with performing only a foraminotomy.

Although the literature lacks evidence of a defined clinical benefit from performing PLF with diskectomy instead of PLF alone, theoretical advantages to removing the anteriorly located disk do exist. First, performing a PLF without diskectomy may result in insufficient indirect root decompression and thus unsatisfactory clinical results and the potential for further surgery. Second, neurologic recovery may be optimized by direct decompression of the root through diskectomy. Finally, with diskectomy, it is possible that recurrent symptoms can be minimized because it involves a direct decompression versus an indirect decompression.

Relatively few studies have directly compared minimally invasive PLF

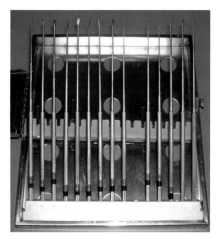

Figure 2 The Rhoton instrument set.

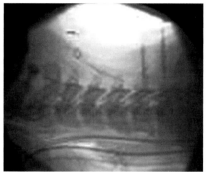

Figure 3 Lateral fluoroscopic image shows C6-7 access with the tubular retractor in final position.

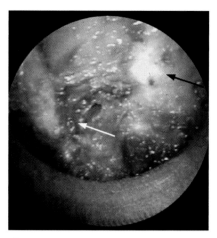

Figure 4 Optimal view following placement of the tubular retractor for a minimally invasive right C5-6 diskectomy. Note that both lateral laminae and the medial half of the facet (black arrow) are visualized. The white arrow indicates the superior articular process.

with open PLF and diskectomy. Studies that evaluated cervical foraminotomy for treatment of radiculopathy have demonstrated rather consistently favorable outcomes. Reports that have compared open with minimally invasive PLF and diskectomy have not demonstrated statistically significant differences in clinical outcomes and have shown that both strategies are efficacious in the treatment of cervical radiculopathy.

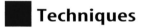

Techniques

Instruments/Equipment Required

The main difference between an open and a minimally invasive posterior cervical diskectomy (PCD) is the access. To perform a minimally invasive posterior decompression, a fixed (ie, nonexpandable) 14- to 16-mm tubular retractor is used. Several tubular systems are available, but none have been shown in the literature to be superior to the rest. A system that uses an articulated arm that is attached to the operating table frame at one end and to the tubular retractor at the other end is ideal. Standard equipment is used for the laminoforaminotomy and diskectomy portions of the procedure. Our preference is to use a

Rhoton microsurgical set for the diskectomy (**Figure 2**).

Procedure

SETUP/PATIENT POSITIONING
There are two options for positioning the patient. One author (K.D.R.) prefers to use Gardner-Wells tongs with traction of 15 to 20 lb suspending the head and neck at a vector to create slight cervical flexion. Another option is to use three-point cranial pins, securing the patient prone to the operating table in slight cervical flexion. Fluoroscopy is used to confirm that the neck is in slight flexion, and the fluoroscope is used throughout the case. The preferred alignment of the cervical spine during the procedure is slightly flexed, to minimize shingling of the facet articular processes and to ensure complete access—and removal—of the superomedial aspect of the superior articular process.

ACCESS
The midline is marked with a vertical line, and a second line 1.5 cm from the midline is then drawn on the surgical side. To determine the incision placement, a 22-gauge spinal needle is placed, under fluoroscopic guidance, perpendicular to the surgical level through this laterally placed line. Once the ideal placement is determined, the incision is made. If a 16-mm tube is to be used, then an

8-mm incision should be made on either side of the needle placement. It is important to make the incision directly over the foramen of interest to facilitate the rest of the case.

Unlike with serial dilation in the lumbar spine, Kirschner wires must not be used in the cervical spine because of the risk of interlaminar space violation. The initial dilator is placed through a small incision made in the deep fascia. The anterior direction is confirmed in the sagittal plane with fluoroscopy and in the coronal plane with direct visualization. Care should be taken not to direct the initial dilator medially because it is narrow enough to violate the interlaminar space. The optimal approach is straight down. Once the dilator is docked on the facet joint of interest, the other dilators are then used to sequentially dilate up to the target diameter, and the final tubular retractor is docked onto the facet and secured rigidly with the articulated arm. If substantial resistance occurs during tissue dilation, the surgeon must ensure that the drape is not entrapped, use saline to decrease the resistance, and, if necessary, enlarge the skin incision slightly. It is important to avoid forcing the dilators or retractors into position because doing so reduces control of the situation and increases the chances of a lateral plunge or medial interlaminar breach. The last dilator should be available throughout the case to use as a wand when adjusting the final retractor, as necessary. **Figure 3** demonstrates the position of the final retractor.

Once the retractor is in place, an operating microscope is brought into position and used during the entire operation. The light source aperture should be adjusted to the diameter of the retractor to minimize glare from the adhesive drape. The optimal view at this point is the medial half of the facet joint and the lateral laminae of the cranial and caudal levels (**Figure 4**). It is important to understand the dimensions of the facet at this point by using a Penfield No. 4 to palpate the lateral border of the lateral masses beyond the lateral border of the tube. This helps avoid iatrogenic instability from excessive facet removal. To perform this surgery minimally invasively, all instruments except for the Rhoton set (ie, the Bovie, bipolar and Penfield No. 4) need to be bayoneted to avoid view occlusion.

The foraminotomy is performed exclusively with a 3-mm diamond or 2.5-mm match-head–tip burr, not with Kerrison rongeurs. We prefer to use a Midas Rex pneumatic drill (Medtronic, Memphis, TN); the elongated curved extension (model TT12C) is necessary to work through the 14- or 16-mm tube without occluding the view. Using Kerrison rongeurs for the foraminotomy is discouraged because of the potential for iatrogenic injury of the nerve root if the instrument is placed into the foramen during decompression. A stenotic foramen often will have axial diameters of 2 to 4 mm, and, considering the bony confines and anterior disk of the foramen, only the nerve root will give way when a Kerrison is placed into it. If a diamond-tip burr is

used, it is important to use near-continuous irrigation of the tip to prevent thermal injury to the nerve root.

LAMINOFORAMINOTOMY

The laminoforaminotomy is performed safely and quickly, following a series of consecutive steps (**Figure 5**). Considering the anatomy of the cervical foramen, for a typical degenerative case, nothing can be compressive to the nerve root lateral to the pedicle. Performing the decompression out to the pedicle will result in a thorough decompression of the root. Therefore, palpation of the caudal pedicle during a PLF without diskectomy marks the termination of the decompression.

The first step of the cervical foraminotomy is removal of the inferomedial half of the inferior articular process. A trough is burred, starting from the laminofacet junction and directed laterally to the midportion of the facet, which also will be in the coronal plane of the caudal pedicle. This trough constitutes the long limb of the L shown in **Figure 5**, *A*. A second trough is then drilled contiguous with but perpendicular to the long limb and is directed inferiorly. Both limbs of the L are deepened sequentially until the resultant inferomedial triangular portion of the inferior articular process is loose and can be removed (**Figure 5**, *B*). Drilling should be confined only to the limbs of the L, and the triangular portion of bone should be preserved and removed en bloc. Bleeding from the cancellous bone is stopped with intermittent application of bone wax or a procoagulant.

Next, the superomedial half of the superior articular process is removed (**Figure 5**, *C* and *D*). This is done in a manner analogous to the previously described technique used to remove the inferomedial half of the inferior articular process. It is extremely important to not drill into this triangular portion of bone; drilling should be confined only to the limbs of the L. This portion of bone is critical in pre-

venting posterior migration of the nerve root, which would make further drilling difficult and dangerous. Once the triangular portion is mobile, it is carefully dissected free of the underlying nerve root and epineural venous plexus using microinstruments. At this time, the caudal pedicle should be palpated with a micro nerve hook or Janetta probe, marking the termination of the decompression (**Figure 5**, *E*).

While drilling the troughs, the epineural venous plexus may be encountered when the anterior cortex is breached. Constant suctioning of the site of bleeding with a 7-French Frazier tip suction, bone wax, and a procoagulant all are useful techniques to use until the drilling is complete. The epineural venous plexus can be well developed but is dealt with easily using a procoagulant and bipolar cautery with irrigation. If a diskectomy is not to be performed after the PLF, we do not expose the root by dissecting and removing the plexus and opening the perineural sheath. If a diskectomy is to be performed, it is important to visualize the root. To do so, the usual microsurgical techniques, with high-power magnification and a procoagulant, are used to minimize bleeding during exposure.

POSTERIOR CERVICAL DISKECTOMY

For lateral disk herniations, it may be advantageous to perform a diskectomy. Access to the disk space is gained through the axilla of the root and lateral dura.

The first step is the removal of the superomedial half of the caudal pedicle to provide more access to the axilla. This is achieved with either a diamond-tip or carbide 2-mm burr with constant protection of the root with a Janetta probe (**Figure 6**). If a diamond tip is used, irrigation also should be used to prevent thermal injury to the root.

A perineural venous plexus of varying degrees of development encom-

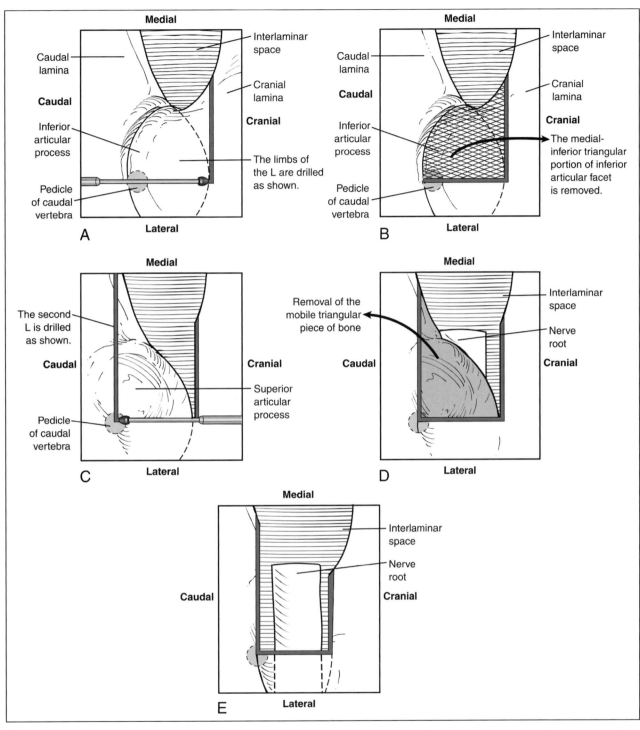

Figure 5 Steps in a posterior cervical laminoforaminotomy. **A,** In step 1, an L is drilled to effectively remove the inferomedial half of the inferior articular process. **B,** In step 2, the triangular portion of bone, which becomes mobile when drilling is complete, is easily removed when the two limbs of the L have been drilled through the anterior cortex. The superior articular process is now visible. **C,** During step 3, another L is drilled as shown. The long limb should extend to the level of the caudal pedicle because this is the point where the decompression is complete. Perineural bleeding can occur as the drill breaches the anterior cortex. The bleeding is controlled with continuous suction with a 7-French Frasier tip with continued drilling and a procoagulant. This step is complete when the medial triangular piece of the superior of bone is mobile. **D,** In step 4, the triangular piece of bone is dissected carefully away from the anterior perineural venous plexus. Bleeding is addressed very effectively with Floseal and gel foam/thrombin. **E,** The completed decompression, after the triangular portion of bone has been removed from the superior articular process.

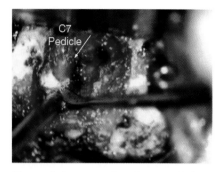

Figure 6 Intraoperative photograph demonstrates the exposure of the pedicle for drilling. The patient's head is to the right. Note that a Janetta probe is used to protect the nerve root and a 7-French Frasier suction can be used to protect the lateral dura.

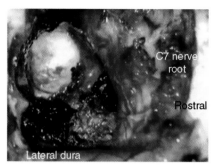

Figure 7 Intraoperative photograph demonstrates the exposure for a minimally invasive posterior left C6-7 diskectomy. The patient's head is to the right. Note the superomedial half of the pedicle has been removed and the C7 nerve root and the lateral dura have been exposed.

passes the root and is contiguous with the epidural plexus. The second step of a diskectomy consists of the ligation of the venous plexus, which provides exposure and visualization of the root and the lateral dura. This is achieved with low-power bipolar electrocautery with irrigation (to prevent adherence of the vessels to the bipolar tips and tearing upon release), microdissection, and liberal use of procoagulants. The importance of visualizing the root and lateral dura cannot be overstated; it ensures the avoidance of an iatrogenic root or dural injury (**Figure 7**). In subannular or subligamentous disk herniations, it can be difficult to discern whether the exposed disk bulge represents dura or anulus/posterior longitudinal ligament. Exposure of the lateral dura eliminates all uncertainty during the anulotomy.

Once the axilla is clearly exposed, the disk is removed with microinstruments. We highly recommend using a Rhoton microsurgical set because it contains all the tools necessary to safely work within this narrow corridor. A micropituitary rongeur is used to retrieve exposed fragments of disk.

The surgical bed is irrigated, and electrocautery or procoagulants are used to address any bleeding. The tubular retractor is removed slowly under microscopic visualization; any

muscular bleeding is addressed with electrocautery.

Wound Closure

The deep fascia is closed with a simple suture, as is the skin. A drain is not necessary.

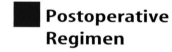

Postoperative Regimen

Most patients can be discharged the day of surgery or the day after. A soft cervical collar is used for comfort for only 1 to 2 days following surgery. After it is discontinued, active range-of-motion exercises are performed as tolerated.

Avoiding Pitfalls and Complications

The surgical errors that cause complications usually arise while obtaining the tubular access or during the decompression.

Complications Related to Access

As with tubular access in the lumbar spine, carefully choosing the site of the incision is critical because if it is too far cranial or caudal the retractor will migrate during the procedure or will not sit flush with the facet, and soft tissue will occlude the view. Therefore, it is important to follow every step in determining the site of the incision from the time the 22-gauge spinal needle is placed perpendicular to the facet of interest. Each error in access obtainment from this point forward is additive and makes the operation more difficult. As mentioned previously, it is critical that the dilators are placed carefully, with visualization and tactile feedback guiding the coronal trajectory and serial fluoroscopic images guiding the sagittal plane trajectory. It is important to remember that even with the placement of dilators, an interlaminar breach is possible (the spine is in flexion for this procedure), *and this can cause a catastrophic neurologic injury.* If the dilators do not pass easily, the situation *must* be rectified to avoid an inadvertent plunge medially or laterally. This can be done by applying saline to the tubes and/or by ensuring that the incision is long enough, that the fascia has been dilated adequately with the Metzenbaum scissors, and that the dilators or final retractor is not binding up on the adhesive drape.

Complications Related to Decompression

Just as in an open foraminotomy, care should be taken to avoid iatrogenic instability of the facet joint. This is accomplished by understanding the anatomy. With minimally invasive surgery, visual feedback is not readily available to assess the dimensions of the lateral masses. Therefore, it is critical to palpate with a bayoneted Penfield No. 4 lateral to the tubular retractor to determine the size. It is important to avoid removing more

Chapter 11

Cervical Laminectomy and Fusion

Raj D. Rao, MD
Ian A. Madom, MD

Indications

Cervical laminectomy is an important tool in the surgeon's armamentarium when dealing with cervical spine pathology. In appropriately selected patients, cervical laminectomy effectively allows for multilevel spinal canal expansion, with limited surgical morbidity. Appropriate and early expansion of the spinal canal allows for restoration of spinal cord morphology, reverses cord edema, and potentially improves cord blood flow—all of which may aid in neurologic recovery.

Posterior decompression techniques in the cervical region are effective in patients who have preoperative preservation of cervical lordosis. Alternatively, the cervical spinal column should have retained mobility that allows internal fixation and fusion in lordosis. Lordosis allows for posterior migration of the cord following the laminectomy and effectively decompresses the spinal cord. The development of postlaminectomy kyphosis is less likely in patients who have preoperative lordosis.

Patients with multilevel pathology at four or more segments of the cervical spine are considered for posterior decompression and fusion. The risks of approach-related dysphagia and voice changes following extensile anterior approaches make a posterior decompression preferable. Patients with marked congenital stenosis of the cervical spinal canal generally require multilevel intervention, so posterior surgical options ought to be considered in these patients.

Posterior approaches also are considered for patients who have undergone previous anterior neck surgery. Scar tissue related to prior intervention can increase the risk of intraoperative complications in such patients.

Contraindications

Cervical laminectomy is ineffective in decompressing the spinal cord in the absence of cervical lordosis or the ability to reconstitute such lordosis by intraoperative mobilization and fixation. It should not be performed without concomitant fusion in patients who are likely to develop postoperative cervical instability or in patients with documented preoperative cervical instability or subluxation. Patients who require wide decompression (including >50% of the facet joints bilaterally) also must undergo cervical fusion. Difficulty with intraoperative positioning of the patient in the prone position may preclude cervical laminectomy. In some of these patients, laminectomy in the sitting position may be an alternative. Finally, laminectomy should not be performed in patients who have axial neck pain without radiculopathy or myelopathy.

Alternative Treatments

When possible, the initial treatment of cervical radiculopathy and myelopathy should be nonsurgical. Anterior surgical intervention for cervical spondylotic conditions is an excellent alternative to cervical laminectomy in many cases. The anterior approach follows an anatomic fascial plane, and access from C2 to T1 can be obtained easily in most individuals. Dysphagia is a relatively frequent occurrence following anterior surgery on the cervical spine, and it is present in up to 50% of individuals one month after surgery. Changes in the patient's voice also may occur occasionally, as a result

Dr. Rao or an immediate family member serves as a board member, owner, officer, or committee member of the North American Spine Society and the Lumbar Spine Research Society. Dr. Madom or an immediate family member has received research or institutional support from Globus Medical.

Table 1 Results of Clinical Studies on Cervical Laminectomy and Fusion

Authors (Year)	Number of Patients	Type of Treatment	Mean Patient Age in Years (Range)	Mean Follow-up (Range)	Fusion Rate	Results
Yasuoka et al (1982)	58	Laminectomy	12 (0-24)	Minimum 5-year follow-up	NR	Postlaminectomy deformity developed in 46% of patients < 15 years of age and 6% of patients 15-24 years
Hamanishi and Tanaka (1996)	69	Wide laminectomy in 69; 34 combined with posterior fusion	61.5 (24-80)	3.5 years (1-10)	80% (27/34 patients)	Improvement in JOA scores: 50.8 ± 30.2% without fusion; 51.2 ± 23.8% with fusion
Kato et al (1998)	44	Laminectomy	57 (39-75)	14.1 years	NR	Mean improvement in JOA score: 40% from 1-5 years, decreased to 30% at last follow-up Deterioration most commonly followed falls and occurred in 3/44 patients
Kumar et al (1999)	25	Laminectomy, fusion, lateral mass fusion	60 (33-79)	47.5 months (25-82)	NR	80% good outcome
Heller et al (2001)	13	Laminectomy, fusion, lateral mass plating	55 (39-78)	25.5 months (9-62)	89% of motion segments (5/13 patients)	Mean Nurick score improved from 2.2 preoperatively to 1.5 postoperatively
Houten and Cooper (2003)	38	Laminectomy, fusion, lateral mass plating	65 (41-86)	30.2 months (6-100)	NR	Mean JOA scores improved from 12.9 to 15.6 in 37 patients
Kuhns et al (2005)	33	Posterior fusion with selective nerve root decompression	47 (28-63)	46 months (20-86)	100%	72% satisfied; 52% mild/no pain

NR = not reported; JOA = Japanese Orthopaedic Association.

of injury to the recurrent or superior laryngeal nerves during the approach. Injuries to the vertebral artery, the thoracic duct, the sympathetic chain, and/or hypoglossal nerves are less frequent but are nonetheless possible complications of the anterior approach. Access to the lower cervical and cervicothoracic spine is difficult in stocky individuals with a short neck. Laminaplasty is an excellent alternative to multilevel laminectomy when posterior decompression of the cervical spinal cord is elected.

Results

The risk of postlaminectomy kyphosis has been reduced to a large degree by using fusion and instrumentation following laminectomy. Laminectomy performed without fusion, particularly in children or young adults, can result in cervical instability, kyphosis, or worsening of the neurologic deficit. The presence of degenerative changes in the cervical spine may, to some degree, protect against the development of instability. Postoperative neck pain is more likely with laminectomy than

with anterior cervical surgery, but it is less likely with laminectomy than with laminaplasty. Neurologic outcomes are better in patients who undergo laminectomy with fusion.

As shown in **Table 1**, fusion rates of up to 100% have been reported after posterior cervical decompression and fusion, with no significant difference between allograft and autograft. More recent studies using stricter fusion criteria have reported fusion rates closer to 62%. Good to excellent satisfaction with respect to postoperative pain has been reported in 72% to 80% of patients. Pain relief at midterm follow-up has been demonstrated in 52% of patients, with only 28% of patients reporting moderate to severe pain after surgery.

The use of instrumentation and fusion following posterior cervical decompression reduces the incidence of postlaminectomy kyphosis. Lateral mass screw instrumentation is now the dominant type of fixation in the cervical spine and has a low incidence of complications when performed appropriately. When performing lateral mass screw instrumentation, there is a 6% incidence of nerve root injury or screw placement in an inadequate position. Screw loosening has been noted in 2% to 6% of cases. The incidence of nerve root injury is lowest when the An modification of the Magerl technique is used for placement of lateral mass screws.

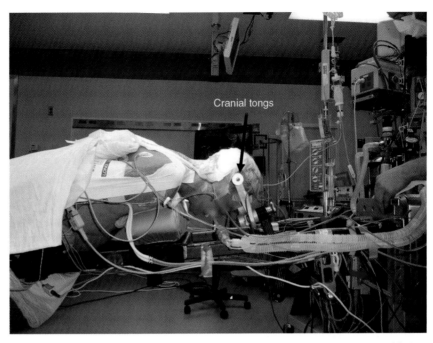

Cranial tongs

Figure 1 Photograph of a patient in the prone position for cervical laminectomy and fusion. The patient's head is secured in cranial tongs and a Mayfield clamp, which is attached to a spinal positioning frame. The arms are taped down securely. The abdomen hangs free between the chest and pelvic pads. The table is tilted in a slight reverse Trendelenburg position.

Techniques

Anesthesia Considerations

The anesthesiologist should be informed if the patient has severe cervical stenosis and myelopathy. Awake intubation and positioning is considered for all such patients. Being awake maintains muscle tone and affords an additional degree of protection for the spinal cord. After confirming preservation of spinal cord function in the final surgical position by asking the patient to move his or her fingers and toes, the patient is anesthetized completely. Hyperextension maneuvers of the neck during intubation may exacerbate myelopathy and should be avoided. Total intravenous anesthesia may be required in patients who are undergoing motor-evoked potential monitoring.

Patient Positioning

Cranial tongs should be applied before the patient is turned prone. Generally, Mayfield cranial tongs are used. The

tongs are applied using sterile technique. Standard sites for the three pins are 1 cm superior to the earlobe and in line with and bifurcated by the tragus. Some surgeons use a halo ring with four pins. The patient is turned prone, and the cranial tongs are secured to a Mayfield clamp that attaches to the surgical table (**Figure 1**). The neck is maintained in a neutral to slightly flexed position. The arms are tucked by the patient's sides; positioning the arms in an abducted position above the level of the shoulder risks traction on the brachial plexus and places the cervical nerve roots in tension. Appropriate padding of all bony prominences and peripheral nerves is essential.

Instruments/Equipment/ Implants Required

Straight and angled curets, Kerrison rongeurs, osteotomes, pituitary rongeurs, Leksell rongeurs, bipolar coagulation, cottonoid patties, and bone

wax are used frequently during cervical laminectomy and should be available during surgery. Currently, most spine surgeons use a high-speed burr to make the primary osteotomies during cervical laminectomy. Mayfield tongs are used to position the patient's head and keep pressure off the face and eyes during surgery. Surgery most often is performed on a spine surgery frame that allows reverse Trendelenburg positioning of the patient while securely stabilizing the torso and extremities and allowing the abdomen to hang free without compression (**Figure 1**). Use of a surgical microscope or operating loupe with a headlight is now standard practice, as these instruments allow improved visualization and accuracy of dissection. Surgeon preference dictates the use of spinal cord monitoring; however, monitoring should be strongly considered in cases of myelopathy and severe degenerative or traumatic stenosis. Baseline somatosensory and motor-evoked potentials before surgery will permit more accurate detection of variation from intraoperative events.

Posterior cervical fusion often is augmented by stabilization of the spinal column using metallic implants. Lateral mass screw–rod constructs are the most common implant used for posterior instrumentation of the cervical spine and provide improved rigidity over interspinous wiring techniques. Lateral mass screws can be used even when the posterior elements are deficient because of trauma, tumors, or prior laminectomy. Lateral mass screws generally are used from C3 to C6, where the lateral masses are well developed. Pedicle screws are used more commonly at C2 and C7, where the pedicles are largest in the cervical spine. Typically, polyaxial screw heads with a 3.5-mm diameter thread and 3.5-mm connecting rod are used. Lateral mass screws are most frequently 14 mm long, whereas pedicle screws are generally 24 mm long. The use of lateral mass screws or pedicle screws in the cervical spine is off-label, although such metallic implants are used frequently by spine surgeons.

Interspinous wiring can be an alternative to lateral mass or pedicle screw fixation in the stabilization of the posterior cervical spine. Although wires provide adequate resistance in flexion, they are not as strong in resisting extension, axial load, rotation, and lateral bending. Commonly used implants are 18- or 20-gauge stainless steel wire or 1- to 1.2-mm titanium braided cable.

Exposure

In most patients, palpation of the prominent C2 and C7 spinous processes allows identification of the midline and assessment of the surgical level. A midline incision is made in the posterior cervical spine, and dissection is carried down to the fascia. The fascia and ligamentum nuchae in the midline are identified, and the super-

ficial soft tissues are stripped off the fascia a short distance from the midline bilaterally. The fascia is incised over the prominence of the spinous process using electrocautery, and further dissection is carried along the spinous processes and lamina in a subperiosteal fashion. After elevation of the paraspinal muscles at all levels desired, deep retractors are positioned to hold the paraspinal muscles apart on either side. Care is taken to preserve the soft tissues over the facet joints until the entire central exposure is performed and the required levels of decompression and fusion are identified. This helps preserve stability and decrease adjacent-level degeneration at levels not included in the decompression. Meticulous dissection and soft-tissue stripping off bone are essential to delineate landmarks required for placement of instrumentation and to provide sufficient surface area for fusion.

Procedure

LAMINECTOMY

A variety of techniques are used to perform decompression, and none has clear advantages with respect to outcome. We recommend that the interspinous ligaments and ligamentum flavum at the proximal and distal extent of the laminectomy be resected as a first step. This is done by penetrating the midline raphe in the ligamentum flavum with an angled 5-0 curet. The ligamentum flavum is stripped off its attachment onto the distal lamina. A 1-mm Kerrison rongeur is used to resect the ligamentum flavum to the medial edge of the facet joint bilaterally.

We then use a high-speed neural burr to create a trough bilaterally at the junction of the lamina and lateral mass at all levels to be included in the laminectomy (**Figure 2**, *A* and *B*). Using a microscope, progress of the burr tip can be followed carefully as it deepens the trough and eventually breaks through the anterior cortex of the lamina. Irrigation and suction are

performed simultaneously to remove bone fragments and facilitate visualization. Residual soft tissue at the base of the trough is cauterized using bipolar coagulation, and it is resected with a 1-mm Kerrison rongeur. The most distal spinous process included is then grasped with a clamp, and gentle posteriorly directed traction is applied to the loose segment. A dental elevator is used to strip any soft-tissue attachments between the posterior aspect of the spinal cord and anterior aspect of the laminae, and the entire laminectomy segment is elevated off the spinal cord en bloc (**Figure 2**, *C*).

An alternative technique for cervical laminectomy includes using a Kerrison rongeur to make the bilateral osteotomy at the junction of the laminae and lateral masses on either side. At all times during the surgical procedure, care should be taken to ensure that instruments are not placed anterior to the lamina, to avoid injury to the spinal cord or nerve roots. Adequacy of decompression can be confirmed by visual confirmation of cord expansion and restoration of cerebrospinal fluid pulsations.

FUSION

When fusion and instrumentation are performed following cervical laminectomy, the most common instrumentation technique used is lateral mass screw and rod stabilization. Lateral mass screws can be used when the posterior elements are deficient (following laminectomy or involving trauma or tumors), and they provide superior biomechanical fixation compared with wiring techniques.

It is essential to create an adequate fusion bed, as this will strongly influence the surgical results. Meticulous dissection of the soft tissues is important to visualize anatomy and identify bony landmarks. Facet joint cartilage and soft tissue should be resected and the posterior bony surfaces decorticated (**Figure 3**, *A*). This can be performed with a 3-mm high-speed burr

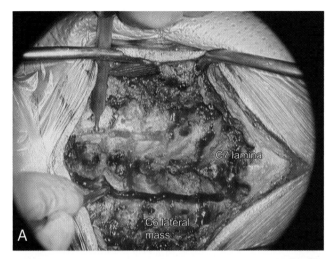

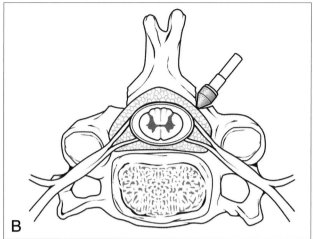

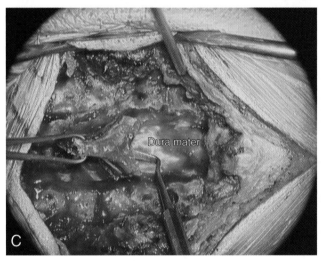

Figure 2 Cervical laminectomy. The patient's head is to the left. **A,** The ligamentum flavum is divided between C2 and C3 and between C7 and T1. Lateral gutters are created at the junction of the lamina and lateral mass on either side using a burr. The photograph shows the creation of lateral mass screw holes before this step, to facilitate better identification of bony landmarks. **B,** Illustration shows the direction of the burr tip during creation of the lateral gutters or troughs on either side of the lamina. **C,** Intraoperative photograph shows how the C7 spinous process is grasped and elevated proximally off the spinal cord to complete the laminectomy. A dental elevator is used to free any residual soft-tissue attachments on the anterior aspect of the laminae.

or with a curet. Identification of screw entry points and trajectory and placement of the implants are better performed with the bony morphology intact. This strategy also reduces bleeding. The resected spinous processes and laminae are stripped of all soft tissue and are morcellized, to provide autograft for fusion. Autologous bone graft obtained from the iliac crest or corticocancellous allograft bone is laid directly onto the bleeding surfaces of the decorticated posterior bone of the lateral masses (**Figure 3**, *B*). Additional graft is inserted directly into the facet joint after resection of all soft tissue and cartilage within the facet joint.

Placement of Screws

LATERAL MASS SCREWS
Adequate exposure of the posterior surface of the lateral mass is essential for safe and appropriate placement of lateral mass screws. The quadrilateral lateral mass is defined superiorly and inferiorly by the articulations above and below, respectively; the medial border is a faint groove at the junction of the lamina and lateral mass; and the lateral border can be palpated. Once the four borders are identified, different techniques are used for screw placement. The Roy-Camille technique uses a starting point at the center of the quadrilateral surface, with the screw directed laterally 10° in

the axial plane and perpendicular to the surface of the lateral mass in the sagittal plane, to exit lateral to the vertebral artery and inferior to the exiting nerve root. The Magerl technique uses a starting point 1 mm medial to the center of the quadrilateral surface. The screw is directed 25° lateral in the axial plane and parallel to the facet joint in the sagittal plane. Lateral fluoroscopy is used to place the screw parallel to and between the articular surfaces of the facet joints. The screw exits lateral to the vertebral artery and superior to the exiting nerve root. This technique was modified by An, who used the same starting point but aimed the

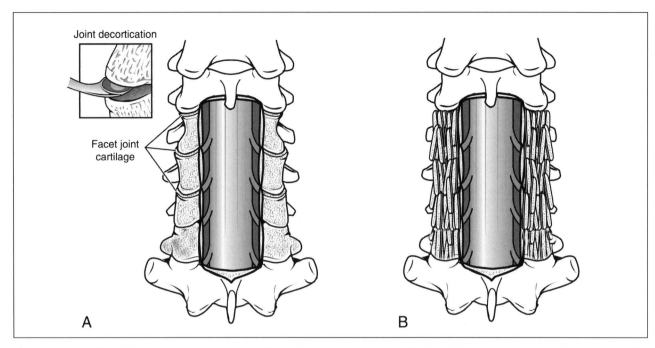

Figure 3 Preparation of the cervical spine for fusion. **A,** Illustration demonstrates decortication of the posterior aspects of lateral masses. The facet joint capsule has been resected, and the posterior third of the facet joint cartilage has been removed with small curets and burrs. **B,** Illustration demonstrates bone-graft strips laid on decorticated surfaces and impacted into the facet joint.

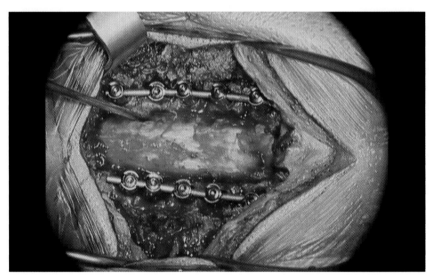

Figure 4 Intraoperative photograph shows lateral mass screws, pedicle screws, and rod construct after decompressive laminectomy from C3 to C7.

screws 30° laterally in the axial plane and 15° superiorly in the sagittal plane, to exit at the intersection of the transverse process and the lateral mass.

Using polyaxial, top-loading screws will allow for small variations in screw placement and makes rod contouring easier. Bicortical screw fixation provides improved biomechanical stability of the fixation, particularly in patients with poor bone quality, but it increases the risk of neurovascular injury (**Figure 4**).

PEDICLE SCREWS
Pedicle screw fixation provides greater biomechanical stability than lateral mass screw fixation, but it carries greater neurovascular risk. The increased strength of pedicle screw fixation allows for stabilization and simultaneous correction of deformity. Pedicle screws should be inserted before decompression to correctly identify bony landmarks. The entry point to the pedicle is 1 to 2 mm inferior to the inferior edge of the inferior articular process and 2 to 3 mm lateral to the midline or 2 to 3 mm medial to the lateral edge of the lateral mass. A high-speed burr is used to create a pilot hole, and a blunt pedicle probe is advanced along the medially angled pedicle. Oblique facet wiring is a less biomechanically stable alternative technique.

Wound Closure
A deep drain may be beneficial in preventing accumulation of a deep hematoma. Watertight closure of the poste-

rior fascia is imperative. This is followed by closure of the subcutaneous tissue, typically with braided, absorbable sutures. An absorbable monofilament suture is our preference for skin closure.

Postoperative Regimen

Patients are placed in a rigid cervical orthosis for 6 weeks postoperatively. When rigid lateral mass fixation has been used, some patients may be placed in a soft collar for 4 weeks postoperatively to allow the soft tissues to heal. This is followed by gradual resumption of the activities of daily living as tolerated by the patient.

Avoiding Pitfalls and Complications

Intraoperative identification of the surgical levels is essential. This is facilitated by intraoperative identification of the large C2 spinous process, the bifid C2 through C6 spinous processes, and the prominent C7 spinous process. Intraoperative radiographs must be obtained to confirm and document the surgical levels.

Bleeding may be controlled by careful dissection, use of bipolar coagulation, and liberal application of bone wax. Placing the patient in the reverse Trendelenburg position is helpful in reducing bleeding. Communication with the anesthesiologist should be undertaken regarding the need to control intraoperative blood pressures and thereby reduce bleeding while simultaneously maintaining adequate systemic and spinal cord perfusion.

Adequate removal of soft tissues from bony surfaces to be fused and removal of articular cartilage from the facet joint will most directly affect the likelihood that a solid fusion mass will form and pseudarthrosis will be avoided.

Preoperative planning is essential. Using CT scans to identify anatomic variations, including vertebral artery aneurysms, and templating of the bony morphology for screw length allow safe placement of lateral mass screws.

Implants are best placed before decompressive laminectomy. The morphology of the posterior elements is more obvious before laminectomy. The intact bony landmarks will help define the quadrilateral surface of the posterior lateral mass and aid in safe screw placement.

When using lateral mass instrumentation, the most proximal and distal screws should be placed first, followed by intervening screws; this allows better alignment of all screws and easier placement of the rod.

Bibliography

Graham AW, Swank ML, Kinard RE, Lowery GL, Dials BE: Posterior cervical arthrodesis and stabilization with a lateral mass plate: Clinical and computed tomographic evaluation of lateral mass screw placement and associated complications. *Spine (Phila Pa 1976)* 1996;21(3):323-329.

Guigui P, Benoist M, Deburge A: Spinal deformity and instability after multilevel cervical laminectomy for spondylotic myelopathy. *Spine (Phila Pa 1976)* 1998;23(4):440-447.

Hamanishi C, Tanaka S: Bilateral multilevel laminectomy with or without posterolateral fusion for cervical spondylotic myelopathy: Relationship to type of onset and time until operation. *J Neurosurg* 1996;85(3):447-451.

Heller JG, Edwards CC II, Murakami H, Rodts GE: Laminoplasty versus laminectomy and fusion for multilevel cervical myelopathy: An independent matched cohort analysis. *Spine (Phila Pa 1976)* 2001;26(12):1330-1336.

Houten JK, Cooper PR: Laminectomy and posterior cervical plating for multilevel cervical spondylotic myelopathy and ossification of the posterior longitudinal ligament: Effects on cervical alignment, spinal cord compression, and neurological outcome. *Neurosurgery* 2003;52(5):1081-1088.

Kato Y, Iwasaki M, Fuji T, Yonenobu K, Ochi T: Long-term follow-up results of laminectomy for cervical myelopathy caused by ossification of the posterior longitudinal ligament. *J Neurosurg* 1998;89(2):217-223.

Komotar RJ, Mocco J, Kaiser MG: Surgical management of cervical myelopathy: Indications and techniques for laminectomy and fusion. *Spine J* 2006;6(6, Suppl):252S-267S.

Kuhns CA, Geck MJ, Wang JC, Delamarter RB: An outcomes analysis of the treatment of cervical pseudarthrosis with posterior fusion. *Spine (Phila Pa 1976)* 2005;30(21):2424-2429.

Kumar VG, Rea GL, Mervis LJ, McGregor JM: Cervical spondylotic myelopathy: Functional and radiographic long-term outcome after laminectomy and posterior fusion. *Neurosurgery* 1999;44(4):771-778.

Rao RD, Currier BL, Albert TJ, et al: Degenerative cervical spondylosis: Clinical syndromes, pathogenesis, and management. *J Bone Joint Surg Am* 2007;89(6):1360-1378.

Rao RD, Marawar SV, Stemper BD, Yoganandan N, Shender BS: Computerized tomographic morphometric analysis of subaxial cervical spine pedicles in young asymptomatic volunteers. *J Bone Joint Surg Am* 2008;90(9):1914-1921.

Roy-Camille R, Saillant G, Mazel C: Internal fixation of the unstable cervical spine by a posterior osteosynthesis with plates and screws, in Sherk HM, ed: *The Cervical Spine*, ed 2. New York, NY, Lippincott, 1989, pp 390-403.

Wiggins GC, Shaffrey CI: Dorsal surgery for myelopathy and myeloradiculopathy. *Neurosurgery* 2007;60(1, Suppl 1):S71-S81.

Xu R, Haman SP, Ebraheim NA, Yeasting RA: The anatomic relation of lateral mass screws to the spinal nerves: A comparison of the Magerl, Anderson, and An techniques. *Spine (Phila Pa 1976)* 1999;24(19):2057-2061.

Yasuoka S, Peterson HA, MacCarty CS: Incidence of spinal column deformity after multilevel laminectomy in children and adults. *J Neurosurg* 1982;57(4):441-445.

Coding

CPT Codes		Corresponding ICD-9 Codes	
22600	Arthrodesis, posterior or posterolateral technique, single level; cervical below C2 segment	723 722.4	721
22614	Arthrodesis, posterior or posterolateral technique, single level; each additional vertebral segment (List separately in addition to code for primary procedure)	723 722.4	721
22840	Posterior non-segmental instrumentation (eg, Harrington rod technique, pedicle fixation across one interspace, atlantoaxial transarticular screw fixation, sublaminar wiring at C1, facet screw fixation) (List separately in addition to code for primary procedure)	723 722.4	721
22842	Posterior segmental instrumentation (eg, pedicle fixation, dual rods with multiple hooks and sublaminar wires); 3 to 6 vertebral segments (List separately in addition to code for primary procedure)	723 722.4	721
22843	Posterior segmental instrumentation (eg, pedicle fixation, dual rods with multiple hooks and sublaminar wires); 7 to 12 vertebral segments (List separately in addition to code for primary procedure)	723 722.4	721
22844	Posterior segmental instrumentation (eg, pedicle fixation, dual rods with multiple hooks and sublaminar wires); 13 or more vertebral segments (List separately in addition to code for primary procedure)	723 722.4	721
63045	Laminectomy, facetectomy and foraminotomy (unilateral or bilateral with decompression of spinal cord, cauda equina and/or nerve root[s], [eg, spinal or lateral recess stenosis]), single vertebral segment; cervical	723 722.4	721
63048	Laminectomy, facetectomy and foraminotomy (unilateral or bilateral with decompression of spinal cord, cauda equina and/or nerve root[s], [eg, spinal or lateral recess stenosis]), single vertebral segment; each additional segment, cervical, thoracic, or lumbar (List separately in addition to code for primary procedure)	723 722.4	721

CPT copyright © 2010 by the American Medical Association. All rights reserved.

Chapter 12

Open-Door Cervical Laminaplasty

Winston Fong, MD
Scott McGovern, MD
Jeffrey C. Wang, MD

◼ Indications

Open-door cervical laminaplasty was developed more than 30 years ago in an attempt to posteriorly decompress multilevel cervical pathology. In 1978, Hirabayashi first reported on the technique known as "expansive open-door laminaplasty," in which the affected cervical vertebrae were stabilized by simple sutures on the hinge side. There have been many modifications to the procedure since that time. A more recent technique for open-door cervical laminaplasty that uses mini titanium plates and allograft spacers to keep the door open is described later in this chapter. To date, no study demonstrates superiority of one technique over another.

Accepted indications for open-door cervical laminaplasty include myelopathy secondary to multilevel congenital stenosis or developmental stenosis caused by spondylosis (**Fig-**ure 1), ossification of the posterior longitudinal ligament, multilevel disk herniations, mass-occupying lesions, or any combination thereof. Open-door cervical laminaplasty should be a primary consideration for cases of multilevel stenosis, as it avoids the morbidity associated with multilevel fusion or laminectomy. Lordotic or neutral alignment of the cervical spine is required for open-door cervical laminaplasty to be successful.

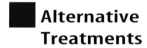

◼ Contraindications

Typically, open-door cervical laminaplasty alleviates spinal cord compression indirectly by expanding the spinal canal, thereby allowing the spinal cord to drift posteriorly away from anterior impinging structures. As such, it is contraindicated in patients with fixed kyphosis. In addition, open-door cervical laminaplasty is contraindicated in patients who have significant preoperative axial neck pain because they tend to have persistent neck pain after undergoing this motion-preserving technique. Furthermore, any condition that results in epidural scarring or adhesions (eg, previous posterior cervical decompressive surgery, ossification of the ligamentum flavum, or prior dorsal epidural infection) might preclude open-door cervical laminaplasty as a treatment option. Relative contraindications to the procedure include one- or two-level disease, severe anterior focal compression of the spinal cord, and a predominance of radicular symptoms.

◼ Alternative Treatments

Nonsurgical management of cervical myelopathy—including continued observation, physical therapy, and oral medications—is generally not recommended. Alternative treatments include multilevel anterior cervical diskectomies/corpectomies with fusion and posterior laminectomy with fusion. The advantages of cervical laminaplasty over the aforementioned

Dr. Wang or an immediate family member serves as a board member, owner, officer, or committee member of the Cervical Spine Research Society and the North American Spine Society; has received royalties from Aesculap/B. Braun, Biomet, Medtronic Sofamor Danek, Zimmer, SeaSpine, Stryker, and Osprey; serves as a paid consultant to or is an employee of Biomet, DePuy, Medtronic Sofamor Danek, Synthes, Stryker, Zimmer, Lanx, and Facet Solutions; serves as an unpaid consultant to Amgen; has received research or institutional support from the AO Foundation; and holds stock or stock options in Pearldiver, Bone Biologics, Axiomed, Flexuspine, Facet Soulutions, VG Innovations, Syndicom, Pioneer, Curative Biosciences, and Invuity. Neither of the following authors nor any immediate family member has received anything of value from or owns stock in a commercial company or institution related directly or indirectly to the subject of this chapter: Dr. Fong and Dr. McGovern.

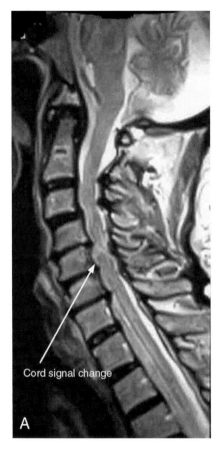

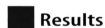

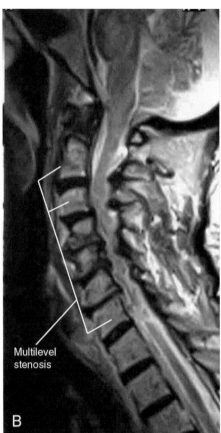

Figure 1 Sagittal T2-weighted MRI scans of the cervical spine demonstrate multilevel spondylosis and stenosis from C2-3 to C6-7. **A,** Cord signal change is evident, most notably at C5-6 (arrow). **B,** Multilevel degenerative changes that produce disk bulging and ligamentum flavum buckling lead to anterior and posterior spinal cord compression respectively, from C2-3 to C6-7. This patient had no neck pain but demonstrated signs of early myelopathy, and thus was a good candidate for open-door cervical laminaplasty.

techniques are that segmental stability is maintained, motion is preserved, and fusion is not required. Before determining the optimal surgical treatment, the pros and cons of each surgical technique should be evaluated with the patient's specific pathology in mind.

Results

Outcomes for open-door cervical laminaplasty typically are quite favorable for patients with conditions that fall within the defined indications for the procedure (**Table 1**). For these patients, preoperative neurologic deterioration is reliably halted, and significant improvements in myelopathy (from 40% to 70% per validated outcome scores) are seen in most patients. Several large studies have

shown that most patients who undergo open-door cervical laminaplasty retain neurologic recovery over the long term. In addition, in studies that compared open-door cervical laminaplasty with anterior or posterior decompression and fusion in patients with multilevel myelopathy and neutral or lordotic cervical spines, neurologic improvements were similar for all procedures, but open-door cervical laminaplasty was associated with a significantly lower incidence of complications.

Technique

Setup/Exposure

The patient is positioned prone, typically on a Jackson table. Rigid fixation of the head with Mayfield tongs is recommended. Electrical monitoring of

somatosensory- and motor-evoked potentials should be considered. As with any surgical case, diligence is necessary to avoid undue pressure or stretch on bony prominences and nerves that could cause sores and iatrogenic nerve palsies. The patient's shoulders may be taped down to facilitate intraoperative imaging of the lower cervical spine (**Figure 2**). Preoperative cervical range of motion should be assessed before general anesthesia is administered. The patient's neck should be positioned in neutral or slight flexion, if tolerated preoperatively. This may "unshingle" the lamina to facilitate its opening and may move the spinal cord away from the posterior elements, thereby making the drilling of the lamina somewhat safer.

A standard midline approach is made over the levels to be decompressed. This is extended down to the

Table 1 Results of Open-Door Laminaplasty

Author(s) (Year)	Number of Patients	Procedure	Mean Patient Age (Range)	Mean Follow-up (Range)	Results
Yonenobu et al (1991)	180	95 laminaplasty 85 laminectomy	56.7 (27-77)	6.1 years (2-16)	Similar rates of functional recovery Laminaplasty associated with fewer complications
Yonenobu et al (1992)	83	42 laminaplasty 41 subtotal corpectomy	56.0 laminaplasty 54.3 subtotal corpectomy	43 months (minimum 24 months)	Similar rates of functional recovery Laminaplasty associated with fewer complications
Heller et al (2001)	26	13 laminaplasty 13 laminectomy and fusion	56 (34-79) laminaplasty 55 (39-78) laminectomy and fusion	26 months (9-62)	Laminaplasty associated with superior clinical results and decreased complications
Satomi et al (2001)	80	204 laminaplasty	54 (16-77)	8 years (5-12)	Maintained neurologic improvement over long term
Wada et al (2001)	47	24 laminaplasty 23 subtotal corpectomy	$(58.5 \pm 11.2)^*$ laminaplasty $(52.7 \pm 7.8)^*$ subtotal corpectomy	12 years (10-14)	Similar maintenance of long-term neurologic improvement Laminaplasty associated with higher rates of axial neck pain but lower operating room time, blood loss, and nonunion
Edwards et al (2002)	26	13 laminaplasty 13 corpectomy	53 (35-67) laminaplasty 53 (39-72) corpectomy	40 months (16-48)	Similar neurologic improvement Laminaplasty associated with lower complications

* Mean ± SD.

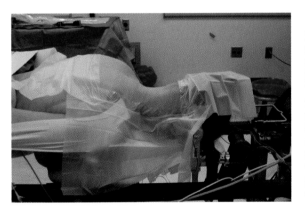

Figure 2 Proper positioning of the patient for the open-door cervical laminaplasty procedure. The patient is placed in the prone position, with the head stabilized in Mayfield tongs and the neck in neutral to slight flexion. The shoulders are taped down to facilitate imaging of the lower cervical spine.

posterior spinous processes. Electrocautery is used to subperiosteally dissect the muscular attachments from the spinous processes and laminae. Special care is used to preserve the musculotendinous attachments to the spinous process of C2, as these are important for maintaining cervical lordosis. Dissection is subsequently taken farther laterally to the lamina-facet border on the hinge side. On the open side, the exposure is extended to the lateral aspect of the lateral masses, taking care not to the damage the facet capsules (**Figure 3**). The appropriate retractors are then placed, and the operating microscope is brought in.

Instruments/Equipment/ Implants Required

We prefer rigid internal fixation with allograft struts to provide immediate stability to our cervical laminaplasty constructs. Titanium plates/screws and precut allograft struts made specifically for open-door cervical laminaplasty are available from several manufacturers. Several alternative fixation methods have been described, including the use of autologous spinous processes as strut grafts, suture anchors, hardware without strut grafts, and strut grafts without hardware.

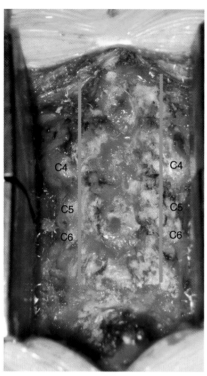

Figure 3 Intraoperative photograph demonstrates the exposure of C3 through C6 in preparation for open-door cervical laminaplasty at those levels. The green lines identify the lamina-facet borders. The facet capsules have been preserved. The spinous processes of C3 through C6 have been removed. The musculotendinous attachments at C2 remain intact.

Procedure

Open-door cervical laminaplasty requires detaching one side of the lamina from the facet, while leaving the opposite side connected (**Figure 4**). Factors such as the side of predominant symptoms, maximum anatomic compression, or the presence of coexisting radiculopathy due to foraminal stenosis influence the decision as to which side is opened. The side of the predominant radicular symptoms typically is the open side, and it easier to perform foraminotomies on the open side. Foraminotomies are performed on the hinge side before expansion of the posterior elements so that the tilted laminae do not obstruct the instruments. Conversely, the foramina

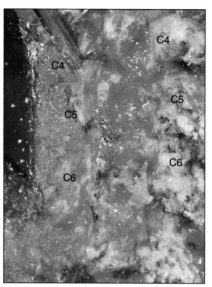

Figure 4 Intraoperative photograph demonstrates completion of the "open" side of the cervical laminaplasty (green arrows). A high-speed air drill was used to thin the lamina to the ligamentum flavum, taking care not to injure the dura. The "hinged" side is still connected.

on the open side are accessed easily after the laminae are elevated (**Figure 5**).

The interspinous ligaments are excised at the interspaces superior and inferior to the levels at which the laminaplasty is being performed. A bone cutter may then be used to resect the spinous processes of the involved levels. Subsequently, the ligamentum flavum at the interspaces superior and inferior to the operated levels are excised bilaterally with the use of a micro Kerrison rongeur to facilitate opening of the posterior arch.

A high-speed air drill with a small burr is used to make troughs bilaterally at the lamina-facet junction. The open side is burred to thin the lamina to the ligamentum flavum while avoiding contact with the dura (**Figure 4**). A micro Kerrison rongeur can be used to complete the cut. The hinge side is burred down to the ventral cortex, leaving it intact. The ligamentum flavum must then be incised carefully on the open side. Hemostasis may be

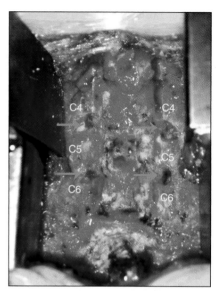

Figure 5 Intraoperative photograph shows where bilateral foraminotomies were performed at C4-5 and C5-6 (green arrows). We routinely perform prophylactic foraminotomies at C4-5 to prevent C5 nerve root palsies. This patient had bilateral C6 radiculopathy, and thus the nerve roots were decompressed at C5-6 as well.

achieved with bone wax and thrombin products. Bipolar cautery should be used to coagulate epidural bleeding. The opening of the lamina is performed by placing curved curets underneath the lamina of the open side and gently manipulating it to the contralateral side. If there is any resistance, the surgeon must check the hinge side to determine if the trough is sufficiently deep. Excessive force should be avoided to prevent breaking the hinge.

Once the lamina has been manipulated into an expanded position, trial spacers are used to determine the proper allograft size by placing them into the expanded lamina-facet gap. The allografts are then attached to the mini plates and inserted so that the notched ends of the graft fit into the cut ends of the lamina and the lateral mass.

The mini plate is centered in the middle of the lamina and lateral mass for ideal placement. A drill bit with a built-in stop is used to prepare the in-

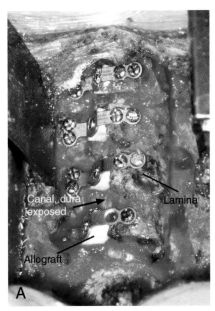
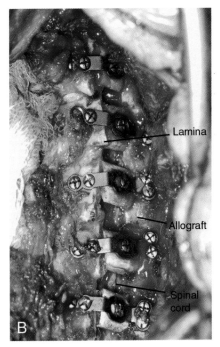
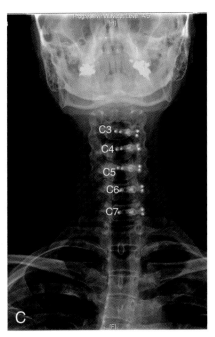

Figure 6 A, Intraoperative photograph shows how premachined allograft struts are used to "prop open" the lamina and expand the canal. The allograft struts are secured in place with titanium plates and screws. **B,** In this intraoperative photograph, rib allograft has been cut to fit under the expanded lamina. The spinal cord can be visualized between the allograft struts. There is now adequate room for the spinal cord. **C,** Postoperative AP radiograph shows a completed C3 through C7 open-door cervical laminaplasty and proper placement of the plates and screws.

sertion sites for the screws. Care must be taken not to alter the plate position while drilling. Proper screw size and direction of placement are essential to avoid violating the facet joints and spinal canal. Two screws are first placed through the plate over the lateral mass to ensure stable purchase in solid bone and to avoid torquing the allograft–plate–host bone interface. Subsequently, one or two screws are placed through the plate into the lamina, depending on the fit of the plate (**Figure 6**). Fluoroscopy may be used to aid and confirm proper placement of hardware (**Figure 6, C**).

Wound Closure

Before closure, the wound is copiously irrigated. The deep fascia is closed over a subfascial drain. The subcutaneous tissue and skin are closed in a typical manner. The patient is treated with antibiotics for 24 hours post-operatively as prophylaxis against infection.

━━━━━━■

Postoperative Regimen

After surgery, the patient is immobilized in a cervical collar for comfort only. The collar typically is worn for several days, but the patient should be weaned from collar use as tolerated to prevent muscle atrophy. Gentle range-of-motion exercises of the neck are encouraged immediately after surgery Flexion/extension radiographs taken 2 weeks postoperatively show maintenance of range of motion at the operated levels (**Figure 7**). Active resistive exercises are started at 3 weeks post-operatively. Driving may commence when the patient has achieved com-fortable and pain-free range of motion of the neck and is no longer being treated with narcotic medications.

━━━━━━■

Avoiding Pitfalls and Complications

One of the main advantages of open-door cervical laminaplasty is that it is associated with fewer complications than other cervical decompression procedures. Proper patient selection is paramount to obtaining good results. Open-door cervical laminaplasty should be considered only for a patient who has multilevel cervical disease, a straight or lordotic spine, and no preoperative axial neck pain. Motor nerve root palsies remain a significant concern and occur in approximately 8% of cases, with C5 being the

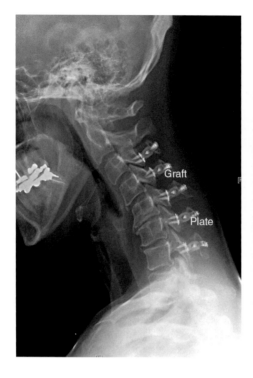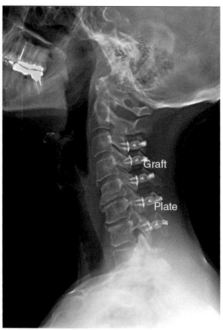

Figure 7 Lateral flexion (**A**) and extension (**B**) radiographs of the cervical spine obtained after open-door cervical laminaplasty show that range of motion has been retained at the surgically repaired levels (C3 through C7).

most commonly affected myotome. Fortunately, most cases of nerve root palsy are temporary. Often, prophylactic selective foraminotomy of the C5 nerve root is performed with open-door cervical laminaplasty; however, this has not been shown to definitively decrease the incidence of C5 nerve root palsy that is associated with the laminaplasty procedure. Finally, attention to good surgical technique will prevent iatrogenic injury.

———————■

■ Bibliography

Edwards CC II, Heller JG, Murakami H: Corpectomy versus laminoplasty for multilevel cervical myelopathy: An independent matched-cohort analysis. *Spine (Phila Pa 1976)* 2002;27(11):1168-1175.

Heller JG, Edwards CC II, Murakami H, Rodts GE: Laminoplasty versus laminectomy and fusion for multilevel cervical myelopathy: An independent matched cohort analysis. *Spine (Phila Pa 1976)* 2001;26(12):1330-1336.

Hirabayashi K: Expansive open-door laminoplasty for cervical spondylotic myelopathy. *Jpn J Surg* 1978;32:1159-1163.

Hirabayashi K, Watanabe K, Wakano K, Suzuki N, Satomi K, Ishii Y: Expansive open-door laminoplasty for cervical spinal stenotic myelopathy. *Spine (Phila Pa 1976)* 1983;8(7):693-699.

Hosono N, Yonenobu K, Ono K: Neck and shoulder pain after laminoplasty: A noticeable complication. *Spine (Phila Pa 1976)* 1996;21(17):1969-1973.

Maeda T, Arizono T, Saito T, Iwamoto Y: Cervical alignment, range of motion, and instability after cervical laminoplasty. *Clin Orthop Relat Res* 2002;401:132-138.

Matsunaga S, Sakou T, Nakanisi K: Analysis of the cervical spine alignment following laminoplasty and laminectomy. *Spinal Cord* 1999;37(1):20-24.

Sasai K, Saito T, Akagi S, Kato I, Ohnari H, Iida H: Preventing C5 palsy after laminoplasty. *Spine (Phila Pa 1976)* 2003;28(17):1972-1977.

Satomi K, Ogawa J, Ishii Y, Hirabayashi K: Short-term complications and long-term results of expansive open-door laminoplasty for cervical stenotic myelopathy. *Spine J* 2001;1(1):26-30.

Shaffrey CI, Wiggins GC, Piccirilli CB, Young JN, Lovell LR: Modified open-door laminoplasty for treatment of neurological deficits in younger patients with congenital spinal stenosis: Analysis of clinical and radiographic data. *J Neurosurg* 1999;90(2, Suppl):170-177.

Wada E, Suzuki S, Kanazawa A, Matsuoka T, Miyamoto S, Yonenobu K: Subtotal corpectomy versus laminoplasty for multilevel cervical spondylotic myelopathy: A long-term follow-up study over 10 years. *Spine (Phila Pa 1976)* 2001; 26(13):1443-1448.

Yonenobu K, Hosono N, Iwasaki M, Asano M, Ono K: Laminoplasty versus subtotal corpectomy: A comparative study of results in multisegmental cervical spondylotic myelopathy. *Spine (Phila Pa 1976)* 1992;17(11):1281-1284.

Yonenobu K, Hosono N, Iwasaki M, Asano M, Ono K: Neurologic complications of surgery for cervical compression myelopathy. *Spine (Phila Pa 1976)* 1991;16(11):1277-1282.

Coding

CPT Codes		Corresponding ICD-9 Codes	
63020	Laminotomy (hemilaminectomy), with decompression of nerve root(s), including partial facetectomy, foraminotomy and/or excision of herniated intervertebral disc, including open and endoscopically-assisted approaches; 1 interspace, cervical	721.1 723.0	722
63035	Laminotomy (hemilaminectomy), with decompression of nerve root(s), including partial facetectomy, foraminotomy and/or excision of herniated intervertebral disc, including open and endoscopically-assisted approaches; each additional interspace, cervical or lumbar (List separately in addition to code for primary procedure)	721.1 723.0	722
63040	Laminotomy (hemilaminectomy), with decompression of nerve root(s), including partial facetectomy, foraminotomy and/or excision of herniated intervertebral disc, reexploration, single interspace; cervical	721.1 723.0	722
63043	Laminotomy (hemilaminectomy), with decompression of nerve root(s), including partial facetectomy, foraminotomy and/or excision of herniated intervertebral disc, reexploration, single interspace; each additional cervical interspace (List separately in addition to code for primary procedure)	721.1 723.0	722
63045	Laminectomy, facetectomy and foraminotomy (unilateral or bilateral with decompression of spinal cord, cauda equina and/or nerve root[s], [eg, spinal or lateral recess stenosis]), single vertebral segment; cervical	721.1 723.0	722
63048	Laminectomy, facetectomy and foraminotomy (unilateral or bilateral with decompression of spinal cord, cauda equina and/or nerve root[s], [eg, spinal or lateral recess stenosis]), single vertebral segment; each additional segment, cervical, thoracic, or lumbar (List separately in addition to code for primary procedure)	724.6	721

Chapter 13

Cervical Laminaplasty: French Door

John G. Heller, MD
James A. Sanfilippo, MD

Indications

Cervical laminaplasty currently is indicated as a posterior approach to relieve multilevel cervical spinal cord compression leading to myelopathy. This includes compression caused by cervical spinal stenosis, an ossified posterior longitudinal ligament, and multilevel subaxial cervical spondylosis. This technique is indicated for patients of all ages, but it may be especially relevant in the younger patient with adequate cervical sagittal alignment and minimal axial neck pain without evidence of instability. Younger patients have a particularly less favorable natural history following multilevel cervical fusions. When necessary, however, the French-door technique may be combined with a fusion. Here the laminas are preserved, creating additional surface area for decortication. The double hinge creates troughs for bone graft placement and a generous fusion bed bilaterally (**Figure 1**). This is in stark contrast to a laminectomy and fusion procedure, in which the only bone remaining to

decorticate is the lateral mass, and the only area left in which to place bone graft is the lateral portion of the lateral mass, outside a fixation device such as a screw-rod construct.

Contraindications

One clear contraindication to cervical laminaplasty is the presence of excessive cervical kyphosis. Having 13° or more of localized cervical kyphosis has been associated with poor surgical outcomes. However, cervical kyphosis of less than 13° has been shown to not prejudice neurologic recovery. Relative contraindications to laminaplasty include mechanical or axial neck pain, ossification of the ligamentum flavum of the yellow ligament, epidural fibrosis, and previous posterior cervical surgery. An additional contraindication to laminaplasty is spondylosis associated with athetoid cerebral palsy, a pathologic entity in which laminaplasty combined with arthrodesis may avoid the risk for instability and

excess motion with the athetoid movements.

Alternative Treatments

The surgical panacea for multilevel cervical myelopathy has yet to be described. Multiple effective procedures currently are available for the treatment of this condition. These options include multilevel anterior cervical decompression with fusion, laminectomy with fusion, and laminaplasty. Whether the spinal cord compression leading to the myelopathy is due to spondylosis, developmental stenosis, ossified posterior longitudinal ligament, or a combination of these pathologic processes, all of these approaches have been described to be safe, with varying rates of success and postoperative complications.

Results

Clinical results reported in the literature over the past 25 years have been promising (**Table 1**). Cervical laminaplasty has been described to be a safe alternative to laminectomy and fusion

Dr. Heller or an immediate family member has received royalties from Medtronic; is a member of a speakers' bureau or has made paid presentations on behalf of Abbott and Medtronic; serves as a paid consultant to or is an employee of Abbott and Medtronic; serves as an unpaid consultant to BioCure; has received research or institutional support from Abbott, Medtronic, and Synthes; and owns stock or stock options in Medtronic. Neither Dr. Sanfilippo nor any immediate family member has received anything of value from or owns stock in a commercial company or institution related directly or indirectly to the subject of this chapter.

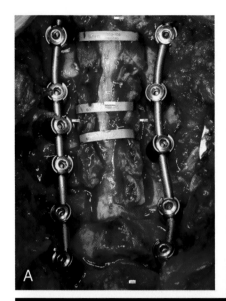

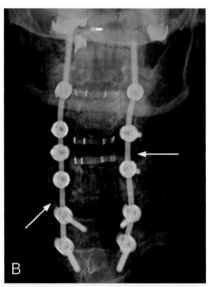

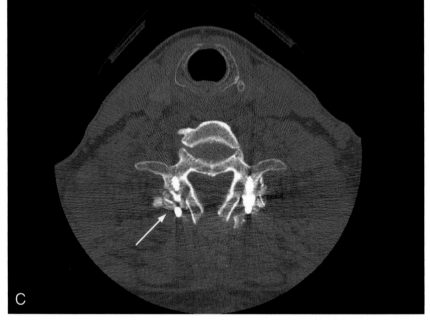

Figure 1 French-door laminaplasty combined with fusion in a patient with multilevel spinal cord compression and subaxial malalignment and instability. **A,** Intraoperative photo of the completed procedure. The patient's head is at the top. **B,** AP radiograph of the same patient 1 year after cervical laminaplasty, demonstrating fusion mass (arrows). **C,** Axial CT scan following cervical laminaplasty, demonstrating healing of the bilateral hinges and lateral fusion mass (arrow).

naplasty has been shown to be at least equivalent in most clinical categories, including improvement in myelopathy, motor deficit, sensory deficit, pain, and gait. Complications commonly associated with laminectomy and fusion, including problems associated with obtaining fusion (eg, pseudarthrosis, broken hardware, and postlaminectomy kyphosis), are avoided with cervical laminaplasty. Similar complications reported with anterior cervical corpectomy and fusion, including dysphagia and dysphonia, also are avoided with the posterior approach used with cervical laminaplasty.

━━━━━━━■

■ Technique

Setup and Patient Positioning

The patient enters the surgical suite on a standard preoperative bed or stretcher. The patient then undergoes induction of general anesthesia and insertion of an endotracheal tube for intubation. If the surgeon opts to use somatosensory-evoked potentials or motor-evoked potentials for spinal cord surveillance, leads are placed at this time. We commonly use spinal cord monitoring for this procedure.

The patient is now turned prone onto a standard operating table, using chest rolls to pad the chest and elevate the torso. Our preferred method is to apply Mayfield tongs before the "flip" to better control the patient's head during the turn. The Mayfield tongs are then connected to the table using the appropriate table attachment. During this positioning, care should be taken to ensure that the patient's head is not rotated and that the patient's neck is maintained in neutral alignment.

With the patient prone and the head controlled, the bed is "broken" to flex the knees 60° to 90°. The bed is then placed in a reverse Trendelenburg position, bringing the posterior

and to anterior cervical decompression and fusion for the treatment of cervical spondylotic myelopathy. Studies have shown that myelopathy has improved in up to 62% of patients, as measured by the Nurick classification system. In other series, the progression of the myelopathy was halted

in all patients treated with French-door laminaplasty. Motor deficits also have improved in these series in up to 93% of patients, whereas sensory deficits improved in 53%.

When compared directly with laminectomy and fusion and anterior cervical corpectomy and fusion, lami-

Table 1 Clinical Results for Cervical Laminaplasty

Authors (Year)	Number of Patients	Procedure or Approach	Mean Patient Age in Years (Range)	Mean Follow-up (Range)	Results
Edwards et al (2000)	18	French-door laminaplasty	54 (34-79)	24 months (18-36)	Progression of myelopathy halted in all cases Patients reported improvement in strength (78%), dexterity (67%), numbness (83%), pain (83%), and gait (67%)
Heller et al (2001)	26	Laminaplasty vs laminectomy and fusion	55 (34-79)	25.5 months (9-62)	Laminaplasty significantly superior to laminectomy and fusion in improvement of myelopathic symptoms and patient subjective symptoms Laminectomy and fusion had significantly more complications, including those associated with fusion and 1 graft harvest
Seichi et al (2001)	60	French-door laminaplasty	55 (37-69)	153 months (120-200)	Relief of myelopathy maintained in 78% of patients at 10-year follow-up Remaining 22% showed deterioration at a mean of 8 years postoperatively, and all patients experiencing deterioration did so following trauma
Edwards et al (2002)	26	Laminaplasty vs anterior cervical corpectomy and fusion	53 (39-72)	40 months (16-58)	Laminaplasty and anterior cervical corpectomy and fusion statistically similar in improvement of myelopathic symptoms Patients undergoing laminaplasty required less postoperative pain medication and experienced fewer complications Complications associated with corpectomy and fusion included pseudarthrosis, dysphagia, and dysphonia, as well as those associated with bone-graft harvest
Maeda et al (2002)	44	Open-door laminaplasty	59 (48-78)	3.2 years (1-9)	Range of motion of the cervical spine decreased by >41% after laminaplasty This loss of motion was seen in conjunction with loss of lordosis
Wang et al (2004)	204	Laminaplasty	63 (36-92)	16 months (Range NR)	127 patients experienced improvement in myelopathic symptoms 74 showed no progression in symptoms; 3 showed mild deteriorations
Sugimoto et al (2007)	18	Open-door laminaplasty	62 (47-78)	2 weeks and 6 months (Mean and range NR)	Cervical rotation after laminaplasty decreased slightly at 2 weeks after surgery, but recovered to almost preoperative levels by 6 months Subaxial rotation (C2 to T1) angles did not significantly decrease following surgery
Suk et al (2007)	85	Open-door laminaplasty	56.7 (35-80)	2 years (Range NR)	Range of motion of the cervical spine decreased by >30% after laminaplasty Cervical kyphosis developed in 11% of the patients Preoperative factors leading to increased postoperative kyphosis are cervical spondylosis, lordosis angle of <10°, and a kyphotic angle during flexion that is larger than a lordotic angle during extension
Takeuchi and Shono (2007)	41	French-door laminaplasty: C3 through C6 vs C3 through C7	69.7 (35-85)	1 year and 2 years (Mean and range NR)	Patients undergoing French-door laminaplasty with maintenance of the C7 spinous process and nuchal ligament attachment experienced fewer axial pain symptoms than those whose C7 spinous process was removed during the procedure

NR = not reported.

surface of the neck parallel to the ground. Using the draw sheet, the arms are now tucked or wrapped to maintain position at the patient's side. At this point, it is important to confirm with the anesthesiologist that all lines are flowing and that the blood pressure cuff, if it is the only method of measuring the patient's pressure, is functioning properly. Now, if the surgeon so chooses, the arms can be taped, pulling the shoulders distally to ensure adequate intraoperative imaging.

Prior to preparation and draping, the neck is flexed slightly, tensioning the posterior cervical musculature and skin, aiding in exposure and closure. This also allows for unshingling of the cervical lamina, facilitating easier identification of landmarks and, later, easier opening of the canal. Additionally, the posterior-superior occipital protuberance must be identified and visualized. The patient's hair needs to be retracted and/or shaved to expose this landmark. The patient is now prepared in the surgeon's preferred method and draped sterilely to maintain exposure of the occipital protuberance, the lateral aspect of the posterior surface of the neck, and the scapular spines bilaterally, ensuring that an appropriate-sized incision can be made without restriction from the surgical drapes.

Exposure

In the classic French-door or double-hinge technique described by Kurokawa and associates, a midline posterior cervical approach is employed to expose the spinous processes, laminae, and medial half of the lateral masses from C2 cranially to T1 caudally. Prior to incision, a skin marker is used to draw the vertical incision in the midline, connecting the C2 spinous process and the T1 spinous process. A scalpel is used to sharply incise the skin and subcuticular layers. A Bovie electrocautery (Bovie Medical, Clearwater, FL) is employed

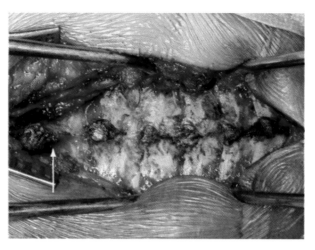

Figure 2 Intraoperative photograph of the full exposure. The patient's head is to the right. The T1 spinous process (arrow) is seen at the extreme left of the wound. The inferior margin of the C2 spinous process is concealed by the overlying skin at the right.

to dissect the subcutaneous tissues in the midline, down to the fascial layer, and then is used to dry the field. Retractors are placed to gently separate the edges and allow for visualization of the midline. The fascia and the cervical musculature are now separated in the midline, using the Bovie and gentle retraction. Once the spinous processes are identified, a metallic "marker" is placed and a cross-table lateral radiograph or lateral C-arm image is used for appropriate level identification.

Once the surgeon is oriented to the appropriate surgical level, the deep paraspinal musculature is elevated off the spinous processes and the lamina bilaterally, using the Bovie and a series of Cobb elevators. The laminae are exposed laterally to the lamina–lateral mass junction, and then the dissection continues laterally, exposing the medial halves of the lateral masses. Care must be taken not to disturb the facet joints and their associated capsules. This is done at each level, from the caudal C2 lamina to the cranial T1 lamina. Meticulous hemostasis is now obtained and needs to be maintained throughout the procedure. The retractors are now positioned deep to maintain the exposure and proper visualization.

More commonly today, the exposure is performed from the inferior portion of C2, exposing only the infe-

riormost portion of the C2 lamina and the medial portion of the C2-C3 joints bilaterally, to either the superior portion of C7 or T1. The actual laminaplasty is performed from C3 to C6, C7, or T1, depending on how caudal the compressive pathology extends and how much decompression is needed to resolve the patient's myelopathy. To ensure complete decompression of the spinal cord, it is a good general rule to include the laminae above and below the level of compressive pathology. Additionally, the attachments of the extensor muscles, namely the semispinalis, are maintained on the posterior elements of C2 (**Figure 2**).

Instruments/Equipment/ Implants Required

Minimal equipment and instrumentation is required to perform cervical laminaplasty. The surgeon will need scalpels, a Bovie, and bipolar electrocautery tools. Cervical retractors, including cerebellar retractors, will be used to hold muscle and tissue apart, thus preserving the exposure. A high-speed burr, with 3-mm diamond and 4-mm round, soft-touch tips, will prove useful. Additionally, some method of maintaining canal expansion must be employed. This will require allograft bone, suture anchors, thin metal wires, or commercially available spacers or plates and their associated instruments.

Postoperative Regimen

Rigidly stabilized patients are immobilized postoperatively in a collar for 12 weeks. A more rigid external orthosis, such as a sternal occipital mandibular immobilizer (SOMI) or halo vest, is used in osteoporotic patients and in those in whom less rigid stabilization has been achieved. In particular, onlay grafting in young children often is accompanied by a Minerva brace or halo. In vertically stable patients with a rod-wire construct, a collar may be adequate. In vertically unstable patients, a halo should be considered unless rigid fixation has been achieved.

Occipitocervical fusion patients should be followed closely. Progressive deformities and neurologic deficits are dealt with more easily when recognized early. The clinician should search for occipital decubiti from greater occipital nerve anesthesia. In early follow-up, especially with elderly patients, limitations in cervical flexion-extension may impact gait stability. Prior to discharge from care, union should be verified with maximum flexion-extension radiographs or CT scan.

Avoiding Pitfalls and Complications

Complication rates vary widely in occipitocervical fusion series, typically as a function of the underlying medical comorbidities. For example, occipitocervical fusion in RA patents historically has been associated with a high incidence of perioperative complications. Modern techniques have reduced the perioperative mortality to between 2% and 10%. Other complications seen more commonly in this group include wound infection and dehiscence and loss of reduction.

The most feared complications involve neurovascular injury. Care is required during the initial subperiosteal dissection to avoid inadvertent penetration into the ligamentum flavum and the spinal canal. Occipital screws appear to be safer than cervical screws, with few reported neurovascular sequelae.

Even more critical is sublaminar wire passage or screw placement. In some cases, upper cervical fixation will benefit from a cannulated drill system, temporary joint fixation with K-wires, or sublaminar C1 wire passage. Fluoroscopic guidance and computer navigation systems have been used to improve the safety of implant placement.

Given the proximity of the internal carotid to the anterior C1 lateral mass, overpenetration must be avoided. If a vertebral artery is injured, a screw should not be placed on the opposite side. In patients with an intact C1 ring, Magerl recommends augmenting the screws with Gallie wiring and fusion. Hooks necessarily encroach on the spinal canal. Hook placement should be avoided at any level with cord edema.

Given the significant arc of flexion-extension motion arising from the occipitocervical junction, fixation and fusion must be undertaken in proper alignment. Proper sagittal alignment is especially important when rigid implants are used. In some cases, decompression is best performed in flexion. Similarly, some pathologies reduce better in flexion and others in extension. Occipitocervical kyphosis must be avoided. Thus, it may be useful to start with the upper cervical spine in slight flexion. Once the screws are in position, alignment must be corrected before final tightening (**Figure 6**).

Intraoperatively, proper alignment may be difficult to assess. Several "occipitocervical angle" measures have been proposed. In one, neutral alignment is defined by the intersection of the McRae line and a line through the superior end plate of C3. In neutral alignment, this angle should be 44°. Occipitocervical distance is obtained by measuring the shortest distance from the superior aspect of the C2 spinous process. Another measure uses a line parallel to the bony palate and the posterior longitudinal line of the C2 vertebra. In 30 healthy volunteers of both sexes and all ages, this angle ranged from 85° to 118°. The mean angle was 97.1° in males and 102.6° in females, with overall mean ± SD of 99.9 ± 8.1°.

A recent study compared the reliability of three techniques used to measure alignment between the occiput and cervical spine. The authors computed mean intraobserver and interobserver intraclass correlation coefficients with the Chamberlain, the McRae, and the McGregor lines and concluded that the McGregor line is the most reproducible and reliable method for measurement of the occipitocervical angle.

Improper final alignment confers several additional risks. First, improper alignment may increase the risk of subsequent subaxial degeneration. In RA patients, malalignment may increase the risk for subaxial subluxations. At the time of the index procedure, all anatomically involved levels should be incorporated in the index surgery.

The rates of postoperative dyspnea and dysphagia can be high even with posterior-only approaches. Recent studies implicate a shallow occiput-C2 angle. Shallow angles reduce the cross-sectional area of the oropharynx.

In a series of occipitocervical fusions in children, transient quadriplegia was seen in one patient. Other problems included fixation failure, pneumonia, wound infection, halo pin infection, skin breakdown under the halo vest, hydrocephalus, and cerebrospinal fluid leak. In children treated before age 6 years, increasing occipitocervical junction lordosis or

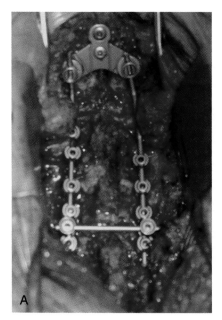

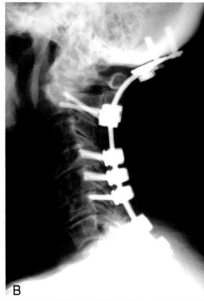

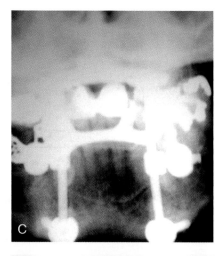

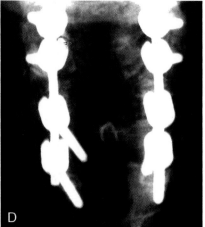

Figure 6 Images demonstrate a long occipitocervicothoracic fusion in an elderly woman with RA who had a history of mild basilar invagination, dens fracture, midcervical stenosis, and a C7-T1 spondylolisthesis. **A,** Intraoperative photograph depicts C2 pars screws placed along with lateral mass screws in the midcervical spine and pedicle screws in the upper thoracic spine. Note the use of a screw-to-rod connector for the more lateral C2 screws. Lateral (**B**) and AP (**C** and **D**) radiographs demonstrate that screw positions at C1, C3, and C7 were skipped to allow a more gradual, gentle rod contour.

"occipitocervical crank-shaft phenomenon" was encountered. The authors recommended fusion in a neutral or slightly flexed position in very young children to account for this predictable increase in lordosis. Other studies have not reported this issue.

Careful exposure of the cervical spine is necessary in all patients but particularly in children; unintended distal extension of the fusion may occur at unnecessarily exposed levels. In adults, pseudarthrosis rates ranged from 0% to 50% but improved with autologous bone grafting and rigid fixation. Occasionally, pseudarthrosis can precipitate further neurologic decline through loss of reduction, instrumentation failure, or cyst formation. Plating systems should be considered strongly if axial control is needed.

Bibliography

Abumi K, Takada T, Shono Y, Kaneda K, Fujiya M: Posterior occipitocervical reconstruction using cervical pedicle screws and plate-rod systems. *Spine (Phila Pa 1976)* 1999;24(14):1425-1434.

Behari S, Nayak SR, Bhargava V, Banerji D, Chhabra DK, Jain VK: Craniocervical tuberculosis: Protocol of surgical management. *Neurosurgery* 2003;52(1):72-81.

Deutsch H, Haid RW Jr, Rodts GE Jr, Mummaneni PV: Occipitocervical fixation: Long-term results. *Spine (Phila Pa 1976)* 2005;30(5):530-535.

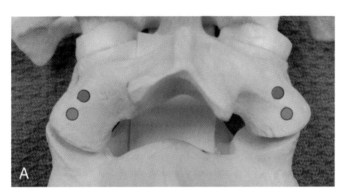

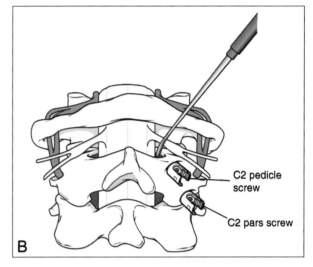

Figure 3 C2 fixation. **A,** The appropriate starting points for C2 pedicle screws (red dots) and C2 pars screws (blue dots) are shown on a model. **B,** Drawing shows a No. 4 Penfield dissector being used to feel the medial border of the C2 pars to guide screw placement.

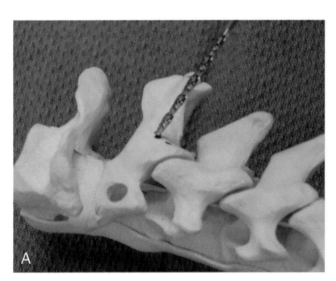

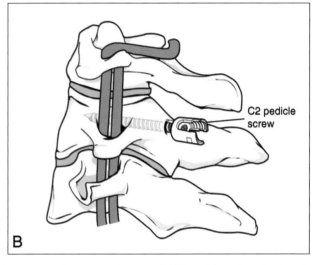

Figure 4 The starting point and cranial-caudal angulation for a C2 pedicle screw are demonstrated on a model (**A**) and shown in a drawing (**B**).

inclination of the pars. A No. 4 Penfield dissector is used to palpate the medial wall of the pars, guide the trajectory of the drill, and prevent a medial cortical breach. A ball-tipped probe is used to check for bony breach. After the screw hole is tapped and reprobed, a 3.5-mm polyaxial screw is then placed within the drill hole along the same trajectory (**Figure 5**). The screw enters the pars at the starting point and remains within the pars. It has a starting point and trajectory similar to that of the C1-C2 transarticular screw, but it is shorter (usually measuring 16 to 18 mm). This length screw stops short of the vertebral artery groove and transverse foramen, minimizing the risk of vertebral artery injury. The maximum possible length of the C2 pars screw can be determined using preoperative CT imaging (**Figure 6**). An example of C2 pars screw use in C1-C2 fusion is shown in Figure 6. Figure 7 shows pars screw use in the fusion of C2 to the subaxial cervical spine.

It is important to obtain and review cervical CT and MRI images as part of preoperative planning to ensure that the pedicle and pars of C2 are of adequate size on both the left and right side of the patient (**Figure 6**). Screw placement on the side of a dominant or anomalous vertebral artery can lead to vertebral artery injury. The

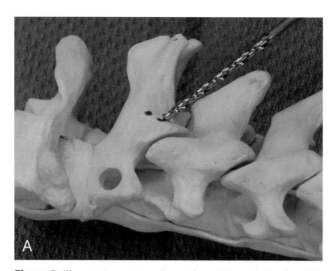

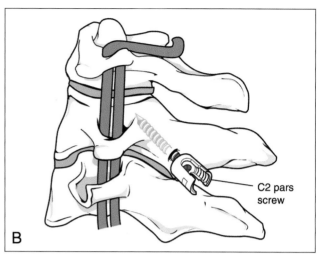

Figure 5 The starting point and cranial-caudal angulation for a C2 pars screw are demonstrated on a model (**A**) and shown in a drawing (**B**).

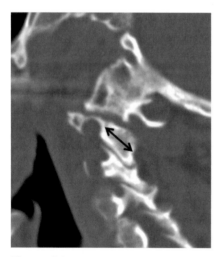

Figure 6 Preoperative parasagittal CT reconstruction image of the cervical spine. The bony area indicated by the double-headed black arrow should be measured prior to insertion of the C2 pars screw to ensure that the screw is the appropriate length and will not cause injury to the vertebral artery.

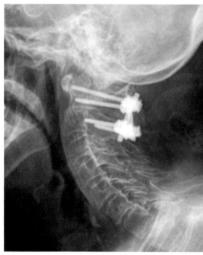

Figure 7 Postoperative lateral radiograph of a patient with a type II dens fracture who underwent posterior C1-C2 fusion with the use of C1 lateral mass screws, C2 pedicle screws, and rods.

vertebral artery is most at risk if drilling, tapping, or screw placement is off in the lateral and caudal direction.

PLACEMENT OF C2 LAMINAR SCREWS
Placement of bilateral, crossing C2 laminar screws was originally described by Wright in 2004 as a form of C2 fixation that avoids the risk of vertebral artery injury. This technique is

useful when abnormal bony or vascular anatomy precludes the placement of either a C2 pedicle or pars screw, or as a salvage technique when an attempt at C2 pedicle or pars screw placement fails.

Bilateral exposure of the C2 spinous process and lamina is needed to place the C2 laminar screw(s). To ensure that there is room within the C2 lamina for two crossing screws,

special attention should be given to the locations (ie, in a superior/inferior direction) within the lamina where each screw will be placed and the trajectory that each screw will take. A 2-mm high-speed burr is used to create a starting point for the laminar screws at the junction of the C2 spinous process and lamina. The starting point on one side is made at the superior aspect of this junction, whereas the starting point on the contralateral side is made at the inferior aspect of the junction (**Figures 8** and **9**). The lamina contralateral to the starting point is then drilled, at the same level in the superior-inferior direction, to a depth of 30 mm. When drilling, the drill should be angled in such a way that it lines up with the natural downslope of the contralateral lamina, erring slightly posterior to the contralateral lamina to avoid a breach into the spinal canal. A ball-tipped probe is used to ensure that there is no ventral breach into the spinal canal. The drill hole is then tapped, and a 4.0-mm × 30-mm polyaxial screw is inserted. This step is repeated for the contralateral side.

Wright's original description of this technique included a series of 10 patients who required C2 fixation, most

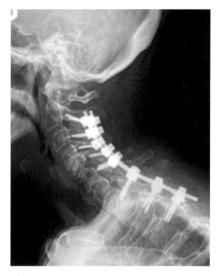

Figure 8 Postoperative lateral radiograph of a patient with cervical stenosis, instability, and myelopathy who underwent a posterior cervical laminectomy from C3 to C7 and posterior spinal fusion from C2 to T3 with the use of C2 pars screws, C3 to C6 lateral mass screws, and T1 to T3 pedicle screws.

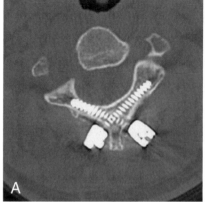

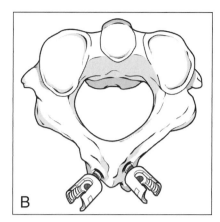

Figure 9 Postoperative axial CT image (**A**) and drawing (**B**) of the C2 vertebra shows the orientation and interlaminar positioning of the bilateral, crossing C2 laminar screws. (Part A is adapted with permission from Wright NM: Posterior C2 fixation using bilateral, crossing C2 laminar screws: Case series and technical notes. *J Spinal Disord Tech* 2004;17:158-162.)

of whom had C1-C2 fusion surgery. All patients in the series underwent surgical treatment without neurologic, vascular, or technical complications. Flexion/extension radiographs demonstrated that all patients had stable C2 fixation at 6-week follow-up. Longer term follow-up was limited in this series. A recent biomechanical study also suggested that bilateral C2 laminar screws provide comparable stability to C2 pedicle screws when used with a C1 lateral mass screw–rod construct to stabilize an unstable C1-C2 segment. Current clinical data on this technique are limited, however, and additional safety and efficacy studies are needed.

Wound Closure

Prior to wound closure, the incision is irrigated copiously with antibiotic/saline solution. A Jackson-Pratt drain is placed deep to the fascia. The ligamentum nuchae is closed in an interrupted fashion using No.1 braided absorbable sutures. The subcutaneous layer is then closed in an interrupted fashion using No. 2-0 braided absorb-

able sutures, and the skin can be closed either in a running or an interrupted fashion using a No. 3-0 or No. 4-0 monofilament suture. The ligamentum nuchae is the thick fascial layer that runs in the midline from the external occipital protuberance down the cervical spine along the tips of the cervical spinous processes. This thick fascia is an attachment site for the paraspinal cervical musculature. If this layer is not securely approximated during the wound closure, the patient may develop postoperative splaying of the paraspinal cervical musculature, prominence of the involved spinous processes, and neck pain.

Postoperative Regimen

The postoperative regimen varies, depending on the type and extent of fusion that is performed. Most patients, particularly those who are elderly or who have significant comorbidities, are sent to a monitored setting for at least 24 hours postoperatively. Bed rest should be avoided, and, if possible, early ambulation with assistance should be encouraged starting on the first postoperative day. Antibiotic

therapy is continued for 24 hours, unless surgery was performed specifically to treat an infection. The drain should be removed on the first postoperative day or when the drainage is less than 30 mL per 8-hour shift.

In general, patients who have undergone C2 fusion procedures are instructed to wear a rigid cervical collar for approximately 6 to 8 weeks. The rigid collar is then replaced by a soft collar (for comfort). Soft collar use is weaned over a 2- to 3-week period, during which time the patient begins a regimen of gentle neck strengthening and range-of-motion exercises. These exercises should be limited, depending on the extent of the surgical fusion (eg, occipitocervical fusion) that was performed. Regular follow-up appointments should be scheduled, during which a clinical examination should be performed and cervical radiographs obtained to assess the progress of the fusion and the integrity of the instrumentation.

Avoiding Pitfalls and Complications

C2 fixation procedures can be technically challenging. Preoperative and intraoperative steps can be taken to minimize the risk of complications, however. First, it is important to review preoperative CT and MRI scans and identify abnormal vertebral artery anatomy. It is essential that the surgeon understands the anatomy of the vertebral artery before C2 screw placement, to minimize the risk of injury. Second, it is important to use careful blunt dissection along the lateral aspect of the C2 lamina. This will minimize the risk of violating the large venous plexus that surrounds the C2 nerve root. If violated, this venous plexus can bleed profusely and complicate placement of the C2 screw. Bipolar cauterization of the venous plexus usually is not successful and actually can make the bleeding worse. If encountered, bleeding from the venous plexus surrounding the C2 nerve root is best addressed by packing the area with thrombin-soaked sterile, absorbable gelatin sponges until adequate hemostasis is achieved. Finally, a recent biomechanical study by Lehman and associates suggested that if there is a breach in the medial cortex or a failure in screw placement when attempting to place a C2 pedicle or a pars screw, either a C2 pedicle screw or a C2 laminar screw should be used. In that study, both of these screws were biomechanically superior to the C2 pars screw in a salvage situation.

—————————■

■ Bibliography

Aryan HE, Newman CB, Nottmeier EW, Acosta FL Jr, Wang VY, Ames CP: Stabilization of the atlantoaxial complex via C-1 lateral mass and C-2 pedicle screw fixation in a multicenter clinical experience in 102 patients: Modification of the Harms and Goel techniques. *J Neurosurg Spine* 2008;8(3):222-229.

Brooks AL, Jenkins EB: Atlanto-axial arthrodesis by the wedge compression method. *J Bone Joint Surg Am* 1978;60(3):279-284.

El Masry MA, El Assuity WI, Sadek FZ, Salah H: Two methods of atlantoaxial stabilisation for atlantoaxial instability. *Acta Orthop Belg* 2007;73(6):741-746.

Gorek J, Acaroglu E, Berven S, Yousef A, Puttlitz CM: Constructs incorporating intralaminar C2 screws provide rigid stability for atlantoaxial fixation. *Spine (Phila Pa 1976)* 2005;30(13):1513-1518.

Grob D, Crisco JJ III, Panjabi MM, Wang P, Dvorak J: Biomechanical evaluation of four different posterior atlantoaxial fixation techniques. *Spine (Phila Pa 1976)* 1992;17(5):480-490.

Harms J, Melcher RP: Posterior C1-C2 fusion with polyaxial screw and rod fixation. *Spine (Phila Pa 1976)* 2001;26(22):2467-2471.

Kim SM, Lim TJ, Paterno J, et al: Biomechanical comparison of anterior and posterior stabilization methods in atlantoaxial instability. *J Neurosurg* 2004;100(3, Suppl Spine):277-283.

Kuroki H, Rengachary SS, Goel VK, Holekamp SA, Pitkänen V, Ebraheim NA: Biomechanical comparison of two stabilization techniques of the atlantoaxial joints: Transarticular screw fixation versus screw and rod fixation. *Neurosurgery* 2005;56(1, Suppl):151-159.

Lehman RA Jr, Dmitriev AE, Helgeson MD, Sasso RC, Kuklo TR, Riew KD: Salvage of C2 pedicle and pars screws using the intralaminar technique: A biomechanical analysis. *Spine (Phila Pa 1976)* 2008;33(9):960-965.

Melcher RP, Puttlitz CM, Kleinstueck FS, Lotz JC, Harms J, Bradford DS: Biomechanical testing of posterior atlantoaxial fixation techniques. *Spine (Phila Pa 1976)* 2002;27(22):2435-2440.

Paramore CG, Dickman CA, Sonntag VK: The anatomical suitability of the C1-2 complex for transarticular screw fixation. *J Neurosurg* 1996;85(2):221-224.

Stulik J, Vyskocil T, Sebesta P, Kryl J: Atlantoaxial fixation using the polyaxial screw-rod system. *Eur Spine J* 2007;16(4):479-484.

Wang MY: Cervical crossing laminar screws: Early clinical results and complications. *Neurosurgery* 2007;61(5, Suppl 2):311-316.

Wright NM: Posterior C2 fixation using bilateral, crossing C2 laminar screws: Case series and technical note. *J Spinal Disord Tech* 2004;17(2):158-162.

Wright NM: Translaminar rigid screw fixation of the axis: Technical note. *J Neurosurg Spine* 2005;3(5):409-414.

Yoshida M, Neo M, Fujibayashi S, Nakamura T: Comparison of the anatomical risk for vertebral artery injury associated with the C2-pedicle screw and atlantoaxial transarticular screw. *Spine (Phila Pa 1976)* 2006;31(15):E513-E517.

Coding

CPT Codes		Corresponding ICD-9 Codes	
22840	Posterior non-segmental instrumentation (eg, Harrington rod technique, pedicle fixation across one interspace, atlantoaxial transarticular screw fixation, sublaminar wiring at C1, facet screw fixation) (List separately in addition to code for primary procedure)	724.6 721	722
22842	Posterior segmental instrumentation (eg, pedicle fixation, dual rods with multiple hooks and sublaminar wires); 3 to 6 vertebral segments (List separately in addition to code for primary procedure)	724.6 721	722
22843	Posterior segmental instrumentation (eg, pedicle fixation, dual rods with multiple hooks and sublaminar wires); 7 to 12 vertebral segments (List separately in addition to code for primary procedure)	722.52 737.30	722
22844	Posterior segmental instrumentation (eg, pedicle fixation, dual rods with multiple hooks and sublaminar wires); 13 or more vertebral segments (List separately in addition to code for primary procedure)	722.52 737.30	722
22851	Application of intervertebral biomechanical device(s) (eg, synthetic cage(s), threaded bone dowel(s), methylmethacrylate) to vertebral defect or interspace (List separately in addition to code for primary procedure)	722.52 737.30	724.6
63050	Laminoplasty, cervical, with decompression of the spinal cord, two or more vertebral segments;	723.0	721.1
63051	Laminoplasty, cervical, with decompression of the spinal cord, two or more vertebral segments; with reconstruction of the posterior bony elements (including the application of bridging bone graft and non-segmental fixation devices (eg, wire, suture, mini-plates), when performed)	723.0	721.1

Chapter 16
C1-C2 Transarticular Fixation

Jason C. Eck, DO, MS
Bradford L. Currier, MD

Indications

C1-C2 arthrodesis using transarticular screws is performed for cases of atlantoaxial instability from a variety of etiologies. These include traumatic injuries, such as odontoid fractures and disruption of the transverse ligament, as well as infection, tumor, rheumatoid arthritis, os odontoideum, and iatrogenic causes.

This technique was first described by Magerl and Seeman in 1987. Prior to that time, atlantoaxial instability typically was treated with a variety of wiring constructs. The major advantage of C1-C2 transarticular screw fixation is that it provides rigid fixation. This has led to increased fusion rates and has eliminated the need for postoperative halo immobilization in most cases. It also allows for atlantoaxial fusion in cases without an intact posterior arch of the atlas, which would be a contraindication for wiring techniques.

Contraindications

Although the C1-C2 transarticular screw technique provides solid fixation for cases of atlantoaxial instability, it is a technically demanding procedure with substantial risks to the neighboring neurovascular structures. There is a wide variation in the normal anatomic location of the vertebral artery with respect to the ideal path for the C1-C2 transarticular screw. The transverse foramen is located in the path of a transarticular screw (and referred to as a "high-riding foramen") on at least one side of the axis in 18% of patients.

The C2 isthmus is the narrowest portion of bone through which the transarticular screw must pass. A 3.5-mm screw typically is used for this procedure, and it is recommended that the C2 isthmus be at least 5 mm in both height and width for this technique. Approximately 10% of patients have a C2 isthmus less than 5 mm in either height or width.

The internal carotid artery (ICA) can be located within 1 mm of the ideal screw exit point on the anterior surface of the C1 lateral mass. The

ICA is at moderate risk of injury from a transarticular screw with bicortical purchase in C1 in 46% of cases and at high risk in 12% of cases on at least one side. If a preoperative CT scan with contrast reveals the ICA is within 2 mm of the anterior cortex of C1 and greater than 4 mm medial to the foramen transversarium, a bicortical screw would be contraindicated on that side. A unicortical screw may be used provided the surgical technique avoids penetrating the anterior aspect of C1 with the drill, tap, or screw.

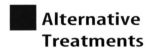

Alternative Treatments

Gallie and Brooks-Jenkins wiring techniques provide technically simple options for C1-C2 stabilization but do not provide rigid fixation and must be combined with postoperative halo immobilization. A C1 lateral mass screw can be secured to a C2 pars interarticularis screw or a C2 laminar screw with a rod. These techniques have a lower reported risk of injury to the vertebral artery, but cost is substantially increased by the additional screws and rods. Transarticular screws also can be inserted through an anterior retropharyngeal approach. This technique has the advantage of avoiding the morbid-

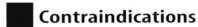

Dr. Eck or an immediate family member is a member of a speakers' bureau or has made paid presentations on behalf of Medtronic. Dr. Currier or an immediate family member serves as a board member, owner, officer, or committee member of the Mayo Clinic; has received royalties from DePuy and Stryker; serves as a paid consultant to or is an employee of DePuy; and has received research or institutional support from Synthes.

Table 1 Results Associated With C1-C2 Transarticular Screws

Authors (Year)	Number of Patients	Indications	Mean Patient Age in Years (Range)	Mean Follow-up (Range)	Fusion Rate	Complications
Grob et al (1991)	161	Varied	49.7 (15-88)	25 months (3-89)	99.4%	Malpositioned screw 15% Implant loosening 1.9% Implant failure 1.9% Vascular injury 0% Hypoglossal nerve injury 0.6% Deep infection 0.6%
Haid et al (2001)	75	Varied	44 (8-76)	29 months (12-66)	96%	Superficial infection 2.7% Transient suboccipital hypesthesia 5.3% Neural injury 0% Vascular injury 0% Implant failure 0%
Reilly et al (2003)	33	Varied	49.9 (21-93)	41 months (21-93)	93.9%	Infection 6% Persistent suboccipital hypesthesia 3%
Fountas et al (2004)	23	Varied	46.3 (19-81)	39.5 months (28-85)	82.6%	Malpositioned screw 8.7% Neural injury 0% Vascular injury 0% Infection 8.7%
Liang et al (2004)	23	Varied	50 (21-84)	38 months (6-53)	95.7%	Persistent suboccipital hypesthesia 8.7% Vertebral artery injury 4.3% Malpositioned screw 4.3%
ElSaghir et al (2005)	57	Rheumatoid arthritis	57 (30-78)	30 months (6-43)	98%	Malpositioned screws 3.5% Implant failure 1.8% Persistent suboccipital hypesthesia 1.8% Infection 3.5% Vascular injury 0% Neural injury 0%
Wang et al (2007)	57	Varied	34.6 (13-66)	47 months (24-76)	100%	Neural injury 0% Vascular injury 0% Malpositioned screws 3.5%

ity of the posterior approach, but it does not allow for concomitant wiring and has less bone surface for achieving fusion.

If only one transarticular screw can be safely inserted, it can be combined with a C1 lateral mass–C2 screw/rod construct on the other side, or a wiring technique, or both. If posterior wiring is combined with a single transarticular screw, the Brooks-Jenkins method is biomechanically superior to the Gallie wiring technique.

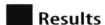

Results

In carefully selected patients, the C1-C2 transarticular screw technique provides a safe and effective method for treating atlantoaxial instability. Reported fusion rates range from 83% to 100% (**Table 1**). The most common serious complication is injury to the vertebral artery, reported in up to 5% of cases. Other complications include malpositioned screws or implant failure (3.5% to 15%), infection (0.6% to 10%), persistent greater occipital neu-

ralgia (0.6% to 10%), and injury to the hypoglossal nerve (0 to 1%).

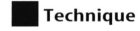

Technique

Setup/Exposure
Preoperative imaging should include a contrast-enhanced CT scan to evaluate the suitability of the C1-C2 transarticular screw technique. **Figure 1** shows the projected path of the transarticular screws. Based on the

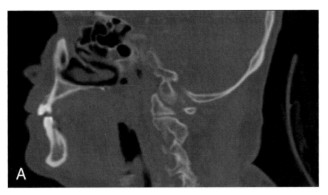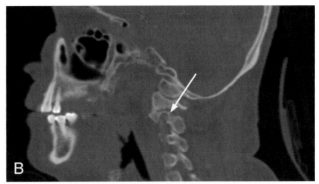

Figure 1 Sagittal CT scans of left (**A**) and right (**B**) sides of the C1-C2 articulation. The right side demonstrates a high-riding foramen transversarium (arrow), making it unsuitable for a C1-C2 transarticular screw.

high-riding foramen transversarium on the right side, the patient would be able to safely tolerate only a left-sided screw (**Figure 1**). The patient is placed in the prone position on a Jackson table (OSI, Union City, CA), with the head securely fixed in a pinion with a Mayfield attachment (Integra Life Sciences Corporation, Plainsboro, NJ) or in traction. The head of the table should be placed on the highest position with the feet on the lowest position, to maximize reverse Trendelenburg positioning to decrease bleeding and make the wound more accessible to the surgical team (**Figure 2**). If intraoperative neuromonitoring is planned, electrophysiology leads should be placed, and adequate baseline measurements should be obtained both before and after final positioning. Special care should be taken to ensure a neutral position of the head without any axial rotation. If the C1-C2 fusion is being extended to the occiput, a neutral occipitocervical angle also is important. This has been defined previously as a mean angle of 44° between a line intersecting the basion and the opisthion and a line parallel to the superior end plate of C3.

Proper positioning is critical to the success of this procedure. AP and lateral fluoroscopic images should be obtained after positioning to ensure adequate visualization as well as reduction of any preexisting defor-

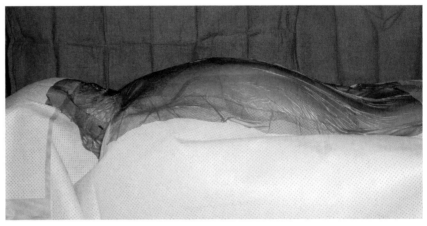

Figure 2 Photograph of patient positioning from the side. The patient should be placed to maximize reverse Trendelenburg positioning.

mity. Additionally, the lateral fluoroscopic view should be used to verify that the appropriate trajectory for the transarticular screw is feasible. The skin incision for the trocar is typically at about the T2 level. The head and neck must be positioned posteriorly enough to allow for the proper trajectory without being limited by the thoracic cavity.

Instruments/Equipment/Implants Required

- One fluoroscopy unit for lateral visualization (a second unit providing AP visualization is optional) or an image guidance system
- Jackson table with pinion head holder and Mayfield attachment or a traction system
- Intraoperative neuromonitoring
- Basic spine instrument set
- Trocar and cannula set
- 2.0-mm burr
- 3.5-mm cortical screws
- Cable system or wires if three-point fixation is desired (recommended)

Procedure

The back of the head and neck should be shaved to allow the occiput and the entire cervical and upper thoracic spine to be in the sterile field. A subcutaneous injection of epinephrine can assist with hemostasis. The large bifid spinous process of C2 is typically palpable. A midline skin incision is made over the C1-C2 level. The midline incision is developed down to the cervical fascia, which is incised in the midline. Self-retaining retractors are placed. The muscles are elevated subperiosteally out to approximately 1.5 cm from the midline, with care taken to protect the attachments of the semispinalis cervicis muscles on the spinous process of C2. If it is necessary to release the insertion of the semispinalis cervicis, consider removing it from the spinous process of C2 with a fleck of bone to enhance the subsequent repair.

The posterior C1 arch is exposed subperiosteally, exercising caution to avoid the vertebral artery on its upper surface and the large venous plexus surrounding the exiting posterior branch of the second spinal nerve. The medial border of the pars interarticularis of C2 is identified (**Figure 3**). The entrance point for the screws is located on the inferior aspect of the C2 inferior facet, several millimeters from the C2-C3 joint space. The distance between the two entrance points is estimated by measuring the distance on an axial image from the preoperative CT scan. This distance is marked on the spine using a caliper and then confirmed by noting the location relative to the medial border of the pars interarticularis of C2. The trajectory of the screw should cause it to pass immediately lateral to this landmark on the axis. Entrance holes for the transarticular screws are then made bilaterally using a 2-mm high-speed burr. Disruption of the C2-C3 facet capsules and interspinous ligament should be avoided.

The lateral fluoroscopic image is then used to identify the appropriate trajectory for the transarticular screws. A caliper can be used to measure the lateral offset for the starting point of the screw. The percutaneous starting point can then be determined by measuring the same distance from the midline because the trajectory of the transarticular screws generally is parallel to the midsagittal plane (**Figure 4**). Small stab incisions are then made bilaterally 1 to 2 cm from the midline at approximately the level of T2. The distance between the stab incisions typically is the same distance as that between the C2 entrance points as determined from the preoperative CT scan. The incisions should be made vertically to allow for adjustments in the entrance point. The sharp trocar is then passed carefully through the stab incision up to the

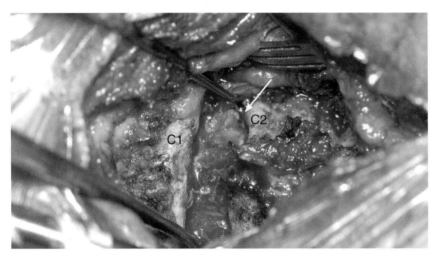

Figure 3 Dissection of the medial border of the pars interarticularis of C2 on the right side (arrow).

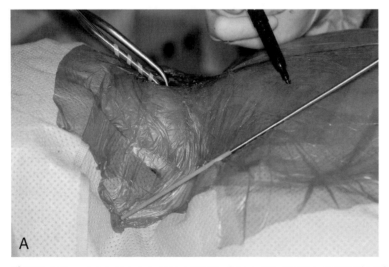
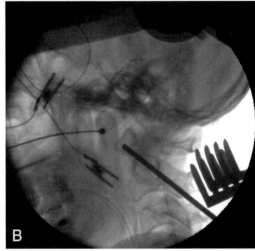

Figure 4 The percutaneous starting point (**A,** shown with marking pen) is identified based on the planned trajectory of the screw using a metal rod overlying the skin while visualizing on lateral fluoroscopy (**B**).

starting point for the screws in C2, where it is docked in the previously prepared hole (**Figure 5**). The trocar should not be passed under the subaxial laminae or through the atlantoaxial membrane as it is advanced to the C2 level. The tip of the trocar can be visualized through the cervical incision as it approaches C2.

The trajectory of the transarticular screw should be parallel to the midsagittal plane and angled cranially to aim for the anterior tubercle of C1 on the lateral image. The cannula is then placed over the trocar. The trocar is removed, and a 2.5-mm drill is passed through the cannula to the screw starting point (**Figure 6**). The trajectory of the drill bit can be extrapolated on the fluoroscopy monitor (**Figure 7**). The drill is advanced across the C1-C2 joint and into the C1 lateral mass under fluoroscopic guidance. It is essential to line up the drill before passing it into C2 because it is difficult to alter the trajectory once a pilot hole has been started. Ideally, C1 and C2 are aligned perfectly before the incision is made.

Occasionally, it is necessary to make intraoperative adjustments to alter the position of C1 relative to C2. This can be accomplished by placing a towel clip or clamp on the spinous process of C2 or the arch of C1 and applying a cranial, caudal, anterior, or posterior-directed force. This maneuver can help reduce C1 relative to C2 or change the trajectory of the transarticular screw path. The technique is fraught with problems, however, and should be used cautiously and only as a last resort. If the position of C1 or C2 must be altered during screw-hole preparation, the exact same position must be maintained until the screw has been seated or the screw will not follow the prepared path.

Once the drill bit has entered the atlas, the image intensifier or image guidance system is used to determine how far anteriorly to pass the drill. The anterior cortex of the C1 lateral mass is penetrated if bicortical C1 fixation is planned, or the drill can stop just short of the anterior cortex for unicortical C1 fixation. A measurement is taken, the hole is tapped, and a 3.5-mm screw is inserted through the

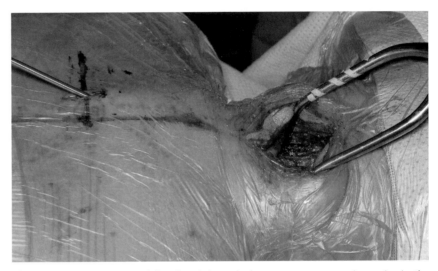

Figure 5 The trocar is carefully placed through the percutaneous starting point in the planned trajectory of the screw (as viewed from the patient's right side).

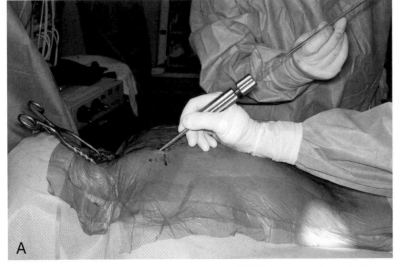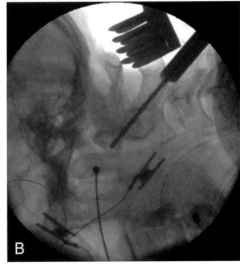

Figure 6 The trocar is removed, and a 2.5-mm drill bit is passed through the cannula to the screw starting point (**A**) and visualized on fluoroscopy (**B**).

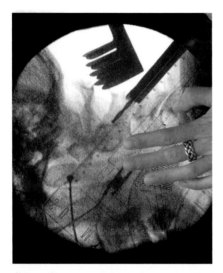

Figure 7 The drill bit is advanced through the trocar under fluoroscopic guidance. The trajectory of the drill bit is extrapolated on the fluoroscopy monitor.

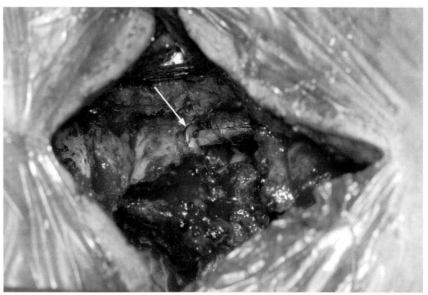

Figure 8 The screw head (arrow) can be directly visualized during the insertion.

cannula. The screw head should be visualized during final seating to prevent fracture of C2 (**Figure 8**). The image intensifier or image guidance system is used to verify proper placement of the screws.

The posterior elements of C1 and C2 are then decorticated, and bone graft is applied (**Figure 9**). This technique can be combined with a posterior wiring construct for additional stability as described in chapter 18. If the semispinalis cervicis was removed for visualization, it should be repaired to the remaining C2 spinous process at this time. Final AP and lateral images should be obtained to verify proper positioning of the instrumentation (**Figure 10**).

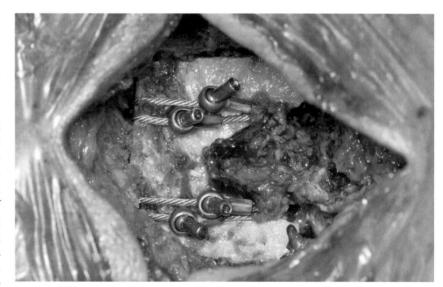

Figure 9 A posterior C1-C2 graft/cable construct is added for more stability.

Wound Closure

The wound is copiously irrigated, and hemostasis is achieved. The wound is closed in layers over a suction drain. The deep facial layer is closed using 1-0 polyglactin suture, the subcutaneous tissues are closed using 2-0 polyglactin, and the skin is closed with 3-0 nylon sutures or a subcuticular closure if the tissues are healthy and the patient is not immunocompromised.

A sterile dressing and a hard cervical collar are then applied.

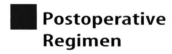

Postoperative Regimen

The patient begins mobilization on postoperative day 1. Deep venous thrombosis prophylaxis is achieved

using mechanical devices. Pain is managed with a patient-controlled analgesia device for the first night, and then patients are converted to oral analgesics. Patients typically remain in the hospital for approximately 3 days.

The patient remains in the hard cervical collar for 3 months postoperatively. At that time, plain radiographs are obtained to verify proper position of the screws and alignment of the spine. Flexion and extension radio-

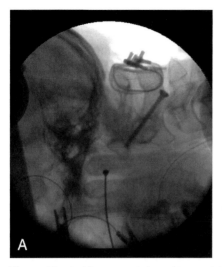 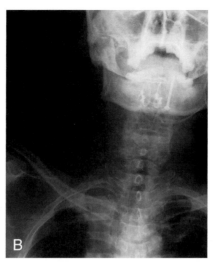

Figure 10 Final fluoroscopic lateral image (**A**) and plain AP radiograph (**B**) of the construct.

graphs verify solid fusion and lack of instability above or below the fusion. During the first 3 months, the patient is instructed to wear the collar at all times and avoid lifting greater than 10 lb. After the 3-month follow-up appointment, the patient is weaned out of the collar and begins isometric neck exercises.

Avoiding Pitfalls and Complications

Posterior C1-C2 transarticular screw fixation is a technically demanding procedure, but it can be performed safely and effectively. We recommend obtaining a preoperative contrast-enhanced CT scan in all cases. This will allow for identification of the vertebral and internal carotid arteries as well as the bone detail for planning the appropriate screw trajectory. If the vertebral artery is high-riding or the isthmus is less than 5 mm in either height or width, we would recommend another technique. If the ICA is located within 2 mm of the anterior cortex of C1 and > 4 mm medial to the foramen transversarium, we recommend placing a unicortical screw.

Although the midpoint of the anterior tubercle of C1 is the target on the lateral image to achieve the correct cephalic angulation of the screw hole, it is not a reliable landmark for the length of the screw hole because of anatomic variation. The front of the anterior tubercle is 5 to 10 mm anterior to the exit point of the drill bit in the lateral mass of C1. The slope of the anterior aspect of the C1 lateral mass is variable and should be examined on an axial CT image of C1 preoperatively. A landmark, such as the anterior aspect of the odontoid or posterior aspect of the anterior tubercle, can be chosen as a reference point when determining the appropriate length of the drill hole and screw on the intraoperative lateral image.

During the exposure, dissection of the semispinalis cervicis muscles off the spinous process of C2 should be avoided, and the C2-C3 facet capsules should be left intact to prevent postoperative risk of kyphosis and adjacent-level degeneration.

The surgery should not be started until adequate fluoroscopic images have been obtained. This includes identifying the anterior tubercle of C1, verifying proper alignment of C1-C2, and demonstrating that the desired screw trajectory is possible through the stab incision without interference from the thoracic cavity.

Transarticular screws and other screw/rod techniques have become useful adjuncts to C1-C2 fusions to allow patients to be mobilized without halo devices. However, if the anatomy is in doubt or the surgeon is not comfortable with the technique, a standard wiring technique, augmented with a postoperative halo immobilization device, is effective and considerably safer.

Bibliography

Currier BL, Maus TP, Eck JC, Larson DR, Yaszemski MJ: Relationship of the internal carotid artery to the anterior aspect of the C1 vertebra: Implications for C1-C2 transarticular and C1 lateral mass fixation. *Spine (Phila Pa 1976)* 2008;33(6): 635-639.

Cyr SJ, Currier BL, Eck JC, et al: Fixation strength of unicortical versus bicortical C1-C2 transarticular screws. *Spine J* 2008;8(4):661-665.

El Saghir H, Boehm H, Greiner-Perth R: Mini-open approach combined with percutaneous transarticular screw fixation for C1-C2 fusion. *Neurosurg Rev* 2005;28(1):59-63.

Fountas KN, Kapsalaki EZ, Karampelas I, et al: C1-C2 transarticular screw fixation for atlantoaxial instability. *South Med J* 2004;97(11):1042-1048.

Grob D, Jeanneret B, Aebi M, Markwalder TM: Atlanto-axial fusion with transarticular screw fixation. *J Bone Joint Surg Br* 1991;73(6):972-976.

Haid RW Jr, Subach BR, McLaughlin MR, Rodts GE Jr, Wahlig JB Jr: C1-C2 transarticular screw fixation for atlantoaxial instability: A 6-year experience. *Neurosurgery* 2001;49(1):65-70.

Liang ML, Huang MC, Cheng H, et al: Posterior transarticular screw fixation for chronic atlanto-axial instability. *J Clin Neurosci* 2004;11(4):368-372.

Magerl F, Seeman PS: Stable posterior fusion of the atlas and axis by transarticular screw fixation, in Kehr P, Werdner PA, eds: *Cervical Spine*. New York, NY, Springer-Verlag, 1987, pp 322-327.

Mandel IM, Kambach BJ, Petersilge CA, Johnstone B, Yoo JU: Morphologic considerations of C2 isthmus dimensions for the placement of transarticular screws. *Spine (Phila Pa 1976)* 2000;25(12):1542-1547.

McGuire RA Jr, Harkey HL: Modification of technique and results of atlantoaxial transfacet stabilization. *Orthopedics* 1995;18(10):1029-1032.

Papagelopoulos PJ, Currier BL, Hokari Y, et al: Biomechanical comparison of C1-C2 posterior arthrodesis techniques. *Spine (Phila Pa 1976)* 2007;32(13):E363-E370.

Paramore CG, Dickman CA, Sonntag VK: The anatomical suitability of the C1-2 complex for transarticular screw fixation. *J Neurosurg* 1996;85(2):221-224.

Reilly TM, Sasso RC, Hall PV: Atlantoaxial stabilization: Clinical comparison of posterior cervical wiring technique with transarticular screw fixation. *J Spinal Disord Tech* 2003;16(3):248-253.

Wang C, Yan M, Zhou H, Wang S, Dang G: Atlantoaxial transarticular screw fixation with morselized autograft and without additional internal fixation: Technical description and report of 57 cases. *Spine (Phila Pa 1976)* 2007;32(6): 643-646.

Coding

CPT Codes		Corresponding ICD-9 Codes	
Posterior Cervical Arthrodesis			
22800	Arthrodesis, posterior, for spinal deformity, with or without cast; up to 6 vertebral segments	737.0 737.3	737.1 737.30
22595	Arthrodesis, posterior technique, atlas-axis (C1-C2)	805.1	805.2
22600	Arthrodesis, posterior or posterolateral technique, single level; cervical below C2 segment	805.1	805.2
22840	Posterior non-segmental instrumentation (eg, Harrington rod technique, pedicle fixation across one interspace, atlantoaxial transarticular screw fixation, sublaminar wiring at C1, facet screw fixation) (List separately in addition to code for primary procedure)	722.52 737.30	724.6
22841	Internal spinal fixation by wiring of spinous processes (List separately in addition to code for primary procedure)	722.52 737.30	724.6
22842	Posterior segmental instrumentation (eg, pedicle fixation, dual rods with multiple hooks and sublaminar wires); 3 to 6 vertebral segments (List separately in addition to code for primary procedure)	722.52 737.30	724.6
22851	Application of intervertebral biomechanical device(s) (eg, synthetic cage(s), threaded bone dowel(s), methylmethacrylate) to vertebral defect or interspace (List separately in addition to code for primary procedure)	722.52 721.1	724.6
Components Referenced in Chapter			
20930	Allograft for spine surgery only; morselized (List separately in addition to code for primary procedure)	721.1 723	722 724.6
20931	Allograft for spine surgery only; structural (List separately in addition to code for primary procedure)	721.1 723.0	722 724.6
20936	Autograft for spine surgery only (includes harvesting the graft); local (eg, ribs, spinous process, or laminar fragments) obtained from same incision (List separately in addition to code for primary procedure)	724.6	722
20937	Autograft for spine surgery only (includes harvesting the graft); morselized (through separate skin or fascial incision) (List separately in addition to code for primary procedure)	724.6	722
20938	Autograft for spine surgery only (includes harvesting the graft); structural, bicortical or tricortical (through separate skin or fascial incision) (List separately in addition to code for primary procedure)	724.6 721.1	722

Chapter 17

Fixation to C1 and C2

Robert A. Hart, MD, MA
Geoffrey Kaung, MD, MS

Indications

Fixation to C1 and C2 is performed for several destabilizing conditions of the atlantoaxial cervical spine. A frequently used technique requires placement of lateral mass screws in C1, with rod fixation to pedicle, pars, or laminar screws in C2 (**Figure 1**). Common indications include type II odontoid fractures, atlantoaxial instability in patients with rheumatoid arthritis, and iatrogenic instability after anterior odontoid resection for the treatment of basilar invagination. Other causes of atlantoaxial instability, such as Down syndrome, also may be treated with this technique. In addition, displaced Jefferson fractures may be treated with open reduction and internal fixation via bilateral C1 lateral mass screws with transverse rod fixation or with concomitant C1-C2 arthrodesis in the event of a ruptured transverse ligament.

Contraindications

Conditions that preclude safe or effective lateral mass screw fixation to C1 include fractures of the C1 lateral masses and significant erosions that obscure bony landmarks, such as erosions that may occur in patients with severe rheumatoid arthritis. Other contraindications include active infection and poor medical condition with inability to tolerate surgery.

Alternative Treatments

C1-C2 fixation also may be performed via transarticular screw placement starting from C2. C1-C2 transarticular fixation most commonly is performed through a posterior approach, although anterior C1-C2 transarticular fixation also has been described. In approximately 20% of patients, transarticular C1-C2 screws cannot be placed safely because of the location of the vertebral artery. Also, this technique requires reduction of the atlantoaxial joint complex before placement of instrumentation.

Posterior wiring procedures, such as Gallie or Brooks techniques, also may be used to stabilize the atlantoaxial complex. These techniques require an intact posterior arch of C1. In addition, they are less biomechanically favorable than screw fixation in rotation and lateral bending; thus, they often require halo stabilization.

Results

Table 1 summarizes the results of several clinical studies that used variations in lateral mass screw placement within C1. Notching the undersurface of the posterior arch of C1 (**Figure 2**) allows a more superior screw placement and has been advocated as a means of avoiding the perineural venous plexus. This reduces blood loss, improves intraoperative visualization, and decreases the potential for postoperative irritation of the greater occipital nerve by the C1 screw. Another potential advantage is reduction of the superior angulation of the screw, thereby decreasing the chance of occipitocervical joint violation.

Dr. Hart or an immediate family member has received royalties from DePuy and SeaSpine; is a member of a speakers' bureau or has made paid presentations on behalf of AO North America, DePuy, Kyphon, and Medtronic; serves as a paid consultant to or is an employee of DePuy and Medtronic; and has received research or institutional support from Acumed, DePuy, and Medtronic. Dr. Kaung or an immediate family member has received research or institutional support from DePuy.

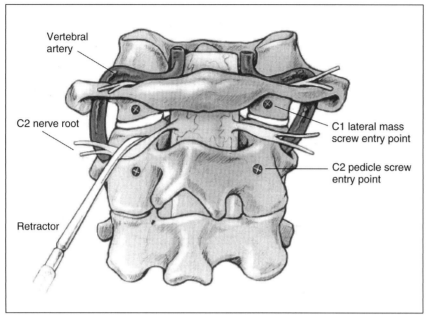

Figure 1 Illustration of the posterior upper cervical spine shows the entry points (marked "×") for the C1 lateral mass screws and C2 pedicle screws used in the polyaxial screw and rod fixation technique. The C1 starting point shown is inferior to the posterior arch of C1. A retractor is shown protecting the C2 nerve root. (Adapted with permission from Harms J, Melcher RP: Posterior C1-C2 fusion with polyaxial screw and rod fixation. *Spine (Phila Pa 1976)* 2001;26(22): 2467-2471.)

A more cranial starting point that allows the screw to be inserted directly through the posterior arch also has been described (**Figure 3**). This theoretically improves the pullout strength of the C1 screw by increasing the length of screw fixation within bone. Morphometric studies have shown, however, that this technique is limited by the size of the posterior arch and is not always feasible. In 709 atlas specimens measured bilaterally, Lee and associates found that only 46.2% had a posterior arch thickness greater than 4 mm, and only 13.7% were greater than 5 mm. Tan and associates found that only 4 of 50 C1 specimens (8%) had a posterior arch thickness less than 4 mm. They also reported that 10 C1 lateral mass screws were successfully placed in 5 patients using this technique. The greatest concern of posterior arch screw placement is the risk of vertebral artery injury within the superior groove, especially

Table 1 Results of Clinical Studies Using Variations in C1 Lateral Mass Screw Placement

Authors (Year)	Number of Patients	Mean Patient Age in Years (Range)	Mean Follow-up (Range)	C1 Screw Entry Point	C1 Screw Trajectory	Complications
Harms and Melcher (2001)	37	49 (2-90)	10 months (0-24)	Middle of junction of posterior arch and midpoint of posteroinferior lateral mass	Slight medialization, parallel to plane of posterior arch	1 deep infection
Goel et al (2002)	160	23 (1.5-79)	42 months (4-168)	Center of posterior lateral mass, 1-2 mm above articular surface	15° medial, 15° superior	18 (11%) C2 sensory loss 6 screws >4 mm anterior cortical protrusion 1 broken screw
Tan et al (2003)	5 patients 50 cadaveric specimens	36 (28-55)	11 months (6-18)	18-20 mm lateral to midline, 2 mm superior to inferior border of posterior arch	Perpendicular to coronal plane, 5° superior	None
Liu et al (2008)	24	63 (16-84)	NR	2-3 mm notch at inferior edge of posterior arch	Based on preoperative CT: 10° medialization, parallel to C1-2 joint space	1 dural tear 1 occipital neuralgia 1 symptomatic occipitocervical joint violation

NR = Not reported.

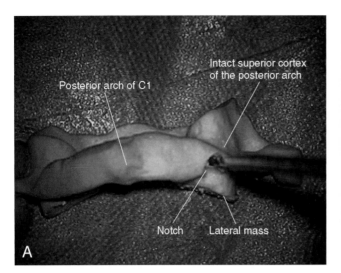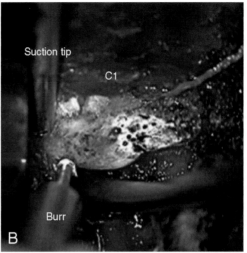

Figure 2 The C1 notching technique. **A,** Notching on the right side is demonstrated in a model. The undersurface of the arch is notched down to the level of the lateral mass without violating the superior cortex. Insertion of the screw into the lateral mass via this notch allows recession of the screw away from the C2 nerve root. By not violating the superior cortex, injury to the vertebral artery can be avoided. **B,** Intraoperative photograph demonstrates notching on the left side. A 2-mm high-speed matchstick burr is used to notch the inferior edge of the posterior arch of C1 to allow better screw placement. The suction tip shown here marks the approximate location of the vertebral artery. (Part A reproduced with permission from Lee MJ, Cassinelli E, Riew KD: The feasibility of inserting atlas lateral mass screws via the posterior arch. *Spine (Phila Pa 1976)* 2006;31(24):2798-2801. Part B adapted with permission from Liu G, Buchowski JM, Shen H, Yeom JS, Riew KD: The feasibility of microscope-assisted "free-hand" C1 lateral mass screw insertion without fluoroscopy. *Spine (Phila Pa 1976)* 2008;33(9):1042-1049.)

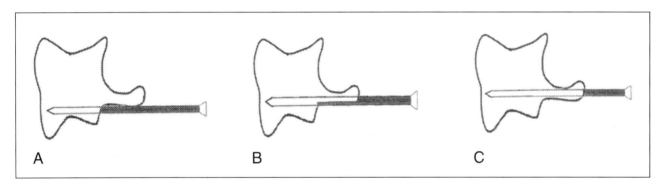

Figure 3 Illustration of C1 lateral mass screw placement. **A,** Lateral mass screw inserted inferior to the posterior arch. **B,** Lateral mass screw inserted partially through the posterior arch via a notching technique. **C,** Lateral mass screw inserted directly through the posterior arch. (Reproduced with permission from Lee MJ, Cassinelli E, Riew KD: The feasibility of inserting atlas lateral mass screws via the posterior arch. *Spine (Phila Pa 1976)* 2006;31(24):2798-2801.)

in the presence of a ponticulus posticus ("little bridge"), an anomalous ossification overlying the groove of the vertebral artery along the posterior arch of C1.

Several biomechanical studies also have been performed to assess the pullout strength of C1 lateral mass screws that were placed using various techniques. Hong and associates showed almost equivalent pullout strength between C1 lateral mass

screws (1718.16 N) and C2 pedicle screws (1631.94 N) in their study. Similarly, Hott and associates demonstrated a mean pullout strength of 667 N using bicortical C1 lateral mass fixation, which was comparable to the pullout strength of C2 pars screws (556 N). In 2007, Eck and associates reported a statistically significant ($P = 0.008$) increase in the pullout strength of C1 lateral mass screws placed with bicortical versus unicorti-

cal purchase. They questioned the necessity of using bicortical fixation routinely, given the greater pullout strength of unicortical C1 lateral mass screws when compared with that of subaxial lateral mass screws reported in other studies, as well as the increased risk of injury to structures anterior to the C1 lateral mass that can occur with bicortical screw placement. In 2009, Ma and associates compared the pullout strength of C1

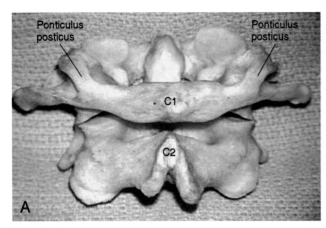 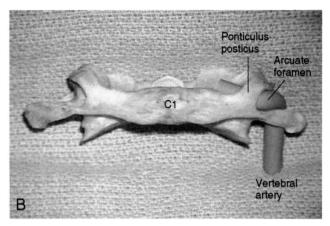

Figure 4 Anterior views of osseous C1 and C2 specimens demonstrate a ponticulus posticus bilaterally (**A**) and the vertebral artery coursing medially within the arcuate foramen and deep to the ponticulus posticus (**B**). (Adapted with permission from Young JP, Young PH, Ackermann MJ, Anderson PA, Riew KD: The ponticulus posticus: Implications for screw insertion into the first cervical lateral mass. *J Bone Joint Surg Am* 2005;87(11):2495-2498.)

screws placed in the lateral mass versus the pedicle (screws placed through the posterior arch) and with unicortical versus bicortical purchase. Unicortical lateral mass screws provided the weakest fixation (mean, 794.5 N) and bicortical pedicle screws the strongest (1757.0 N), whereas the pullout strengths of bicortical lateral mass screws and unicortical pedicle screws were equivalent (1243.8 N and 1192.5 N, respectively). The investigators also advocated placement of unicortical pedicle screws in C1 as an alternative to placement of bicortical C1 lateral mass screws.

■———————■

■ Technique

Setup/Exposure

Awake fiberoptic intubation is recommended in cases of cervical instability. We also recommend routine monitoring of somatosensory-evoked potentials and motor-evoked potentials, with baseline recordings obtained before and just after prone positioning of the patient.

The patient is positioned prone on a Jackson table with the abdomen free. The head is stabilized in radiolucent Mayfield tongs. The arms are tucked at the sides and secured with towel clips. Under lateral fluoroscopic guidance, the head is positioned in slight flexion, balancing optimal reduction of C1 to C2 against favorable surgical access to the region. The base of the skull is shaved, and the posterior cervical spine is prepared from above the external occipital protuberance down to the upper thoracic spine, depending on the amount of exposure desired. The posterior iliac crest also may be prepared if autograft harvest or bone marrow aspiration is desired.

Palpable landmarks through the skin include the external occipital protuberance and the spinous process of C2. The posterior ring of C1 itself is not palpable. A standard midline approach is performed. It is helpful to stay within the midline raphe to avoid excessive bleeding from the posterior musculature. The spinous process of C2 is easily recognized as the most prominent bifid spinous process in the upper cervical spine. Care should be taken to preserve the inferior semispinalis attachments to this structure. Exposure of the posterior ring of C1 should proceed with caution from the midline protuberance. The vertebral artery travels laterally along the supe-

rior edge of the posterior arch of C1 to the lateral mass, where it enters the foramen transversarium and extends inferiorly. Therefore, dissection along the superior ridge of C1 beyond 1.5 cm from the midline should be avoided. In up to 15% of patients, a ponticulus posticus overlies the groove for the vertebral artery, thereby creating an arcuate foramen (Figures 4 and 5). This anatomic variant should not be mistaken for a wide posterior arch, as using the ponticulus posticus as the starting point for screw placement increases the risk of injury to the vertebral artery.

Instruments/Equipment/Implants Required

The availability of bipolar electrocautery for hemostasis is required. Hemostatic agents, such as thrombin-soaked gel foam or commercially available hemostatic matrix products, are helpful if venous bleeding is encountered around the C2 nerve root.

Fixation within the lateral mass of C1 requires a standard 1- or 2-mm high-speed burr, a hand drill with adjustable stop, a tap, and 3.5- or 4.0-mm polyaxial screws. Because the entry point of the C1 screw often lies significantly more anterior than that

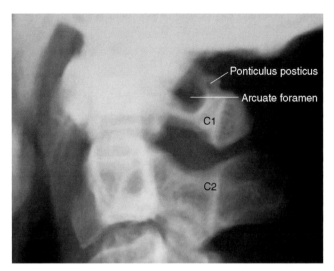

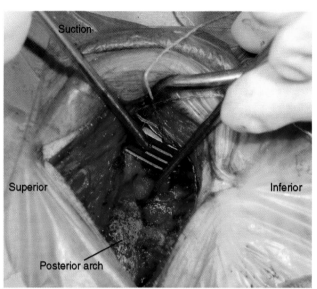

Figure 5 Lateral radiograph of the cervical spine demonstrates an arcuate foramen of C1 and a ponticulus posticus. (Adapted with permission from Young JP, Young PH, Ackermann MJ, Anderson PA, Riew KD: The ponticulus posticus: Implications for screw insertion into the first cervical lateral mass. *J Bone Joint Surg Am* 2005;87(11): 2495-2498.)

Figure 6 Intraoperative photograph shows palpation of the starting point of a C1 lateral mass screw just below the C1 arch on the right side of the patient. (Courtesy of C. D. Riew, MD.)

of the C2 screw, most manufacturers produce screws with an 8- to 10-mm unthreaded portion of the shank that remains superficial to the C1 lateral mass; this allows easier attachment to C2 screws via a rod-based system and is intended to prevent irritation of the C2 nerve root.

Procedure

The lateral mass of C1 is identified using blunt dissection with a No. 4 Penfield elevator just inferior to the C1 ring and approximately 2 to 3 cm lateral to the midline. The starting point of the screw lies in the middle of the C1 lateral mass in the coronal plane, which is palpable as the most prominent landmark on the rounded surface of the lateral mass (**Figure 6**). An alternative starting point in patients with a sufficiently thick posterior arch is on the inferior portion of the arch itself, just superior to the lateral mass. Before attempting to use this starting point, it is crucial that the surgeon verifies that the ring is of sufficient size to avoid injury to the vertebral artery.

A 1- or 2-mm burr is used to score the starting point. The trajectory for screw placement is slightly medialized (5° to 10°) and parallel to the posterior arch in the sagittal plane (**Figure 3**). In some cases, access to the starting point on the lateral mass can be improved by notching the inferior border of the C1 ring with a burr or a 2-mm Kerrison rongeur; this facilitates screw placement along an ideal trajectory.

A No. 2 Penfield elevator is placed at the medial border of the lateral mass to protect the spinal cord, and a similar instrument (a No. 4 or No. 3 Penfield elevator) is placed laterally to protect the vertebral artery. These retractors also pull the C2 nerve root inferiorly, so it is out of danger. A hand drill is then used to insert a drill bit approximately 1 cm, and the trajectory is confirmed using AP and lateral fluoroscopic visualization. Although some authors advocate bicortical placement, we place unicortical screws because this avoids risk to anterior structures such as the internal carotid artery and the hypoglossal nerve (**Figure 7**). A depth gauge is used to probe the tract and to measure

its length. The hole is tapped at its entry point, and an appropriate length 3.5-mm polyaxial screw is then placed.

If fusion of the C1-C2 facet joints is required, decortication and placement of a bone graft may be performed by dissecting superiorly along the C2 isthmus to reach the joint. Alternatively, a corticocancellous bone graft can be compressed against the C1 and C2 laminae using a cable or wire tightened transversely between the pair of rods connecting the C1 and C2 screws (**Figure 8**).

Wound Closure

The wound is closed in layers. The fascial layer should be approximated with heavy No. 0 absorbable sutures in interrupted figure-of-8 fashion to obtain a watertight closure. A subfascial suction drain is placed, and it is typically removed on the first postoperative day. No. 2-0 absorbable sutures and staples are used to close subcutaneous tissue and skin.

——■

Postoperative Regimen

Patients are placed in either a rigid or a soft cervical collar for comfort and to prevent extremes of motion. Upright AP and lateral cervical radiographs are obtained during hospitalization. The patient is encouraged to mobilize as soon as possible. Discharge from the hospital occurs when pain is well controlled and the patient can mobilize easily. Patients with spinal cord injuries or severe preoperative myelopathy should be considered for admission to an intensive care unit for postoperative observation and airway management.

Avoiding Pitfalls and Complications

The greatest dangers in C1 fixation are injuries to the vertebral artery and the spinal cord. As discussed previously, dissection along the posterior arch of C1 should avoid the superior ridge beyond 1.5 cm from the midline.

A ponticulus posticus may be mistaken for a broad posterior arch; screw placement in this situation can lead to vertebral artery injury. The presence of an arcuate foramen, through which the vertebral artery runs, can be identified by careful examination of preoperative lateral radiographs or reconstructed sagittal CT images. The thickness of the arch that is inferior to the vertebral artery groove should be measured preoperatively on a sagittal CT reconstruction, independent of the presence of an arcuate foramen. A

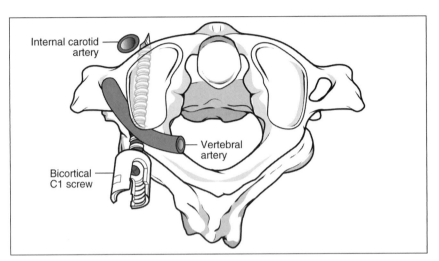

Figure 7 Axial diagram shows the risk of injury to the internal carotid artery with bicortical C1 screw placement. Also shown is the course of the vertebral artery along the superior edge of the posterior arch of C1.

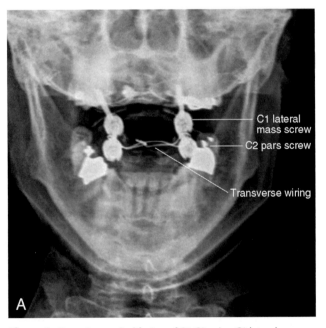 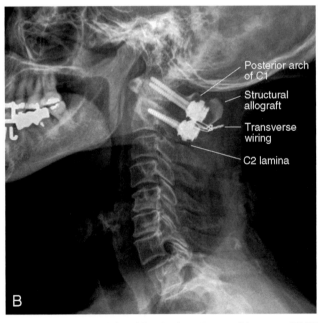

Figure 8 Posterior cervical fusion of C1-C2 using C1 lateral mass screws and C2 pars screws with rod fixation in a 69-year-old woman. AP (**A**) and lateral (**B**) radiographs are shown. Structural allograft and bone morphogenetic protein-2 were placed between the posterior arch of C1 and the lamina of C2, and the graft was compressed with transverse wiring between the rods.

dense perineural venous plexus is present between the lateral masses of C1 and C2. Hemostasis can be maintained with a combination of bipolar electrocautery and hemostatic agents if needed. This plexus may be avoided altogether by using a starting point on the inferior portion of the C1 ring; however, as already described, this starting point should be used only when the ring is sufficiently thick to avoid injury to the vertebral artery.

Gentle inferior retraction of the C2 nerve root should prevent injury, although routine transection also has been described. This produces postoperative occipital numbness and, in our experience, is generally not necessary. Using a screw with a smooth proximal shank may reduce the potential for postoperative irritation of the nerve root.

Injuries to structures anterior to the C1 vertebra, including the internal carotid artery and the hypoglossal nerve, are possible with an anterior cortical breach. This can be prevented by avoiding bicortical screw placement.

Bibliography

Currier BL, Maus TP, Eck JC, Larson DR, Yaszemski MJ: Relationship of the internal carotid artery to the anterior aspect of the C1 vertebra: Implications for C1-C2 transarticular and C1 lateral mass fixation. *Spine (Phila Pa 1976)* 2008;33(6): 635-639.

Currier BL, Todd LT, Maus TP, Fisher DR, Yaszemski MJ: Anatomic relationship of the internal carotid artery to the C1 vertebra: A case report of cervical reconstruction for chordoma and pilot study to assess the risk of screw fixation of the atlas. *Spine (Phila Pa 1976)* 2003;28(22):E461-E467.

Eck JC, Walker MP, Currier BL, Chen Q, Yaszemski MJ, An KN: Biomechanical comparison of unicortical versus bicortical C1 lateral mass screw fixation. *J Spinal Disord Tech* 2007;20(7):505-508.

Goel A, Desai KI, Muzumdar DP: Atlantoaxial fixation using plate and screw method: A report of 160 treated patients. *Neurosurgery* 2002;51(6):1351-1357.

Goel A, Laheri V: Plate and screw fixation for atlanto-axial subluxation. *Acta Neurochir (Wien)* 1994;129(1-2):47-53.

Harms J, Melcher RP: Posterior C1-C2 fusion with polyaxial screw and rod fixation. *Spine (Phila Pa 1976)* 2001;26(22): 2467-2471.

Hong X, Dong Y, Yunbing C, Qingshui Y, Shizheng Z, Jingfa L: Posterior screw placement on the lateral mass of atlas: An anatomic study. *Spine (Phila Pa 1976)* 2004;29(5):500-503.

Hott JS, Lynch JJ, Chamberlain RH, Sonntag VK, Crawford NR: Biomechanical comparison of C1-2 posterior fixation techniques. *J Neurosurg Spine* 2005;2(2):175-181.

Lee MJ, Cassinelli E, Riew KD: The feasibility of inserting atlas lateral mass screws via the posterior arch. *Spine (Phila Pa 1976)* 2006;31(24):2798-2801.

Liu G, Buchowski JM, Shen H, Yeom JS, Riew KD: The feasibility of microscope-assisted "free-hand" C1 lateral mass screw insertion without fluoroscopy. *Spine (Phila Pa 1976)* 2008;33(9):1042-1049.

Ma XY, Yin QS, Wu ZH, et al: C1 pedicle screws versus C1 lateral mass screws: Comparisons of pullout strengths and biomechanical stabilities. *Spine (Phila Pa 1976)* 2009;34(4):371-377.

Melcher RP, Puttlitz CM, Kleinstueck FS, Lotz JC, Harms J, Bradford DS: Biomechanical testing of posterior atlantoaxial fixation techniques. *Spine (Phila Pa 1976)* 2002;27(22):2435-2440.

Tan M, Wang H, Wang Y, et al: Morphometric evaluation of screw fixation in atlas via posterior arch and lateral mass. *Spine (Phila Pa 1976)* 2003;28(9):888-895.

Yeom JS, Buchowski JM, Park KW, Chang BS, Lee CK, Riew KD: Undetected vertebral artery groove and foramen violations during C1 lateral mass and C2 pedicle screw placement. *Spine (Phila Pa 1976)* 2008;33(25):E942-E949.

Young JP, Young PH, Ackermann MJ, Anderson PA, Riew KD: The ponticulus posticus: Implications for screw insertion into the first cervical lateral mass. *J Bone Joint Surg Am* 2005;87(11):2495-2498.

Coding

CPT Codes		Corresponding ICD-9 Codes	
22595	Arthrodesis, posterior technique, atlas-axis (C1-C2)	170.2 714.30 714.32	714.0 714.31 733.82
22840	Posterior non-segmental instrumentation (eg, Harrington rod technique, pedicle fixation across one interspace, atlantoaxial transarticular screw fixation, sublaminar wiring at C1, facet screw fixation) (List separately in addition to code for primary procedure)	170.2 342.9 343	342.1 342.90 343.0
22841	Internal spinal fixation by wiring of spinous processes (List separately in addition to code for primary procedure)	170.2 342.9 343	342.1 342.90 343.0
20936	Autograft for spine surgery only (includes harvesting the graft); local (eg, ribs, spinous process, or laminar fragments) obtained from same incision (List separately in addition to code for primary procedure)	170.2 733.13	724.6 737.30

CPT copyright © 2010 by the American Medical Association. All rights reserved.

Chapter 18

Posterior Cervical Wiring Technique

Sanford E. Emery, MD, MBA

Indications

For decades, cervical wiring was the sole method of internal fixation in the posterior cervical spine. Since the 1990s, wiring has been used primarily as an adjunct to more rigid fixation methods, including screws, rods, and occipital plates. The two main functions of wiring are to augment modern stabilization techniques and hold in place corticocancellous bone grafts used for arthrodesis. Posterior wiring may be indicated for the subaxial spine, C1-C2, and occipitocervical procedures.

Contraindications

Posterior cervical wiring has very few contraindications. In the subaxial spine, the absence of spinous processes (such as in postlaminectomy patients) will preclude the common interspinous wiring method. In these patients, a facet wiring technique can be performed; however, this technique is rarely, if ever, used today and is mentioned only for historical purposes. Osteoporotic posterior elements make it more difficult to successfully use wiring techniques, but this is not a

contraindication. Indeed, any sublaminar wiring technique (typically under the C1 ring and/or under the C2 lamina) requires adequate room in the spinal canal to avoid neurologic injury. This most often is an issue with a fixed C1 on C2 subluxation in a rheumatoid patient, where the space available for the cord at the C1 level can be severely compromised.

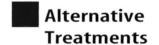
Alternative Treatments

More rigid methods of internal fixation have largely replaced wiring as a stand-alone method for posterior cervical fusion procedures. Lateral mass screws with rods are used today in the subaxial (below C2) spine (**Figure 1**). C1-C2 fusions typically are performed with transarticular screws (**Figure 2**), polyaxial lateral mass/pedicle screws (**Figure 3**), or C2 intralaminar screw fixation (**Figure 4**). Wiring is still often used with C1-C2 constructs to stabilize bone blocks, ensuring graft contact to the C1 ring and posterior element of C2. Occipital plates with screw/rod distal fixation have become the procedure of choice for occipitocervical fusions (**Figure 5**). Occipital

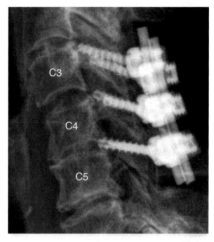

Figure 1 Lateral radiograph demonstrates lateral mass screws for posterior cervical fixation.

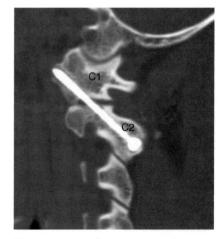

Figure 2 Sagittal CT image with C1-C2 transarticular screw fixation.

Dr. Emery or an immediate family member has received research or institutional support from DePuy and Medtronic Sofamor Danek.

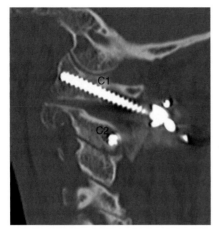

Figure 3 Sagittal CT image shows C1 lateral mass fixation with a polyaxial screw for C1-C2 fixation.

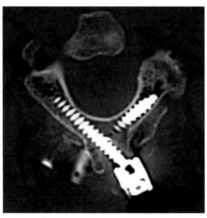

Figure 4 Cross-sectional CT image demonstrates intralaminar screw fixation of C2.

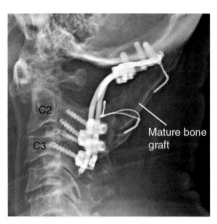

Figure 5 Lateral plain radiograph demonstrates occipitocervical fusion with skull plating, rod-screw construct, and wiring of a bone graft at 1-year follow-up. Note the graft incorporation to the skull and C2.

Table 1 Published Studies on Results of Posterior Cervical Wiring

Author(s) (Year)	Number of Patients	Procedure or Approach	Mean Patient Age in Years (Range)	Mean Follow-up (Range)	Fusion/Success Rate	Results
McAfee et al (1991)	37	Occipitocervical fusion with wiring plus bone graft	54 (24-78)	2 years, 10 months (range NR) Only 5 patients with follow-up <2 years	85% fusion rate	72% improved neurologically Better results with preoperative reduction of basilar invagination
Taggard et al (2004)	27	Posterior C1-C2 fusion; transarticular screws versus wiring plus halo	54 (21-82)	31 months (12-92)	Transarticular screws: fusion rate = 93% Wiring: fusion rate = 38%	No neurologic or vascular complications Clinical outcomes not assessed
Nockels et al (2007)	69	Occipitocervical fusion with rigid instrumentation	51 (11-90)	37 months (6-66)	97% fusion rate	In 87% of patients, myelopathy improved
Epstein (2008)	35	Subaxial posterior cervical fusion with wiring, bone graft	65 (range NR); SD = 10.4	Minimum 1 year (SF-36 and radiographs)	100% fusion rate	29 good to excellent 6 fair to poor

NR = not reported, SF-36 = Short Form 36.

wiring techniques can still be used to attach corticocancellous struts for arthrodesis if desired.

Currently, posterior cervical fixation techniques employing screw/rod/plate constructs are not approved by the US Food and Drug Administration in this setting and represent an "off-label" use.

Results

As reported in the literature, fusion in the subaxial spine has a high success rate using wire plus corticocancellous blocks or simple wiring and pure cancellous bone chips. Arthrodesis of C1-C2 and occipitocervical procedures using wire techniques alone are more challenging, with acceptable results suggested in the literature,

but they are considered inferior to more rigid means of internal fixation (**Table 1**).

Techniques
Setup/Exposure
The intraoperative setup and exposure for wiring techniques is the same

as for other methods of posterior cervical fusion. Typically, the patient is placed in a rigid head-holder device, with careful positioning (usually avoiding hyperextension) so as not to compromise the spinal canal. A midline incision with elevation of the paraspinal muscles off the posterior elements is followed by placement of deep retractors.

Instruments/Equipment/Implants Required

Typically, 20-gauge stainless steel wire is used for subaxial, C1-C2, and occipitocervical wiring procedures. Commonly, 22-gauge wires are used to wire in subaxial corticocancellous bone grafts in the Bohlman triple-wire technique. Many surgeons today prefer braided cable constructs instead of wire. Either can be successful, but cables have memory and at times can protrude into the dorsal aspect of the spinal canal if any loosening occurs over time.

Procedure

For the triple-wire technique used in the subaxial spine (**Figure 6**), a small hole is made near the base of the spinous process of the involved levels. Typically, this hole is started with a burr and completed with a towel clamp. The 20-gauge wire is passed through the spinous process, looped over the top (or bottom) of the spinous process and through the hole a second time, and then pulled tight. The loop helps distribute the stress on the bone to improve fixation and minimize the risk of cutout. The wire is then passed through the adjacent spinous process (and more, depending on the length of the fusion) in a similar looped fashion. The wire can then be tightened by twisting the ends and trimming the excess. The 22-gauge wires can be used to wire down corticocancellous rectangular blocks onto the lamina if desired, or bone chips can simply be packed over roughened laminar surfaces.

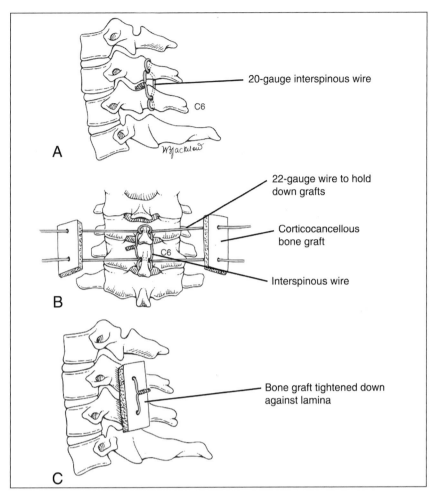

Figure 6 Illustration of the triple-wire technique for the subaxial spine. **A,** A 20-gauge interspinous wire is placed at the base of the spinous processes. **B,** Rectangular corticocancellous bone grafts are captured using 22-gauge wire on each spinous process. **C,** The grafts are tightened down on top of the lamina. (Adapted with permission from Heller JG, Klekamp JW, Blechner MG: Posterior cervical instrumentation, in Emery SE, Boden SD, eds: *Surgery of the Cervical Spine*. Philadelphia, PA, WB Saunders, 2003, p 64.)

For C1-C2 wiring, the modified Gallie technique requires passage of a wire under C1, feeding the ends through the looped tip, and cinching it down onto the C1 ring. Care must be taken not to push the stiff wire down into the spinal canal when performing this technique. A second wire is then used in the base of the C2 spinous process. These wires are fed through corticocancellous blocks and tightened (**Figures 7 and 8**). Alternatively, a Brooks wiring technique requires passing C1 and C2 sublaminar wires on the right and left sides and then twisting these down to press trapezoidal-shaped corticocancellous bone grafts onto the lamina of C1 and C2 (**Figure 9**).

Wire fixation to the skull typically involves making a unicortical tunnel near the inion, which is approximately 3 cm below the external occipital protuberance. This wire is looped onto itself and fed through the tunnel again. The outer cortex of the skull is strong bone, and excellent fixation usually can be achieved. The ends of this wire are passed through corticocancellous blocks, and wiring is

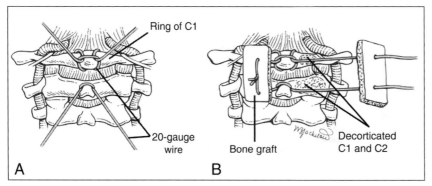

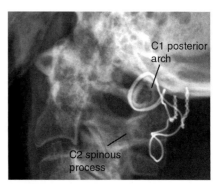

Figure 7 Drawings of the modified Gallie wiring technique for C1-C2 fixation and arthrodesis. **A**, A 20-gauge wire is passed under the C1 lamina, looped through itself, and pulled tight. A second 20-gauge wire is placed at the base of the C2 spinous process. **B**, Rectangular corticocancellous bone grafts are tightened down onto the lamina. (Reproduced with permission from Heller JG, Klekamp JW, Blechner MG: Posterior cervical instrumentation, in Emery SE, Boden SD, eds: *Surgery of the Cervical Spine*. Philadelphia, PA, WB Saunders, 2003, p 60.)

Figure 8 Lateral radiograph of the cervical spine shows healed C1-C2 fusion using modified Gallie wiring plus bone grafting.

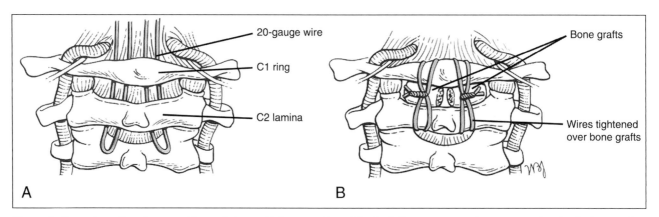

Figure 9 Illustration of Brooks-type wiring technique with bone grafting of C1-C2. **A,** Two 20-gauge wires are passed under the lamina of C1 and C2. **B,** Corticocancellous bone graft blocks are placed between the C1 and C2 lamina, and the wires are tightened. Grafts need to be trapezoidal in shape so they do not slip anteriorly into the spinal canal. (Adapted with permission from Heller JG, Klekamp JW, Blechner MG: Posterior cervical instrumentation, in Emery SE, Boden SD, eds: *Surgery of the Cervical Spine*. Philadelphia, PA, WB Saunders, 2003, p 61.)

performed under C1 and/or through C2 as described above. Twisting the wires down onto the block grafts provides stability for the grafts and the construct itself (**Figures 10 and 11**). If care is taken with the placement of some occipital plate designs on the skull, the surgeon can still wire corticocancellous iliac grafts and achieve good bony contact (**Figure 12**).

Wound Closure

Wound closure is performed in layers, with loose approximation of the paraspinal muscle and tight closure of

the fascial layer, followed by subcutaneous and skin closure, typically over a drain. Care should be taken to reattach the musculature to the C2 spinous process (if it is not involved in the fusion) to minimize the risk of postoperative kyphosis.

Postoperative Regimen

Because wiring techniques alone are stable but not rigid, the typical choice

of postoperative immobilization is between a hard collar and a halo vest. If wiring is used as an adjunct to more rigid internal fixation, the choice usually is between a soft collar and hard collar. Between 6 and 8 weeks of immobilization typically are recommended for successful arthrodesis; however, the exact procedure, bone quality, and overall stability of the construct may allow shorter or dictate longer periods of postoperative protection.

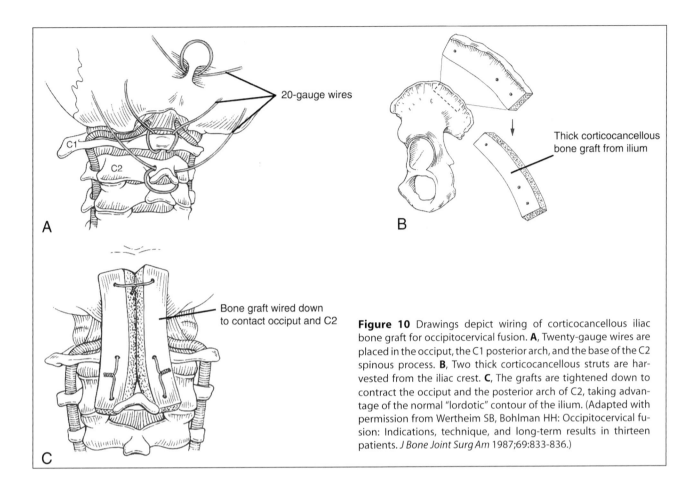

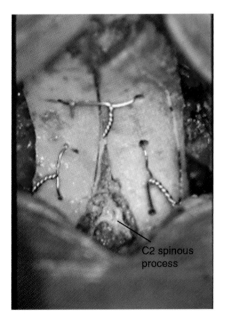

Figure 10 Drawings depict wiring of corticocancellous iliac bone graft for occipitocervical fusion. **A,** Twenty-gauge wires are placed in the occiput, the C1 posterior arch, and the base of the C2 spinous process. **B,** Two thick corticocancellous struts are harvested from the iliac crest. **C,** The grafts are tightened down to contract the occiput and the posterior arch of C2, taking advantage of the normal "lordotic" contour of the ilium. (Adapted with permission from Wertheim SB, Bohlman HH: Occipitocervical fusion: Indications, technique, and long-term results in thirteen patients. *J Bone Joint Surg Am* 1987;69:833-836.)

Figure 11 Intraoperative photograph of wired iliac struts for an occipitocervical fusion procedure. The patient's head is at the top.

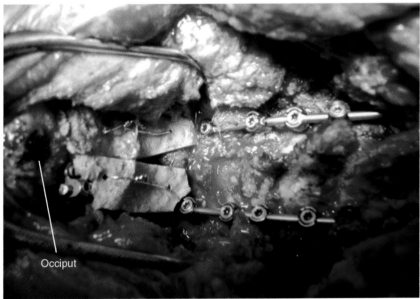

Figure 12 Intraoperative photograph of wired occipitocervical bone graft with underlying plate-rod-screw internal fixation. The patient's head is to the left.

Avoiding Pitfalls and Complications

As with most spine procedures, attention to detail is mandatory. Passing sublaminar wires under C1 is facilitated by first making a tract using tiny angled curets. A small blunt nerve hook helps retrieve the leading loop of the wire. If spinous process drill holes are too close to the lamina, the wire can be inadvertently passed into the spinal canal. Overtightening of wire constructs can cut through the corticocancellous bone blocks or through the posterior elements. In the subaxial spine, overtightening of midline wires theoretically can cause narrowing of the foramen and radiculopathy; initial placement of lateral mass screw-rod constructs followed by wire tightening can avoid this potential problem. With posteriorly displaced odontoid fractures, the Brooks-type wiring technique should be used with care because wire tightening will tend to pull back the ring of C1 and increase fracture displacement. A thorough understanding of spinal anatomy is needed for these procedures, including knowledge of cranial venous sinus locations when performing occipital fixation.

————————■

Bibliography

An HS, Gordin R, Renner K: Anatomic considerations for plate-screw fixation of the cervical spine. *Spine (Phila Pa 1976)* 1991;16(10, Suppl):S548-S551.

Brooks AL, Jenkins EB: Atlanto-axial arthrodesis by the wedge compression method. *J Bone Joint Surg Am* 1978;60(3): 279-284.

Clark CR, Goetz DD, Menezes AH: Arthrodesis of the cervical spine in rheumatoid arthritis. *J Bone Joint Surg Am* 1989; 71(3):381-392.

Deutsch H, Haid RW Jr, Rodts GE Jr, Mummaneni PV: Occipitocervical fixation: Long-term results. *Spine (Phila Pa 1976)* 2005;30(5):530-535.

Epstein NE: An argument for traditional posterior cervical fusion techniques: Evidence from 35 cases. *Surg Neurol* 2008; 70(1):45-52.

Gallie WE: Fractures and dislocations of the cervical spine. *Am J Surg* 1939;46:495-499.

Ghanayem AJ, Leventhal M, Bohlman HH: Osteoarthrosis of the atlanto-axial joints: Long-term follow-up after treatment with arthrodesis. *J Bone Joint Surg Am* 1996;78(9):1300-1307.

Grob D, Jeanneret B, Aebi M, Markwalder TM: Atlanto-axial fusion with transarticular screw fixation. *J Bone Joint Surg Br* 1991;73(6):972-976.

Harms J, Melcher RP: Posterior C1-C2 fusion with polyaxial screw and rod fixation. *Spine (Phila Pa 1976)* 2001;26(22): 2467-2471.

Heller JG, Carlson GD, Abitbol JJ, Garfin SR: Anatomic comparison of the Roy-Camille and Magerl techniques for screw placement in the lower cervical spine. *Spine (Phila Pa 1976)* 1991;16(10, Suppl):S552-S557.

McAfee PC, Cassidy JR, Davis RF, North RB, Ducker TB: Fusion of the occiput to the upper cervical spine: A review of 37 cases. *Spine (Phila Pa 1976)* 1991;16(10, Suppl):S490-S494.

Nockels RP, Shaffrey CI, Kanter AS, Azeem S, York JE: Occipitocervical fusion with rigid internal fixation: Long-term follow-up data in 69 patients. *J Neurosurg Spine* 2007;7(2):117-123.

Taggard DA, Kraut MA, Clark CR, Traynelis VC: Case-control study comparing the efficacy of surgical techniques for C1-C2 arthrodesis. *J Spinal Disord Tech* 2004;17(3):189-194.

Wertheim SB, Bohlman HH: Occipitocervical fusion: Indications, technique, and long-term results in thirteen patients. *J Bone Joint Surg Am* 1987;69(6):833-836.

Wright NM: Posterior C2 fixation using bilateral, crossing C2 laminar screws: Case series and technical note. *J Spinal Disord Tech* 2004;17(2):158-162.

Coding

CPT Codes		Corresponding ICD-9 Codes	
Posterior Cervical Wiring			
22326	Open treatment and/or reduction of vertebral fracture(s) and/or dislocation(s), posterior approach, one fractured vertebra or dislocated segment; cervical	805.1 805.3 805.5	805.2 805.4 805.6
22328	Open treatment and/or reduction of vertebral fracture(s) and/or dislocation(s), posterior approach, one fractured vertebra or dislocated segment; each additional fractured vertebra or dislocated segment (List separately in addition to code for primary procedure)	805.1 805.3 805.5	805.2 805.4 805.6
22800	Arthrodesis, posterior, for spinal deformity, with or without cast; up to 6 vertebral segments	737.0 737.3	737.1 737.30
22595	Arthrodesis, posterior technique, atlas-axis (C1-C2)	805.1	805.2
22600	Arthrodesis, posterior or posterolateral technique, single level; cervical below C2 segment	805.1	805.2
22840	Posterior non-segmental instrumentation (eg, Harrington rod technique, pedicle fixation across one interspace, atlantoaxial transarticular screw fixation, sublaminar wiring at C1, facet screw fixation) (List separately in addition to code for primary procedure)	722.52 737.30	724.6
22841	Internal spinal fixation by wiring of spinous processes (List separately in addition to code for primary procedure)	722.52 737.30	724.6
22842	Posterior segmental instrumentation (eg, pedicle fixation, dual rods with multiple hooks and sublaminar wires); 3 to 6 vertebral segments (List separately in addition to code for primary procedure)	722.52 737.30	724.6
22851	Application of intervertebral biomechanical device(s) (eg, synthetic cage(s), threaded bone dowel(s), methylmethacrylate) to vertebral defect or interspace (List separately in addition to code for primary procedure)	722.52 721.1	724.6
Components Referenced in Chapter			
20930	Allograft for spine surgery only; morselized (List separately in addition to code for primary procedure)	721.1 723	722 724.6
20931	Allograft for spine surgery only; structural (List separately in addition to code for primary procedure)	721.1 723.0	722 724.6
20936	Autograft for spine surgery only (includes harvesting the graft); local (eg, ribs, spinous process, or laminar fragments) obtained from same incision (List separately in addition to code for primary procedure)	724.6	722
20937	Autograft for spine surgery only (includes harvesting the graft); morselized (through separate skin or fascial incision) (List separately in addition to code for primary procedure)	724.6	722
20938	Autograft for spine surgery only (includes harvesting the graft); structural, bicortical or tricortical (through separate skin or fascial incision) (List separately in addition to code for primary procedure)	724.6 721.1	722

Chapter 19
Occipitocervical Fusion

Lee H. Riley III, MD
A.F. Pull ter Gunne, MD
A. Jay Khanna, MD, MBA

◼ Indications

Occipitocervical fusion is indicated for occipitocervical instability and deformity due to trauma to the occipitocervical joint, inflammatory conditions of the upper cervical spine, infection, tumors, congenital anomalies, and iatrogenic instability from cervical decompression. Pain from malunion of fractures of the atlas or occipital condyles also is an indication for fusion. Patients with atlantoaxial instability who are not candidates for atlantoaxial fixation because of anatomic considerations or in whom previous attempts at C1-C2 fusion have failed also may require occipitocervical fusion.

◼ Contraindications

Occipitocervical fusion in the growing child may lead to secondary spinal deformities from continued growth. This potential late sequela needs to be balanced against the long-term benefits of fusion.

◼ Alternative Treatments

Halo bracing may be an alternative to fusion for some occipitocervical and upper cervical fractures, but it is associated with a high incidence of nonunion and malunion requiring surgery. Halo brace treatment is not indicated in occipitocervical dislocations that are highly unstable and require urgent, rigid internal fixation and fusion.

◼ Results

Studies have shown that 50% of cervical flexion/extension occurs at the occiput-C1 joint, and 50% of axial rotation occurs at the C1-C2 joint. Therefore, fusion to the occiput results in a loss of 50% of both normal flexion/extension and axial rotation of the cervical spine. Rigid fixation provides immediate stability and lessens the need for supplemental external fixation. It also improves the fusion rate and reduces rehabilitation time. Neurologic deterioration is halted as a result of both direct decompression and rigid stabilization. Reported fusion rates with rigid occipitocervical fixation vary from 80% to 100% (Table 1).

◼ Techniques

Setup
Prone positioning for occipitocervical fusion in a patient with cervical instability or critical stenosis requires careful planning and teamwork that begins before induction of anesthesia and intubation. A patient with an unstable spine, compromised neurologic function, or severe cord compression may require awake intubation and po-

Dr. Riley or an immediate family member serves as a board member, owner, officer, or committee member of LifeNet Health; serves as a paid consultant to or is an employee of AO, DePuy, and Spinal Kinetics; has received research or institutional support from AO, Blackstone Medical, DePuy, Mitek, the Orthopaedic Scientific Research Foundation, Smith & Nephew, Stryker, Synthes, Wright Medical Technology, and Zimmer; and owns stock or stock options in Spinal Kinetics. Dr. Khanna or an immediate family member is a member of a speakers' bureau or has made paid presentations on behalf of AOSpine North America; serves as a paid consultant to or is an employee of Blackstone Medical, Kyphon, and Zimmer; and has received research or institutional support from Blackstone Medical and Zimmer. Neither Dr. Pull ter Gunne nor any immediate family member has received anything of value from or owns stock in a commercial company or institution related directly or indirectly to the subject of this chapter.

Table 1 Posterior Occipitocervical Fusion Results

Authors (Year)	Number of Patients	Approach	Mean Age in Years (Range)
Hamblen (1967)	13	Posterior	39 (5-63)
Heywood et al (1988)	14	Posterior	NR
Elia et al (1992)	27	Posterior	48 (13-77)
Lieberman and Webb (1998)	13	Posterior	58 (18-78)
Heidecke et al (1998)	14	Posterior	41 (19-68)
Zimmermann et al (2002)	20	Posterior	61 (40-76)
Matsunaga et al (2003)	19	Posterior	NR
Kalra et al (2007)	54	Anterior/posterior	31 (3-65)
Fenoy et al (2008)	234	Posterior: 183 Anterior/posterior: 51	36 (2.5-86)

NR = not reported.

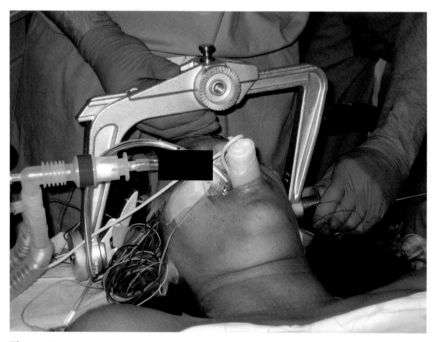

Figure 1 Photograph shows placement of a Mayfield frame to secure the head and allow precise positioning of the occipitocervical spine.

sitioning to minimize the risk of neurologic injury. Secure control of the head and neck is required during positioning in the prone position.

Mayfield tongs are placed with the patient supine. The single pin is positioned above the ear, in line with the bony external auditory canal. The double pins are placed at the same level on the opposite side. The anterior aspect of the frame should be located over the forehead with 1 to 2 inches of space between the frame and the forehead so that the forehead does not rest on the frame. The frame is then tightened to the required pressure using the tightening knob (**Figure 1**).

During the turning process, the head and neck should be maintained in the neutral position at all times. The patient is carefully turned prone on either chest rolls or a Wilson frame. We prefer the Wilson frame because it

Table 1 *(continued)*

Mean Follow-up (Range)	Fusion Rate	Results
4 years, 10 months (4 months–15 years, 2 months)	100%	Presenting symptoms: 8 relieved, 4 decreased, 1 deteriorated Neurologic function: 4/8 relieved, 3/8 decreased, 1/8 deteriorated
NR	86%	Presenting symptoms: 12/14 decreased Neurologic function: 7/8 improved
NR	89%	Neurologic function: 9/11 improved, 2/11 no change
24 months minimum in 12/13 patients	92%	Neurologic function: 12 improved, 1 no change
20 months (12-48)	100%	Neurologic function: 3/4 relieved, 1/4 improved
6.3 months (0.5-23)	95%	Presenting symptoms: decreased pain in all 20 Neurologic function: 3/5 decreased, 2/5 no improvement
116 months (36-216)	95%	Neurologic function: 13 improved, 5 no change, 1 deteriorated
18 months (2-84)	80%	Neurologic function: 24 improved, 18 stabilized, 4 deteriorated, 2 died, 6 lost to follow-up
20.2 months (1- 120)	97%	Presenting symptoms: 215 improved, 16 no improvement, 3 unknown

provides good decompression of the abdomen and chest, is adjustable, and readily maintains its position. A Jackson table can also be used for prone positioning.

The head and neck are then placed in a functional position that allows the patient to look down to see the feet when using stairs and up to see shelves above the head. Rotation should be neutral, and forward thrust of the head and neck should be avoided. Axial rotation and head tilt are assessed by ensuring that the ears and the shoulders are parallel. Neutral axial rotation is confirmed by making sure the nose and chin are in line with the sternal notch. Flexion/extension and forward thrust are assessed by looking at the patient from the side and looking at the overall alignment of the head and neck with the shoulders, trunk, hips, and knees.

The forehead, eyes, and axilla should be free of pressure. The elbows are padded to prevent injury to the ulnar nerve. The arms are tucked at the side in the neutral position. Mild traction is applied to the shoulders, and the shoulders are taped to the side. The knees are flexed using a wedge and padded with pillows and foam. The table is placed in a 30° reverse Trendelenburg position to minimize venous bleeding (**Figure 2**). Finally, a lateral radiograph is obtained as a final confirmation of position.

Instruments/Equipment/ Implants Required

Many cervical fixation systems currently are available, several of which are specially adapted for use in occipitocervical spine fusions. Lateral mass screw fixation systems, with special screws for placement into C1 and C2, are readily available. Occipital plates for direct fixation to the occiput allow the use of larger, more cortical screws, primarily in the midline, where the oc-

ciput is the thickest and perhaps allows for the strongest fixation. Transition plates that transform the rods at the opposite end also are available; these plates facilitate connection of the occipital area to the cervical spine. Wiring techniques also are commonly used, either to supplement occipitocervical fixation or as the primary fixation.

Exposure

The inion and the spinous processes of C2, C7, and T1 are the most prominent palpable landmarks in the midline of the posterior cervical spine and can be used to plan the incision (**Figure 3**). Bupivacaine with epinephrine is infiltrated into the skin and subcutaneous tissues in the midline, along the length of the planned incision. The skin incision is then made in the midline from 1 cm superior to the inion inferiorly to the inferior extent of the fusion. The incision is carried

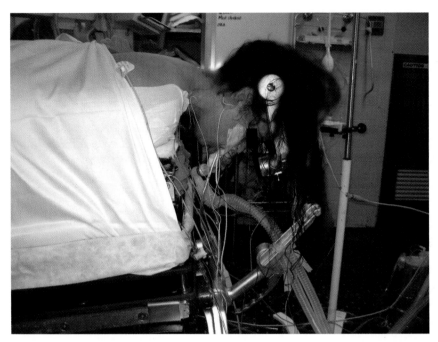

Figure 2 Photograph of a patient in a 30° reverse Trendelenburg position with the head and neck in a functional position.

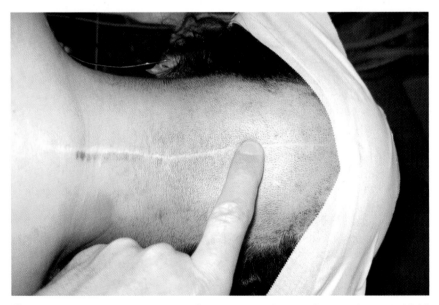

Figure 3 Photograph shows palpation of the inion to confirm its inclusion in the surgical field.

omy of this region. The course of the vertebral artery is highly variable and needs to be studied on the preoperative CT and MRI scans. The large gap between the laminae of C2, C1, and the occiput can be inadvertently entered with a Cobb or Bovie electrosurgical generator (Bovie Medical, Clearwater, FL). A large venous plexus surrounds the medial aspect of the C1-C2 facet joint capsule and C2 isthmus. Careful subperiosteal dissection and irrigating bipolar forceps are used to minimize bleeding from this region. The vertebral artery course at the level of the C1 lamina needs to be known. Dissection generally should not extend more than 1.5 cm lateral to the midline in adults (1 cm in children).

Dissection of the occiput should extend to the occiput and laterally to the lateral extent of the caudal exposure. Self-retaining cerebellar retractors, both articulating and nonarticulating, can be used to maintain exposure.

Procedure

INSTRUMENTATION TECHNIQUE
A variety of occipital cervical fixation techniques can be used. Specific techniques may be contraindicated in some patients because of anatomic variations. Variations in the location and size of the vertebral foramen of C1 and C2 can prevent placement of C1 screws (**Figure 4**), transarticular C1-C2 screws, and C2 pedicle screws. The thickness of the lamina of C2 may not allow translaminar screw placement. A sagittal reconstruction CT scan of the occiput and cervical spine should be obtained to provide a thorough understanding of the anatomy of the occiput and upper cervical spine and ensure that the safest and most effective fixation technique is used.

C2 Pedicle Screw Insertion
The starting point for the C2 pedicle screw is in the upper inner quadrant of the lateral mass of C2. The medial border and superior and inferior margins

down to the spinous processes with electrocautery. A subperiosteal dissection is then made using electrocautery and a large Cobb elevator. Caution must be exercised to avoid entering the canal with the dissection because the laminae may not overlap below C2 and do not overlap above it. Dissection is begun at the C2-C3 level and carried inferiorly to the inferior extent of the exposure and laterally to the lateral aspect of the lateral masses.

Exposure of the occipitocervical and atlantoaxial region is more difficult and carries a greater risk of complications because of the unique anat-

178 © 2011 American Academy of Orthopaedic Surgeons

eral fluoroscopic imaging of the lower cervical spine (**Figure 6**). The cranial end of the bandage must be applied on the acromion to obtain sufficient pulling force.

A skin incision longer than that required for a standard spinous process wiring is made. The cranial adjacent lamina of the uppermost fixed vertebra should be exposed entirely, taking care to protect the cranial facet joint capsule. The paravertebral muscles are dissected laterally to expose the lateral margins of the articular masses completely for exact determination of the screw insertion point.

Instruments/Equipment/ Implants Required

Screws having 3.5-, 4.0-, and 4.5-mm diameters, suitable for the pedicle size of each vertebra, are recommended. The length of the screw typically is 20 or 22 mm for C3 through C7. A screw length greater than or equal to 24 mm is required to penetrate the anterior cortex of the vertebral body and increase the screw stability of C2. A constrained type of locking mechanism connecting the screws and plates/rods is essential for this procedure to obtain a rigid stabilizing effect and deformity correction capability.

Procedure

SCREW PLACEMENT

Manual Screw Insertion

The points of screw penetration of the lateral mass for the C3 through C7 pedicles are slightly lateral to the center of the articular mass and close to the inferior margin of the inferior articular process of the cranially adjacent vertebra. The shape and size of the lateral mass are variable in each vertebra and in each individual patient, however. Therefore, the surgeon must review CT scans carefully before screw insertion.

The cranial margin of the lamina of C2 is the landmark for the point of screw penetration for C2. To confirm

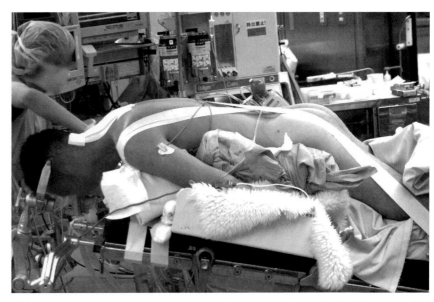

Figure 6 Clinical photograph demonstrates patient positioning. The shoulders are pulled caudally by a heavy bandage for intraoperative lateral fluoroscopic imaging of the lower cervical spine.

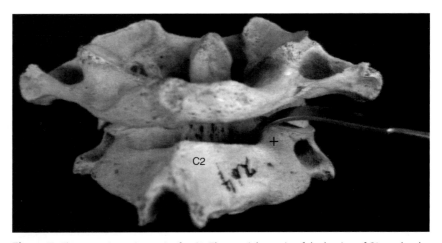

Figure 7 The screw insertion point for C2. The cranial margin of the lamina of C2 can be the landmark for the point of screw penetration for C2 (cross). To confirm the screw insertion points in C2, a small spatula can be inserted into the spinal canal along the cranial margin of the C2 lamina to the medial surface of the pedicle of C2.

the screw insertion points in C2, a small spatula can be inserted into the spinal canal along the cranial margin of the C2 lamina to the medial surface of the pedicle of C2 (**Figure 7**). The angle of the C2 pedicle axis to the sagittal plane is 15° to 25° in the transverse plane.

The lateral margin of the articular mass of the cervical spine has a notch approximately at the level of the

pedicle. The pedicles are located slightly below the lateral vertebral notch at C2, at the notch at C3 through C6, and at or slightly above the notch at C7 (**Figure 8**). The points of screw penetration for the C3 through C7 pedicles are slightly lateral to the center of the articular mass and close to the inferior margin of the inferior articular process of the cranially adjacent vertebra. Craniocaudal

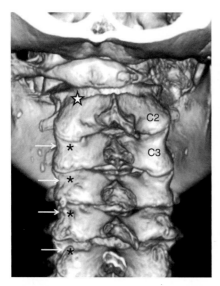

Figure 8 Three-dimensional CT reconstruction shows screw insertion points for C2 (white star) and for C3 through C7 (asterisks). The lateral margin of the articular mass of the cervical spine has a notch (white arrows). The pedicles are located slightly below the lateral vertebral notch at C2, at the notch at C3 through C6, and at or slightly above the notch at C7. Screw insertion points (asterisks) are 2 to 4 mm medial to the notch.

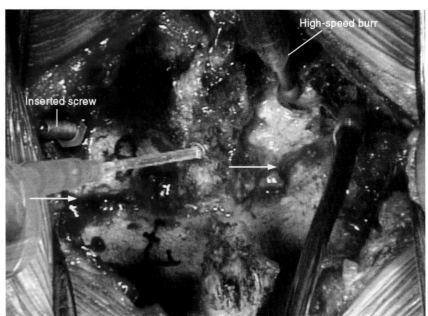

Figure 9 Intraoperative photograph shows the creation of a funnel-shaped screw insertion hole using a high-speed burr. White arrows indicate the facet joints.

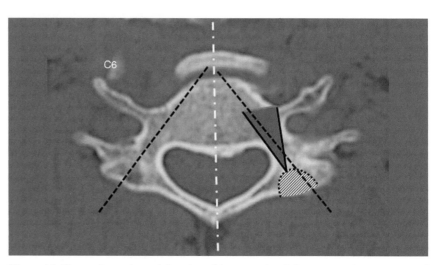

Figure 10 The starting point and direction of the cervical pedicle screw are shown on an axial CT scan. The dashed and dotted white line indicates the midline. The two dashed black lines indicate the anatomic axis of the pedicle. The semicircular shaded area denotes the excised outer portion of the articular mass. Through funnel-shaped resecting of the articular mass toward the entrance of the pedicle cavity using a high-speed burr, the starting point of the screw approaches the entrance of the pedicle cavity. As a consequence, the surgeon obtains more freedom in the screw insertion angle. The triangular area between the two black lines indicates the possible screw insertion direction.

orientation of the screw insertion point can be confirmed by a lateral image intensifier. We usually create a funnel-shaped hole at the screw insertion point using a high-speed burr (**Figure 9**). The sagittal plane angle for the insertion of the screw changes, depending on the spinal level. It increases from the C2 level to the C5 level. Pedicle screw insertion requiring a large angle in the sagittal plane can be difficult. Because of the short length of the cervical pedicle axis, however, the screw can be inserted at a smaller angle than the angle of anatomic axis. We usually insert screws with an angle of 25° to 45° to the sagittal plane for the pedicle from C3 to C7. By making the funnel-shaped hole bigger and deeper with a curet or high-speed burr, the surgeon can see the medial cortex of the posterior portion of the pedicle and the pedicle cavity directly in most cases. This funnel-shaped resection of the outer portion of the articular mass toward the entrance of the pedicle cavity allows more freedom and potential angulation for the positioning of the screw (**Figure 10**). After creating the insertion hole, a small pedicle probe, tap, and screws are inserted into the pedicle with the help of a lateral image intensifier to confirm the direction and insertion depth. We recommend

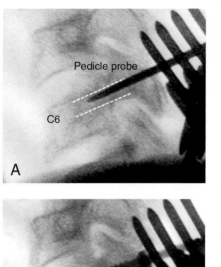

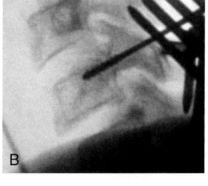

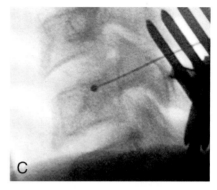

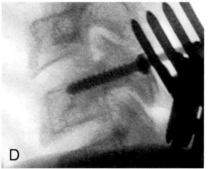

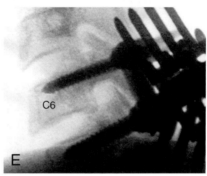

Figure 11 Lateral intraoperative fluoroscopic images demonstrate regulation of pedicle probe insertion using lateral C-arm fluoroscopy. **A,** The dashed white lines indicate the cranial and caudal margins of the pedicle. The pedicle probe, tap, and screws must be advanced between the two lines. **B,** Tapping of the pedicle. **C,** Sounding of the pedicle. We recommend using a pedicle sounder to confirm the proper creation of the screw insertion path after probing and tapping. **D,** Screw insertion. **E,** Longitudinal screw connection with a plate.

confirming the proper creation of the screw insertion path after probing and tapping using a pedicle sounder (**Figure 11,** *A* through *D*).

The intended angle of screw insertion in the sagittal plane is parallel to the upper end plate for pedicles C5 through C7 and is in a slightly cephalad direction in C2 through C4, according to the angulation in the sagittal plane. The C2 screw usually is perpendicular to the anterior surface of the vertebral body.

Computer-Assisted Screw Insertion

The technology of computer navigation continues to develop in the field of spine surgery. Current computer-assisted image guidance systems navigate only a screw guide tube at the insertion point of the bone surface, however, and do not guide the actual tip of the pedicle probe, tap, or screw within the pedicle. Therefore, such systems do not enhance safety or accuracy when placing pedicle screws. We have developed a new computer-assisted guidance system for cervical pedicle

screws. This system facilitates obtaining real-time, three-dimensional instrument/screw tip information at each step (probing, tapping, and screw insertion into the vertebra) and is useful in improving the safety and accuracy of pedicle screw placement in the cervical spine. Further modifications and developments in the technology will increase its safety and refine surgical techniques.

LONGITUDINAL CONNECTION USING A PLATE/ROD

Prior to plate or rod application, a dorsal decompression by laminaplasty or laminectomy is recommended for a patient with a narrow spinal canal to avoid possible neurologic deterioration created when the vertebral alignment is changed after longitudinal connection of the screws. The lateral masses and laminae must be decorticated, and bone chips obtained from the spinous processes and laminae must be placed. In the final stage of instrumentation, inserted screws are connected with a plate or a rod (**Figure 11,** *E*). Simple plate fixation is pre-

ferred for one- or two-segment fixation (**Figure 12**). The alignment of the screw head in the coronal plane may be off in multilevel fixation. Therefore, a rod with a screw rather than a plate is recommended for multilevel fixation over three segments (**Figure 13**). Plates and rods are contoured in the sagittal plane with the expected correction of kyphotic deformity. Correction of the kyphosis is performed by tightening the nuts or by rotating the rods using rod holders. As a consequence, the posterior part of the cervical spine can be shortened. Therefore, surgeons must be careful to avoid excessive shortening of the posterior part of the spine because of the potential for the development of a nerve root lesion by foraminal stenosis.

Wound Closure

One or two deep drains are placed on the lamina or on the exposed nerve tissue. Layered subcutaneous suturing and ordinary skin closure are performed.

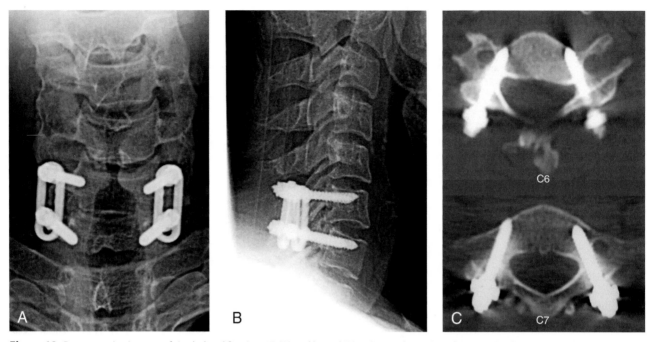

Figure 12 Postoperative images of single-level fixation. AP (**A**) and lateral (**B**) radiographs and axial CT scan (**C**) demonstrate the proper screw insertion points and directions.

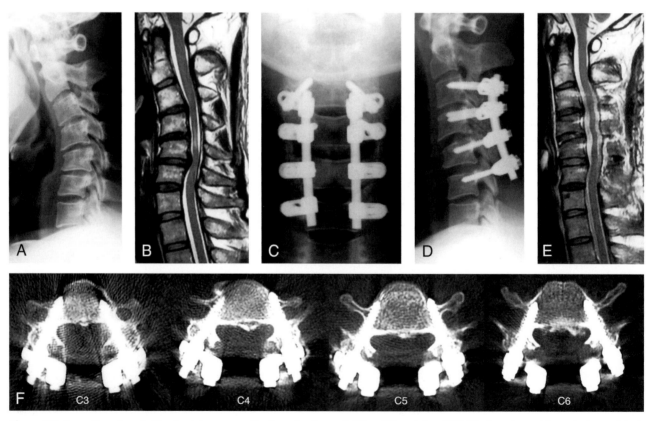

Figure 13 Correction of cervical kyphosis in preoperative lateral radiograph (**A**) and T1-weighted MRI (**B**) of a patient with cervical spondylosis with kyphosis who developed cervical myelopathy. Correction of the kyphosis and spinal cord compression by laminectomy were undertaken. AP (**C**) and lateral (**D**) radiographs demonstrate proper screw insertion and correction of the kyphosis. **E,** Postoperative T1-weighted MRI shows sufficient spinal cord decompression. **F,** Postoperative CT images show proper pedicle screw placement in each vertebra.

Postoperative Regimen

Postoperative immobilization varies according to the number of spinal segments fixed, the patient's general condition, the stability of the inserted screws, the extent of osteoporosis, and other factors. Generally, patients who required fixation of one to three motion segments wear a short, soft neck collar postoperatively for 2 to 3 weeks. A Philadelphia collar is applied for 2 to 3 months in patients with severe osteoporosis and in those who underwent fixation of four or more motion segments. More rigid postoperative external supports, including halo-vest immobilization, typically are not used. All patients are permitted to ambulate or sit up in bed the day after surgery unless contraindicated by their general condition. Patients who had jobs with low physical demands preoperatively can return to their original jobs 3 to 6 weeks after surgery, before bony union is complete. Patients whose preoperative work entailed a heavy physical demand can return to their jobs 2 to 3 months after surgery.

Avoiding Pitfalls and Complications

Pedicle screw fixation is a useful procedure for reconstruction of the cervical spine in patients with various kinds of disorders. Surgeons must keep in mind, however, that cervical pedicle screw placement is limited by anatomic variation of the pedicle and the vertebral artery. Possible complications directly attributable to pedicle screw fixation in the cervical spine include nerve root injury from a cranially or caudally dislodged screw, vertebral artery injury or obstruction from a laterally perforated screw, and dural injury or spinal cord injury from a screw that strays out medially. Nerve root complication by iatrogenic foraminal stenosis, not directly related to screw insertion, is another possible neural complication caused by correction of a kyphotic or translational deformity.

Complications associated with cervical pedicle screw fixation cannot be completely eliminated; they can be minimized, however, by sufficient preoperative imaging studies of the pedicles, thorough knowledge of local anatomy, and strict control of screw placement during surgery.

Bibliography

Abumi K, Itoh H, Taneichi H, Kaneda K: Transpedicular screw fixation for traumatic lesions of the middle and lower cervical spine: Description of the techniques and preliminary report. *J Spinal Disord* 1994;7(1):19-28.

Abumi K, Kaneda K, Shono Y, Fujiya M: One-stage posterior decompression and reconstruction of the cervical spine by using pedicle screw fixation systems. *J Neurosurg* 1999;90(1, Suppl):19-26.

Abumi K, Shono Y, Ito M, Taneichi H, Kotani Y, Kaneda K: Complications of pedicle screw fixation in reconstructive surgery of the cervical spine. *Spine (Phila Pa 1976)* 2000;25(8):962-969.

Abumi K, Shono Y, Kotani Y, Kaneda K: Indirect posterior reduction and fusion of the traumatic herniated disc by using a cervical pedicle screw system. *J Neurosurg* 2000;92(1, Suppl):30-37.

Abumi K, Shono Y, Taneichi H, Ito M, Kaneda K: Correction of cervical kyphosis using pedicle screw fixation systems. *Spine (Phila Pa 1976)* 1999;24(22):2389-2396.

Abumi K, Takada T, Shono Y, Kaneda K, Fujiya M: Posterior occipitocervical reconstruction using cervical pedicle screws and plate-rod systems. *Spine (Phila Pa 1976)* 1999;24(14):1425-1434.

Bozbuga M, Ozturk A, Ari Z, Sahinoglu K, Bayraktar B, Cecen A: Morphometric evaluation of subaxial cervical vertebrae for surgical application of transpedicular screw fixation. *Spine (Phila Pa 1976)* 2004;29(17):1876-1880.

Heller JG, Silcox DH III, Sutterlin CE III: Complications of posterior cervical plating. *Spine (Phila Pa 1976)* 1995;20(22):2442-2448.

Hojo Y, Ito M, Abumi K, et al: A late neurological complication following posterior correction surgery of severe cervical kyphosis. *Eur Spine J* 2010 Oct. 9 [Epub ahead of print].

Johnston TL, Karaikovic EE, Lautenschlager EP, Marcu D: Cervical pedicle screws vs. lateral mass screws: Uniplanar fatigue analysis and residual pullout strengths. *Spine J* 2006;6(6):667-672.

Karaikovic EE, Daubs MD, Madsen RW, Gaines RW Jr: Morphologic characteristics of human cervical pedicles. *Spine (Phila Pa 1976)* 1997;22(5):493-500.

Karaikovic EE, Kunakornsawat S, Daubs MD, Madsen TW, Gaines RW Jr: Surgical anatomy of the cervical pedicles: Landmarks for posterior cervical pedicle entrance localization. *J Spinal Disord* 2000;13(1):63-72.

Kast E, Mohr K, Richter HP, Börm W: Complications of transpedicular screw fixation in the cervical spine. *Eur Spine J* 2006;15(3):327-334.

Kotani Y, Abumi K, Ito M, Minami A: Improved accuracy of computer-assisted cervical pedicle screw insertion. *J Neurosurg* 2003;99(3, Suppl):257-263.

Reinholt M, Magerl F, Rieger M, Blauth M: Cervical pedicle screw placement: Feasibility and accuracy of two insertion techniques based on morphometric data. *Eur Spine J* 2007;16(1):46-56.

Yoshimoto H, Sato S, Hyakumachi T, Yanagibashi Y, Masuda T: Spinal reconstruction using a cervical pedicle screw system. *Clin Orthop Relat Res* 2005;431:111-119.

Yukawa Y, Kato F, Yoshihara H, Yanase M, Ito K: Cervical pedicle screw fixation in 100 cases of unstable cervical injuries: Pedicle axis views obtained using fluoroscopy. *J Neurosurg Spine* 2006;5(6):488-493.

Coding

CPT Codes		Corresponding ICD-9 Codes	
20930	Allograft for spine surgery only; morselized (List separately in addition to code for primary procedure)	721.1 723	722 724.6
20931	Allograft for spine surgery only; structural (List separately in addition to code for primary procedure)	721.1 723.0	722 724.6
20936	Autograft for spine surgery only (includes harvesting the graft); local (eg, ribs, spinous process, or laminar fragments) obtained from same incision (List separately in addition to code for primary procedure)	724.6	722
20937	Autograft for spine surgery only (includes harvesting the graft); morselized (through separate skin or fascial incision) (List separately in addition to code for primary procedure)	724.6	722
20938	Autograft for spine surgery only (includes harvesting the graft); structural, bicortical or tricortical (through separate skin or fascial incision) (List separately in addition to code for primry procedure)	724.6 721.1	722
22326	Open treatment and/or reduction of vertebral fracture(s) and/or dislocation(s), posterior approach, one fractured vertebra or dislocated segment; cervical	805.1 805.3 805.5	805.2 805.4 805.6
22328	Open treatment and/or reduction of vertebral fracture(s) and/or dislocation(s), posterior approach, one fractured vertebra or dislocated segment; each additional fractured vertebra or dislocated segment (List separately in addition to code for primary procedure)	805.1 805.3 805.5	805.2 805.4 805.6
22800	Arthrodesis, posterior, for spinal deformity, with or without cast; up to 6 vertebral segments	737.0 737.3	737.1 737.30
22595	Arthrodesis, posterior technique, atlas-axis (C1-C2)	805.1	805.2
22600	Arthrodesis, posterior or posterolateral technique, single level; cervical below C2 segment	805.1	805.2
22840	Posterior non-segmental instrumentation (eg, Harrington rod technique, pedicle fixation across one interspace, atlantoaxial transarticular screw fixation, sublaminar wiring at C1, facet screw fixation) (List separately in addition to code for primary procedure)	722.52 737.30	724.6
22842	Posterior segmental instrumentation (eg, pedicle fixation, dual rods with multiple hooks and sublaminar wires); 3 to 6 vertebral segments (List separately in addition to code for primary procedure)	722.52 737.30	724.6
22851	Application of intervertebral biomechanical device(s) (eg, synthetic cage(s), threaded bone dowel(s), methylmethacrylate) to vertebral defect or interspace (List separately in addition to code for primary procedure)	722.52 721.1	724.6

CPT copyright © 2010 by the American Medical Association. All rights reserved.

Chapter 22
Cervical Osteotomy

Edward D. Simmons, MD, CM, MSc, FRCSC

Indications

The primary indication for cervical spine osteotomy is fixed flexion deformity with impairment of the frontal visual field and difficulty with personal hygiene and activities of daily living. Difficulty with swallowing also is common. Most patients who present with these findings have a history of ankylosing spondylitis that has progressed to an ossified spine with a fixed deformity at the cervicothoracic junction. These patients have a high incidence of previously undiagnosed cervical spine fracture, usually near the cervicothoracic junction, often from minor traumatic events (**Figure 1**). The incidence of an earlier cervical spine fracture in patients presenting with rigid fixed cervical flexed deformities has been found to be 35%. These patients can be mistakenly diagnosed as having a cervical "strain" and are placed in a soft collar. The cervical spine then will gradually assume a flexed position over the ensuing weeks and months, with the fracture healing in fixed deformity.

Cervical osteotomy carries certain risks; the most obvious are neurologic, including possible quadriparesis.

Nerve root irritation is the most common potential complication. Other potential complications include air embolism (related to the sitting position), loss of correction, stroke, and infection. The patient must have a severe enough deformity to warrant undergoing the procedure and must be able to cope with the postoperative regimen.

Contraindications

Well-defined contraindications include deformities that are not severe enough to warrant undergoing the procedure or medical comorbidities that would make it risky for a patient to undergo the procedure. The procedure also is contraindicated when the deformity is flexible and passively correctable.

A cervical flexion deformity of less than 30° generally does not warrant osteotomy correction unless a lumbar spine deformity or hip flexion contracture deformity is present, which creates a malaligned sagittal balance, resulting in a functional handicap. The patient's entire sagittal alignment must

be assessed, not just the cervicothoracic junction (see chin-brow–to–vertical diagram in **Figure 2**). A deformity often is present to some degree in the lumbar spine, usually a loss of lumbar lordosis that gives rise to a slightly flexed position through the lumbar spine. This, in combination with the cervical spine flexion deformity, can result in significant sagittal plane malalignment and an inability to maintain level vision. If the lumbar spine deformity is the greater of the two deformities, then it would be more appropriate to undertake lumbar spine osteotomy rather than cervical osteotomy. If the cervical spine clearly has the primary deformity, and the amount of malalignment is great enough to cause a major handicap, then cervical osteotomy may be indicated.

Other contraindications include spinal canal stenosis that is significant enough to prevent the osteotomy from being performed safely. Also, the vertebral arteries must be assessed with CT to ensure that their normal entry point at C6 is present (**Figure 3**).

Alternative Treatments

In spinal conditions (other than ankylosing spondylitis) that do not result in an ossified rigid spine, other

Dr. Simmons or an immediate family member owns stock or stock options in Abbott, Amgen, Alphatec Spine, Genzyme, Johnson & Johnson, Novartis, and Proctor & Gamble.

Portions of this chapter are adapted with permission from Simmons ED, DiStefano RJ, Zheng Y, Simmons EH: Thirty-six years experience of cervical extension osteotomy in ankylosing spondylitis: Techniques and outcomes. Spine (Phila Pa 1976) 2006;31(26):3006-3012.

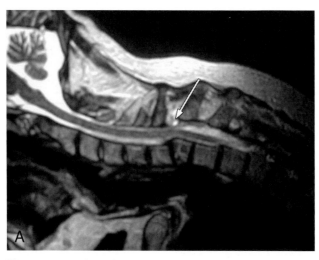
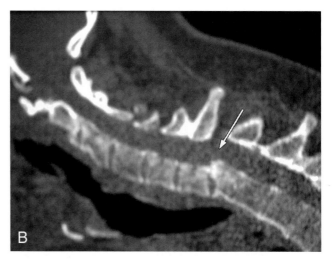

Figure 1 Sagittal MRI (**A**) and CT scan (**B**) of a patient with fixed flexion deformity of the cervical spine reveal signs of a previously undiagnosed fracture at C6-7 (arrows). (Adapted with permission from Simmons ED, DiStefano RJ, Zheng Y, Simmons EH: Thirty-six years experience of cervical extension osteotomy in ankylosing spondylitis: Techniques and outcomes. *Spine (Phila Pa 1976)* 2006;31(26):3006-3012.)

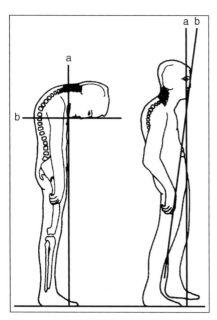

Figure 2 Drawing shows the proper clinical assessment of flexion deformity. The intersection of lines *a* and *b* forms the chin-brow–to–vertical angle. (Adapted with permission from Simmons EH: The cervical spine in ankylosing spondylitis, in Bridwell KH, DeWald RL, eds: *The Textbook of Spinal Surgery*, ed 2. Philadelphia, PA, Lippincott-Raven, 1997, p 1136.)

options for correction may include releases, traction, and fixation without osteotomy in the corrected position. For patients with the typical fixed flexion deformity of the cervical spine

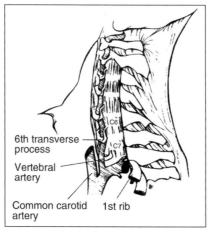

Figure 3 Drawing from a lateral view shows the entry of the vertebral artery at C6. (Adapted with permission from Simmons EH: The cervical spine in ankylosing spondylitis, in Bridwell KH, DeWald RL, eds: *The Textbook of Spinal Surgery*, ed 2. Philadelphia, PA, Lippincott-Raven, 1997, p 1144.)

who have no mobility, such as patients with ankylosing spondylitis, alternative treatments do not exist, aside from activity modification (eg, no driving if the visual field is inadequate). Most of these patients do not have pain because the ankylosing spondylitis usually has progressed to its end point, with major inflammatory pain no longer present.

Results

The results of cervical osteotomy have proven to be quite good (**Table 1**) as long as complications can be avoided. In a long-term review by Simmons and associates of 131 cases of cervical extension osteotomy for ankylosing spondylitis, very good correction was obtained, with a low incidence of serious complications. In this series, 2 patients had significant neurologic complications, and 18 patients had problems with transient C8 radiculopathy. The incidence of pseudarthrosis was 4.6%, with 6 confirmed pseudarthroses requiring further revision fusion. Two patients succumbed to myocardial infarction in the early postoperative period, and 1 patient died of a pulmonary embolism at 30 days postoperatively. The remaining patients went on to successful fusion, and no recurrence of deformity was noted. Because the spine is completely ossified above and below the site of the osteotomy, this is what one would expect because no area exists in which deformity can recur. The possibility of fracture from fairly minor trauma remains because of the generalized osteopenia and lever arm forces

Table 1 Results of Cervical Spine Osteotomy

Author(s) (Year)	Number of Patients	Procedure or Approach	Mean Patient Age in Years (Range)	Mean Follow-up (Range)	Fusion Success Rate	Results
Urist (1958)	1	Cervical posterior	44	12 weeks	NR	Correction maintained
Law (1959)	2	Cervical (3-4 level)	41 (33-49)	NR	NR	1 good 1 death
Simmons (1977)	42	Cervical posterior	NR	4 years (1-4)	96	Good
Savini et al (1988)	1	Posterior Simmons method	42	2 years	100	Good
Bhojraj et al (1993)	1	Anterior and posterior	27	3 years	100	Good
Shimizu et al (1996)	1	Posterior prone Hartshill rectangle	46	3.75 years	100	Good
McMaster (1997)	15	Cervical posterior	48 (35-67)	18 months (9 months to 3 years)	NR	3 neurologic deficits 1 quadriplegic
Mehdian et al (1999)	1	Posterior with internal fixation	39	18 months	100	Good
Taggard & Traynelis (2000)	7	Posterior fracture fixation	60 (44-83)	NR	100	Good
Simmons et al (2006)	131	Posterior	50 (30-79)	9.7 years (2-23)	97	Good Complications: 7 perioperative mortalities 2 paraparesis 18 transient C8 radiculopathies

NR = not reported.

present; however, the risk of fracture is no greater than it was preoperatively. The current technique, with resection of the C7 pedicle and increased lateral mass bony resection, has resulted in a reduced incidence of C8 radiculopathy postoperatively.

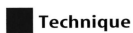

Technique

Setup/Exposure

In the operating room, a cranial halo and vest are applied. The patient is then seated in a modified dental chair, and the posterior neck and lower occipital area are shaved, prepared, and draped. An overhead beam and posts are used to place an adhesive transparent plastic drape (**Figure 4**). The patient's chest is fitted with a Doppler monitor to detect any potential air embolism, a potential risk of surgery in the sitting position. A large sponge is always kept immersed in a basin of saline for placement in the wound if an air embolism is detected on the Doppler. The patient is given some intra-venous sedation throughout the procedure but is conscious and breathing on his or her own, with oxygen delivered via a nasal cannula and monitored by the anesthesiologist. Infiltration of 1% bupivacaine is then introduced into the skin and subcutaneous tissues over the area of the planned surgical incision, which is in the midline from the upper cervical area down to the T2 area. A midline incision is then made through the skin and subcutaneous tissues. Further local anesthesia infiltration is used

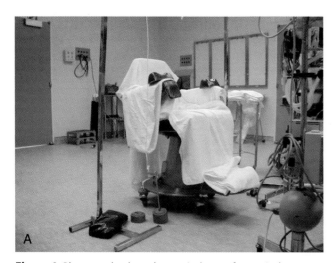 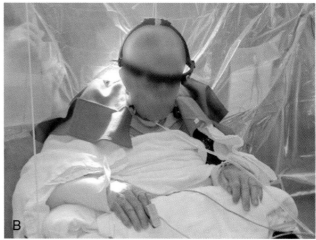

Figure 4 Photographs show the surgical setup for cervical osteotomy, with dental chair (**A**) and plastic drape (**B**). (Panel A is reproduced with permission from Simmons ED, DiStefano RJ, Zheng Y, Simmons EH: Thirty-six years experience of cervical extension osteotomy in ankylosing spondylitis: Techniques and outcomes. *Spine (Phila Pa 1976)* 2006;31(26):3006-3012.)

along the periosteum over the tips of the spinous processes and laminae. Subperiosteal elevation of the paraspinal muscles is then performed in a routine fashion, with further local anesthesia used as needed. The posterior elements of the spine are then cleaned of all soft tissue with visualization down to the T2 level. The last bifid spinous process, which is at the C6 level, is identified. A lateral radiograph is taken to confirm the levels. It is extremely important that the osteotomy be performed at the C7-T1 junction because this is below the entry level of the vertebral arteries and above the thoracic spine. The spinal canal is fairly spacious at this level, which allows correction of the deformity with enough room to accommodate the spinal cord without compromise or disrupting the vertebral artery complex. If the osteotomy is done below T1 in error, then no correction will be attainable because the rigid thoracic cage and rib structures will not allow any correction.

Instruments/Equipment Required

The following instruments and equipment should be on hand for cervical osteotomy: Cobb periosteal elevator, Kerrison and Leksell rongeurs, dural seekers, a dental chair, a Doppler monitoring device, a cranial halo and vest, and overhead traction.

Procedure

Once the correct level has been determined, bone removal can begin. The spinous process of C7 is removed with rongeurs, and the lamina is thinned out. The fragments of bone that are removed are kept for the autologous bone graft at the end of the procedure. Kerrison rongeurs are used to remove the entire posterior arch of C7, along with most of the inferior arch of C6 and approximately 50% of the superior arch of T1. The remaining arch of T1 and C6 also is beveled and undercut to allow ample room for the spinal cord during the extension osteoclasis maneuver. The C7-T1 lateral masses are resected widely. A preoperative calculation can be made of the amount of bone that should be removed based on the deformity that is present; however, in general, enough bone must be removed to provide abundant room for the exiting C8 nerve roots. C8 radiculopathy is the most common postoperative complication, and ample bony resection will minimize the incidence of this complication.

Initially, I carried out the procedure leaving most of the C7 pedicle intact. In recent years, however, I have modified the procedure to involve resection of the C7 pedicle (**Figure 5**, *A*) to allow even more room for C8 nerve roots (**Figure 5**, *B*). This has reduced the incidence of C8 radiculopathy considerably. A dural seeker is used to probe the spinal canal. The patient experiences no pain while the bone is being removed because no pain nerve endings are present in the bone itself. The patient will not perceive pain on slight touching of the posterior thecal sac of the spinal cord but will have discomfort or radicular symptoms if the C8 nerve dorsal root ganglion is touched. When the dural seeker probes the C8 nerve roots, some symptoms may be elicited, such as tingling or slight discomfort in a C8 distribution in the upper extremity; this actually is another confirmation that the correct level is being addressed.

Once the posterior bony resection has been completed (**Figure 5**, *C* and *D*), including complete resection of the C7-T1 lateral masses, then no remaining posterior bony structures remain to impede extension of the spine. If the patient had any prior cervical spine surgery, then careful neurolysis of the thecal sac must be performed before undertaking the extension maneuver. Deep sutures are inserted into the deep fascia because it is much easier to close the incision following the extension maneuver if the sutures are placed ahead of time. Standing behind the patient, the surgeon has very good control of the head and neck. The inline cervical traction is now released. The surgeon firmly grasps the halo in both hands, carefully supporting the head and neck, and then, in a very controlled fashion, brings the neck back into extension. The neck is brought back in a gentle extension arc, not simply pulled straight backward. The surgeon must remember that the neck is rotating in an extension arc through the osteotomy site, and no other forces should be applied that would cause any displacement of the osteotomy site. This arc provides an osteoclasis of the anterior aspect of the spine that often is palpable by the surgeon during the extension maneuver. In most cases, the amount of force needed is fairly mild to moderate. If undue force appears to be necessary, the surgeon must confirm that the osteotomy was performed at the correct level. If the osteotomy was done below C7-T1, then no extension will be attainable. The surgical team would then have to repeat the procedure at the correct site.

Once the neck is brought into the corrected position, the surgeon carefully holds the head and neck while unscrubbed assistants assess the rotation, lateral tilt, and sagittal plane position of the head and neck. A position of 10° of flexion is desirable because it allows the patient to sit and read at a desk and see the floor ahead while walking. The dura must be free to glide underneath the laminae of C6 and T1 as the extension maneuver is performed, and this must be determined beforehand. Once the appropriate position of the neck has been determined, the uprights to the vest are attached to the anterior aspect of the halo. The bone graft is then packed

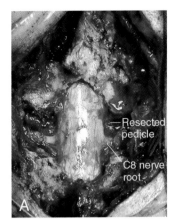
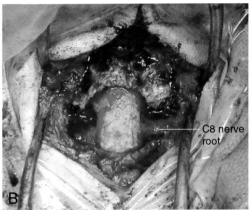
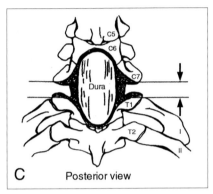
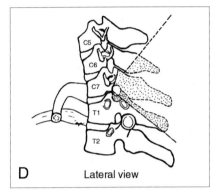

Figure 5 Intraoperative photographs and anatomic drawings show the resection area for posterior cervical osteotomy. The patient's head is at the top. Note that ample room is provided for the exiting C8 nerve roots. The resection is shown partially finished (**A**) and completed (**B**). In **C,** the arrows indicate the gap needed for the exiting C8 nerve roots. In **D,** the dotted areas inside the dashed lines represent areas of bone resection (Panels **A** and **B** adapted and panel **C** reproduced with permission from Simmons EH: The cervical spine in ankylosing spondylitis, in Bridwell KH, DeWald RL, eds: *The Textbook of Spinal Surgery,* ed 2. Philadelphia, PA, Lippincott-Raven, 1997, p 1143. Panel **D** reproduced with permission from Simmons ED, DiStefano RJ, Zheng Y, Simmons EH: Thirty-six years experience of cervical extension osteotomy in ankylosing spondylitis: Techniques and outcomes. *Spine (Phila Pa 1976)* 2006;31(26):3006-3012.)

into the osteotomy site, over both posterolateral surfaces.

Wound Closure

A suction drain is inserted, and the deep fascial sutures are tied down. Subcutaneous sutures are then used, followed by staples for the skin. Once the wound is closed, the posterior halo vest uprights are attached, securing the halo to the vest with the neck in the corrected position. The brief-acting anesthetic agent will have worn off by this point, so the neurologic status of the patient can be evaluated. The patient is then helped up to a standing position and assisted to walk

a few steps to a bed. A regular bed or a circoelectric bed can be used.

Some authors have suggested undertaking instrumentation in these cases; however, in most instances, following the correction of the deformity, very little room to facilitate instrumentation exists. In addition, the landmarks are quite obscure, the bone is extremely osteopenic, and even if instrumentation was used, halo vest immobilization would still be necessary for postoperative care because the instrumentation would be too weak to withstand daily physiologic forces on its own. This is an important point because these cases are different from

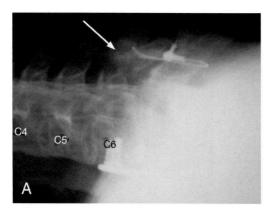 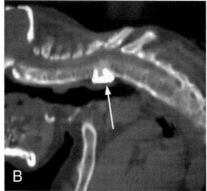 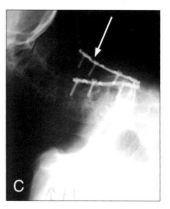

Figure 6 Failed internal fixation following cervical osteotomy. The patient's head is to the left. **A,** Lateral radiograph shows failed internal fixation (arrow) at the osteotomy site. Note the flexed kyphotic position of the neck and the avulsed spinous process of C6. **B,** Sagittal CT demonstrates a failed internal fixation at C7-T1 (arrow). **C,** Lateral radiograph depicts a failed posterior fixation and loss of correction. Note plate pull-out (arrow) with recurrent flexion deformity at C5 through T1.

other spinal conditions, in which mobility above the surgical site is still present. In these cases, the neck is completely rigid above the osteotomy site and all of the forces are concentrated at the osteotomy site, with the weight of the head creating a significant lever arm. I have been referred several cases in which instrumentation has been used without halo vest immobilization and early postoperative failure has occurred (**Figure 6**).

Postoperative Regimen

The patient is mobilized on postoperative day 1, with ambulation as tolerated. Physical and occupational therapy are begun in the hospital, to educate the patient appropriately. Standard halo pin care is performed. At 4-month follow-up, radiographs are taken and a CT study is conducted to evaluate the healing of the bone graft at the osteotomy site. The halo vest usually can be removed at this time, and a cervical orthosis can be used for an additional 6 weeks. **Figures 7 and 8** show two patients who underwent cervical osteotomy.

Avoiding Pitfalls and Complications

Neurologic injury is the most important complication to avoid. Careful consideration must be given to preoperative planning and assessment. A preoperative CT scan should be done to assess the spinal canal and vertebral arteries. Intraoperatively, the surgeon must be absolutely certain that the osteotomy is being done at the C7-T1 level and not above it. I am aware that some surgeons try to carry out slight correction in the cervical spine above C7-T1; however, in most of these cases, the deformity is quite severe, and the amount of correction necessary cannot be done at levels above C6 because of the presence of the vertebral arteries. I have found that placing the patient in the sitting position is best for this procedure because it permits very careful control of the head-neck axis and appropriate positioning of the patient. Because most of these patients present with large fixed cervical deformities, positioning in the standard prone fashion is not technically feasible and certainly makes the surgery much more difficult to carry out. In addition, the head and neck cannot be controlled as well during the extension maneuver with the pa-

tient lying in the standard prone position.

The bone resection must be adequate to allow ample room for the spinal cord centrally; this is done by removing enough of the C6 and T1 laminae and by undercutting and beveling the remaining laminae. In addition, the C7-T1 lateral masses must be resected widely, along with the C7 pedicle, to allow ample room for the exiting C8 nerve roots. Care must be taken to ensure that no dural adhesions are present before carrying out the osteoclasis extension maneuver.

Postoperatively, the patient must be immobilized in the halo vest for 4 months; other forms of immobilization are inadequate. Instrumentation has not been necessary to ensure a high fusion rate in these patients, and I believe that the extra time needed to insert the instrumentation—and the potential complications risked—do not warrant its use in these cases. Even when instrumentation is used, I strongly recommend that a halo vest also be used for 4 months. Therefore, little benefit is to be gained from using instrumentation—only increased risks.

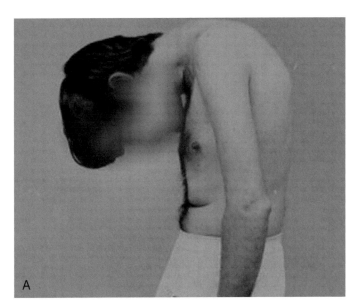

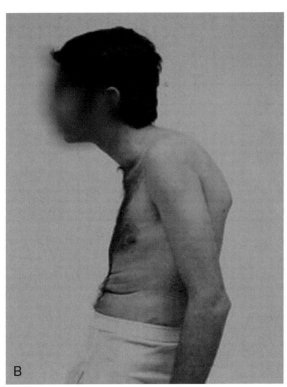

Figure 7 Clinical photographs of a patient with a severe, fixed chin-on-chest deformity that impaired both swallowing and the visual field. **A,** Preoperative photograph. **B,** The same patient following extension osteotomy.

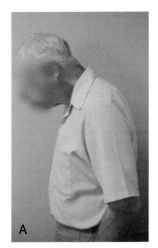

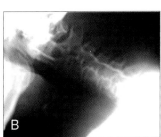

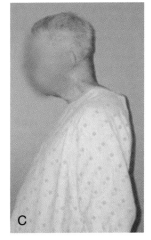

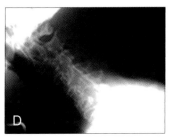

Figure 8 Images of a patient with a fixed flexion deformity of the cervical spine. Preoperative lateral clinical photograph (**A**) and radiograph (**B**). Postoperative lateral clinical photograph (**C**) and radiograph (**D**) of the same patient. (Reproduced with permission from Simmons ED, DiStefano RJ, Zheng Y, Simmons EH: Thirty-six years experience of cervical extension osteotomy in ankylosing spondylitis: Techniques and outcomes. *Spine (Phila Pa 1976)* 2006;31(26):3006-3012.)

Bibliography

Bhojraj SY, Dasgupta D, Dewoolkar LV: One-stage "front" and "back" correction for rigid cervical kyphosis: A safer technique of correction for a rare case of adult-onset Still's disease. *Spine (Phila Pa 1976)* 1993;18(13):1904-1908.

Harris AG, Heron JS, Renwick WA: Anaesthesia for posterior cervical osteotomy. *Can Anaesth Soc J* 1975;22(1):84-90.

Hunter T, Dubo H: Spinal fractures complicating ankylosing spondylitis. *Ann Intern Med* 1978;88(4):546-549.

Law WA: Osteotomy of the cervical spine. *J Bone Joint Surg Br* 1959;41:640-641.

McMaster MJ: Osteotomy of the cervical spine in ankylosing spondylitis. *J Bone Joint Surg Br* 1997;79(2):197-203.

Mehdian SM, Freeman BJ, Licina P: Cervical osteotomy for ankylosing spondylitis: An innovative variation on an existing technique. *Eur Spine J* 1999;8(6):505-509.

Olerud C, Frost A, Bring J: Spinal fractures in patients with ankylosing spondylitis. *Eur Spine J* 1996;5(1):51-55.

Savini R, Di Silvestre M, Gargiulo G: Cervical osteotomy by the Simmons method in the treatment of cervical kyphosis due to ankylosing spondylitis: Case report. *Ital J Orthop Traumatol* 1988;14(3):377-383.

Shimizu K, Matsushita M, Fujibayashi S, Toguchida J, Ido K, Nakamura T: Correction of kyphotic deformity of the cervical spine in ankylosing spondylitis using general anesthesia and internal fixation. *J Spinal Disord* 1996;9(6):540-543.

Simmons ED, DiStefano RJ, Zheng Y, Simmons EH: Thirty-six years experience of cervical extension osteotomy in ankylosing spondylitis: Techniques and outcomes. *Spine (Phila Pa 1976)* 2006;31(26):3006-3012.

Simmons ED, Simmons EH: Ankylosing spondylitis, in Farcy JPC, ed: *Spine: State of the Art Reviews.* Philadelphia, PA, Hanley & Belfus, 1994, vol. 8, no. 3, pp 589-603.

Simmons EH: Kyphotic deformity of the spine in ankylosing spondylitis. *Clin Orthop Relat Res* 1977;128(128):65-77.

Simmons EH: Ankylosing spondylitis: Surgical considerations, in Rothman RH, Simeone FA, eds: *Spine.* Philadelphia, PA, Saunders, 1992, pp 1447-1511.

Simmons EH: The surgical correction of flexion deformity of the cervical spine in ankylosing spondylitis. *Clin Orthop Relat Res* 1972;86:132-143.

Smith-Petersen MN, Larson CB, Aufranc OE: Osteotomy of the spine for correction of flexion deformity in rheumatoid arthritis. *Clin Orthop Relat Rest* 1969;66:6-9.

Taggard DA, Traynelis VC: Management of cervical spinal fractures in ankylosing spondylitis with posterior fixation. *Spine (Phila Pa 1976)* 2000;25(16):2035-2039.

Urist MR: Osteotomy of the cervical spine: Report of a case of ankylosing rheumatoid spondylitis. *J Bone Joint Surg Am* 1958;40(4):833-843.

Zigler J, Rockowitz N, Capen D, Nelson R, Waters R: Posterior cervical fusion with local anesthesia: The awake patient as the ultimate spinal cord monitor. *Spine (Phila Pa 1976)* 1987;12(3):206-208.

Coding

CPT Codes		Corresponding ICD-9 Codes	
22210	Osteotomy of spine, posterior or posterolateral approach, one vertebral segment; cervical	720.0 737.10 737.12	733.81 737.11 737.20
22216	Osteotomy of spine, posterior or posterolateral approach, one vertebral segment; each additional vertebral segment (List separately in addition to primary procedure)	720.0 737.10 737.12	733.81 737.11 737.20
20661	Application of halo, including removal; cranial	805.02 805.04 805.06	805.03 805.05 805.07

Minimally Invasive Posterior Cervical Lateral Mass Fusion

James P. Lawrence, MD, MBA
Alan S. Hilibrand, MD

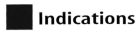 Indications

Minimally invasive surgical (MIS) techniques, which reduce the degree of surgical exposure and the degree of muscle retraction and injury, continue to evolve. These approaches take advantage of improved instrumentation, fluoroscopic visualization, and magnification with either loupes or a microscope. In the cervical spine in particular, MIS techniques may provide a benefit by reducing the degree of surgical exposure and iatrogenic muscular injury. Posterior minimally invasive lateral mass fusion may be used to treat fractures of the articular processes or subluxation and/or dislocation of the facet joints, or it may be used as the posterior component of a combined anterior-posterior procedure in which posterior arthrodesis is required without the need for a midline decompression.

Contraindications

A formal open procedure should be used in patients requiring a central decompression procedure because of the greater vulnerability of the exposed spinal cord to iatrogenic injury. Although a formal laminectomy may be performed with MIS techniques, the passage of instruments over the exposed dura to perform a stabilization procedure introduces additional risk when performed with limited visualization. In addition, the MIS approach is suitable only for levels in the subaxial spine, from C3 through C7. The upper cervical spine (occiput to C2) has a unique anatomy that requires substantially different screw direction and length than that used in the lower cervical spine. At the cervicothoracic junction, the difficulty in obtaining adequate fluoroscopic visualization may make it difficult to routinely use a minimally invasive posterior approach.

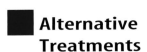 Alternative Treatments

The technique of anterior decompression and arthrodesis is commonly used to establish neural element decompression and segmental stability in the setting of degenerative disease and/or traumatic injuries of the cervical spine. In the setting of traumatic or degenerative instability requiring a posterior approach, open posterior lateral mass fusion with instrumentation is widely practiced. In some cases, posterior arthrodesis can provide more rigid fixation than anterior arthrodesis by restoring the posterior tension band. Patients with severe injuries to the cervical vertebral column, such as fracture-dislocations, may benefit from a combined approach with both anterior and posterior instrumentation. The technique of posterior lateral mass screw and plate or rod fixation focuses on the safe placement of lateral mass screws based on surface landmarks to avoid injury to the vertebral artery and nerve roots. MIS posterior lateral mass fusion uses the same technique but allows delivery of all instruments through a tubular retractor system using fluoroscopy and magnification.

Results

The results of three clinical studies on the use of MIS techniques in posterior cervical lateral mass fusion are summarized in **Table 1**. Wang and

Dr. Lawrence or an immediate family member serves as a paid consultant to or is an employee of Gentis Corporation. Dr. Hilibrand or an immediate family member has received royalties from Biomet, Zimmer, Stryker, and Aesculap/B. Braun; has received research or institutional support from Medtronic, DePuy, Stryker, Osteotech, and Synthes; and owns stock or stock options in Amedica, Vertiflex, Nexgen, Benvenue Medical, Pioneer Surgical, Life Spine, Paradigm Spine, Promethean Surgical Devices (PSD), and Syndicom.

Table 1 Results of MIS Techniques in Posterior Cervical Lateral Mass Fusion

Authors (Year)	Number of Patients	Procedure	Mean Age in Years	Follow-up	Fusion Success	Results
Wang et al (2003)	3	2 anterior-posterior, 1 posterior alone	40	Minimal	NR	Technically feasible
Fong and Duplessis (2005)	2	Anterior-posterior arthrodesis	40	Minimal	NR	Technically feasible
Wang and Levi (2006)	18	14 anterior-posterior, 4 posterior alone	41	At least 2 years	100%	2 converted to open surgical procedures

associates published the initial report in 2003 describing the use of MIS techniques to facilitate posterior lateral mass arthrodesis. This original case series included three patients who had sustained traumatic injuries—a C4-C5 facet fracture with anterolisthesis and C5 radiculopathy, a C3-C4 unilateral facet fracture with subluxation, and a neurologically intact patient with C3-C4 bilaterally jumped facets. The first two patients underwent anterior decompression and arthrodesis at the level of injury, which was supplemented posteriorly with lateral mass arthrodesis using a screw-rod construct via a MIS technique using a tubular retractor system. The third patient was treated exclusively through a posterior approach, in which the authors removed the superior articular facet bilaterally, reduced the facet dislocation, and then performed an arthrodesis through the tubular retractor. The follow-up period was brief, but they noted an absence of postoperative complications and concluded that this method of treatment was technically feasible.

Fong and Duplessis published a case series involving two patients, one with a C5-C6 facet subluxation and the other with a C7 burst fracture with an incomplete spinal cord injury and focal kyphosis at C5-C6 resulting from a flexion-distraction injury. Both patients underwent anterior decompression and arthrodesis and received supplementary posterior fixation through this posteriorly based MIS approach. Again, there was minimal follow-up, and no data are available on the clinical and radiographic outcomes.

The only report with short- and intermediate-term follow-up was published by Wang and Levi in 2006. They reviewed the outcomes of 18 patients treated by posterior MIS techniques who were followed for at least 2 years. Radiographic follow-up consisted of flexion-extension radiographs and CT scans obtained at an unspecified time postoperatively. The patient group was heterogeneous, consisting of 10 patients with traumatic injuries, 4 with pseudarthrosis, 2 with metastatic lesions, 1 with cervical myelopathy, and 1 with vertebral osteomyelitis. Fourteen of the 18 patients (78%) had anterior-posterior treatment, and 4 had posterior-alone treatment. The procedures for 2 of the 18 patients (11%) were converted to an open approach because of poor fluoroscopic visualization at the inferior end of the construct. Two (11%) complications occurred in the group, including one superficial wound infection and one patient with persistent iliac crest bone graft site pain after grafting for the treatment of a pseudarthrosis. CT scans demonstrated fusion in all cases.

Techniques

Setup/Exposure

The patient is positioned prone with the head stabilized in Mayfield tongs. The operating table may be rotated 180° to facilitate an easier approach with the fluoroscopy unit, with care taken to extend the appropriate respiratory tubing and intravenous access lines. Lateral fluoroscopy is used to identify the appropriate bony anatomy, specify the surgical level, confirm the posture of the cervical spine, and guide reduction through manipulation of the Mayfield tongs. Fluoroscopy also is used to localize the incision, guide the dilating retractors, and place the instrumentation.

After the skin is infiltrated with local anesthetic, a 2.0-cm midline skin incision is made to introduce a set of tubular dilator retractors. Sharp incision of the muscular fascia can facilitate an easier passage of the retractor to rest on the surgical lateral masses. Usually a single midline skin incision is followed by two paramedian fascial incisions, each biased just lateral to the spinous processes. This provides the best trajectory across the lateral mass for screw placement.

Instruments/Equipment/Implants Required

Instruments and equipment required for this procedure include a fluoroscope, a tubular/minimally invasive retractor system with lighting, an ap-

Chapter 24

Thoracic Pedicle Screw Fixation

Sigurd Berven, MD
Anthony Gibson, MBBS

Indications

Thoracic spine fixation with pedicle screws is an important and useful technique in spinal surgery. Multiple options exist for thoracic spine fixation, including wires, hooks, and pedicle screws. The choice of fixation anchor is made on a case-by-case basis depending on the specific goals of the surgery. Important considerations in choosing a thoracic spine fixation technique include bone density, cost, individual surgeon experience, and the need to correct deformity in the sagittal or coronal plane. Thoracic pedicle screws have specific value in deformity correction, tumor reconstruction, and stabilization of the spine for traumatic and degenerative conditions. Examples of thoracic pedicle screw applications and constructs are shown in **Figure 1**, and examples of the use of thoracic pedicle screws in deformity and tumor treatment are shown in **Figure 2**. Thoracic pedicle screws have significant advantages over hooks and wires in the

spine with good bone density. These advantages include rigid three-column fixation of the spine; direct derotation of apical segments in deformity; powerful segmental correction; and effective fixation after laminotomy, osteotomy, or loss of integrity of posterior elements. Significant variability exists in the choice of thoracic fixation anchors.

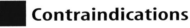

Contraindications

Thoracic pedicle screws require accurate placement with an end point that is anterior to the neural elements and in the area of the great vessels. Thoracic pedicle fixation may be contraindicated in patients with dural ectasia or exceptionally narrow pedicles (Lenke type D). In these cases, the primary fixation of the screw is in the vertebral body rather than the cortical boundaries of the pedicle. Patients with anterior column deficiency and osteolysis or bone loss involving the

pedicle also may have inadequate bone stock for thoracic pedicle fixation.

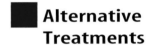

Alternative Treatments

Alternatives to thoracic pedicle fixation include fixation with hooks or wires. Hooks and wires may be placed in the sublaminar space, around transverse processes, or around spinous processes. In bone of poor mineral density, spinous process wires and pedicle or laminar hooks have demonstrated better fixation than pedicle screws as measured by pullout strength. Sublaminar hooks and wires require penetration into the epidural space for insertion and may incur significant risk to the neural elements. Fixation with hooks or wires is limited to the posterior column; thus, control of the anterior column of the spine is reduced, as is derotation and deformity correction.

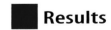

Results

The value of thoracic pedicle screws can be measured by comparing pull-

Dr. Berven or an immediate family member has received royalties from Scientx and Pioneer; is a member of a speakers' bureau or has made paid presentations on behalf of DePuy, Kyphon, Medtronic Sofamor Danek, and Osteotech; serves as a paid consultant to or is an employee of DePuy, Kyphon, Medtronic Sofamor Danek, and Osteotech; and has received research or institutional support from DePuy and Medtronic Sofamor Danek. Neither Dr. Gibson nor any immediate family member has received anything of value from or owns stock in a commercial company or institution related directly or indirectly to the subject of this chapter.

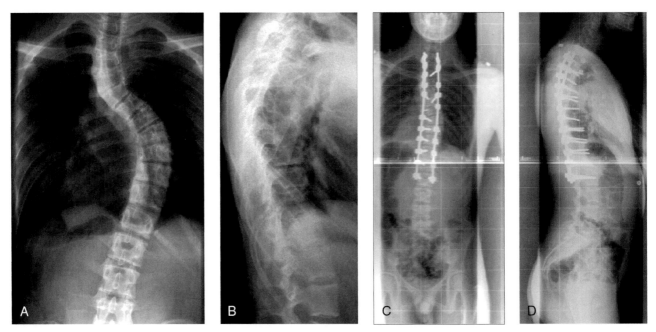

Figure 1 Applications of thoracic pedicle screws. Preoperative AP (**A**) and lateral (**B**) radiographs demonstrate a scoliotic deformity. Postoperative AP (**C**) and lateral (**D**) radiographs show correction of the deformity using a thoracic pedicle screw system extending from T4 to L2.

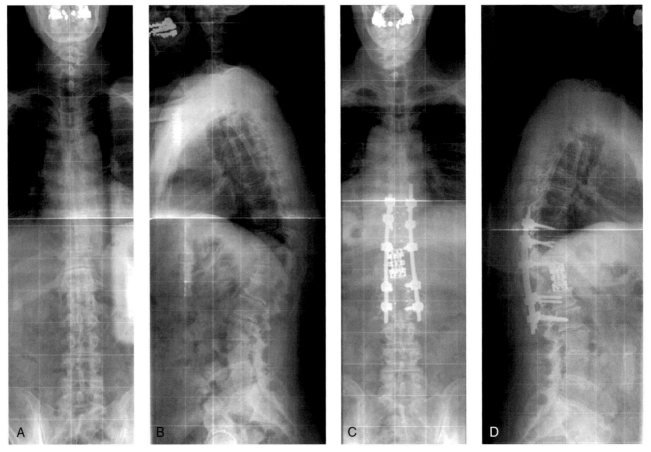

Figure 2 Preoperative AP (**A**) and lateral (**B**) radiographs show tumor involvement at level T12. Postoperative AP (**C**) and lateral (**D**) radiographs show excision of this region and insertion of an expandable cage along with rigid fixation using a thoracic pedicle screw construct from T9 to L2.

Table 1 Biomechanical Data

Authors (Year)	Number of Pullout Tests	Mean Pullout Force (N)	
		Hooks	**Screws**
Liljenqvist et al (2001)	90	T4-T8 = 321 T9-T12 = 600	T4-T8 = 531 T9-T12 = 807
Gayet et al (2002)	98	1150 ± 350	4-mm screws = 820 ± 418 5-mm screws = 1396 ± 435
Hackenburg et al (2002)	72	T4-T8 = 337.1 T9-T12 = 541.3	T4-T8 = 583.2 T9-T12 = 696.9
Cordista et al (2006)	100	577 (pedicle claw)	309

out strength, construct rigidity, and deformity correction of thoracic screws versus alternative methods of fixation. Biomechanical and radiographic studies of these parameters demonstrate that in bone of normal density, screws have more rigid fixation and better capacity for correction of deformity than hooks or wires. Other outcome parameters of interest include differences in the number of levels that require instrumentation for correction and differences in clinical outcomes between fixation types.

Biomechanical Data

Biomechanical studies demonstrate that screws have a higher longitudinal pullout strength compared with hooks. In bone of normal density at levels T4-T8, the pullout strength of screws is greater than that of hooks (531 N versus 321 N) and at levels T9-T12, the absolute values are higher for both (807 N versus 600 N). The pullout strength of thoracic pedicle screws at all levels is significantly affected by screw diameter and bone mineral density. In bone with poor mineral density, thoracic pedicle screws have been shown to have compromised pullout, with a bone mineral density of less than 100 mg/mL hydroxyapatite, neutralizing any advantage that thoracic pedicle screws have over hooks at higher densities. **Table 1**

summarizes biomechanical data on thoracic pedicle screws and hooks.

Radiographic Data

Thoracic pedicle screws are powerful tools for radiographic correction of spinal deformity, including rotation and Cobb-angle measurements. Thoracic pedicle constructs result in improved major curve correction and spontaneous correction of secondary curves compared with hooks. Apical rotation also is better with thoracic pedicle screws than with hooks or hybrid constructs. Results of retrospective studies in patients with idiopathic scoliosis have demonstrated major curve corrections between 55.8% and 80.6% for thoracic pedicle screw constructs, producing an improved correction in every study compared to hook/screw constructs. Results for hooks and hybrid constructs demonstrate 50% to 71.3% correction. Importantly, at 2-year follow-up, hook constructs have been shown to be consistently less effective than thoracic pedicle screw constructs. Loss of correction was around 5% in screw constructs but 8% to 10% in hook constructs. **Table 2** summarizes the literature on curve correction with pedicle screw and alternative constructs.

The safety of placement of thoracic pedicle screws is an important consideration in determining their value in comparison with laminar hooks. The

literature covering the accuracy of screw placement demonstrates that screw malposition is more common in deformed spines than in spines without significant rotation. In large-scale studies, screw malposition rates are between 1.5% and 43%. Neurologic complications are the major concern in placing thoracic pedicle screws around the spinal cord. Rates of neural injury, including direct nerve injury and spinal cord injury, have been reported to be between 0% and 0.9%.

Clinical Outcomes

Little evidence has been produced to show that the improved biomechanical and radiographic outcomes of thoracic pedicle screws (compared with hooks and wires) are reflected in clinical outcomes. No difference in function, pain, or revision rates has been demonstrated effectively. The value of improved correction on patient satisfaction or change in health-related quality of life also has not been demonstrated. Thus, the question of whether the better correction is of benefit to the patient remains controversial.

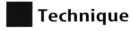

■ Technique

Setup/Exposure
Preoperative planning is an important step in preparing for surgical strate-

Table 2 Radiographic Results of Fixation With Hooks Versus Pedicle Screws

Authors (Year)	Number of Cases and Type of Fixation	Mean Patient Age in Years	Mean Follow-up	Major Curve Correction	% Correction Loss	Results
Suk et al (1995)	31 hooks 23 screws in hook pattern 24 segmental pedicle screws	16.3	Minimum 2 years	Hooks: 55% Screws in hook pattern: 66% Segmental screws: 72%	Hooks: 6% Screws in hook pattern: 2% Segmental screws: 1%	3% malposition No major neurologic complications
Liljenqvist et al (2002)	49 hooks 50 screws	17.3	83 months	Hooks: 51.7% Screws: 55.8%	Hooks: 6.5% Screws: 3.6%	No major neurologic complications
Kim et al (2004)	26 hooks 26 screws	14.8 (hooks) 14.2 (screws)	2 years	Hooks: 50% Screws: 76%	Hooks: 8% Screws: 5.4%	No major neurologic complications
Dobbs et al (2006)	32 hooks 34 screws	13.9 (hooks) 13.8 (screws)	2 years	Hooks: 45% Screws: 56% (Cobb-angle correction)	Hooks: 11% Screws: 3%	No major neurologic complications
Kim et al (2006)	29 hybrid 29 screws	14.8	2 years	Hybrid: 56% Screws: 70%	Hybrid: 9% Screws: 2.4%	No major neurologic complications
Bess et al (2007)	28 hooks 28 screws	49	3.6 years	Hooks: 36% Screws: 41%	Hooks: 2 years, 2%; 4.8 years, 7% Screws: 2 years, 3%; 2.5 years, 0%	No major neurologic complications
Lehman et al (2008)	57 screws 73 hybrid constructs	NR	1 year	Hooks: Lenke 1A, 71.3% Screws: Lenke 1A, 80.6%	2.5°	NR

NR = not reported.

gies in the thoracic spine. The size and trajectories of pedicles and the availability of posterior elements for alternative fixation must be assessed before exposure of the spine. Preoperative plain radiographs and CT scans may be most useful for the preoperative planning of thoracic fixation. Surgical techniques may involve the use of intraoperative navigation with fluoroscopy or CT guidance or the "free-hand" technique based on identifiable anatomic landmarks. T1-T2 and T10-T12 generally are the largest pedicles, whereas pedicles T3-T9 may be less than 4 mm in diameter. In patients with spinal deformity, great variations in pedicle morphometry can be observed. The pedicles on the concave side of the deformity may have a considerably smaller working diameter than those on the convex side, and this may create difficulty in navigating the concave pedicles in deformity. Daubs and associates have classified pedicle types into four categories: A through D, with type A pedicles characterized by a large, cancellous diameter, and type D pedicles characterized by a cortical pedicle without a cancellous portion. The recognition of pedicle types is important in determining a preoperative strategy and in anticipating the need for alternative fixation.

A meticulous exposure of the spine is important for accurate screw placement. The goals of the exposure are to uncover the transverse processes, the facet joints, and the pars interarticularis of the spine. A partial facetectomy to remove the inferior portion of the thoracic facet joint is important in identifying an accurate starting site for thoracic pedicle screws (**Figure 3**). Landmarks for placement of thoracic pedicle screws include the lateral aspect of the pars interarticularis, the transverse processes, and the superior facet joint.

Instruments/Equipment Required

In addition to the normal sterile surgical set used for spine surgery, the most important instruments for this procedure are a curved gear shift probe (pedicle finder), a ball-tip probe, a screw probe (tap), and a screw insertion set matched to the patient's anatomy. Several different sets are made specifically for this purpose, and selection is made according to surgeon preference and suitability for the case. Rods and rod cutters will be required for placement toward the end of surgery, and a rod-bending set will be used to gain correction to the desired angle.

Procedure
Placement of thoracic pedicle screws and construct completion may be considered in six steps.

IDENTIFICATION OF A STARTING POINT
The entry point for thoracic pedicle screws is determined by orientation in the cranial to caudal direction and in the medial to lateral trajectory. At T1, T2, T10, T11, and T12, the starting point for thoracic screws is at the proximal third of the transverse process and at the lateral margin of the pars interarticularis. From T3 to T9, the thoracic pedicle starting point is more cranial and begins above the ridge between the top of the transverse process and the superior facet, with a medial to lateral position at the lateral half of the articular surface of the superior facet.

CREATING A STARTING SITE AND PROBING THE PEDICLE
An awl or a 4- to 5-mm ball-tip burr may be used to create a starting point for the pedicle finder or the gearshift tool. Starting at a vertebra with neutral rotation will improve accuracy and establish a reference point for subsequent pedicles. The cancellous soft spot of the pedicle is identifiable by a vascular "blush" or source of bleeding.

The pedicle probe or gearshift tool is advanced in a medial to lateral direction according to the thoracic level and the rotation of the spine (**Figure 4**, *A*). In the nonrotated spine, T12 has 0° of axial angulation, and there is a progressively more lateral to medial orientation of the thoracic pedicles until L5 caudal and T1 cranial, in which the angle is 25° or more.

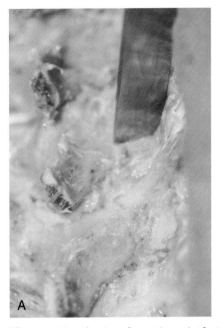 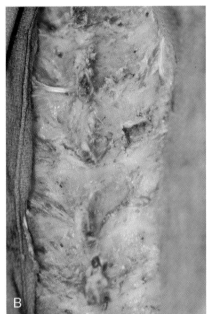

Figure 3 Identification of a starting point for thoracic pedicle screw insertion. **A,** Exposure of the superior facet of T7 using an osteotome. **B,** Exposure of the posterior elements in the thoracic spine required for placement of pedicle screws.

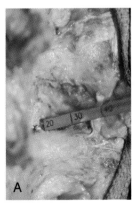 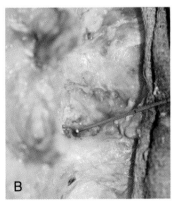 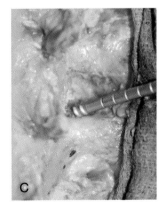 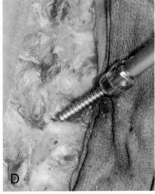

Figure 4 Insertion of thoracic pedicle screws (posterior view). **A,** The pedicle is probed down to a depth of 20 mm using a "gearshift" pedicle probe. **B,** The cancellous tunnel is examined on all four sides with a ball-tip probe to check for medial perforation in the first 20 mm, the section closest to the spinal cord. **C,** The tunnel is tapped. Undertapping by 0.5 to 1 mm increases the pullout strength of the pedicle. **D,** The screw is inserted along the trajectory of the tap probe.

Advancing the pedicle finder with the convexity of the tool pointing medially will minimize the risk of perforation of the medial wall of the pedicle. Once the pedicle finder is at a 20-mm depth, the instrument may be removed and reoriented to point medially to guide the probe toward the center of the vertebral body anterior to the spinal canal.

PALPATION

To check for perforation of the pedicle wall, a blunt-end ball-tip probe is passed down and should encounter bony wall on all four sides and at the end of the cancellous tunnel (**Figure 4**, *B*). In the first 20 mm of the tract, the medial wall is adjacent to the spinal canal, and this region should be palpated particularly carefully for any signs of perforation. The hole in the pedicle also should be visualized for any signs of bleeding or cerebrospinal fluid leakage. The appropriate length of the pedicle screw may be measured from the ball tip at the level of the entry site when the ball tip is at the anterior cortex of the vertebral body. Lateral or medial perforation of the pedicle may be corrected by redirecting the pedicle probe.

TAPPING

Undertapping the pedicle by 0.5 to 1 mm improves the pullout strength of the pedicle (**Figure 4**, *C*). After tapping the pedicle, the integrity of the cortical walls may be confirmed with the ball-tip probe. Palpation of cortical threads in continuity should demonstrate intact bone circumferentially. Screw insertion follows the trajectory of the tap and probe. The first few turns of insertion are performed with minimal force to ensure that the screw follows the tapped path because undue force may cause misdirection (**Figure 4**, *D*).

CONFIRMATION OF SCREW PLACEMENT

Radiography and neural monitoring are useful in confirming thoracic pedicle screw placement. Intraoperative fluoroscopy or plain films will demonstrate pedicle screw position. Screw length and sagittal trajectory is measured on the lateral view, and the accuracy of the starting point and the axial trajectory is measured on the PA view. If the distal screw tip crosses the midline of the vertebral body on a neutral view of the vertebra, the screw may have penetrated the medial wall of the pedicle. An en face radiographic view of the pedicle is a sensitive technique that can determine the position of the pedicle screw relative to the cylinder of the pedicle and can be useful in determining a start site before screw placement.

The use of neuromonitoring in confirming the accuracy of the thoracic screw placement is limited. Evoked stimulation of pedicle screws with distal electromyographic recording may demonstrate medial breach of the pedicle screw encroaching into the canal. The measurement of electromyographic signals from thoracic myotomes may improve the sensitivity of the technique. A clear threshold for normal or intraosseous values has not been established in the thoracic spine, but thresholds less than 8 mA are suspicious for medial or inferior cortical perforation.

CORRECTION

The rod connecting the pedicle screws is the tool used for correcting spinal deformity with segmental fixation. In the spine with hypokyphosis, placement of the rod at the concave side with convex apical pressure of the open screws allows for improved correction of apical rotation and restoration of kyphosis. In contrast, in the kyphotic thoracic spine, placement of the convex rod with segmental compression may be a more effective technique for sagittal plane correction. Using fixed-axis screws at the apex of the deformity improves the ability to derotate the spine.

Wound Closure

Wound closure is an important part of the surgical procedure, and inadequate wound closure may lead to wound dehiscence and infection. Irrigation of the surgical field before bone grafting is useful in reducing the risk of infection. No evidence exists to support the use of pulsatile lavage over a slow-flow method. The use of antibiotics within the irrigant also is not supported by level I evidence in the spine. The thoracic spine is closed in 5 layers, with a running or interrupted No. 0 or No. 1 suture in the thoracodorsal facia, followed by a No. 0 suture in the subcutaneous layer. The deep dermal layer is closed with 2-0 interrupted deep dermal sutures, and the skin may be closed with a subcuticular suture or with staples or nylon. The role of subfacial or subcutaneous drainage is not well established.

——————■

■ Postoperative Regimen

Thoracic fixation with pedicle screws is a stable technique of spinal immobilization, and a brace generally is not required. A brace may be used to control noninstrumented portions of the spine or in cases in which the fixation is compromised by poor bone quality or limited fixation points. Mobilization after surgery improves recovery time and may limit complications, including deep vein thrombosis and wound compromise. Most patients may transfer out of bed to a chair on the day after surgery and progress rapidly to independent ambulation. Preoperative function is an important predictor of postoperative mobility.

The mechanical prophylaxis used to prevent deep vein thrombosis includes compression stockings, sequential compression pumps, and early mobilization. Pain control may include an epidural catheter, patient-controlled analgesia, or oral medications.

Avoiding Pitfalls and Complications

Accurate placement of thoracic pedicle screws creates an optimal construct for stabilizing the thoracic spine. In patients with small pedicles (Lenke types C and D) and those with significant rotational deformity, complete intraosseous screw placement may be compromised. Familiarity with osseous anatomy is the most valuable tool for avoiding complications of screw placement. Intraoperative radiography, including fluoroscopy, or computer-assisted navigation may be useful in improving the accuracy of screw placement.

The technique described in this chapter is a transosseous placement technique in which a cancellous channel is navigated with the pedicle probe. In patients with a narrower pedicle, the screw trajectory may traverse from being in the bone at the transverse process and pedicle junction, to being out of bone lateral to the pedicle, and moving back into bone at the junction of the pedicle and vertebral body. This "in out in" technique increases the functional working diameter for screw insertion. The technique increases the relative area so as to take into account the rib head and the pedicle diameter. Width increases on average from between 4.6 and 8.5 mm to between 12.6 and 17.9 mm, providing a much greater area for screw placement. The technique results in a slight compromise in pullout strength compared with completely

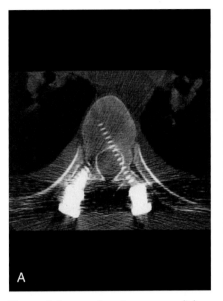 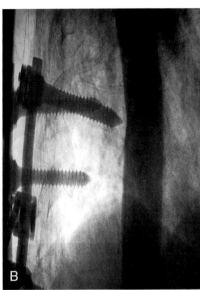

Figure 5 Images show improper pedicle screw placement. **A,** Axial CT fluoroscopic image demonstrates medial wall penetration. **B,** Contrast radiograph demonstrates vascular abutment. Damage to major vessel is a serious but rare complication of thoracic pedicle screw use.

intraosseous screws, but it is particularly useful in patients with very narrow or completely cortical pedicles.

The misplacement of pedicle screws in the thoracic spine may lead to significant consequences, including neural damage, vascular injury, pneumothorax, and gastrointestinal compromise. Inferior malpositions are the most common (as high as 49% of all malpositions), followed by lateral, superior, and medial malpositions. Medial malpositions are the most likely to compromise neural structures, as shown in **Figure 5**, A. No reliable epidural space exists between the pedicle and the dura medially. Superiorly, a safe zone is present from 1.5 to 3.9 mm; inferiorly, the safe zone is variable and may range from 1.7 to 2.8 mm. Neural complications are rarely found in the literature, with estimates of prevalence ranging from 0% to 0.9%.

Vascular injury also is a complication of three-column fixation with thoracic pedicle screws. In scoliosis patients, the aorta is positioned more laterally and posteriorly relative to the vertebral body compared with patients having normal spines, and the aorta is at greater risk of puncture by a misplaced screw (**Figure 5**, B). This has significant consequences because the surgeon must take care to avoid lateral misplacement of screws on the left and concave sides of the thoracic deformity. It has even been shown that up to 12% of vertebral body screws placed posteriorly form a contour in the aorta; however, none of these gave rise to any vascular complications at 2-year follow-up after surgery. The role of screw removal for screws adjacent to the great vessels remains unknown.

■ Bibliography

Bess RS, Lenke LG, Bridwell KH, Cheh G, Mandel S, Sides B: Comparison of thoracic pedicle screw to hook instrumentation for the treatment of adult spinal deformity. *Spine (Phila Pa 1976)* 2007;32(5):555-561.

Coe JD, Warden KE, Herzig MA, McAfee PC: Influence of bone mineral density on the fixation of thoracolumbar implants: A comparative study of transpedicular screws, laminar hooks, and spinous process wires. *Spine (Phila Pa 1976)* 1990;15(9):902-907.

Cordista A, Conrad B, Horodyski M, Walters S, Rechtine G: Biomechanical evaluation of pedicle screws versus pedicle and laminar hooks in the thoracic spine. *Spine J* 2006;6(4):444-449.

Daubs MD, Kim YJ, Lenke LG: Posterior spinal fusion with pedicle screws, In Tolo V, Skaggs D, eds: *Master Techniques in Orthopaedic Surgery: Pediatric Orthopaedics.* New York, NY, Lippincott Williams & Wilkins, 2008.

Dobbs MB, Lenke LG, Kim YJ, Kamath G, Peelle MW, Bridwell KH: Selective posterior thoracic fusions for adolescent idiopathic scoliosis: Comparison of hooks versus pedicle screws. *Spine (Phila Pa 1976)* 2006;31(20):2400-2404.

Ebraheim NA, Jabaly G, Xu R, Yeasting RA: Anatomic relations of the thoracic pedicle to the adjacent neural structures. *Spine (Phila Pa 1976)* 1997;22(14):1553-1557.

Gayet LE, Pries P, Hamcha H, Clarac JP, Texereau J: Biomechanical study and digital modeling of traction resistance in posterior thoracic implants. *Spine (Phila Pa 1976)* 2002;27(7):707-714.

Hackenberg L, Link T, Liljenqvist U: Axial and tangential fixation strength of pedicle screws versus hooks in the thoracic spine in relation to bone mineral density. *Spine (Phila Pa 1976)* 2002;27(9):937-942.

Kim YJ, Lenke LG, Bridwell KH, Cho YS, Riew KD: Free hand pedicle screw placement in the thoracic spine: Is it safe? *Spine (Phila Pa 1976)* 2004;29(3):333-342.

Kim YJ, Lenke LG, Cho SK, Bridwell KH, Sides B, Blanke K: Comparative analysis of pedicle screw versus hook instrumentation in posterior spinal fusion of adolescent idiopathic scoliosis. *Spine (Phila Pa 1976)* 2004;29(18):2040-2048.

Kim YJ, Lenke LG, Kim J, et al: Comparative analysis of pedicle screw versus hybrid instrumentation in posterior spinal fusion of adolescent idiopathic scoliosis. *Spine (Phila Pa 1976)* 2006;31(3):291-298.

Lehman R Jr, Lenke L, Kuklo T, Richards BS, Bridwell K: Comparative analysis between Lenke type 1A-, B-, and C-curve patterns: Pedicle screw vs. hybrid constructs. Which maintains correction better? *Proceedings of the NASS 23rd Annual Meeting/Spine J* 2008;8(5, suppl):162S-163S.

Lenke LG, Kuklo TR, Ondra S, Polly DW Jr: Rationale behind the current state-of-the-art treatment of scoliosis (in the pedicle screw era). *Spine (Phila Pa 1976)* 2008;33(10):1051-1054.

Liljenqvist U, Hackenberg L, Link T, Halm H: Pullout strength of pedicle screws versus pedicle and laminar hooks in the thoracic spine. *Acta Orthop Belg* 2001;67(2):157-163.

Liljenqvist U, Lepsien U, Hackenberg L, Niemeyer T, Halm H: Comparative analysis of pedicle screw and hook instrumentation in posterior correction and fusion of idiopathic thoracic scoliosis. *Eur Spine J* 2002;11(4):336-343.

O'Brien MF, Lenke LG, Mardjetko S, et al: Pedicle morphology in thoracic adolescent idiopathic scoliosis: Is pedicle fixation an anatomically viable technique? *Spine (Phila Pa 1976)* 2000;25(18):2285-2293.

Sucato DJ, Duchene C: The position of the aorta relative to the spine: A comparison of patients with and without idiopathic scoliosis. *J Bone Joint Surg Am* 2003;85-A(8):1461-1469.

Suk SI, Kim WJ, Lee SM, Kim JH, Chung ER: Thoracic pedicle screw fixation in spinal deformities: Are they really safe? *Spine (Phila Pa 1976)* 2001;26(18):2049-2057.

Suk SI, Lee CK, Kim WJ, Chung YJ, Park YB: Segmental pedicle screw fixation in the treatment of thoracic idiopathic scoliosis. *Spine (Phila Pa 1976)* 1995;20(12):1399-1405.

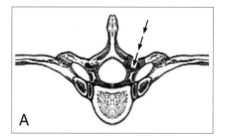 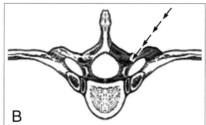 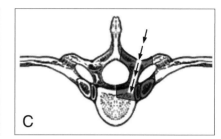

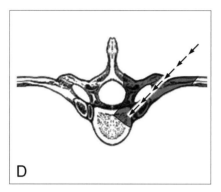 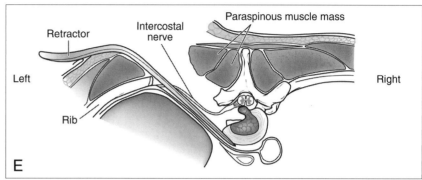

Figure 3 Illustrations depict the trajectories of the five variants of posterolateral approaches for the treatment of thoracic disk herniations. **A,** The traditional transfacet pedicle-sparing approach. **B,** The modified transfacet pedicle-sparing approach (including complete facetectomy and midline-sparing partial laminectomy) described by Bransford and associates. **C,** The transpedicular approach. **D,** The costotransversectomy approach. **E,** The lateral extracavitary approach. (Panels **A** through **D** adapted with permission from Bransford R, Zhang F, Bellabarba C, Konodi M, Chapman JR: Early experience treating thoracic disc herniations using a modified transfacet pedicle-sparing decompression and fusion. *J Neurosurg Spine* 2010;12:221-231.)

verse ligaments, thus freeing the transverse process from the underlying rib. The neurovascular bundle is protected as the rib is dissected subperiosteally with a Cobb elevator. The ribs are then cut 5 cm lateral to the costotransverse junction. Soft-tissue attachments between the rib and the vertebral body are then incised, and the rib is excised and morcellized for use as bone graft. The pleura is then dissected bluntly off the anterolateral vertebral bodies if anterior access to the disk space and adjacent vertebral bodies is required. This also allows for anterior retraction of the pleura and a more horizontal line of sight and approach to the anterior spinal canal. The intercostal bundle is identified and followed medially to identify the neural foramen. The remainder of the decompression and fusion is then performed as described for the transfacet approach.

For a more extensive anterior decompression, such as a corpectomy, the technique differs somewhat. A temporary rod is connected to the pedicle screws contralateral to the planned costotransversectomy approach. This temporary stabilization avoids any movement that may jeopardize the spinal cord because the spine gradually becomes circumferentially destabilized during the course of the decompression. In addition, if a corpectomy is planned, an additional rib generally will need to be resected for each additional disk level requiring exposure. On the contralateral side, before placement of the temporary rod, facetectomies are performed at the disk levels adjacent to the planned corpectomy, followed by diskectomy using a reverse-angled curet and pituitary rongeur. Resection of the pedicle with a high-speed burr is followed by longitudinal osteotomy of

the posterolateral cortex extending between the two disk spaces. On the side of the costotransversectomy, reconstruction of the corpectomy defect normally requires sacrificing the thoracic nerve root corresponding to the planned corpectomy level. The nerve root is ligated before being transected to avoid CSF leakage and is incised proximal to the dorsal root ganglion to avoid painful neuroma formation. Following exposure of the vertebral body, decompression can be performed anteriorly and posteriorly. The corpectomy entails performing diskectomies adjacent to the vertebral body in question or performing a transverse bony resection adjacent to the disk herniation in the case of a partial corpectomy and subsequently performing the bulk of the intervening bony resection with rongeurs or a high-speed drill. If necessary, the anterior cortex can be removed with a Kerrison

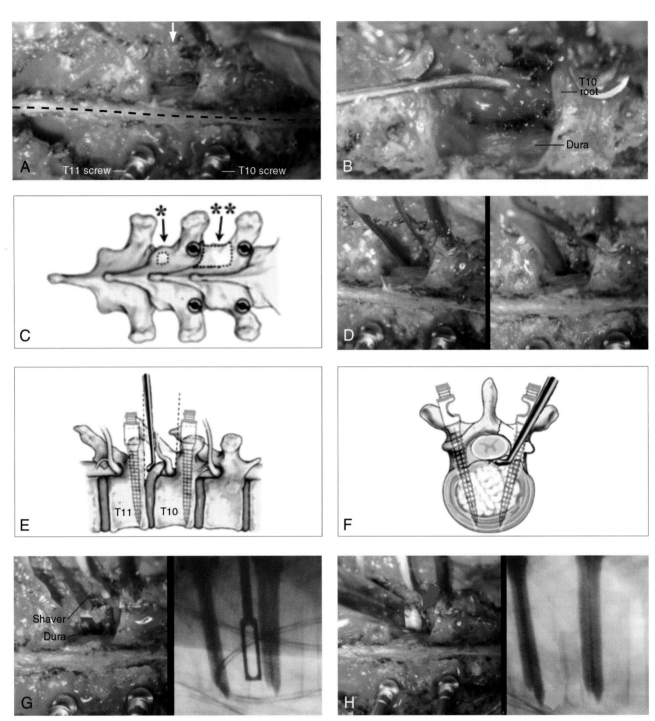

Figure 4 The modified transfacet approach. Intraoperative photographs demonstrate, after pedicle screw placement, the complete facetec-tomy (from pedicle to pedicle) (**A**) and midline-sparing partial laminectomy (**B**) that are performed to expose the thecal sac, the nerve root, and the herniated disk (indicated in panel B by a Penfield No. 4 dissector). The arrow indicates the facetectomy, and the dashed line indicates the midline. **C,** Drawing depicts the posterior elements of the thoracic spine. The single asterisk indicates the area of facet removal as described by Stillerman and associates, in their transfacet pedicle-sparing approach. The double asterisks indicate the extent of bone removal in the modification described by Bransford and associates. **D,** Distraction is applied between the pedicles with a lamina spreader (left), and the disk material is removed with pituitary forceps (right) to create a central cavity into which prominent disk material can be pushed using reverse-angle curets placed carefully within the plane between the anterior dura and the herniated disk (**E** and **F**). Interbody fusion is then performed through the posterolateral approach. **G,** An intraoperative image (left) and lateral fluoroscopy (right) of the posterior spine show end-plate preparation. **H,** Placement of the interbody spacer (arrow) is shown in an intraoperative image of the posterior spine (left) and a lateral fluoroscopic view (right). (Adapted with permission from Bransford R, Zhang F, Bellabarba C, Konodi M, Chapman JR: Early experience treating thoracic disc herniations using a modified transfacet pedicle-sparing decompression and fusion. *J Neurosurg Spine* 2010;12:221-231.)

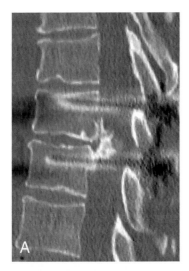

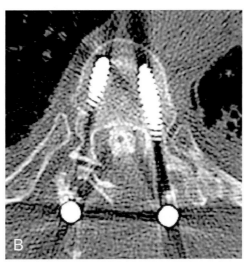

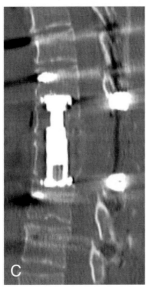

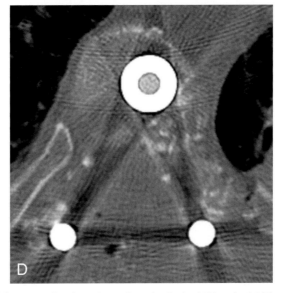

Figure 5 Images of a patient with progressive thoracic myelopathy. Sagittal (**A**) and axial (**B**) CT scans demonstrate a large, central, calcified thoracic disk protrusion following an attempt at decompression using a transfacet approach at another institution. The original decompression had been abandoned because of worrisome intraoperative electrodiagnostic changes with CSF leakage. Sagittal (**C**) and axial (**D**) CT images obtained following a two-level corpectomy through a costotransversectomy approach show that adequate decompression was achieved.

transverse angle of approach to the anterior spinal canal. The indications for its use are similar to those described for costotransversectomy. The primary difference is that the plane of the approach is lateral to the paraspinous muscles, unlike the previously described exposures in which the plane of dissection courses medial to the paraspinous musculature. Following a midline or paramedian incision, a subcutaneous flap is developed, exposing the midline and lateral edge of the paraspinous muscles. The thoracodorsal fascia is incised longitudinally in a paramedian location, approximately 5 cm lateral to the midline, over the lateral aspect of the paraspinous muscles. In the upper thoracic spine, the upper back musculature, including the trapezius, latissimus dorsi, and rhomboids, must be either elevated from the midline as a flap or split along their fibers to access the underlying posterior rib cage lateral to the paraspinous muscles. The erector spinae muscles are then dissected from lateral to medial off the posterior rib cage. The paraspinal muscles are then retracted to the contralateral side. Placement of posterior instrumentation also requires the paraspinal muscles to be dissected off the midline structures. The posteromedial 8 to 10 cm of one of the ribs is resected, and the technique then proceeds in a manner similar to that described previously for the costotransversectomy approach.

Wound Closure

Wound closure is generally performed by approximating the thoracodorsal fascia, subcutaneous tissue, and dermis with braided absorbable suture. This is followed by a running subcuticular closure using absorbable monofilament suture and wound closure glue.

rongeur. Finally, the plane between the anterior dura and the posterior vertebral cortex is developed, and reverse-angled curets are used to push the posterior cortex and the attached annular and disk tissue anteriorly into the corpectomy defect, where it can be retrieved easily. The anterior column can then be reconstructed with structural allograft or a cage and morcellized bone graft.

Lateral Extracavitary Approach

The lateral extracavitary approach (**Figure 3**, *E*) is a variation of the costotransversectomy that allows a more directly lateral approach to the vertebral body and therefore an even more

Postoperative Regimen

For the costotransversectomy and far lateral approaches, in which the dissection proceeds along the pleura, it is imperative to obtain an upright AP chest radiograph in the recovery area to evaluate for pneumothorax. Postoperative care generally involves early mobilization without bracing. Perioperative antibiotics, wound suction drains, and urinary catheters are normally discontinued within 24 hours of surgery. Hardware placement and successful excision of a calcified disk can be assessed with a postoperative CT scan. The adequacy of neural decompression can be further assessed by myelography or MRI in patients with persistent neurologic deficits. Routine upright plain radiographs are obtained before discharge and at 6 weeks, 3 months, 6 months, and 1 year postoperatively to assess alignment, hardware position and integrity, and consolidation of the fusion. The presence of radiolucencies surrounding instrumentation or structural graft and changes in alignment of 5° or greater may herald a pseudarthrosis or failure of fixation that may require additional investigation.

Avoiding Pitfalls and Complications

Misidentification of the Surgical Level

Wrong-level surgery occurs with relatively greater frequency in the thoracic spine than in the lumbar spine, primarily because of landmarks that are less easily identifiable and a failure to recognize transitional intervertebral levels. Although probably underreported in the literature, it has been reported with similar frequency in both anterior and posterolateral approaches. The risk of this complication can be minimized by cross-referencing plain radiographs with neuroimaging studies such as MRI or CT myelography to help identify ambiguous numbering sequences. Other useful techniques include preparation of a wide surgical field that allows for multineedle localization from a reliable landmark such as the sacrum, counting ribs, and observing the location of the targeted disk pathology relative to other obvious radiographic findings such as large osteophytes. The use of preoperative CT-guided needle localization of the desired level has recently been advocated as a means of ensuring that the appropriate level is targeted.

Inadequate Decompression

Because the posterolateral approaches do not provide as direct a visualization of the central spinal canal as the anterior transthoracic approach, incomplete decompression has been described as a potential complication. Various techniques can help identify the adequacy of decompression intraoperatively. They range in sophistication from identification of a residual prominence by palpating the spinal canal anterior to the dura with a curved elevator to intraoperative ultrasound or myelography. In addition, postoperative imaging studies should be scrutinized to ensure the adequacy of decompression in patients with persistent neurologic abnormalities.

CSF Leakage

One of the primary causes of CSF leakage is the presence of intradural thoracic disk herniation, which has been reported in up to 12% of cases. Dense calcification within the disk is known to be an associated factor, making CT myelography useful in identifying disks with a strong likelihood of intradural extension. Although the best approach to calcified thoracic disks remains undetermined, an advantage to the posterolateral approaches is the low likelihood of CSF-pleural fistulas compared with the transthoracic approach.

Pleural Defects

Pleural defects have been reported in up to 13% of posterolateral approaches, generally from costotransversectomy or lateral extracavitary approaches. Avoiding pleural defects is achieved by meticulous identification of pericostal and perivertebral tissue planes. Intraoperatively, filling the wound with saline before closure and observing for air bubbles can help identify small pleural defects. Pleural defects are best repaired intraoperatively, if possible, which often avoids the need for a thoracostomy tube. For unrepairable defects, although placement of a thoracostomy tube is a reasonable approach, our experience, which has been supported by several authors, is that minor pleural defects usually do not require thoracostomy tube placement. An alternative approach is to obtain an upright postoperative chest radiograph to confirm the presence of a pneumothorax before placing a chest tube. Because of the potential for an unrecognized pleural tear, routinely obtaining an upright chest radiograph to look for a pneumothorax in the immediate postoperative period is a safe practice after a costotransversectomy or a lateral extracavitary approach has been performed.

Intercostal Neuralgia

Intercostal neuralgia has been reported infrequently after posterolateral approaches. In cases where the nerve root is transected to provide exposure for the anterior reconstruction of a corpectomy defect through a costotransversectomy or lateral extracavitary approach, neuralgia can be avoided by sectioning the nerve root proximal to the dorsal root ganglion.

Postoperative Instability

Postoperative instability has been reported following posterolateral decompression procedures without arthrodesis. This potential problem can be avoided by performing routine arthrodesis at the level of disk resection when the approach has involved considerable facet or vertebral body resection. This generally is the case in all approaches described, other than a more conservative transpedicular approach. The exposure required to safely complete the decompression procedure generally allows for safe interbody fusion, which can be readily supplemented by posterior instrumentation through these versatile approaches.

Spinal Cord Ischemia

Because of the potential for spinal cord infarction caused by interruption of the radicular arterial blood supply to the spinal cord during a posterolateral decompressive procedure, some authors have advocated the use of preoperative angiography when treating pathology between T8 and L1 to ensure the absence of significant radiculomedullary arterial blood supply coursing through the foramen at the operative level. This is a controversial issue, particularly because no such catastrophic vascular event has been reported in the treatment of thoracic disk disease through a posterolateral approach.

Bibliography

Bilsky MH: Transpedicular approach for thoracic disc herniations. *Neurosurg Focus* 2000;9(4):e3.

Bransford RJ, Zhang F, Bellabarba C, Konodi M, Chapman JR: Early experience treating thoracic disc herniations using a modified transfacet pedicle-sparing decompression and fusion. *J Neurosurg Spine* 2010;12(2):221-231.

Bransford RJ, Zhang F, Bellabarba C, Lee MJ: Treating thoracic disc herniations: Do we always have to go anteriorly? *Evidence Based Spine-Care Journal* 2010;1(1):21-28.

Chen TC: Surgical outcome for thoracic disc surgery in the postlaminectomy era. *Neurosurg Focus* 2000;9(4):e12.

Delfini R, Di Lorenzo N, Ciappetta P, Bristot R, Cantore G: Surgical treatment of thoracic disc herniation: A reappraisal of Larson's lateral extracavitary approach. *Surg Neurol* 1996;45(6):517-523.

Dickman CA, Rosenthal D, Regan JJ: Reoperation for herniated thoracic discs. *J Neurosurg* 1999;91(2, suppl):157-162.

Dietze DD Jr, Fessler RG: Thoracic disc herniations. *Neurosurg Clin N Am* 1993;4(1):75-90.

Dinh DH, Tompkins J, Clark SB: Transcostovertebral approach for thoracic disc herniations. *J Neurosurg* 2001;94 (1, suppl):38-44.

Fessler RG, Sturgill M: Review: Complications of surgery for thoracic disc disease. *Surg Neurol* 1998;49(6):609-618.

Le Roux PD, Haglund MM, Harris AB: Thoracic disc disease: Experience with the transpedicular approach in twenty consecutive patients. *Neurosurgery* 1993;33(1):58-66.

Maiman DJ, Larson SJ, Luck E, El-Ghatit A: Lateral extracavitary approach to the spine for thoracic disc herniation: Report of 23 cases. *Neurosurgery* 1984;14(2):178-182.

McCormick WE, Will SF, Benzel EC: Surgery for thoracic disc disease: Complication avoidance. Overview and management. *Neurosurg Focus* 2000;9(4):e13.

Ridenour TR, Haddad SF, Hitchon PW, Piper J, Traynelis VC, VanGilder JC: Herniated thoracic disks: Treatment and outcome. *J Spinal Disord* 1993;6(3):218-224.

Simpson JM, Silveri CP, Simeone FA, Balderston RA, An HS: Thoracic disc herniation: Re-evaluation of the posterior approach using a modified costotransversectomy. *Spine (Phila Pa 1976)* 1993;18(13):1872-1877.

Singounas EG, Kypriades EM, Kellerman AJ, Garvan N: Thoracic disc herniation: Analysis of 14 cases and review of the literature. *Acta Neurochir (Wien)* 1992;116(1):49-52.

Stillerman CB, Chen TC, Couldwell WT, Zhang W, Weiss MH: Experience in the surgical management of 82 symptomatic herniated thoracic discs and review of the literature. *J Neurosurg* 1998;88(4):623-633.

Coding

CPT Codes		Corresponding ICD-9 Codes	
22532	Arthrodesis, lateral extracavitary technique, including minimal discectomy to prepare interspace (other than for decompression); thoracic	721.1 722.51 805.2	721.41 733.13 806.21
22534	Arthrodesis, lateral extracavitary technique, including minimal discectomy to prepare interspace (other than for decompression); thoracic or lumbar, each additional vertebral segment (List separately in addition to code for primary procedure)	733.13 805.4	805.2
22842	Posterior segmental instrumentation (eg, pedicle fixation, dual rods with multiple hooks and sublaminar wires); 3 to 6 vertebral segments (List separately in addition to code for primary procedure)	342.1 342.90 343.0	342.9 343 343.1
22843	Posterior segmental instrumentation (eg, pedicle fixation, dual rods with multiple hooks and sublaminar wires); 7 to 12 vertebral segments (List separately in addition to code for primary procedure)	170.2 342.9 343	342.1 342.90 343.0
22844	Posterior segmental instrumentation (eg, pedicle fixation, dual rods with multiple hooks and sublaminar wires); 13 or more vertebral segments (List separately in addition to code for primary procedure)	170.2 342.9 343	342.1 342.90 343.0
63055	Transpedicular approach with decompression of spinal cord, equina and/or nerve root(s) (eg, herniated intervertebral disc), single segment; thoracic	722.11 722.72	722.51
63057	Transpedicular approach with decompression of spinal cord, equina and/or nerve root(s) (eg, herniated intervertebral disc), single segment; each additional segment, thoracic or lumbar (List separately in addition to code for primary procedure)	722.11 722.52 723.0	722.51 722.72 724.02
63064	Costovertebral approach with decompression of spinal cord or nerve root(s) (eg, herniated intervertebral disc), thoracic; single segment	722.11	722.72
63066	Costovertebral approach with decompression of spinal cord or nerve root(s) (eg, herniated intervertebral disc), thoracic; each additional segment (List separately in addition to code for primary procedure)	722.11 723.0	722.72
63101	Vertebral corpectomy (vertebral body resection), partial or complete, lateral extracavitary approach with decompression of spinal cord and/or nerve root(s) (eg, for tumor or retropulsed bone fragments); thoracic, single sgement	170.2 806.21 806.23	806.20 806.22 806.24
63103	Vertebral corpectomy (vertebral body resection), partial or complete, lateral extracavitary approach with decompression of spinal cord and/or nerve root(s) (eg, for tumor or retropulsed bone fragments); thoracic or lumbar, each additional segment (List separately in addition to code for primary procedure)	733.13 805.4	805.2

CPT copyright © 2010 by the American Medical Association. All rights reserved.

Chapter 26

The Costotransversectomy Approach for Vertebrectomy

Michael D. Daubs, MD
Michael L. Fernandez, MD

Indications

A costotransversectomy approach allows nearly circumferential access to the anterior thoracic spine. Complete decompression of the neural elements, reconstruction, and stabilization of the anterior column are possible with this approach, which is suitable for all levels of the thoracic spine and can be used for several spinal conditions, including thoracic disk herniations, fractures, tumor, infection, and deformity. It offers many advantages over the anterior approach, especially in the cervicothoracic junction and the upper thoracic spine, where the anterior approach can be technically difficult. In most of the destabilizing conditions of the thoracic spine, kyphosis (a collapsed vertebral segment) is a major issue. When approached anteriorly, the apex of the kyphosis is located deep in the wound, where direct visualization can be difficult. If approached posteriorly, through the costotransversectomy approach, the apex of the kyphosis is directed posteriorly, in the same direction as the approach, which makes it

more easily visualized and decompressed away from the spinal cord.

Although this approach is a major reconstruction procedure with its own inherent risks, it may be tolerated better than a traditional transthoracic approach in patients with significant cardiopulmonary conditions. It also has the benefit of being a single-stage procedure, in which both decompression and stabilization can be performed simultaneously through one approach. In addition, it does not require the added expertise of an approach surgeon.

Contraindications

The costotransversectomy vertebrectomy is a complex spinal reconstructive surgery in which significant blood loss can occur. Patients with severe comorbidities may not be able to tolerate the procedure. A relative contraindication to this approach is a central lesion (tumor, fracture fragments, abscess) that causes narrow, focal, ventral cord compression. The com-

pressing anterior lesion can be difficult to visualize posteriorly around the thecal sac. A direct anterior approach may be better indicated in this scenario.

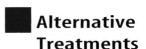

Alternative Treatments

A thoracic vertebrectomy through an open transthoracic or thoracoscopic approach followed by posterior instrumentation and stabilization, when indicated, has been the traditional approach for many thoracic conditions and remains a viable and safe alternative. Depending on the community standards and the expertise of the primary surgeon, this approach may require the additional skills of an approach surgeon.

Results

Although very few studies have specifically evaluated the performance and outcomes of a total thoracic vertebrectomy through a costotransversectomy approach, several studies have described using this approach in addressing various spinal pathologies.

Dr. Daubs or an immediate family member serves as a paid consultant to or is an employee of Synthes and has received research or institutional support from Stryker. Dr. Fernandez or an immediate family member has received research or institutional support from AO and DePuy.

Table 1 Results of Thoracic Spine Procedures Through a Costotransversectomy Approach

Authors (Year)	Number of Patients	Approach	Mean Patient Age in Years (Range)	Mean Follow-up in Months (Range)	Fusion Success Rate	Results
Smith et al (2005)	16	Costotransversectomy	12 (4-16)	60.1 (24-144)	81.3%	13 satisfactory 2 fair 1 poor
Jain et al (2007)	16 (9 pts >1 yr follow-up)	Costotransversectomy	15.6 (3-38)	13.2 (3-36)	100% in 9 pts at 1-year follow-up	Mean kyphosis correction: 27.3°
Wong et al (2007)	5 (4 pts >7 years follow-up)*	Modified costotransversectomy	53.2 (42-60)	105 (84-120)	100% in 4 pts at follow-up	2 patients with neurologic improvement No neurologic deterioration
Abdullah et al (2008)	1	Costotransversectomy	56	1.5	NR	"Good"
Jain et al (2008)	2	Costotransversectomy	58 (57-59)	28 (27-29)	NR	Patients returned to full activities
Kamat et al (2008)	8	Transpedicular, unilateral/bilateral	51 (25-74)	(6-27)	NR	At follow-up, 7 patients without symptoms†

NR = not reported.
* 1 patient died 5 months postoperatively, secondary to chest infection (excluded). Remaining 4 patients had >7 yrs follow-up.
† 1 patient died from progression of neoplastic process.

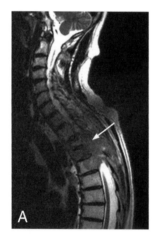 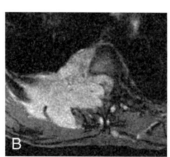 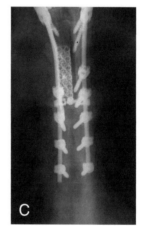 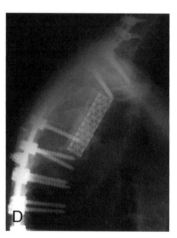

Figure 1 Images of a patient with metastatic lung adenocarcinoma invading T3, T4, and T5. **A,** Sagittal MRI demonstrates the pathology (arrow). **B,** Axial MRI shows invasion of the tumor into the thoracic spinal canal. AP (**C**) and lateral (**D**) radiographs obtained following a debulking of the tumor through a costotransversectomy approach with vertebrectomy of T3, T4, and T5, thoracic pedicle screw instrumentation, cervical lateral mass fixation, and anterior column reconstruction with a methylmethacrylate-reinforced titanium mesh cage.

The results of these studies vary, depending on the underlying pathology and the indication for the costotransversectomy. The successful resection of solitary and multiple upper thoracic malignant tumors, osteomyelitis, spinal tuberculosis, and kyphotic deformities has been reported by several authors (**Table 1**). Overall, the results are good, with noted advantages, especially in the upper thoracic spine, where anterior approaches can be more difficult (**Figure 1**). Eliminating the need for both an anterior and a posterior approach in cases that require posterior fixation also is an advantage.

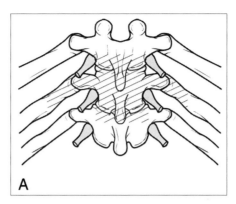

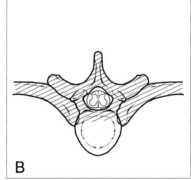

A   B

Figure 2 Illustrations show posterior (**A**) and axial (**B**) views of the thoracic spine. Shaded areas indicate areas of bone that are resected during the costotransversectomy approach.

■ Technique

Setup/Exposure

The patient is placed prone on a radiolucent Jackson table. The table should allow 360° fluoroscopic exposure of the spine. The table also should allow rotation to "airplane" the patient from the left and right so visualization can be facilitated as needed. The cervical spine is stabilized with three-point Mayfield tongs or Gardner-Wells tongs with 10 to15 lb of traction. The patient's arms are well padded. The arms are tucked at the side for a vertebrectomy in the upper thoracic spine; they are placed in the 90/90 position for a procedure in the mid and lower thoracic spine. Intraoperative neurologic monitoring is recommended. Autologous blood salvage with a cell saver device is used in the setting of trauma and deformity correction.

A midline incision is performed through the skin and subcutaneous tissue to the spinous processes and posterior fascia. Using the standard posterior approach to the thoracic spine, the paraspinal muscles are dissected subperiosteally away from the midline, exposing the lamina and transverse processes. At the level of the planned vertebrectomy, the rib is exposed posteriorly and laterally approximately 5 cm.

Instruments/Equipment/ Implants Required

Pedicle screw fixation typically is used, but thoracic hook instrumentation can be equally effective. Kerrison, pituitary, and large bone rongeurs are required. Long-handled small, medium, and large curets (anterior spine instruments) are helpful for resecting disk and bone fragments. Depending on surgeon comfort, a high-speed burr also can be used for bone resection.

Thin-blade, footed impactors aid in the final removal of the posterior wall of the vertebral body. Rib dissectors and a rib cutter are used for the partial rib resection. Reconstruction of the resected vertebral body requires a large structural autograft or allograft segment (femur, humerus, or multiple fibulas), a mesh titanium or polyetheretherketone cage, or an expandable cage. In a patient with a malignant tumor resection in whom life expectancy is limited, polymethylmethacrylate also may be used for structural support. A surgeon headlamp is very helpful for illumination during the vertebral body resection.

Procedure

Following the initial exposure, posterior thoracic pedicle screws are placed using the freehand technique. Pedicle screw position is confirmed with plain radiographic or fluoroscopic imaging. The planned area of bone resection is shown in **Figure 2**. A wide, complete laminectomy is performed using a high-speed burr for initial thinning of the lamina and a Kerrison rongeur for completion. The transverse processes and ribs are dissected circumferentially with a small curved curet, periosteal dissector, or rib dissector. The pleura is carefully dissected ventrally, away from the rib. The rib is cut 4 to 5 cm lateral from the costovertebral joint using a rib cutter or high-speed

burr. The rib is dissected from the costovertebral joint attachment using curets and cautery and removed en bloc. Removal of the rib and transverse process allows access to the lateral vertebral wall (**Figure 3**, *A*). With the pleura carefully dissected away, the vertebral wall is dissected subperiosteally to the anterior wall of the vertebral body, using a small Cobb elevator or periosteal dissector. A small, malleable retractor is placed anteriorly along the vertebral body to retract and protect the pleura and vascular structures (**Figure 3**, *B*). At this point in the procedure, the dura is widely exposed, and the lamina, pars interarticularis, and facet joints have been removed. The thoracic pedicle is intact and the thoracic nerve roots are exposed. The thoracic nerve roots are tied off with No. 2-0 silk sutures placed proximal and distal to the dorsal root ganglion (DRG) and resected with a No. 15 scalpel distal to the DRG. This allows full access to the lateral vertebral body and the cranial and caudal disk space. The disk is incised with a No. 10 scalpel. Pituitary rongeurs and curets are used to excise the disk.

Vertebral body resection is begun by removing the lateral wall of the pedicle and proceeds ventromedially into the vertebral body. A high-speed burr is used to take down the lateral cortical vertebral wall and cancellous body (**Figure 4**). Long anterior instru-

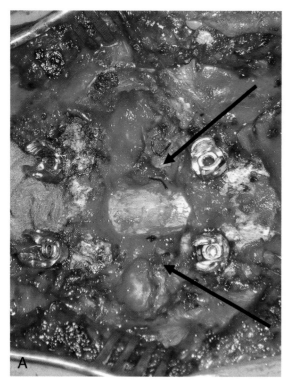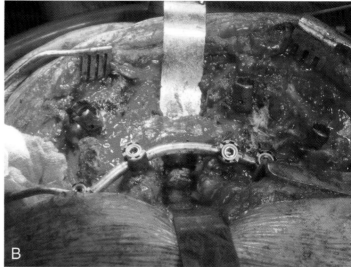

Figure 3 Intraoperative photographs show surgical steps in preparation for vertebrectomy. The patient's head is to the right. **A,** The thoracic spine is shown following a complete laminectomy and resection of the facets, pars interarticularis, transverse process, and rib. The thoracic nerve roots have been resected and tied off (arrows). **B,** Malleable retractors are placed anteriorly around the vertebral body to protect the anterior vascular structures during the vertebrectomy. A temporary rod also has been inserted for temporary stabilization.

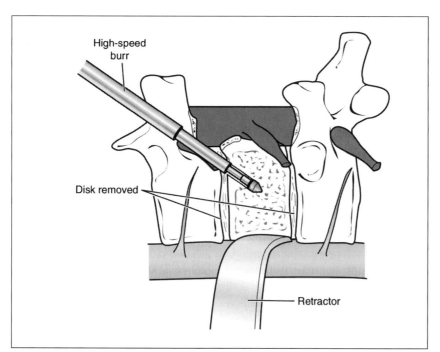

Figure 4 Illustration shows a high-speed burr removing cortical bone from the lateral vertebral wall during the initial steps of the vertebrectomy.

ments that typically are used in anterior thoracic and lumbar procedures (angled and straight curets and large pituitary rongeurs or bone biters) are helpful during the disk and vertebral body resection to ensure good control and leverage (**Figure 5,** *A*).

The dissection above is performed bilaterally. Working on one side while the contralateral side is packed off with large cottonoids and a viscous hemostatic solution helps reduce blood loss. As the vertebral body resection proceeds from each side toward the midline, a cavity is eventually created with a thin anterior and posterior wall remaining. It is important to place a temporary rod in position before the final resection of the anterior and posterior wall, or sooner, depending on the stability of the vertebral body, to prevent sudden collapse of the vertebral body and potential neurologic injury. The anterior

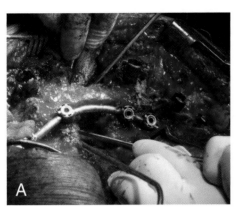
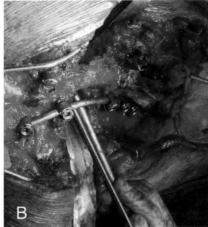
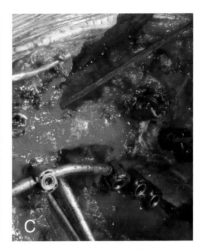

Figure 5 Intraoperative photographs show further bone removal during vertebrectomy. The patient's head is to the right. **A,** Resection of cancellous bone from the vertebral body with a long-handled curet. The vertebral body is almost completely removed. The thecal sac is untouched while the decompression is performed, as a result of the wide exposure. Note the temporary rod that has been placed to prevent translation across the vertebrectomy site. A high-speed burr is used to remove the remaining cancellous bone (**B**) and thin the cortical walls (**C**).

wall can be resected completely by using the high-speed burr to thin the cortical surface down to the anterior longitudinal ligament (ALL), or via initial thinning with the burr followed by complete resection using a Kerrison ronguer. The malleable retractors should be positioned anterior to the ALL to protect the anterior vascular structures. The posterior wall is excised by a gradual thinning that is performed from the anterior side. Curets or a high-speed burr can be used to perform the thinning (**Figure 5,** *B* and *C*). Tilting the table slightly away from the side on which the surgeon is working can aid in visualizing the posterior wall during the resection. A flat-footed Woodson dural dissector is used to palpate the posterior wall and develop an interval between the ventral surface of the dura, the posterior longitudinal ligament (PLL), and the posterior wall. When the posterior wall has been thinned adequately, a footed impactor is used to tamp down the wall into the vertebral body cavity (**Figure 6**). The remnants of the posterior wall, which can be at the far cranial and caudal ends, can be excised with Kerrison rongeurs as needed.

Once the vertebral body, including the posterior wall, has been removed,

the initial correction of deformity is performed with in situ bending of the rods (**Figure 7**). Then an intervertebral support device (eg, mesh cage, expandable cages, PMMA cement block, allograft or autograft strut) can be placed. Placing the cage into the interbody space at this point prevents potential overshortening of the posterior column and spinal cord. Expandable cages have an advantage because they can be inserted in the contracted position when they are small and then expanded as needed if further correction is achieved with the sagittal in situ benders (**Figure 8**). The space available to insert the devices from the posterolateral position is limited. If an expandable cage is not available, distraction can be performed through the pedicle screws to allow insertion, followed by compression to help lock in the device. The bone-screw interface must be monitored closely during compressive or distractive maneuvers to avoid loss of fixation. Bone graft and bone graft substitutes may be placed in and around the cage to promote bony fusion (**Figure 9**).

Wound Closure

Wound closure is performed following thorough irrigation. The wound is

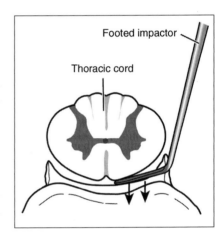

Figure 6 Illustration shows a footed impactor with a thin blade inserted between the dura and the posterior wall. Ventral manual pressure or mallet impaction is used to collapse the posterior vertebral wall into the vertebrectomy cavity.

closed in layers. First, the posterior fascia is closed with heavy suture material (No. 1 absorbable braided suture). Next, the subcutaneous layer is closed with a No. 2-0 absorbable braided suture. The skin is closed with either a running No. 3-0 absorbable monofilament suture or No. 3-0 nylon. Depending on the pathology, a drain (either above or below the fascia) may be used. A drain is highly recommended for this procedure to

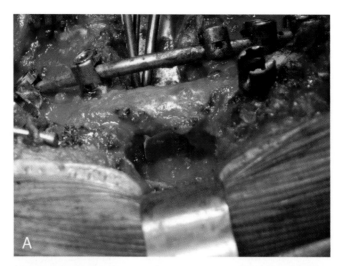

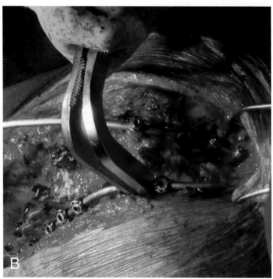

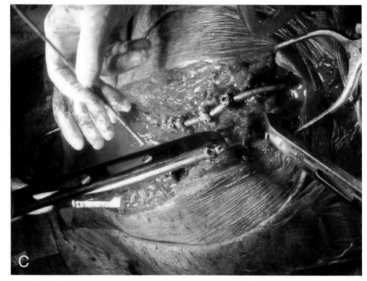

Figure 7 Intraoperative photographs demonstrate initial correction of deformity. The patient's head is to the right. **A,** The vertebral body, including the posterior wall, has been removed. **B,** Coronal benders are used to correct the deformity in the coronal plane. **C,** Sagittal benders are used to correct the sagittal plane deformity.

help prevent the formation of a hematoma, which can drain into or around the pleural space.

Postoperative Regimen

Patients routinely are placed in the surgical intensive care unit or intermediate care unit overnight and transferred to a floor unit as soon as they are deemed stable. Patients are mobi-

lized on postoperative day 1. Routine chest radiographs should be performed postoperatively in the recovery room, on postoperative day 1, and as indicated thereafter to evaluate for pneumothorax or pleural effusion. Chest tube placement may be necessary if a large pleural effusion or pneumothorax develops. Patients are encouraged to be as active as possible but should avoid heavy lifting, twisting, or bending at the waist. External bracing is not used routinely. Patients are discharged on average 5 to 7 days after

surgery, when their pain is well controlled with oral medication and physical therapy deems the patient safe for independent ambulation.

Avoiding Pitfalls and Complications

Thoracic costotransversectomy vertebrectomy is a highly technical procedure that requires a significant amount of preoperative planning. A

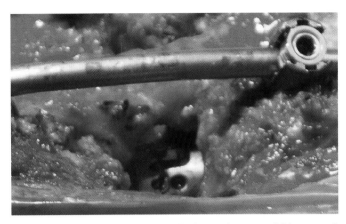

Figure 8 Intraoperative photograph shows the expandable cage after placement in the vertebral body defect. (The patient's head is to the right.) The cage is expanded to touch the end plate of the cranial and caudal vertebral body. As the kyphotic deformity is corrected with in situ bending in the sagittal plane, the cage is gradually expanded to fill the defect.

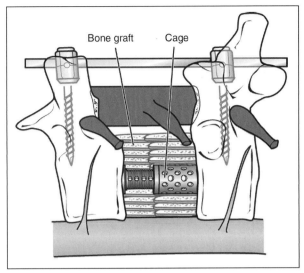

Figure 9 Illustration shows reconstruction of the anterior column with an expandable titanium cage.

thorough review of the preoperative CT and MRI images is necessary to discern the extent of the pathology and its involvement with surrounding soft-tissue structures. The approach is circumferential, although it is started posteriorly. Most spine surgeons are familiar with the posterior approach, and this familiarity is an advantage when gaining experience with this procedure.

The major pitfalls to avoid are neurologic injury, blood loss, and pleural tears. Neurologic injury is best prevented by using neurologic monitoring, maintaining normotensive blood pressure, performing a wide laminectomy and decompression to avoid any unnecessary thecal sac retraction, using a temporary rod to stabilize the spine as the decompression progresses, and carefully removing the posterior wall with controlled posterior-to-anterior impaction. Extensive blood loss can be avoided through careful subperiosteal dissection, especially laterally, where the segmental vessels arise. The segmentals can be dissected laterally and retracted with the periosteum. If the vessels do bleed, they should be identified early and clipped or tied off. Constant packing with a liquid hemostatic agent and large, wide cottonoids or lap sponges also is helpful during the vertebrectomy. Careful technique with a curet or rib dissector while clearing the pleura from around the rib and slow dissection along the lateral vertebral wall should be used to avoid entering the pleural cavity. If tearing does occur, the tear can be closed with a No. 2-0 absorbable braided suture placed around a red rubber catheter attached to a large syringe. As the purse-string closure is tightened, the syringe is used to remove air from the pleural cavity to avoid a pneumothorax. If a pneumothorax does develop, a chest tube will be necessary. Patients should be warned of this possibility preoperatively. Pleural effusions also can develop. If no respiratory compromise or distress is present, pleural effusions can be managed nonsurgically. If they are large, however, chest tube insertion may be required. Postoperative chest radiographs should be performed routinely, especially if any signs of respiratory distress are present.

■

Bibliography

Abdullah SH, Ata OA, El-Adwan N: Thoracic spinal epidural abscess caused by Salmonella typhi. *Neurol Med Chir (Tokyo)* 2008;48(3):140-142.

Fessler RG, Sturgill M: Review: Complications of surgery for thoracic disc disease. *Surg Neurol* 1998;49(6):609-618.

Jain AK, Maheshwari AV, Jena S: Kyphus correction in spinal tuberculosis. *Clin Orthop Relat Res* 2007;460:117-123.

Jain S, Sommers E, Setzer M, Vrionis F: Posterior midline approach for single-stage en bloc resection and circumferential spinal stabilization for locally advanced Pancoast tumors: Technical note. *J Neurosurg Spine* 2008;9(1):71-82.

Kamat A, Gilkes C, Barua NU, Patel NR: Single-stage posterior transpedicular approach for circumferential epidural decompression and three-column stabilization using a titanium cage for upper thoracic spine neoplastic disease: A case series and technical note. *Br J Neurosurg* 2008;22(1):92-98.

Sciubba DM, Gallia GL, McGirt MJ, et al: Thoracic kyphotic deformity reduction with a distractible titanium cage via an entirely posterior approach. *Neurosurgery* 2007;60(4 Suppl 2):223-231.

Smith JT, Gollogly S, Dunn HK: Simultaneous anterior-posterior approach through a costotransversectomy for the treatment of congenital kyphosis and acquired kyphoscoliotic deformities. *J Bone Joint Surg Am* 2005;87(10):2281-2289.

Wong YW, Leong JC, Luk KD: Direct internal kyphectomy for severe angular tuberculous kyphosis. *Clin Orthop Relat Res* 2007;460:124-129.

Coding

CPT Codes		Corresponding ICD-9 Codes	
20931	Allograft, structural, for spine surgery only (List separately in addition to code for primary procedure)	170.2 733.13	724.6 733.81
22532	Arthrodesis, lateral extracavitary technique, including minimal discectomy to prepare interspace (other than for decompression); thoracic	721.2 722.51 805.2	721.41 733.13 806.21
22534	Arthrodesis, lateral extracavitary technique, including minimal discectomy to prepare interspace (other than for decompression); thoracic or lumbar, each additional vertebral segment (List separately in addition to code for primary procedure)	733.13 805.4	805.2
22610	Arthrodesis, posterior or posterolateral technique, single level; thoracic (with or without lateral transverse technique)	170.2 738.4 806.20	737.39 756.12 806.21
22614	Arthrodesis, posterior or posterolateral technique, single level; each additional vertebral segment (List separately in addition to code for primary procedure)	170.2 722.52 737.39	722.10 724.02 738.4
22840	Posterior non-segmental instrumentation (eg, Harrington rod technique, pedicle fixation across one interspace, atlantoaxial transarticular screw fixation, sublaminar wiring at C1, facet screw fixation) (List separately in addition to code for primary procedure)	170.2 342.9 343	342.1 342.90 343.0
22841	Internal spinal fixation by wiring of spinous processes (List separately in addition to code for primary procedure)	170.2 342.9 343	342.1 342.90 343.0
22842	Posterior segmental instrumentation (eg, pedicle fixation, dual rods with multiple hooks and sublaminar wires); 3 to 6 vertebral segments (List separately in addition to code for primary procedure)	342.1 342.90 343.0	342.9 343 343.1

Lagrone MO, Bradford DS, Moe JH, Lonstein JE, Winter RB, Ogilvie JW: Treatment of symptomatic flatback after spinal fusion. *J Bone Joint Surg Am* 1988;70(4):569-580.

Alexander WA: Lumbar spinal osteotomy. *J Bone Joint Surg Br* 1959;41-B(2):270-278.

Lichtblau PO, Wilson PD: Possible mechanism of aortic rupture in orthopaedic correction of rheumatoid spondylitis. *J Bone Joint Surg Am* 1956;38-A(1):123-127.

McMaster MJ: A technique for lumbar spinal osteotomy in ankylosing spondylitis. *J Bone Joint Surg Br* 1985;67(2): 204-210.

Ponte A: Posterior column shortening for Scheuermann's kyphosis: An innovative one-stage technique, in Haher TR, Merola AA, eds: *Surgical Techniques for the Spine*. New York, NY, Thieme Verlag, 2003, pp 107-113.

Ponte A, Vero B, Siccardi GL: Surgical treatment of Scheuermann's hyperkyphosis, in Winter RB, ed: *Progress in Spinal Pathology: Kyphosis*. Bologna, Italy, Aulo Gaggi, 1984, pp 75-80.

Simmons EH: Kyphotic deformity of the spine in ankylosing spondylitis. *Clin Orthop Relat Res* 1977;128:65-77.

Smith-Petersen MN, Larson CB, Aufranc OE: Osteotomy of the spine for correction of flexion deformity in rheumatoid arthritis. *Clin Orthop Relat Res* 1969;66:6-9.

van Royen BJ, de Kleuver M, Slot GH: Polysegmental lumbar posterior wedge osteotomies for correction of kyphosis in ankylosing spondylitis. *Eur Spine J* 1998;7(2):104-110.

Coding

CPT Codes		Corresponding ICD-9 Codes	
22212	Osteotomy of spine, posterior or posterolateral approach, one vertebral segment; thoracic	737.10 737.40	737.41
22216	Osteotomy of spine, posterior or posterolateral approach, one vertebral segment; each additional vertebral segment (List separately in addition to primary procedure)	737.10 737.40	737.41
20900	Bone graft, any donor area; minor or small (eg, dowel or button)	715	733
20902	Bone graft, any donor area; major or large	715	733
20903	Allograft for spine surgery only; morselized (List separately in addition to code for primary procedure)	721.1 723	722 724.6
20931	Allograft for spine surgery only; structural (List separately in addition to code for primary procedure)	721.1 723.0	722 724.6
20936	Autograft for spine surgery only (includes harvesting the graft); local (eg, ribs, spinous process, or laminar fragments) obtained from same incision (List separately in addition to code for primary procedure)	724.6	722
20937	Autograft for spine surgery only (includes harvesting the graft); morselized (through separate skin or fascial incision) (List separately in addition to code for primary procedure)	724.6	722
20938	Autograft for spine surgery only (includes harvesting the graft); structural, bicortical or tricortical (through separate skin or fascial incision) (List separately in addition to code for primary procedure)	724.6 721.1	722
22800	Arthrodesis, posterior, for spinal deformity, with or without cast; up to 6 vertebral segments	342.1 342.90 343.0	342.9 343 343.1
22802	Arthrodesis, posterior, for spinal deformity, with or without cast; 7 to 12 vertebral segments	342.1 342.90 343.0	342.9 343 343.1
22804	Arthrodesis, posterior, for spinal deformity, with or without cast; 13 or more vertebral segments	342.1 342.90 343.0	342.9 343 343.1
22808	Arthrodesis, anterior, for spinal deformity, with or without cast; 2 to 3 vertebral segments	342.1 342.90 343.0	342.9 343 343.1
22810	Arthrodesis, anterior, for spinal deformity, with or without cast; 2 to 3 vertebral segments	342.1 342.90 343.0	342.9 343 343.1
22812	Arthrodesis, anterior, for spinal deformity, with or without cast; 8 or more vertebral segments	342.1 342.90 343.0	342.9 343 343.1
22840	Posterior non-segmental instrumentation (eg, Harrington rod technique, pedicle fixation across one interspace, atlantoaxial transarticular screw fixation, sublaminar wiring at C1, facet screw fixation) (List separately in addition to code for primary procedure)	722.52 737.30	724.6
22842	Posterior segmental instrumentation (eg, pedicle fixation, dual rods with multiple hooks and sublaminar wires); 3 to 6 vertebral segments (List separately in addition to code for primary procedure)	722.52 737.30	724.6

CPT Codes		Corresponding ICD-9 Codes	
	Coding (continued)		
22843	Posterior segmental instrumentation (eg, pedicle fixation, dual rods with multiple hooks and sublaminar wires); 7 to 12 vertebral segments (List separately in addition to code for primary procedure)	722.52 737.30	724.6
22844	Posterior segmental instrumentation (eg, pedicle fixation, dual rods with multiple hooks and sublaminar wires); 13 or more vertebral segments (List separately in addition to code for primary procedure)	722.25 737.30	724.6
22851	Application of intervertebral biomechanical device(s) (eg, synthetic cage(s), threaded bone dowel(s), methylmethacrylate) to vertebral defect or interspace (List separately in addition to code for primary procedure)	722.52 721.1	724.6

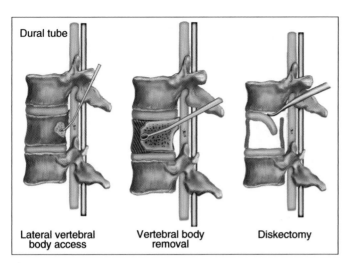

Figure 3 Illustration depicts vertebral body corpectomy and diskectomy. Decancellation begins with the lateral vertebral body and then proceeds through the entire cancellous channel of the body, leaving a thin rim of the anterior as well as posterior body wall. Diskectomies are then performed both above and below the vertebral excision.

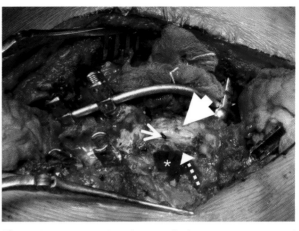

Figure 4 Intraoperative photograph demonstrates near-total decancellation of the T12 vertebral body (asterisk). A thin rim of the posterior body wall is marked by the dashed arrow. The T12 nerve root on the right was ligated and divided (small arrow). The large arrow marks the dural sac.

the thoracic spine than when performing similar procedures in the lumbar spine. For a scoliotic or kyphoscoliotic deformity, resecting the apical concave pedicle can be quite challenging because it is very cortical. In a pure scoliotic deformity, the entire spinal cord/dural sac is resting on the medial concave pedicle, which does not have any anterior vertebral body associated with it as the body is swung lateral and posterior in its rotated position on the convexity. As previously discussed, using a small, high-speed drill is helpful to carefully burr away the cortical bone along this concave region. Thus, in scoliosis and kyphoscoliosis deformities, the majority of the vertebral body will be removed from the convexity of the deformity because that is where the vertebral body is located. We prefer to perform the concave resection of the pedicle before the convex removal so as to minimize bleeding into this dependent concave region. This also allows the concave spinal cord to transpose somewhat more medially and remove tension before going to the convexity for completion of the corpectomy. The entire body is removed except for the ante-

rior shell, as we like to keep a thin rim of bone intact on the anterior longitudinal ligament for fusion purposes. If this anterior bone is thick and cortical, then it must be thinned to allow easy closure of the resection area (**Figure 4**).

Thoracic diskectomies are completed above and below the resected body to expose the adjacent vertebral body end plates. As with any corpectomy, care should be taken to avoid violating the adjacent end plates (**Figure 3**). Overly aggressive diskectomies and end-plate disruption can lead to interbody cage subsidence and loss of correction.

The final aspect of the vertebral resection before correction is removal of the posterior vertebral body wall. The dura must be circumferentially inspected and freed of any attachments, which would include the anterior epidural venous plexus, the posterior longitudinal ligament, or osteophytes that typically arise at the bone-disk interface. The dissection in the anterior spinal canal between the dura and the posterior vertebral wall can cause significant blood loss. Epidural bleeding can be controlled with bipolar cautery

and/or a combination of topical hemostatic agents. Once the dura is completely freed from any anterior connection, the eggshell-thin posterior vertebral body wall can be tamped away from the spinal cord into the corpectomy defect with reverse-angled curets, spondylophyte impactors, Woodson elevators, or a specialized posterior wall impactor (**Figure 5, A**). Deliberate dural inspection should follow the removal of the posterior vertebral body; if any points of compression or attachment are found, they should be removed.

At this point, the resection is complete and closure of the defect and deformity correction can take place via compression (**Figure 5, B**). The spinal column is always shortened, not lengthened, with convex compression as the initial and primary correcting technique. Again, before and throughout closure, the surgeon should circumferentially inspect the dura and anticipate any potential points of compression, addressing them before and during reduction.

Correction typically is performed either with pedicle screws directly, in primary cases where a good bony grip

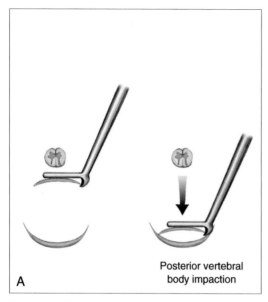

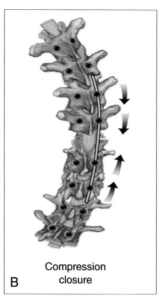

Figure 5 Illustrations show impaction of the posterior wall of the vertebral body into the defect created using a specialized posterior vertebral body impaction device (**A**) and correction of the deformity using compression (**B**).

of the vertebrae is found, or in a construct-to-construct closure mechanism, using dominoes at the apex of the resection area. In this method, closing is performed from a construct rod above to a construct rod below to distribute the forces of correction over several pedicle screw levels. It is imperative to compress slowly, as subluxation and/or dural impingement can occur along the way. In any deformity that has a degree of kyphosis, we recommend placing an anterior structural cage once the spine has been corrected between 50% and 75% to prevent overshortening of the deformity (**Figure 6**). The interbody device also acts as a hinge to provide further kyphosis correction. Typically, the spinal column will be shortened by 1 to 1.5 cm. A cage of appropriate height and

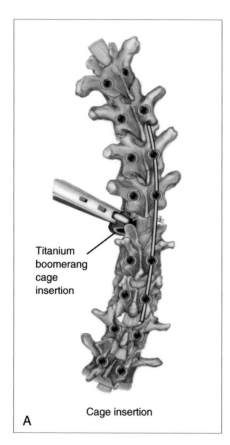

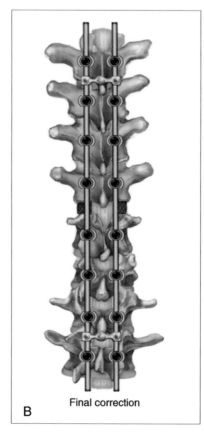

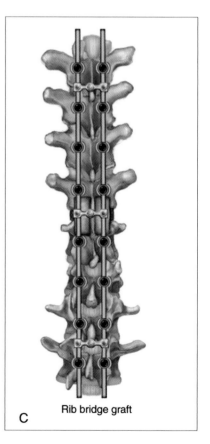

Figure 6 Following approximately 50% to 75% closure, a cage or structural bone graft is templated and placed anteriorly into the anterior column defect. Final correction is performed with the cage to lock it in place anteriorly. Temporary rods are replaced by permanent rods, and then the ribs previously excised are bivalved and then placed, cancellous surface down, from the lamina above to the lamina below to cover the laminectomy defect once complete freedom of the dura is confirmed circumferentially.

length is then inserted, and further closure and compression on the cage is performed as a final correction maneuver (**Figure 7**, *A*). Once closure of the VCR has been completed, a permanent contralateral rod is placed. The temporary closing rod is removed and a permanent, final rod is placed on the ipsilateral side. Appropriate compression and distraction forces, in situ contouring, and other correction techniques may be performed, always being mindful of any resultant effect on the resected area and spinal cord with respect to subluxation, dural impingement, or unloading of the anterior interbody cage. Alignment is confirmed by intraoperative radiographs once reduction is complete and final circumferential dural inspection is performed to confirm a capacious spinal canal and dura that is free of impingement. If the spinal alignment is satisfactory, split-thickness rib autograft is placed over the laminectomy defect and secured to the rods using sutures or a cross-link (**Figure 6**). When placing the rib struts, care must be taken not to induce any spinal cord compression in the region of the osteotomy where the dura is already redundant from the closure (**Figure 7**, *B*).

Wound Closure

After completing the final inspection of the dura and instrumentation, the wound is irrigated with saline. The posterior spine and facet joints are decorticated with a high-speed burr, and a copious amount of locally harvested bone graft is placed. Subfascial and suprafascial hemovac drains are brought out through separate stab incisions and the wound is closed in layers with interrupted absorbable su-

tures. The skin is reapproximated and sterile dressings are applied.

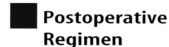

Postoperative Regimen

Once closure is completed, the patient is turned supine on the bed and allowed to emerge from anesthesia for an appropriate wake-up test before leaving the operating room. The patient is monitored in the intensive care unit for at least 24 hours. Most patients sit on the side of the bed on postoperative day 1, and they are encouraged to get out of bed into a chair by postoperative day 2. Patients are started on a diet of ice chips and advanced as tolerated with the return of bowel function. If a patient is found to have soft bone at the time of surgery or required cervicothoracic fusion, a custom brace is used for 3 months.

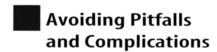

Avoiding Pitfalls and Complications

Posterior thoracic VCR is a highly technical, demanding procedure even in the most experienced hands. We recommend the use of multimodality neurophysiologic monitoring that includes motor-tract monitoring. In our experience, patients who lose NMEP data do so most commonly during the actual spinal shortening and correction. Another common reason for lost NMEP data has been spinal subluxation, which can occur before, during, or even after the corrective procedure.

The spine is rendered extremely unstable during this posterior reconstruction, and thus it is imperative to regain primary stability with a dural sac that is free from compression and not excessively shortened anteriorly (during kyphotic reconstructions). Restoring appropriate anterior height via a larger anterior cage has restored the lost NMEP data. To date, we have not had a patient who was normal neurologically before the procedure suffer a spinal cord deficit following a posterior thoracic VCR.

We feel strongly about the importance of maintaining normotensive anesthesia during correction and closure of these deformities. A mean arterial pressure of at least 75 to 80 mm Hg during this time is recommended. Occasionally, this will require the adjunctive use of dopamine as a low-dose inotrope. Often blood products will be given even if the hematocrit seems adequate, because a fair amount of hemodilution occurs over the course of these procedures, depending on the amount of fluids provided by anesthesia.

When performed as described, a posterior thoracic VCR allows for complete resection of all vertebral elements, including 360° neural decompression, and provides for simultaneous control of the spinal column. This technically demanding yet powerful procedure can result in dramatic radiographic and clinical correction of severe spinal deformities (**Figures 8** and **9**). It has replaced separate anterior and posterior approaches for all of our pediatric and adult patients with severe spinal deformities.

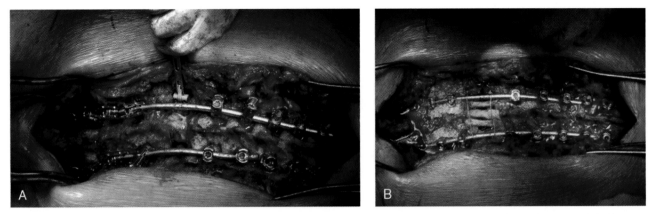

Figure 7 Intraoperative photographs show final correction and grafting. **A,** Placement of the titanium cage from the patient's left after 75% closure of the osteotomy. Note the use of bilateral rods during partial reduction and the improvement in kyphosis. **B,** After circumferential dural inspection, the previously harvested rib grafts are placed from the lamina above to the lamina below to cover the laminectomy defect.

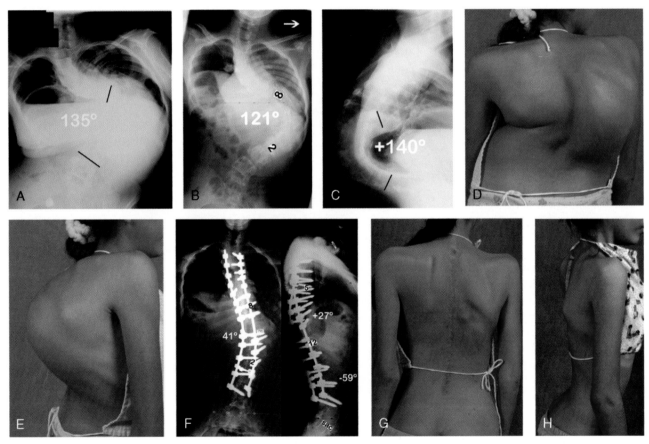

Figure 8 Severe idiopathic kyphoscoliosis in an 18-year-old girl. Preoperative AP (**A**) and side-bending AP (**B**) and lateral (**C**) radiographs and clinical photographs taken from the back (**D**) and side (**E**) of the patient depict 135° of coronal plane deformity, which side-bent to only 121°, and 140° of thoracic kyphosis, creating a combined 275° of biplanar deformity. The patient was treated with preoperative halo-gravity traction, then a single-level T11 posterior vertebral column resection. **F,** Postoperative AP and lateral radiographs show correction in the coronal plane to 41° and in the sagittal plane to 27°. Postoperative clinical photographs demonstrate the marked correction of the severe truncal deformity, as seen from the back (**G**) and side (**H**). (Reproduced with permission from Lenke LG, Sides BA, Koester LA, Hensley M, Blanke KM: Vertebral column resection for the treatment of severe spinal deformity. *Clin Orthop Relat Res* 2010;468:687-699.)

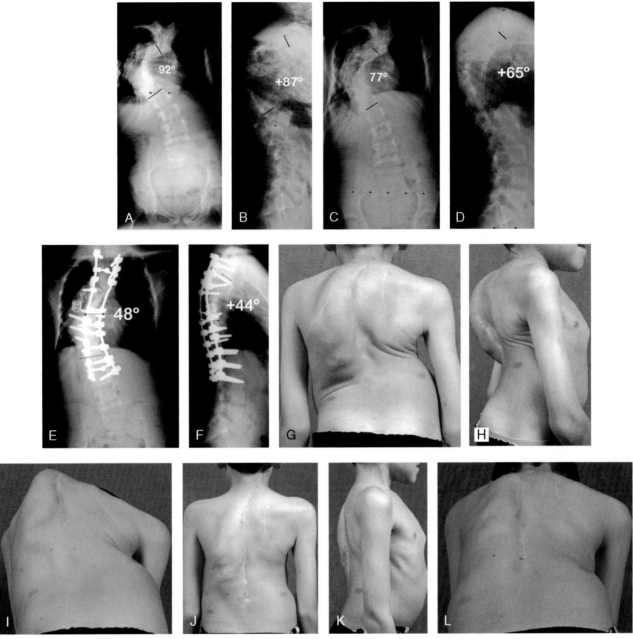

Figure 9 Thoracic kyphoscoliosis in a 10-year-old boy with neurofibromatosis who underwent several earlier anterior and posterior spinal fusion attempts. Preoperative AP (**A**) and lateral (**B**) radiographs depict a progressive 92° coronal plane deformity and 87° sagittal plane deformity, creating a combined 179° of kyphoscoliosis. Preoperative AP (**C**) and lateral (**D**) radiographs obtained after placement of 20 lb of halo-gravity traction. The coronal plane corrected to 77° of deformity and the sagittal plane to 65° of deformity. AP (**E**) and lateral (**F**) radiographs taken 2 years postoperatively show realignment in both planes after treatment with a three-level VCR and a posterior spinal fusion from T1 to L3. Preoperative (**G** through **I**) and postoperative (**J** through **L**) clinical photographs demonstrate the marked correction of the severe truncal deformity. In the preoperative views, note the prior posterior skin as well as bilateral anterior thoracotomy incisions from the prior unsuccessful circumferential attempts at spine fusion. The marked improvement in thoracic prominence is due to spine correction only, because previously the patient had undergone a convex thoracoplasty at another institution.

Bibliography

Boachie-Adjei O, Bradford DS: Vertebral column resection and arthrodesis for complex spinal deformities. *J Spinal Disord* 1991;4(2):193-202.

Bradford DS, Tribus CB: Vertebral column resection for the treatment of rigid coronal decompensation. *Spine (Phila Pa 1976)* 1997;22(14):1590-1599.

Bridwell KH: Decision making regarding Smith-Petersen vs. pedicle subtraction osteotomy vs. vertebral column resection for spinal deformity. *Spine (Phila Pa 1976)* 2006;31(19 suppl):S171-S178.

Kim YJ, Lenke LG, Bridwell KH, Cho YS, Riew KD: Free hand pedicle screw placement in the thoracic spine: Is it safe? *Spine (Phila Pa 1976)* 2004;29(3):333-342.

Leatherman KD: Abstract: Resection of vertebral bodies. *J Bone Joint Surg Am* 1969;5(1):206.

Lenke LG, O'Leary PT, Bridwell KH, Sides BA, Koester LA, Blanke KM: Posterior vertebral column resection for severe pediatric deformity: Minimum two-year follow-up of thirty-five consecutive patients. *Spine (Phila Pa 1976)* 2009;34(20): 2213-2221.

Lenke LG, Sides BA, Koester LA, Hensley M, Blanke KM: Vertebral column resection for the treatment of severe spinal deformity. *Clin Orthop Relat Res* 2010;468(3):687-699.

Suk SI, Chung ER, Kim JH, Kim SS, Lee JS, Choi WK: Posterior vertebral column resection for severe rigid scoliosis. *Spine (Phila Pa 1976)* 2005;30(14):1682-1687.

Suk SI, Chung ER, Lee SM, Lee JH, Kim SS, Kim JH: Posterior vertebral column resection in fixed lumbosacral deformity. *Spine (Phila Pa 1976)* 2005;30(23):E703-E710.

Suk SI, Kim JH, Kim WJ, Lee SM, Chung ER, Nah KH: Posterior vertebral column resection for severe spinal deformities. *Spine (Phila Pa 1976)* 2002;27(21):2374-2382.

Wang Y, Zhang Y, Zhang X, et al: A single posterior approach for multilevel modified vertebral column resection in adults with severe rigid congenital kyphoscoliosis: A retrospective study of 13 cases. *Eur Spine J* 2008;17(3):361-372.

Coding

CPT Codes		Corresponding ICD-9 Codes	
20937	Autograft for spine surgery only (includes harvesting the graft); morselized (through separate skin or fascial incision) (List separately in addition to code for primary procedure)	170.2 733.13 737.30	724.6 733.81
22212	Osteotomy of spine, posterior or posterolateral approach, one vertebral segment; thoracic	720.0 737.10 737.12	733.81 737.11 737.20
22216	Osteotomy of spine, posterior or posterolateral approach, one vertebral segment; each additional vertebral segment (List separately in addition to primary procedure)	720.0 737.10 737.12	733.81 737.11 737.20
22612	Arthrodesis, posterior or posterolateral technique, single level; lumbar (with or without lateral transverse technique)	170.2 721.42 722.10	721.3 722.0 737.39
22614	Arthrodesis, posterior or posterolateral technique, single level; each additional vertebral segment (List separately in addition to code for primary procedure)	170.2 722.52 737.09	722.10 724.02 738.4
22842	Posterior segmental instrumentation (eg, pedicle fixation, dual rods with multiple hooks and sublaminar wires); 3 to 6 vertebral segments (List separately in addition to code for primary procedure)	342.1 342.90 343.0	342.9 343 343.1
22843	Posterior segmental instrumentation (eg, pedicle fixation, dual rods with multiple hooks and sublaminar wires); 7 to 12 vertebral segments (List separately in addition to code for primary procedure)	170.2 342.9 343	342.1 342.90 343.0
22844	Posterior segmental instrumentation (eg, pedicle fixation, dual rods with multiple hooks and sublaminar wires); 13 or more vertebral segments (List separately in addition to code for primary procedure)	170.2 342.9 343	342.1 342.90 343.0
63087	Vertebral corpectomy (vertebral body resection), partial or complete, combined thoracolumbar approach with decompression of spinal cord, cauda equina or nerve root(s), lower thoracic or lumbar; single segment	170.2 721.41 722.72	567.31 721.42 722.73
63088	Vertebral corpectomy (vertebral body resection), partial or complete, combined thoracolumbar approach with decompression of spinal cord, cauda equina or nerve root(s), lower thoracic or lumbar; each additional segment (List separately in addition to code for primary procedure)	170.2 721.41 722.72	567.31 721.42 722.73

Chapter 29
Pedicle Subtraction Osteotomy

Serena S. Hu, MD
Murat Pekmezci, MD

▉ Indications

Sagittal plane deformity may develop secondary to ankylosing spondylitis or after a fusion, most classically after Harrington distraction instrumentation, but it may also occur with osteoporotic compression fractures or degenerative disk disease. Some patients may respond to physical therapy, particularly if flexibility is present in the spine below the fused segments, but most patients with fixed sagittal deformity need surgical correction. Several types of osteotomies can be used to address sagittal deformity; this chapter addresses pedicle subtraction osteotomy (PSO).

PSO was initially described by Thomasen in 1985 and is being used with increasing frequency. It involves excision of the posterior elements as well as the bilateral pedicles and a posterior-based wedge from the vertebral body. PSO provides correction via a closing-wedge osteotomy that hinges at the anterior longitudinal ligament and shortens the length of the spinal column when the defect is closed. It is a technically complex procedure with high complication rates because of the proximity of the neural elements and great vessels and because it is usually performed in patients who have had one or more prior spinal fusions. The reported average correction achieved per level of PSO ranges from 26° to 41°. Because PSO provides a significant amount of correction, one level usually is enough to achieve the desired correction (**Figure 1**). It also can be used as a tool to correct coronal plane deformity by performing an asymmetric resection (**Figure 2**). Additional modifications of the PSO have been reported. One modification involves removing the upper end plate, disk, and lower end plate of the vertebra above to improve correction at each level. A recent modification that can allow more angular correction involves opening of the anterior column in addition to closure of the posterior elements. For such cases, we prefer to use a cage filled with bone to support the anterior column.

Selection of the osteotomy level is an important step in the planning of the PSO and depends on several factors, such as risk of neurologic injury, the magnitude of correction, the number of fixation points, and the location of the deformity. The spinal cord ends at the level of L1 and the size of the spinal canal increases distally, thus theoretically the risk of neurologic injury is relatively smaller at levels distal to L1. Despite the larger canal/neural element ratio, however, a higher incidence of neurologic complications at L4 and L5 have been reported. Therefore, with regard to the risk of neurologic injury, the preferable PSO site would be at the L2 or L3 vertebra. As the level of osteotomy is moved distally, the amount of translation achieved at the C7 vertebra by a similar wedge removal is greater. For example, a PSO at L5 would provide better correction than a similarly sized PSO at L2. On the other hand, because PSO destabilizes all three columns of the spine, it also is important to achieve adequate fixation points proximal and distal to the osteotomy. We recommend at least three bilateral fixation points proximal and distal to the osteotomy level.

The principles of deformity correction may lead the surgeon to consider correctional osteotomy at the apex of the deformity. Because of neurologic considerations and correction of a desired amount of sagittal imbalance, however, the surgeon may instead perform the PSO at a more distal level.

Dr. Hu or an immediate family member is a member of a speakers' bureau or has made paid presentations on behalf of Synthes and DePuy, serves as a paid consultant to or is an employee of Pioneer, and has received research or institutional support from DePuy and Metronic Sofamor Danek. Neither Dr. Pekmezci nor any immediate family member has received anything of value from or owns stock in a commercial company or institution related directly or indirectly to the subject of this chapter.

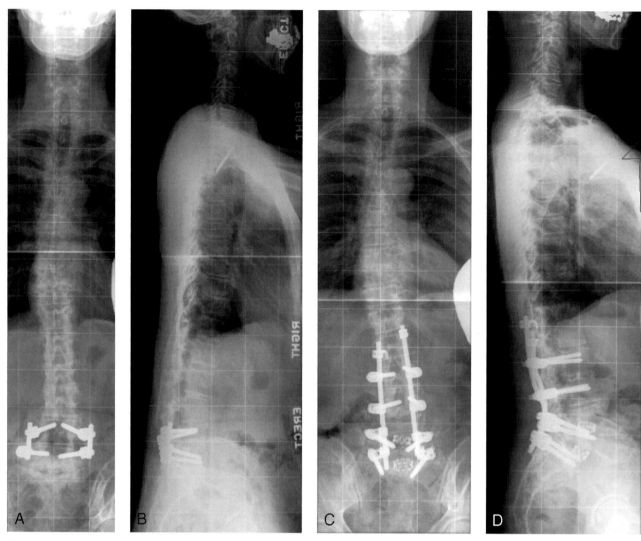

Figure 1 Radiographs of a 65-year-old woman who initially had a T4-L4 posterior spine fusion and later had extension of the fusion to L5 with a segmental spinal instrumentation system. Preoperative AP (**A**) and lateral (**B**) full spine views show sagittal imbalance. Postoperative AP (**C**) and lateral (**D**) full spine views show improved sagittal balance following an L4 PSO.

This may result in a zig-zag appearance in the sagittal plane; however, it has been shown that this secondary deformity is not generally felt by the patient. In summary, the level of the osteotomy should be selected on a case-by-case basis, considering the criteria mentioned previously.

PSO is indicated for patients who have substantial fixed sagittal imbalance (>10 to 12 cm), patients who have had an earlier circumferential fusion or an equivalent disease process (eg, ankylosing spondylitis) that precludes a Smith-Petersen osteotomy (SPO), and

patients who have a sharp angular kyphotic deformity. A one-level PSO usually provides adequate correction. If the preoperative sagittal imbalance exceeds 25 cm or the goal of deformity correction is >70°, however, then more than one PSO can be considered.

Contraindications

An absolute contraindication to PSO is existing anterior instrumentation at the level of the intended osteotomy. In

addition, the surgeon may prefer alternative procedures for patients with anterior pseudarthrosis, patients who are physiologically elderly or have significant comorbidities such as diabetes or cardiopulmonary disease, patients with a history of psychiatric disorders, patients who need only 10° to 20° of correction or have only 4 to 7 cm of sagittal imbalance for which an SPO would provide satisfactory results, and patients with poor family or social support.

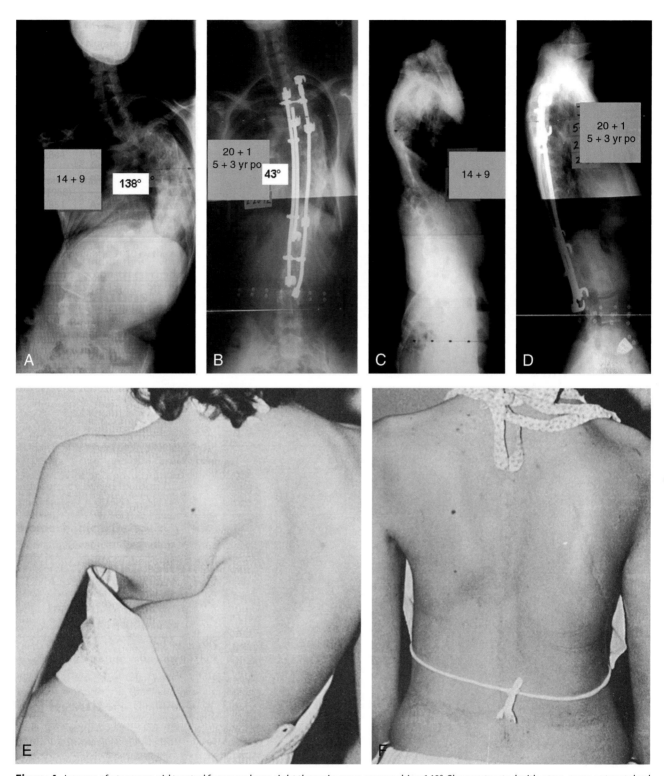

Figure 4 Images of a teenage girl treated for a very large right thoracic curve approaching 140°. She was treated with a two-segment vertebral column resection and long instrumented fusion. The order of treatment was preliminary halo traction, then thoracotomy and two-level corpectomies anteriorly, followed by additional halo traction, and finally the ultimate posterior instrumented fusion. Weight-bearing AP preoperative (**A**) and postoperative (**B**) and lateral preoperative (**C**) and postoperative (**D**) radiographs and clinical photographs taken from the back preoperatively (**E**) and postoperatively (**F**) demonstrate the dramatic improvement in the spinal curvature in this patient. The patient gained 5 inches in trunk height, and pulmonary functions increased by 30% in spite of the thoracotomy.

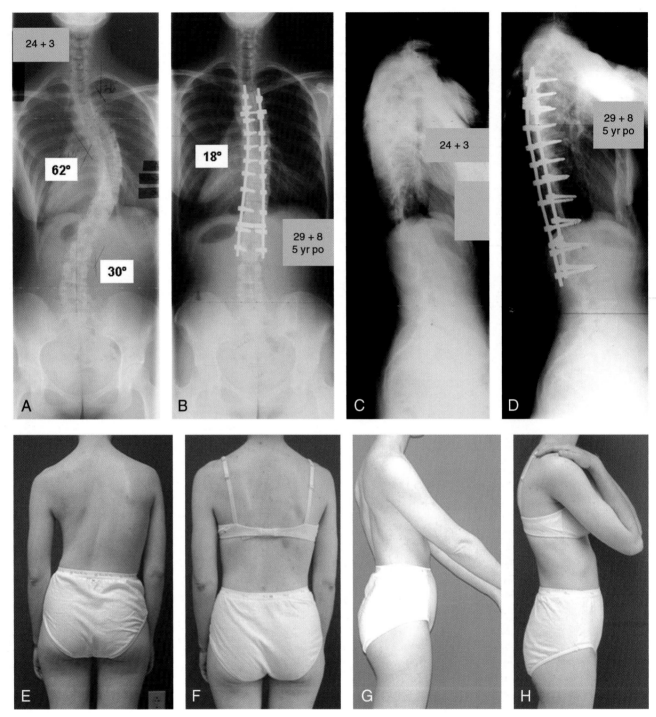

Figure 5 Images of a young woman with a substantial right thoracic curve with limited flexibility. She was treated with pedicle screw implants. A combination of in situ contouring of the concave rod and apical vertebral derotation accomplished the correction. Weight-bearing AP preoperative (**A**) and postoperative (**B**) and lateral preoperative (**C**) and postoperative (**D**) radiographs and clinical photographs taken from the back preoperatively (**E**) and postoperatively (**F**) and side preoperatively (**G**) and postoperatively (**H**) demonstrate the substantial improvement in the curve. Her SRS-30 outcome scores, converted to a 100-point scale, were 82 preoperatively and 88 at 5-year follow-up.

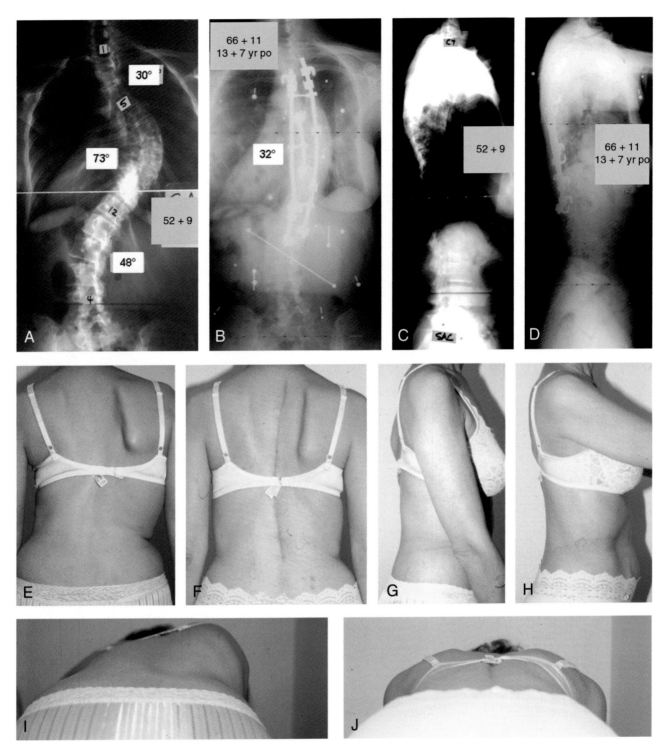

Figure 6 Images of a progressive thoracic curve with a much smaller lumbar curve in a middle-aged woman. Degenerative changes were present in all segments of the lumbar curve; MRI showed disk degeneration at all levels from T12 to the sacrum. The patient reported no pain from the lumbar curve, but she was dissatisfied with the progressive deformity in the thoracic spine. She was treated with a hook-only construct and a thoracoplasty. Weight-bearing AP preoperative (**A**) and postoperative (**B**) and lateral preoperative (**C**) and postoperative (**D**) radiographs and clinical photographs taken from the back preoperatively (**E**) and postoperatively (**F**), from the side preoperatively (**G**) and postoperatively (**H**), and bending preoperatively (**I**) and postoperatively (**J**) demonstrate the postoperative correction in the coronal and axial planes with maintenance of the sagittal plane. Her SRS-22 outcome scores at 14-year follow-up were 25/25 for pain, 23/25 for function, 30/30 for self-image, 23/25 for mental health, and 10/10 for satisfaction. A good result can be achieved with hooks. Thoracoplasty, at times, can be an appropriate treatment in an adult.

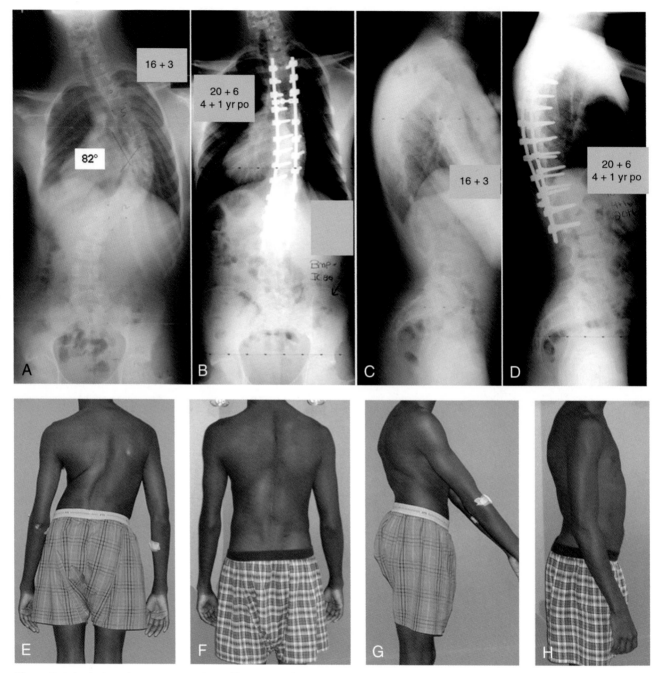

Figure 7 A single thoracic curve greater than 80° in a teenage boy. His right shoulder was dramatically higher than his left. This curve corrected by only 15° on various side bending, stretch, and push-prone maneuvers. Without pedicle screw implants, formal anterior releases or thoracoscopic releases would have been indicated. He was treated with pedicle screws implants and radical facetectomies. Weight-bearing PA preoperative (**A**) and postoperative (**B**) and lateral preoperative (**C**) and postoperative (**D**) radiographs and clinical photographs taken from the back preoperatively (**E**) and postoperatively (**F**) and side preoperatively (**G**) and postoperatively (**H**) demonstrate the very satisfactory correction that was achieved. More correction might have been achieved if the construct was carried one or two levels higher.

staging of corrections over time. We find that having pedicle screws at all levels facilitates correction by allowing force to be applied from segment to segment. Vertebral column resection often has a role in treating curves over 120°, particularly if the curve also is hyperkyphotic. As pedicle screw techniques and vertebral column resection techniques improve, anterior and posterior surgery will be needed less frequently (**Figure 7**).

Setup

Neurophysiologic monitoring, consisting of somatosensory-evoked potentials and some form of motor tract monitoring, is used in all patients. Patients are positioned prone on a Jackson table, with all bony prominences padded carefully. The abdomen is allowed to hang free to minimize epidural venous pressure. For standard idiopathic scoliosis cases in which the anticipated surgical duration is 3 to 4 hours, a prone view is used. If a longer surgery with potentially greater blood loss is expected, tongs or a halo is used.

Instrumentation

Many implant possibilities are reasonable for the correction of a thoracic curve. Multiple hooks, such as first-generation Cotrel-Doubosset instrumentation, combined with sublaminar Luque wires or spinous process Wisconsin wires can provide a good-quality correction. Many surgeons prefer a hybrid construct composed of hooks above, screws below, and wires in the middle. The construct gaining increasing popularity is the one using mostly pedicle screws.

It appears that more correction is possible using pedicle screw implants. The amount of true derotation that is achieved with the pedicle screw technique remains somewhat debatable, however. It is not entirely clear how much of the additional correction obtained is from the use of pedicle screws per se or from the use of a fixation point at every level of the spine. Clearly, pedicle screws often result in a significant enough correction that the need for thoracoplasty or anterior releases is dramatically reduced in many cases.

Stainless steel is by far the most common metal used for the treatment of thoracic scoliosis. Stainless steel rods have ideal stiffness and lack the notch sensitivity of titanium. The obvious limitation of stainless steel implants is streak artifact that renders postoperative MRI of limited value. We use 5.5-mm rods in most patients; however, either smaller or larger diameter rods are preferable at times, depending on the pathoanatomy of the deformity and the size of the patient.

Procedure

After a routine iodine-based scrub and paint preparation, the skin is incised. A subperiosteal dissection of the posterior spinal elements is then performed using a combination of Cobb elevators and bovie electrocautery. Level locationalization is determined with the aid of intraoperative radiography or fluoroscopy. After exposure is completed, the posterior elements of the levels to be fused are further denuded of any residual soft tissue using large curets. A ½-inch straight osteotome and mallet are then used to perform inferior facetectomies at all levels included in the fusion except, of course, the most distal segment. Intra-articular cartilage is scraped off using a small curet. Inferior facetectomies are performed for three reasons: to harvest local autograft, to increase the rate of facet fusion by the removal of cartilage and arthrodesis of the joint spaces, and to better visualize anatomic landmarks for proper pedicle screw placement.

Using posterior element topography, segmental pedicle screws are then placed using a straight, blunt-tipped gearshift and free-hand technique. Screws are typically placed at every level on the concavity of the curve and at most levels along the convexity. To limit the occurrence of junctional problems, it has become the preference of the senior author (K.H.B) to place a unilateral pedicle hook at the proximal segment on the side of the main thoracic curve convexity. This technique invariably necessitates omitting the screw at the level below the hook to seat the hook comfortably and avoid implant crowding. As the screws are placed, intermittent fluoroscopic checks are performed. When all fixation points are in proper position, the correcting rod is placed. In most idiopathic scoliosis cases, in which the thoracic sagittal plane is either normal or hypokyphotic, the correcting rod is on the concavity.

Using the principles of correction outlined above (depending on curve type), the deformity is then corrected. An intraoperative radiograph is obtained and scrutinized carefully. If the surgeon is satisfied with the correction, then the set screws are broken off and the spine is arthrodesed. The gold standard in achieving fusion has always been the use of iliac bone, rib bone, or both if thoracoplasty has been performed. Like many surgeons throughout the country, we have been trying to minimize the violation of the rib cage and the ilium. Morbidity is associated with iliac harvesting and, if the patient ever needs a long fusion to the sacrum, having the ilium available for pelvic fixation is important. The ability to achieve stable sacropelvic fixation is compromised by iliac harvesting, so we now do everything possible to avoid taking iliac bone. Using pedicle screw implants leaves more surface area for fusion and allows greater decortication than can be accomplished when hooks or sublaminar wires are used.

We usually begin by resecting all the spinous processes, except those at the very top and bottom of the construct/instrumented fusion. An osteotome and mallet are then used to raise flaps of bone just as described with the initial Moe fusions using Harrington instrumentation. The bone thus obtained, added to the previously excised inferior facets, typically totals 40 to 70 mL of local autologous bone graft. Next, a high-speed burr is used to thoroughly decorticate the entire exposed posterior bed. We do not hesitate to supplement the bone graft material with morcellized fresh frozen femoral head allograft and biologic products, even those that are not US Food and Drug Administration

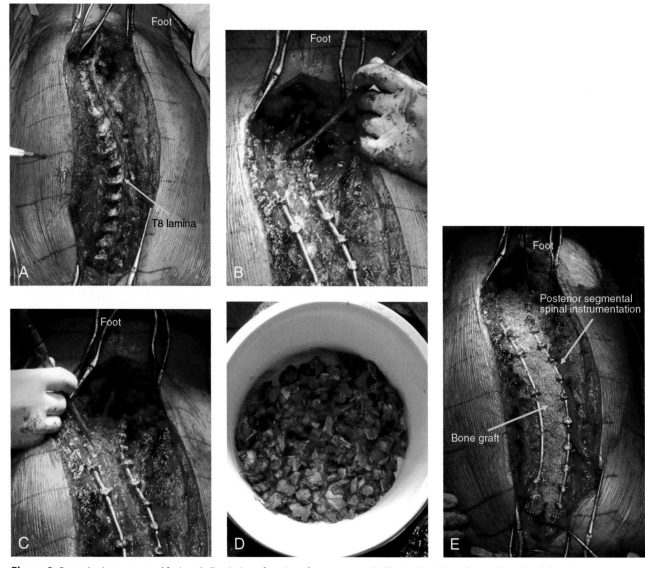

Figure 8 Posterior instrumented fusion. **A,** Depiction of a spine after exposure. **B,** The implants have been placed and the spinous processes excised. Flaps of bone are raised with an osteotome and mallet. **C,** Posterior elements are decorticated with a high-speed burr. **D,** A large quantity of autologous bone has been generated. **E,** The appearance of the spine after the graft has been applied. The graft will typically include 50 mL of local bone, 50 mL of morcellized fresh frozen femoral head allograft, and a substantial quantity of compression-resistant matrix (CRM) sponges soaked with biologic proteins. The CRM sponge is a compression-resistant matrix of collagen sponge impregnated with tricalcium phosphate and hydroxyapatite.

(FDA)-approved for posterior use. Some preliminary reports suggest that this approach accomplishes a higher fusion rate than the more traditional approach, which relies entirely on iliac bone and a more limited local harvest without fresh frozen femoral head allograft or biologic supplementation (**Figure 8**).

Wound Closure

The wound is closed in layers over drains using a combination of 1-0 and 2-0 absorbable sutures. A subcuticular 3-0 monofilament suture is used to achieve a cosmetic skin closure. Adhesive strips are placed on the skin edges, and a sterile dressing composed of gauze and tape is applied.

Postoperative Regimen

Pediatric patients routinely spend a night in the intensive care unit after surgical correction of thoracic scoliosis. Adult patients often are sent to the floor after surgery; however, occasionally they are sent to the intensive care unit, if the surgery results in substantial blood loss or if significant preoperative medical comorbidities are present. As discussed earlier, patients are helped to stand on the morning after surgery so the surgeon can assess balance. We frequently encourage patients to ambulate with the aid of a walker as soon as the day after surgery. Drains usually are removed on the third postoperative day. Weight-bearing long-cassette radiographs and clinical photographs are obtained a week after surgery, when patients return to the office for a wound check.

Avoiding Pitfalls and Complications

Complications that occur with an exquisitely low prevalence following thoracic scoliosis surgery include neurologic injury and wound infection. As stated previously, neurologic injury can be minimized with very large curves if preoperative halo traction is used and slower, more gradual realignment is achieved, particularly in cases of severe kyphosis. A more common pitfall that can occur when surgery is performed by inexperienced surgeons is suboptimal coronal or sagittal balance. The surgeon must pay close attention to shoulder balance and resist the temptation to achieve perfect correction of the main thoracic curve at the expense of postoperative shoulder asymmetry. In patients with false double major curves, it is important to leave some residual tilt to the lower instrumented vertebra so that there is a harmonious coronal transition into the lumbar curve. Thorough preoperative assessment of the sagittal plane also is of great importance in avoiding junctional problems.

Bibliography

Bradford DS, Tay BK, Hu SS: Adult scoliosis: Surgical indications, operative management, complications, and outcomes. *Spine (Phila Pa 1976)* 1999;24(24):2617-2629.

Bridwell KH: Decision making on anterior versus posterior versus combined approaches for idiopathic adolescent scoliosis, in Kim DH, Betz RR, Huhn SL, Newton PO, eds: *Surgery of the Pediatric Spine.* New York, NY, Thieme, 2008, pp 669-681.

Bridwell KH, Hanson DS, Rhee JM, Lenke LG, Baldus C, Blanke K: Correction of thoracic adolescent idiopathic scoliosis with segmental hooks, rods, and Wisconsin wires posteriorly: It's bad and obsolete, correct? *Spine (Phila Pa 1976)* 2002; 27(18):2059-2066.

Bridwell KH, McAllister JW, Betz RR, Huss G, Clancy M, Schoenecker PL: Coronal decompensation produced by Cotrel-Dubousset "derotation" maneuver for idiopathic right thoracic scoliosis. *Spine (Phila Pa 1976)* 1991;16(7): 769-777.

Bridwell KH, Shufflebarger HL, Lenke LG, Lowe TG, Betz RR, Bassett GS: Parents' and patients' preferences and concerns in idiopathic adolescent scoliosis: A cross-sectional preoperative analysis. *Spine (Phila Pa 1976)* 2000;25(18):2392-2399.

Dobbs MB, Lenke LG, Walton T, et al: Can we predict the ultimate lumbar curve in adolescent idiopathic scoliosis patients undergoing a selective fusion with undercorrection of the thoracic curve? *Spine (Phila Pa 1976)* 2004;29(3):277-285.

Kim YJ, Lenke LG, Bridwell KH, Kim KL, Steger-May K: Pulmonary function in adolescent idiopathic scoliosis relative to the surgical procedure. *J Bone Joint Surg Am* 2005;87(7):1534-1541.

King HA, Moe JH, Bradford DS, Winter RB: The selection of fusion levels in thoracic idiopathic scoliosis. *J Bone Joint Surg Am* 1983;65(9):1302-1313.

Lenke LG, Betz RR, Bridwell KH, et al: Intraobserver and interobserver reliability of the classification of thoracic adolescent idiopathic scoliosis. *J Bone Joint Surg Am* 1998;80(8):1097-1106.

Lenke LG, Bridwell KH, O'Brien MF, Baldus C, Blanke KM: Recognition and treatment of the proximal thoracic curve in adolescent idiopathic scoliosis treated with Cotrel-Dubousset instrumentation. *Spine (Phila Pa 1976)* 1994;19(14):1589-1597.

Lowe T, Berven SH, Schwab FJ, Bridwell KH: The SRS classification for adult spinal deformity: Building on the King/Moe and Lenke classification systems. *Spine (Phila Pa 1976)* 2006;31(19, Suppl):S119-S125.

Luhmann SJ, Lenke LG, Kim YJ, Bridwell KH, Schootman M: Thoracic adolescent idiopathic scoliosis curves between 70 degrees and 100 degrees: Is anterior release necessary? *Spine (Phila Pa 1976)* 2005;30(18):2061-2067.

Coding

CPT Codes		Corresponding ICD-9 Codes	
20930	Allograft for spine surgery only; morselized (List separately in addition to code for primary procedure)	170.2 733.13	724.6 733.81
20931	Allograft for spine surgery only; structural (List separately in addition to code for primary procedure)	170.2 733.13	724.6 733.81
20936	Autograft for spine surgery only (includes harvesting the graft); local (eg, ribs, spinous process, or laminar fragments) obtained from same incision (List separately in addition to code for primary procedure)	170.2 733.13	724.6 737.30
20937	Autograft for spine surgery only (includes harvesting the graft); morselized (through separate skin or fascial incision) (List separately in addition to code for primary procedure)	170.2 733.13	724.6 733.81
20938	Autograft for spine surgery only (includes harvesting the graft); structural, bicortical or tricortical (through separate skin or fascial incision) (List separately in addition to code for primary procedure)	170.2 733.13	724.6 733.81
22802	Arthrodesis, posterior, for spinal deformity, with or without cast; 7 to 12 vertebral segments	342.1 342.90	342.9 343
22804	Arthrodesis, posterior, for spinal deformity, with or without cast; 13 or more vertebral segments	342.1 342.90	342.9 343
22808	Arthrodesis, anterior, for spinal deformity, with or without cast; 2 to 3 vertebral segments	342.1 342.90	342.9 343
22810	Arthrodesis, anterior, for spinal deformity, with or without cast; 4 to 7 vertebral segments	342.1 342.90	342.9 343
22812	Arthrodesis, anterior, for spinal deformity, with or without cast; 8 or more vertebral segments	342.1 342.90	342.9 343
22840	Posterior non-segmental instrumentation (eg, Harrington rod technique, pedicle fixation across one interspace, atlantoaxial transarticular screw fixation, sublaminar wiring at C1, facet screw fixation) (List separately in addition to code for primary procedure)	170.2 342.9	342.1 342.90
22841	Internal spinal fixation by wiring of spinous processes (List separately in addition to code for primary procedure)	170.2 342.9	342.1 342.90

Chapter 31
Transthoracic Diskectomy: Anterior Approach

Anthony Rinella, MD
Alex Gitelman, MD

◼ Indications

Thoracic disk herniations are more challenging to diagnose than their cervical or lumbar counterparts. Early symptoms often are subtle and therefore may lead to a delay in diagnosis. Symptoms can vary from atypical pain patterns to severe myelopathy. Modern imaging techniques provide excellent visual information about the thoracic spine; however, the high rate of asymptomatic herniations and the broad range of other diagnoses that can produce similar symptoms make diagnosing a symptomatic thoracic disk herniation difficult. Depending on the location of the herniation, one of several techniques—laminectomy, laminoforaminotomy, transpedicular, costotransversectomy, or transthoracic—can be used (**Figure 1**). The transthoracic technique is performed from an anterior approach, and the others are performed from a posterior approach. Central herniations typically require a transthoracic approach, which is the focus of this chapter.

Surgical treatment is indicated if 4 to 6 weeks of nonsurgical management fails to provide relief or if the patient has severe radiculopathy or myelopathy. A less aggressive approach may be acceptable in children because the natural history of the disorder appears to be different in youth. Similarly, lateral disk herniations causing radicular symptoms alone may benefit from continued observation, depending on the degree of pain. Thoracic diskectomy for axial pain may offer less predictable outcomes than for neural compression because most thoracic disk herniations are asymptomatic, and muscular tenderness alone is common. When thoracic myelopathy is present, patients with mild presentations and early treatment typically have better outcomes than those with more serious or longstanding deficits, especially if ossification of the posterior longitudinal ligament is present.

◼ Contraindications

Poor overall health and/or poor cardiopulmonary status, particularly in the absence of myelopathy, are contraindications to surgical treatment. This is especially true when a thoracotomy is considered, or when an extended surgery in the prone position is expected. In particular, the inability to tolerate one-lung ventilation is a contraindication. A relative contraindication is a lateral soft-disk herniation (which can be approached posteriorly).

◼ Alternative Treatments

The treatment protocols for acute thoracic disk herniations are similar to those for lumbar disk herniations. When axial back pain symptoms predominate, activity modification, nonsteroidal anti-inflammatory drugs (NSAIDs), and physical therapy are indicated. Muscle relaxants also may be beneficial. When radicular symptoms are significant, corticosteroids, administered orally or by epidural injection, may be beneficial. Bracing has a very limited role because it may lead to deconditioning.

The natural history of thoracic disk herniations is similar to that of herni-

---

Dr. Rinella or an immediate family member is a member of a speakers' bureau or has made paid presentations on behalf of Medtronic and Stryker and serves as a paid consultant to or is an employee of Zimmer Spine. Neither Dr. Gitelman nor any immediate family member has received anything of value from or owns stock in a commercial company or institution related directly or indirectly to the subject of this chapter.

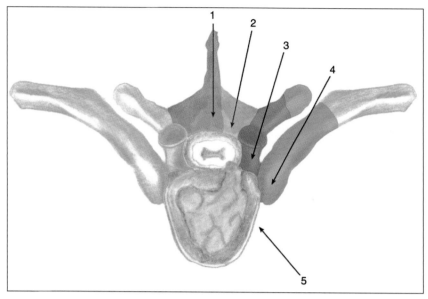

Figure 1 Drawing demonstrates surgical approaches for thoracic disk herniation surgery. **1** and **2** are used for laminectomy. **2** also is used for laminoforaminotomy. **3** is used for pediculofacetectomy through the transpedicular approach. **4** is used for costotransversectomy. A more lateral resection of the rib than that shown here allows a more acute approach to the dorsal disk; this is called a lateral extracavitary approach. **5** is used for the transthoracic approach.

ations of the cervical and lumbar spine. Time and nonsurgical management usually improve mild symptoms. The symptoms of patients with lower extremity symptoms or frank myelopathy, however, tend to progress at a variable rate.

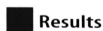

Results

Treatment of thoracic disk herniations with an anterior approach, either transthoracic or by costotransversectomy, is fairly reliable in achieving good relief of symptoms in most patients (Table 1). Thoracoscopy was first reported as a treatment for this disease in 1995, and later data demonstrated up to 84% patient satisfaction and 70% long-term clinical success. This approach was noted to result in a shorter intensive-care unit stay, a shorter chest-tube drainage time, and a more rapid return to work compared with the thoracotomy approach. On the other hand, thoracoscopy has a

higher rate of intercostal neuralgia and visceral injury from trochar placement. Soft, flexible ports may help to minimize postoperative intercostal neuralgia.

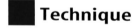

Technique

Setup/Exposure/Patient Positioning

The choice of approach depends on the location of the herniation. Lateral herniations (**Figure 2**) can be managed with a posterior approach. Central herniations (**Figure 3**) are most commonly managed with an anterior transthoracic approach with or without thoracoscopic assistance. The anterior approach is the only method by which the ventral spinal cord can be visualized directly. From a technical perspective, the anterior approach allows excellent exposure of the T4-5 to T11-12 intervertebral disks. Multiple levels can be accessed, and the entire disk can be visualized. The disadvan-

tages include the necessity of entering the chest cavity and the need for placing a postoperative chest tube. Furthermore, because most of the disk must be removed to perform the decompression, fusion often is necessary. It is difficult to access the upper thoracic disks via this approach because of the position of the mediastinal structures, and any posterior compression must be addressed separately through a posterior approach. Some authors recommend preoperative angiography to determine the location of the artery of Adamkiewicz and other major blood vessels. These vessels can be protected by careful dissection and by avoiding significant dissection in the intervertebral foramina, however.

For this procedure, the patient is placed in the lateral decubitus position with an axillary roll placed under the axilla in contact with the table. The chest is prepared for open thoracotomy whether an endoscopic or an open procedure is planned in the event that conversion to the thoracotomy is needed. It can be helpful to flex the table downward to allow expansion of the thorax. Double-lumen endotracheal tubes allow collapse of the ipsilateral lung and ventilation of the contralateral lung.

A lateral fluoroscopic image is obtained before making the incision, which is centered over the affected disk space in a curvilinear fashion between the ribs. Typically, the rib is one or two levels above the affected disk. In the upper thoracic spine, the scapula may limit the exposure. In the upper chest, a right-side approach helps avoid the mediastinal structures. In the lower thoracic spine, a left-side approach is preferable because it is easier to mobilize the aorta than the vena cava.

Electrocautery is used to dissect the muscles off the superior aspect of the rib to avoid injury to the intercostal neurovascular bundle, which runs along the inferior aspect of the rib. The parietal pleura is then divided,

Table 1 Results of Treatment of Thoracic Disk Disease Via a Transthoracic Approach

Authors (Year)	Number of Patients	Approach or Technique	Mean Patient Age in Years (Range)	Mean Follow-up in Months (Range)	Results/Comments
Anterior					
Crafoord et al (1958)	1	Transthoracic	36	NR	T10-11 disk herniation Rapid resolution of symptoms
Bohlman and Zdeblick (1988)	19	Transthoracic vs costotrans-versectomy	36 (25-73)	48	22 disks in 19 patients 11 patients costotransversectomy, 8 patients transthoracic 16 patients good or excellent results, 1 fair, 1 poor No differences between approach and outcomes
Currier et al (1994)	19	Transthoracic	46 (19-74)	12 minimum	22 disks in 19 patients 6 excellent results, 6 good, 3 fair, 3 poor
Regan et al (1995)	12	Transthoracic vs thoracoscopy	42 (32-55)	NR	All patients treated with thoracoscopy 5 of 12 had disk herniations No outcomes data
Stillerman et al (1998)	71	Transthoracic vs transfacet vs extracavitary vs transpedicular	48 (19-75)	12+	82 disks in 71 patients Improvements: pain (87%), hyperreflexia (95%), sensory (84%), bowel/bladder (76%), motor (58%) Complications 15%
Anand and Regan (2002)	100	Thoracoscopy	42 (22-76)	48 (2-6)	117 disks in 100 patients 84% overall subjective patient satisfaction rate 70% long-term clinical success rate
Posterior					
Patterson and Arbit (1978)	3	Transpedicular	46	NR	Inferior facet of the superior vertebra resected in addition to the superior facet of the inferior vertebra and superior portion of the pedicle 3 patients with excellent recovery: T1-2 (1), T8-9 (2)
Arce and Dohrmann (1985)	218	Laminectomy vs posterolateral vs lateral vs thoracic	45	NR	280 patients studied for demographic purposes 218 cases reviewed for clinical outcomes Laminectomy: 42% success rate, 16% asymptomatic, 32% made worse, 10% unchanged, 4% died Higher success rates for posterolateral, lateral, and transthoracic approaches
Le Roux et al (1993)	20	Transpedicular	44	12	All patients either asymptomatic or improved after surgery 18 returned to work

NR = not reported.

and thoracotomy retractors are placed. Resection of the medial 2 cm of the rib in contact with the disk space allows visualization of the pedicle and easier access to the neuro-foramina and spinal canal. Partial resection of the pedicle can increase visualization of the spinal canal. The resected rib material may be used as autologous bone graft.

Instruments/Equipment Required

The transthoracic approach is best performed on a radiolucent table using a headlight system with surgical

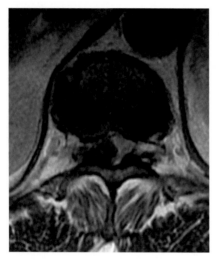

Figure 2 T2-weighted MRI sequence demonstrates a large right-side herniation at T11-12. The position of the disk made the approach through an anterior or posterior laminoforaminotomy possible.

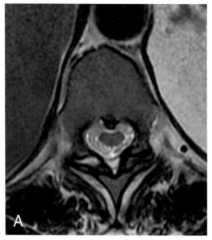
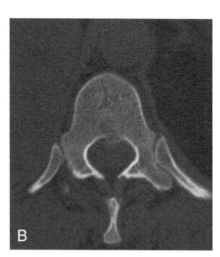

Figure 3 Images demonstrate a central thoracic disk herniation. **A,** Area of low signal intensity on T2-weighted MRI indicates the herniation. **B,** CT scan of the same level confirms that the disk is calcified. The central position of this herniation makes a transthoracic approach the best option.

loupes or an operating microscope. A full set of thoracotomy retractors and instruments, a high-speed drill and long spinal instruments (curets, Cobb elevators, Kerrison and pituitary rongeurs), as well as an anterior spinal fixation system and an interbody fusion device should be available. Fluoroscopy or intraoperative portable radiography is required for localization and evaluation of the position of the instrumentation.

Procedure

The ipsilateral lung is collapsed by the anesthesiologist, and the parietal pleura over the spinal column is divided in a U fashion. Care is taken to avoid injury to the underlying segmental vessels and the sympathetic chain. The disk level is verified by using a bayoneted spinal needle and fluoroscopy. The disk is then marked, and the spinal needle is removed. The sympathetic chain over the symptomatic disk may need to be divided; however, the segmental vessels should be left intact if only a single-level diskectomy is to be performed. The segmental vessels may need to be sacrificed if a corpectomy is needed.

The rib head is then removed with Cobb elevators and curets, uncovering the pedicle of the inferior vertebrae. A high-speed burr is used to thin the pedicle as much as possible, and the remaining pedicle wall is removed with a Kerrison rongeur. The spinal canal and the dura are then exposed; loupes or microscope magnification may be used to improve visualization. The high-speed burr is then used to drill down the superior and inferior end plates around the disk, and the diskectomy and decompression are performed with microcurets and pituitary rongeurs.

If fusion is necessary, it may be performed using the resected rib as autograft; depending on the size of the vertebral resection, a cage may need to be used. A screw-plate or screw-rod internal fixation device is then implanted.

Role of Fusion

Considerable dispute exists within the spine literature as to when fusion is necessary after thoracic diskectomy.

Common indications are instability or Scheuermann disease. Relative indications are multiple-level resections or single-level diskectomies that require wide facet excisions. This is especially true at the thoracolumbar junction because of the transitional anatomy and high force concentration that are present. The stability imparted by the ribs and sternum makes it unclear exactly when fusion is necessary, especially among the levels with true ribs. Therefore, the decision should be based on the surgeon's opinion of the instability imparted by the procedure.

Wound Closure

A chest tube is inserted before closure and is connected to suction. Multilayer closure is performed, and a sterile dressing is placed around the wound site and the chest tube site. A separate drain is not necessary because the chest tube also functions as a drain.

■ Postoperative Regimen

The chest tube that was connected to suction during surgery may be switched to a water seal and then removed once the lung is reinflated and fluid drainage and pneumothorax are resolved. Serial chest radiographs are needed to help with chest tube management. Postoperative radiographs are obtained to confirm the proper position of the instrumentation. With rigid internal fixation, a brace rarely is needed, and the patient is mobilized with assistance as soon as he or she is able to tolerate it.

■ Avoiding Pitfalls and Complications

Preoperative planning is extremely important, because access to the herniation must be achieved without manipulation of the spinal cord. Furthermore, it must be very clear preoperatively at what level the herniation resides, especially if the imaging studies do not include a cervical or lumbar vertebra for counting purposes. Calcified disks or disk fragments may have dural adhesions. Equally important is adequate intraoperative localization of the thoracic level. PA and lateral radiographs are recommended to ensure that the correct level is identified.

Intraoperatively, the lung may be reinflated briefly every 30 minutes to reduce the incidence and severity of postoperative atelectasis.

Inappropriately angled screws may violate the spinal canal, risking spinal cord injury. The risk is increased if the patient shifts during the procedure. This risk may be minimized by confirming that the patient is in the absolute lateral position before insertion of internal fixation.

If a dural leak is encountered during the procedure, it should be repaired with fine sutures; fibrin glue may be used to augment the repair. Lumbar drain placement should be considered in cases of large dural tears.

■ Bibliography

Aizawa T, Sato T, Sasaki H, et al: Results of surgical treatment for thoracic myelopathy: Minimum 2-year follow-up study in 132 patients. *J Neurosurg Spine* 2007;7(1):13-20.

Anand N, Regan JJ: Video-assisted thoracoscopic surgery for thoracic disc disease: Classification and outcome study of 100 consecutive cases with a 2-year minimum follow-up period. *Spine (Phila Pa 1976)* 2002;27(8):871-879.

Arce CA, Dohrmann GJ: Herniated thoracic disks. *Neurol Clin* 1985;3(2):383-392.

Arce CA, Dohrmann GJ: Thoracic disc herniation: Improved diagnosis with computed tomographic scanning and a review of the literature. *Surg Neurol* 1985;23(4):356-361.

Awwad EE, Martin DS, Smith KR Jr, Baker BK: Asymptomatic versus symptomatic herniated thoracic discs: Their frequency and characteristics as detected by computed tomography after myelography. *Neurosurgery* 1991;28(2):180-186.

Bohlman HH, Zdeblick TA: Anterior excision of herniated thoracic discs. *J Bone Joint Surg Am* 1988;70(7):1038-1047.

Brown CW, Deffer PA Jr, Akmakjian J, Donaldson DH, Brugman JL: The natural history of thoracic disc herniation. *Spine (Phila Pa 1976)* 1992;17(6, Suppl)S97-S102.

Crafoord C, Hiertonn T, Lindblom K, Olsson SE: Spinal cord compression caused by a protruded thoracic disc: Report of a case treated with antero-lateral fenestration of the disc. *Acta Orthop Scand* 1958;28(2):103-107.

Currier BL, Eismont FJ, Green BA: Transthoracic disc excision and fusion for herniated thoracic discs. *Spine (Phila Pa 1976)* 1994;19(3):323-328.

Dickman CA, Rosenthal D, Regan JJ: Reoperation for herniated thoracic discs. *J Neurosurg* 1999;91(2 Suppl):157-162.

Hodgson AR, Stock FE: Anterior spinal fusion: A preliminary communication on the radical treatment of Pott's disease and Pott's paraplegia. *Br J Surg* 1956;44(185):266-275.

Le Roux PD, Haglund MM, Harris AB: Thoracic disc disease: Experience with the transpedicular approach in twenty consecutive patients. *Neurosurgery* 1993;33(1):58-66.

Oskouian RJ, Johnson JP: Endoscopic thoracic microdiscectomy. *J Neurosurg Spine* 2005;3(6):459-464.

Patterson RH Jr, Arbit E: A surgical approach through the pedicle to protruded thoracic discs. *J Neurosurg* 1978;48(5):768-772.

Regan JJ: Percutaneous endoscopic thoracic discectomy. *Neurosurg Clin N Am* 1996;7(1):87-98.

Regan JJ, Mack MJ, Picetti GD III: A technical report on video-assisted thoracoscopy in thoracic spinal surgery: Preliminary description. *Spine (Phila Pa 1976)* 1995;20(7):831-837.

Stetkarova I, Chrobok J, Ehler E, Kofler M: Segmental abdominal wall paresis caused by lateral low thoracic disc herniation. *Spine (Phila Pa 1976)* 2007;32(22):E635-E639.

Stillerman CB, Chen TC, Couldwell WT, Zhang W, Weiss MH: Experience in the surgical management of 82 symptomatic herniated thoracic discs and review of the literature. *J Neurosurg* 1998;88(4):623-633.

Stillerman CB, Weiss MH: Management of thoracic disc disease. *Clin Neurosurg* 1992;38:325-352.

Wood KB, Blair JM, Aepple DM, et al: The natural history of asymptomatic thoracic disc herniations. *Spine (Phila Pa 1976)* 1997;22(5):525-530.

Wood KB, Garvey TA, Gundry C, Heithoff KB: Magnetic resonance imaging of the thoracic spine: Evaluation of asymptomatic individuals. *J Bone Joint Surg Am* 1995;77(11):1631-1638.

Coding

CPT Codes		Corresponding ICD-9 Codes	
63064	Costovertebral approach with decompression of spinal cord or nerve root(s) (eg, herniated intervertebral disc), thoracic; single segment	722.11	722.72
63066	Costovertebral approach with decompression of spinal cord or nerve root(s) (eg, herniated intervertebral disc), thoracic; each additional segment (List separately in addition to code for primary procedure)	722.11 723.0	722.72
22556	Arthrodesis, anterior interbody technique, including minimal discectomy to prepare interspace (other than for decompression); thoracic	721.2 722.51	721.41 733.13

CPT copyright © 2010 by the American Medical Association. All rights reserved.

Chapter 32
Anterior Thoracoscopic Diskectomy and Release

Peter O. Newton, MD
Eric S. Varley, DO

Indications

Anterior thoracoscopic surgery has been used to successfully treat a wide range of spinal deformities. Posterior instrumentation and fusion remains the gold standard for spinal deformity correction, but anterior thoracoscopic release and diskectomy are useful adjunctive techniques in carefully selected patients. The goal of thoracoscopic anterior release is to improve the flexibility of rigid motion segments within the curve, thus producing greater correction. A thoracoscopic anterior diskectomy offers the potential advantage of reduced chestwall morbidity compared with an open thoracotomy. A steep learning curve is required for mastering this technique, but the advantages of thoracoscopic anterior surgery, including lower pulmonary morbidity, less postoperative pain, access to more vertebral levels, improved cosmesis, and prevention of crankshaft deformity, are worth the effort. Thoracoscopic anterior release and diskectomy have the same indications as an open anterior technique, with additional consideration given to pulmonary function. These indications include the correction of scoliosis, kyphosis, and congenital deformity. For larger, more rigid curves greater than 75° with flexibility less than 50%, anterior thoracoscopic diskectomy and release may help gain needed spinal mobility for curve correction and reduce the risk of crankshaft deformity (**Figure 1**). Modern posterior pedicle screw instrumentation systems are capable of deformity correction in these severe cases; however, an anterior release still may be indicated to optimize coronal and axial plane correction, improve sagittal alignment by increasing thoracic kyphosis, and prevent crankshaft growth (**Figure 2**). These indications must be weighed in the context of the patient's needs and the surgeon's experience with the procedure.

———————————————■

Dr. Newton or an immediate family member serves as a board member, owner, officer, or committee member of the Pediatric Orthopaedic Society of North America and the Scoliosis Research Society; has received royalties from DePuy; is a member of a speakers' bureau or has made paid presentations on behalf of DePuy; serves as a consultant to or is an employee of DePuy; has received research or institutional support from the National Institutes of Health (NIAMS & NICHD), DePuy, Axial Biotech, Alphatech Spine, and Zimmer; owns stock or stock options in Nuvasive; and has received nonincome support (such as equipment or services), commercially derived honoraria, or other non–research-related funding (such as paid travel) from DePuy Spine. Neither Dr. Varley nor any immediate family member has received anything of value from or owns stock in a commercial company or institution related directly or indirectly to the subject of this chapter.

Contraindications

Impaired preoperative pulmonary function and abnormalities of the intrathoracic viscera are two contraindications to anterior thoracoscopic surgery. The pulmonary status must allow single-lung ventilation and be free from intrathoracic pleural adhesions from previous thoracotomy procedures or pulmonary infections (**Figure 3**). A minimum of 2 to 3 cm of working space between the rib cage and the spinal column also is required to provide adequate visualization. If the distance is less than 2 cm, then thoracoscopy is not recommended. Additionally, a patient who weighs less than 30 kg (66 pounds) is a relative contraindication because the relative benefits of a minimally invasive technique seem to be reduced in children. Successful thoracoscopic surgical techniques depend on proper visualization and adequate lung function; any condition in which either of these two parameters is compromised is a contraindication to this technique.

———————————————■

Alternative Treatments

In patients with the previously mentioned contraindications, the surgeon

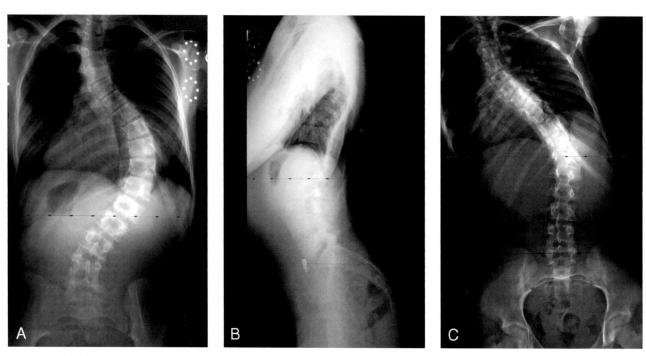

Figure 1 AP (**A**), lateral (**B**), and AP side-bending (**C**) radiographs of a right Lenke 2AN curve with a large thoracic coronal Cobb angle and less than 50% flexibility on side bending, all of which are indications for a thoracoscopic anterior release and diskectomy.

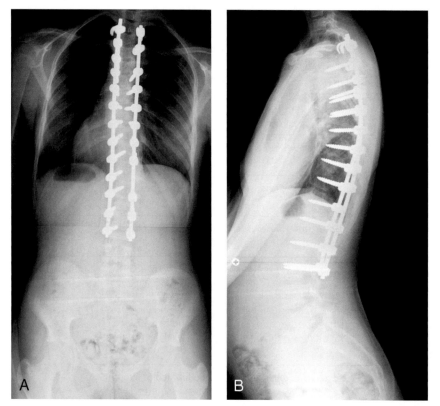

Figure 2 Postoperative AP (**A**) and lateral (**B**) radiographs of a patient who underwent thoracoscopic anterior spinal release and diskectomy before posterior spinal instrumentation and fusion, allowing optimal three-plane correction.

must decide whether an open thoracotomy or a posterior-only approach is appropriate. A posterior-only approach may include osteotomies and anterior column resections. The removal of these structures provides greater spinal flexibility and thus may preclude the need for an anterior release. The value of a careful and thorough multilevel diskectomy cannot be overstated in the treatment of large sweeping thoracic curves or in patients at particular risk of pseudarthrosis.

Results

Anterior thoracoscopic spine surgery has been shown to be a valuable technology in addressing spinal deformity. This technique allows direct access to the anterior stabilizing structures of the spine, enables mobilization of a rigid deformity, and provides a large surface for arthrodesis. The advantages of this technique are reduced

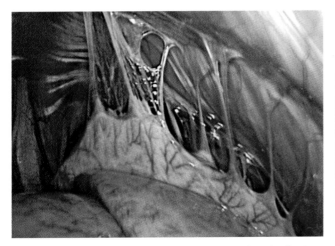

Figure 3 Intraoperative endoscopic view shows pleural adhesions preventing retraction of the lung tissue.

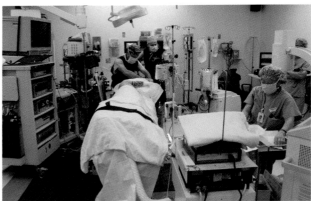

Figure 4 Operating room setup for anterior thoracoscopy. The video monitor is placed posterior to the patient with the harmonic scalpel generator, the electrocautery device, suction/irrigation equipment, and the cell saver positioned at the head of the table on either side of the anesthesiologist.

blood loss and minimization of trauma to the chest-wall musculature; the main disadvantage is an increase in surgical time (**Table 1**). Posterior instrumentation alone allows for a similar correction rate, but the advantages of anterior release and diskectomy in improving curve flexibility and preventing crankshaft deformity have been demonstrated in the literature. The indications for thoracoscopic release and diskectomy continue to evolve, requiring the surgeon to make an optimal recommendation for each patient based on surgeon experience and patient needs.

Technique

The patient and the surgical team should be aware of and prepared for a possible conversion to an open thoracotomy procedure. A well-trained surgical staff and an anesthesiologist experienced in single-lung ventilation also are essential for optimal patient positioning, visualization, and ventilation maintenance.

The patient is placed under general endotracheal anesthesia using a double-lumen endotracheal tube to allow single-lung ventilation. Bron-chial endoscopy is used to confirm the accuracy of the endotracheal tube placement and ensure that the lung is sufficiently deflated to provide optimal visualization of the spine. Spinal cord monitoring also is performed for the vertebrae controlling the upper and lower extremities.

Setup/Exposure

The operating room is set up with the video monitor aligned properly and oriented across the patient to allow access to the spine from the most intuitive viewing perspective. The harmonic scalpel generator, the electrocautery device, suction/irrigation equipment, and the cell saver are positioned at the head of the table on either side of the anesthesiologist (**Figure 4**). The patient is then placed on a radiolucent table in the lateral decubitus position, with the legs scissored and padded properly to prevent pressure on the peroneal nerve. Care must be taken to position the patient in a direct lateral orientation on the table so that the surgeon, who, with the assistant, is positioned anterior to the patient, is properly oriented to the spine. An axillary roll is then placed under the chest with one arm secured with tape and the free arm held loosely on a pillow to allow manipulation of the scapula.

The thoracoscopic portal placement is determined by the type of deformity being treated and the number of levels being released. The location of the portals is determined by fluoroscopic identification to provide access to all motion segments to be treated (**Figure 5**). Three to four portals typically are placed along the anterior axillary line for exposure and release of the anterior spine (**Figure 6**). These anterior portals allow greater exposure of the concave aspects of the deformity during disk excision and retraction of the great vessels than portals placed more posteriorly.

Instruments/Equipment/ Implants Required

The equipment needed for thoracoscopic surgery includes a high-quality endoscope and a three-chip video system to ensure good visualization. The endoscope should be equipped with angled viewing ranging from 0° to 45°. Endoscopic retractors for the lung diaphragm, peanut dissectors, a suction/irrigation pump, and a harmonic scalpel all are required. For the disk excision, surgical tools common to open spine surgery (including rongeurs, curets, and end-plate

Table 1 Summary of Results of Thoracoscopic Procedures

Authors (Year)	Number of Patients	Procedure	Mean Patient Age in Years (Range)	Mean Follow-up in Years (Range)	Results
Niemeyer et al (2000)	29	AR + PISF	16 (5-26)	2 (1-4)	51% coronal Cobb angle correction* 6 pulmonary complications 188 min surgical time (for AR only)
Lenke et al (2004)	21	AR + AISF	13 (9-17)	2.3 (2-5)	62% coronal Cobb angle correction No pulmonary complications reported Surgical time NR
Newton et al (2005)	112	AR + PISF	13 (2-28)	3 (2-7)	55% coronal Cobb angle correction 15 pulmonary complications 160 min surgical time (for AR only)
Lonner et al (2006)	28	AR + AISF	14.6 (10-17)	2.6 (2-4)	54.5% coronal Cobb angle correction 3 pulmonary complications 360 min surgical time
Cheung et al (2007)	11	AR + PISF	16.5 (11.9-35.5)	5.6 (2.2-8.1)	39% coronal Cobb angle correction No pulmonary complications reported 258 min surgical time
Norton et al (2007)	45	AR + AISF	14 (11.1-17.4)	4.6 (2-8)	67% coronal Cobb angle correction 3 pulmonary complications 346 min surgical time
Newton et al (2008)	25	AR + AISF	13 (10-16)	5.3 (4.6-6.7)	52% coronal Cobb angle correction No pulmonary complications reported Surgical time NR
Lonner et al (2009)	26	AR+ AISF	14.8 (10.2-18.6)	2.2 (2-4)	58.1% coronal Cobb angle correction No pulmonary complications 334 min surgical time

AR = anterior release, PISF = posterior instrumentation and spinal fusion, AISF = anterior instrumentation and spinal fusion, NR = not reported.

*Coronal Cobb angle correction = (postoperative Cobb angle) ÷ (preoperative Cobb angle) × 100.

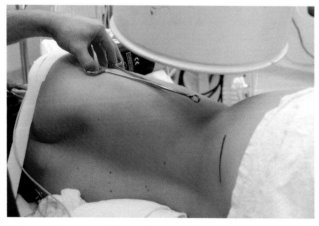

Figure 5 Photograph shows the patient in a direct lateral position with the anatomic landmarks identified with fluoroscopy.

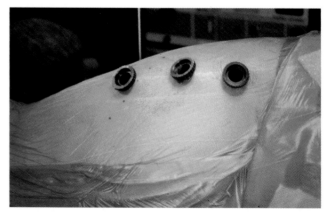

Figure 6 Intraoperative photograph of the patient placed in the lateral position with three portals shown oriented along the anterior axillary line for exposure and release of the anterior spine.

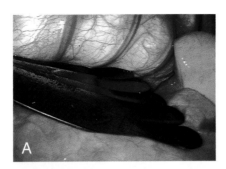
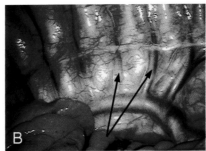

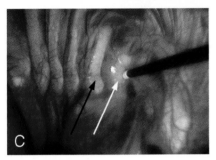
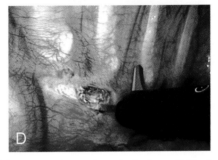
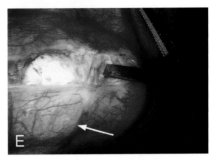

Figure 7 Intraoperative endoscopic views of thoracoscopic anterior spinal release. **A,** The fan retractor on the lung. **B,** The deflated lung is shown, with the azygous vein and segmental vessels (arrows) clearly displayed. **C,** Correct identification of the vertebral levels to be released relies on rib counting from the first rib (white arrow), which is less obvious than the second rib (black arrow) and requires palpation with a peanut dissector. **D,** The harmonic scalpel divides the pleura. **E,** Once the pleura is divided, the harmonic laparoscopic coagulating shears are applied to a 5-mm length of a segmental vessel (arrow) to coagulate the vessel before it is divided.

shavers) are available in long versions for endoscopic use.

Procedure

After portals are established through the chest wall, complete lung deflation is confirmed. Care must be taken when placing the inferior portals to avoid the site at which the diaphragm inserts into the chest wall. Initial exposure of the spine often requires gentle retraction of the lung with an endoscopic fan retractor until it becomes completely atelectatic (**Figure 7,** *A*). The vasculature, including the azygous vein and subclavian artery, is identified before introducing the surgical instruments to prevent inadvertent injury (**Figure 7,** *B*). The vertebral levels are confirmed by identifying the first rib partially hidden beneath the subclavian artery and counting down distally (**Figure 7,** *C*). Pleural dissection then may be performed longitudinally over the length of the spine (**Figure 7,** *D*). As the pleura is dissected, the segmental vessels are divided using harmonic

laparoscopic coagulating shears to allow greater anterior spinal exposure for circumferential annular release and disk excision. To achieve optimal hemostasis, the harmonic scalpel is used over a 3- to 5-mm length of each segmental vessel (**Figure 7,** *E*). Following the division of the pleura, any remaining areolar tissue is divided, and packing sponges are used to create a space between the anterior spine and the pleura. Blunt circumferential exposure of the spine should be completed before disk excision. If distal exposure to the T12-L1 disk space is required, the longitudinal pleural incision may be extended with division and inferior retraction of the diaphragm insertion. Blunt dissection is then used to strip the diaphragm off the anterior spine, exposing the L1 vertebra. Exposure distal to L1 is not practical with this approach.

Disk excision is initiated by performing a circumferential annulotomy with the ultrasonic blade of the harmonic scalpel (**Figure 8,** *A*). Endo-

scopic rongeurs are first used to excise the most anterior and concave aspects of the intervertebral disk (**Figure 8,** *B*). The diskectomy should then proceed toward the convex rib head. An angled curet or rongeur may be used to remove the superior and inferior cartilage end plates from the vertebra. Awareness of the diskectomy path is vital to avoid damage to the neural elements as well as to prevent excess bone excision, which will cause increased bleeding and suboptimal visualization. The key to a comprehensive diskectomy is optimal visualization deep into the disk space; it not only allows complete removal of all disk tissue but also prevents injury to the posterior longitudinal ligament and neural elements (**Figure 8,** *C*). Bleeding from the bone can be limited by using the avascular plane of dissection between the cartilage end plate and the vertebral body in skeletally immature patients. Once the diskectomy is complete, bone graft (allograft or autograft) is placed (**Figure 8,** *D*). The

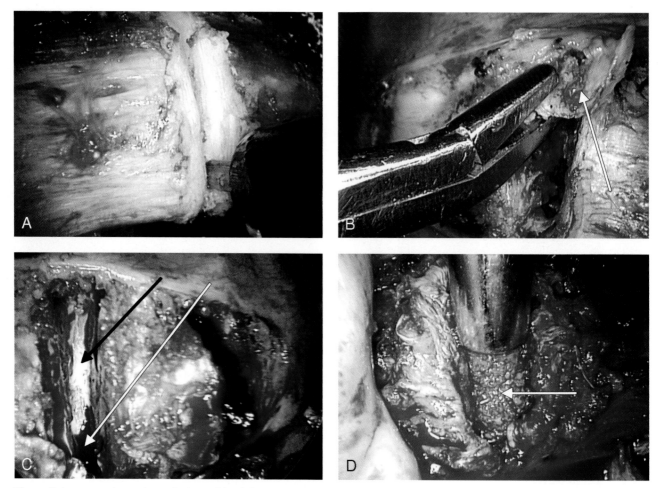

Figure 8 Intraoperative endoscopic views of the diskectomy. **A,** The disk incision is performed with a harmonic scalpel. **B,** The removal of disk tissue (arrow) is performed with an endoscopic rongeur. **C,** A complete disk excision (white arrow) demonstrates the intact posterior longitudinal ligament (black arrow). **D,** Morcellized autologous iliac crest bone graft (arrow) is placed in the disk space to ensure a solid fusion.

bone graft may be delivered into the disk space with an endoscopic plunger.

Wound Closure

The thoracoscopic procedure is completed by reapproximation and closure of the pleura using an endoscopic suturing device. Beginning at the distal site of the pleural or diaphragm incision, the suture needle is passed through both sides of the tissue. Once passed, an externally tied knot is slid down and secured (**Figure 9,** *A*). This suturing device provides a simple method of performing a running closure of the pleura by allowing a double-ended needle to be passed

from one jaw to the other (**Figure 9,** *B*). Once the pleura has been closed, the portals are removed, and the collapsed lung is reinflated by applying gradual positive-pressure ventilation. Lung reinflation is observed and confirmed endoscopically. The anesthesiologist should suction the trachea and the bronchi to reduce the risk of postoperative atelectasis; this is especially important in a long procedure and in the dependent lung because mucous congestion may be significant. The portals are then closed, beginning with the fascia and continuing superficially to the subcutaneous tissue, and then the skin. A chest tube is then inserted through an inferior

portal, tunneled subcutaneously to enter the chest more proximally, and secured with a purse-string closure.

Postoperative Regimen

The postoperative regimen varies, depending on whether anterior and posterior procedures are staged. In general, following posterior instrumentation, the patient is mobilized to a chair on postoperative day 1 or 2. The chest tube is removed when the drainage is less than 1 mL/kg in an 8- to 12-hour period; this typically oc-

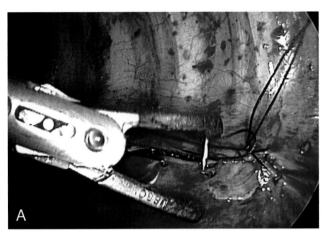
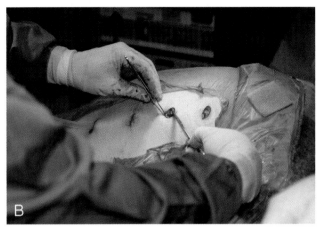

Figure 9 Wound closure. **A,** An endoscopic suturing device completes the reapproximation and closure of the pleura with an internally tied knot. **B,** Clinical photograph demonstrates how the portals are closed and the skin is reapproximated, with a chest tube placed in the inferior portal secured by a purse-string closure.

curs between the second and fourth postoperative day. Aggressive respiratory therapy is recommended, including incentive spirometry, chest percussion therapy, and early mobilization.

Avoiding Pitfalls and Complications

The potential complications of thoracoscopic surgery are essentially the same as those of an open anterior spinal procedure; they include possible injury to the cardiovascular system, major vessels, the lung, the diaphragm, the thoracic duct, or the spinal cord.

The greatest risk of iatrogenic injury is posed by suboptimal endoscopic visualization. Inadequate lung deflation and excessive bleeding are the most common causes of poor visualization. Minimizing each source of

bleeding with prompt and judicious use of electrocautery, ultrasonic coagulation, bone waxing, and early diskspace bone grafting is critical for maintaining optimal visualization, particularly in the later stages of the procedure. Proper camera/endoscope orientation also is necessary and requires having an assistant who is familiar with endoscopic procedures. The working instrument (harmonic scalpel, rongeur, or curet) should be placed in the portal that is aligned most closely with the disk. An angled endoscope placed one portal above or below will allow visualization directly into the depths of the disk space.

Additionally, before introducing the endoscope, direct sighting down a thoracic portal is an expedient means of ensuring that no lung tissue is in the surgical path and that the portal is positioned correctly. The instruments can then more easily be placed directly into the area of interest once the sur-

geon has been oriented by this "sneak peek."

An injury to the thoracic duct can be recognized intraoperatively by the presence of a cloudy fluid accumulation. Damage to the thoracic duct may be repaired by either suture or clip ligation of the vessels. If a chylous effusion develops postoperatively, a nonfat diet and a possible thoracic duct ligation must be considered.

Injury to the spinal cord may result from direct trauma during the diskectomy or from vascular insufficiency occurring after segmental vessel ligation. To prevent vascular insufficiency, an attempt to maintain key segmental vessels should be considered in high-risk cases, such as revision, congenital deformity, or kyphosis. Neuromonitoring and temporary vessel clipping also are recommended in high-risk cases.

Bibliography

Cheung KM, Wu JP, Cheng QH, Ma BS, Gao JC, Luk KD: Treatment of stiff thoracic scoliosis by thoracoscopic anterior release combined with posterior instrumentation and fusion. *J Orthop Surg* 2007;2:16.

Early SD, Newton PO, White KK, Wenger DR, Mubarak SJ: The feasibility of anterior thoracoscopic spine surgery in children under 30 kilograms. *Spine (Phila Pa 1976)* 2002;27(21):2368-2373.

Lenke LG, Betz RR, Harms J, et al: Adolescent idiopathic scoliosis: A new classification to determine extent of spinal arthrodesis. *J Bone Joint Surg Am* 2001;83-A(8):1169-1181.

Lenke LG, Newton PO, Marks MC, et al: Prospective pulmonary function comparison of open versus endoscopic anterior fusion combined with posterior fusion in adolescent idiopathic scoliosis. *Spine (Phila Pa 1976)* 2004;29(18):2055-2060.

Lonner BS, Auerbach JD, Estreicher M, et al: Video-assisted anterior thoracoscopic spinal fusion versus posterior spinal fusion: A comparative study utilizing the SRS-22 outcome instrument. *Spine (Phila Pa 1976)* 2009;34(2):193-198.

Lonner BS, Kondrachov D, Siddiqi F, Hayes V, Scharf C: Thoracoscopic spinal fusion compared with posterior spinal fusion for the treatment of thoracic adolescent idiopathic scoliosis. *J Bone Joint Surg Am* 2006;88(5):1022-1034.

Newton PO, Parent S, Marks M, Pawelek J: Prospective evaluation of 50 consecutive scoliosis patients surgically treated with thoracoscopic anterior instrumentation. *Spine (Phila Pa 1976)* 2005;30(17, Suppl):S100-S109.

Newton PO, Upasani VV, Lhamby J, Ugrinow VL, Pawelek JB, Bastrom TP: Surgical treatment of main thoracic scoliosis with thoracoscopic anterior instrumentation: A five-year follow-up study. *J Bone Joint Surg Am* 2008;90(10):2077-2089.

Newton PO, White KK, Faro F, Gaynor T: The success of thoracoscopic anterior fusion in a consecutive series of 112 pediatric spinal deformity cases. *Spine (Phila Pa 1976)* 2005;30(4):392-398.

Niemeyer T, Freeman BJ, Grevitt MP, Webb JK: Anterior thoracoscopic surgery followed by posterior instrumentation and fusion in spinal deformity. *Eur Spine J* 2000;9(6):499-504.

Norton RP, Patel D, Kurd MF, Picetti GD, Vaccaro AR: The use of thoracoscopy in the management of adolescent idiopathic scoliosis. *Spine (Phila Pa 1976)* 2007;32(24):2777-2785.

Papin P, Arlet V, Marchesi D, Laberge JM, Aebi M: Treatment of scoliosis in the adolescent by anterior release and vertebral arthrodesis under thoracoscopy: Preliminary results. *Rev Chir Orthop Reparatrice Appar Mot* 1998;84(3):231-238.

Reddi V, Clarke DV Jr, Arlet V: Anterior thoracoscopic instrumentation in adolescent idiopathic scoliosis: A systematic review. *Spine (Phila Pa 1976)* 2008;33(18):1986-1994.

Son-Hing JP, Blakemore LC, Poe-Kochert C, Thompson GH: Video-assisted thoracoscopic surgery in idiopathic scoliosis: Evaluation of the learning curve. *Spine (Phila Pa 1976)* 2007;32(6):703-707.

Wong HK, Hee HT, Yu Z, Wong D: Results of thoracoscopic instrumented fusion versus conventional posterior instrumented fusion in adolescent idiopathic scoliosis undergoing selective thoracic fusion. *Spine (Phila Pa 1976)* 2004;29(18):2031-2038; discussion 2039.

Coding

CPT Codes		Corresponding ICD-9 Codes	
22808	Arthrodesis, anterior, for spinal deformity, with our without cast; 2 to 3 vertebral segments	342.1 342.90 343.0	342.9 343 343.1
22810	Arthrodesis, anterior, for spinal deformity, with or without cast; 4 to 7 vertebral segments	342.1 342.90 343.0	342.9 343 343.1
22812	Arthrodesis, anterior, for spinal deformity, with or without cast; 8 or more vertebral segments	342.1 342.90 343.0	342.9 343 343.1
22845	Anterior instrumentation; 2 to 3 vertebral segments (List separately in addition to code for primary procedure)	170.2 342.9 343	342.1 342.90 343.0
22846	Anterior instrumentation; 4 to 7 vertebral segments (List separately in addition to code for primary procedure)	170.2 342.9 343	342.1 342.90 343.0
22847	Anterior instrumentation; 8 or more vertebral segments (List separately in addition to code for primary procedure)	170.2 342.9 343	342.1 342.90 343.0
20930	Allograft, morselized, or placement of osteopromotive material, for spine surgery only (List separately in addition to code for primary procedure)	170.2 733.13 737.30	724.6 733.81
20931	Allograft, structural, for spine surgery only (List separately in addition to code for primary procedure)	170.2 733.13	724.6 733.81
20936	Autograft for spine surgery only (includes harvesting the graft); local (eg, ribs, spinous process, or laminar fragments) obtained from the same incision (List separately in addition to code for primary procedure)	170.2 733.13	724.6 737.30
20937	Autograft for spine surgery only (includes harvesting the graft); morselized (through separate skin or fascial incision) (List separately in addition to code for primary procedure)	170.2 733.13 737.30	724.6 733.81
20938	Autograft for spine surgery only (includes harvesting the graft); structural, bicortical or tricortical (through separate skin or fascial incision) (List separately in addition to code for primary procedure)	170.2 733.13	724.6 733.81

CPT copyright © 2010 by the American Medical Association. All rights reserved.

Chapter 33
Thoracoscopic Corpectomy and Fusion

Rudolf W. Beisse, MD

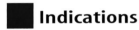

Indications

For certain types of fractures, tumors, and infection of the thoracolumbar spine associated with extensive destruction or defects of the vertebral body and the intervertebral disks, reconstruction of the load-bearing anterior spine is required to restore mobility and avoid loss of correction.

The anterior thoracoscopic approach, usually in combination with posterior instrumentation, is indicated for the following conditions: (1) fractures and unstable injuries located at the thoracolumbar junction from T11 to L2 (**Figure 1**); (2) fractures classified as A1.3, A2, A3, B, and C according to the AO classification of spine fractures with significant curvature of 20° or more in the sagittal or coronal plane (with type B and C fractures, posterior in addition to anterior instrumentation is mandatory; with the other types, it is optional); (3) posttraumatic, degenerative, or tumor-related narrowing of the spinal canal; (4) diskoligamentous segmental instability; (5) posttraumatic defor-

mity (anterior release and reconstruction); and (5) spondylodiskitis.

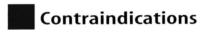

Contraindications

Thoracoscopic procedures are contraindicated in patients with cardiopulmonary insufficiency, acute posttraumatic respiratory failure, or coagulopathy. In patients with previous surgical interventions or infectious diseases of the lung and the mediastinum, extensive adhesions might be a relative contraindication for thoracoscopy.

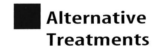

Alternative Treatments

Anterior reconstructive procedures in the anterior column of the thoracolumbar spine can be performed via either a conventional open or a mini-

open approach using microsurgical techniques. Posterolateral approaches, either unilateral or bilateral, also are appropriate for accessing the anterior column, but they usually are associated with higher approach-related morbidity because of the extensive exposure of the spine, spinal canal, and ribs that is associated with the ligature of roots.

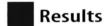

Results

In the management of spinal trauma, single posterior-only stabilizing and reconstructive techniques, even those using transpedicular bone grafting, have been shown to be insufficient in many cases, resulting in severe loss of correction of a previously achieved reduction. The anterior column supports almost 80% of body weight in the upright position. Several studies have demonstrated that surgical reconstruction of the load-bearing anterior column, including corpectomy, vertebral body replacement, and instrumentation, leads to a significantly better outcome in terms of the fusion rate and maintenance of correction (**Table 1**).

The influence of minimally invasive surgical techniques on the outcomes of patients with sports injuries to the spine was analyzed in a series of more than 1,500 patients who under-

Dr. Beisse or an immediate family member has received royalties from Aesculap Medical, is a member of a speakers' bureau or has made paid presentations on behalf of Aesculap Medical, and serves as a paid consultant to or is an employee of Aesculap Medical.

Portions of this chapter were adapted with permission from Beisse R: Endoscopic surgery on the thoracolumbar junction of the spine. Eur Spine J 2006;15:687-704.

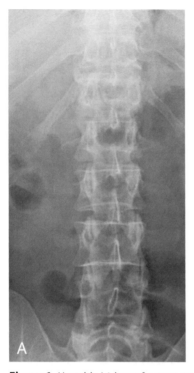 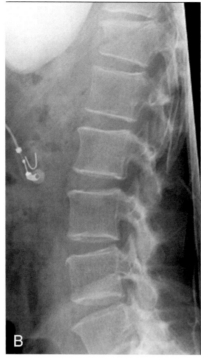 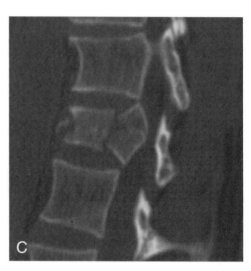

Figure 1 Unstable L1 burst fracture, type A 2.3 (AO classification), with spinal canal compromise. AP (**A**) and lateral (**B**) radiographs of the thoracolumbar junction demonstrate a discrete loss of height in L1, mainly in the anterior part of the vertebral body. **C,** The full extent of the injury is shown in a 2-dimensional CT reconstruction, which demonstrates a severe protrusion of the posterior wall, narrowing of the spinal canal, and a split fracture of the vertebral body in the sagittal plane.

went thoracoscopic surgery from 1996 through 2011 at the Trauma Center in Murnau, Germany, and the Orthopaedic Hospital of Munich. Of these 1,500 patients, data on 96 patients with spinal injuries between T3 and L2 were recorded in a 2-year period. A neurologic deficit was present in 15% of the patients, according to the Frankel scale. An injury at the thoracolumbar junction between T11 and L2 was present in 66% of the patients. In 19% of the patients, the injury was categorized as stable, and nonsurgical treatment was indicated. In 21% of the patients, posterior-only reduction and stabilization was performed. In 62% of the patients, posterior and thoracoscopic anterior reconstruction was performed, and in 14%, anterior-only thoracoscopic reconstruction was performed. At 2-year follow-up, loss of correction measured 0.5° in the group of posterior and anterior reconstruction patients and 5.5° in patients

treated nonsurgically, which was almost the same as the 4.5° loss of correction measured after single posterior-only reduction and stabilization. Two years after injury, 91% of the patients had resumed sports activity, 84% with similar frequency and 68% with the same intensity.

In a two-institution study of 212 patients with unstable spine injuries treated thoracoscopically at the Trauma Center in Murnau and at Stanford University, complete fusion was observed at 1-year follow-up in 85% of the fractures treated with anterior-only techniques and in 90% of the fractures treated with posterior and anterior techniques. Mean follow-up time was 3.9 years. Reconstruction of the spine profile was successful in more than 90% of the cases.

Initially, the mean operating time was 3.5 hours for a bisegmental reconstruction at the thoracolumbar junction including partial vertebrectomy,

vertebral body replacement, and anterior instrumentation. The time for the portion devoted to the approach to the retroperitoneal section ranged from 10 to 20 minutes, including the suture of the diaphragm. Passing the learning curve and using instruments and implants specially developed for the thoracoscopic technique shortened the mean operating time significantly, to 90 to 120 minutes.

Technique

Instruments/Equipment/Implants Required

For image transmission, we use a rigid 30° endoscope connected to a xenon light source and a 3-chip HDTV camera. The image is transmitted onto three flat-screen HDTVs mounted on a movable endoscopy tower positioned at the foot of the operating table. The

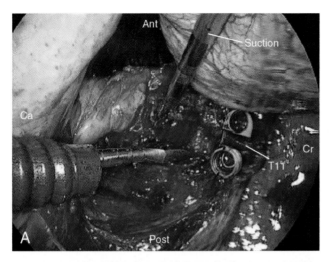

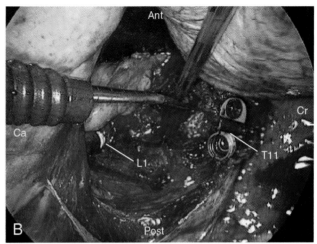

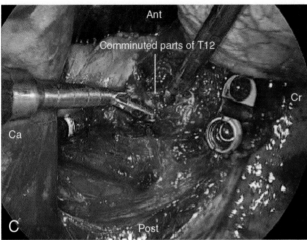

Figure 6 Partial corpectomy and decompression. **A,** A posterior osteotomy of the vertebral body is performed following the (virtual) connecting line between the two screws at their posterior alignment. **B,** An anterior osteotomy is performed, following the line of the anterior boundary of the screws. **C,** A partial corpectomy and posterior wall resection are performed using rongeurs and a high-speed drill. Ant = anterior, Ca = caudal, Cr = cranial, Post = posterior.

body and the disks are exposed with the rasp.

PARTIAL CORPECTOMY AND DECOMPRESSION

The extent of the planned partial vertebrectomy is defined with an osteotome, starting with the posterior osteotomy (**Figure 6**, *A*), followed by an anterior osteotomy using a slightly angled osteotome to avoid injury to the greater vessels in front (**Figure 6**, *B*). The disk spaces are opened to define the borders. After resection of the intervertebral disk(s), the fragmented parts of the vertebra are removed carefully with rongeurs. Radical removal of nonfractured parts of the vertebral body should be avoided. If decompression of the spinal canal is neces-

sary, the lower border of the pedicle should first be identified with a blunt hook. The base of the pedicle is then resected in a cranial direction with a Kerrison rongeur, and the thecal sac can be identified. Then the posterior fragment that occupies the spinal canal can be removed (**Figure 6**, *C*).

BONE GRAFTING

When using a bone graft for vertebral body replacement, the graft bed is prepared, and the length and the depth of the graft bed are measured with a caliper. When a monosegmental fusion is planned, a tricortical bone graft is taken from the iliac crest. If the bone graft is longer than 2 cm, the iliac crest is reconstructed using a titanium plate. The bone graft is prepared for

insertion and mounted on a graft holder. The cortical bone is perforated with several burr holes to facilitate vascular ingrowth and new bone formation. The working portal is removed, and a speculum is inserted. This allows the insertion of a bone graft up to 1.5 cm in length into the thoracic cavity. If the bone graft is longer, it is inserted without using the speculum, but with Langenbeck hooks. In such cases, the graft is mounted on the graft holder inside the thoracic cavity. The bone graft is inserted by press-fit into the graft bed.

VERTEBRAL BODY REPLACEMENT

For vertebral body replacement, especially in bisegmental reconstructions, I use a hydraulic distractible cage. The

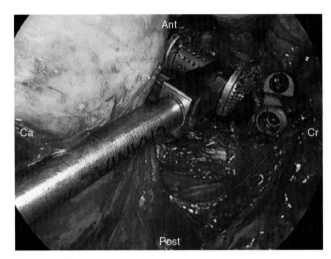

Figure 7 Vertebral body replacement with a distractible titanium cage. The cage is inserted in a central position within the vertebral body defect and checked fluorographically in both planes. Ant = anterior, Ca = caudal, Cr = cranial, Post = posterior.

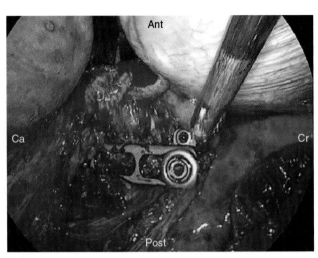

Figure 8 The anterior instrumentation is completed using a constraint plate system. Ant = anterior, Ca = caudal, Cr = cranial, Post = posterior.

titanium cage comes with fully adaptable end plates to reduce the risk of subsidence. Before the vertebral replacement device is implanted, a probe hook is used under fluoroscopic control to verify that the implant site has been prepared to the correct size and depth and is clean.

Two Langenbeck hooks are inserted into the incision for the working portals, and the incision is widened slightly. The vertebral body replacement is then gradually introduced through the chest wall into the thoracic cavity and positioned over the defect in the vertebral body with a holder (**Figure 7**). Another check is made that no soft tissue, in particular the ligated segment vessels, has slipped between the corpectomy defect and the vertebral body replacement. With carefully regulated blows on a tamper and under fluoroscopic control, the vertebral body replacement is implanted into the planned central position in the vertebral body and distracted. The implant is surrounded with the spongiosa harvested from the partial corpectomy. An antibiotic medium (eg, gentamicin collagen) can be added to the spongiosa.

After the corpectomy defect zone has been filled with spongiosa, it is covered with a fibrin fleece.

ANTERIOR INSTRUMENTATION
Because the screws and clamping elements that came with the implant were placed into position before beginning the partial corpectomy, the plate now just has to be fastened and the anterior screws of the four-point fixation inserted. The distance between the screws is defined with a special measuring instrument to select a plate of the correct length. This is introduced lengthwise into the thoracic cavity through the incision for the working portal, laid onto the clamping elements using a holding forceps, and fixed with nuts with a starting torque of 15 Nm. The plate can be brought into direct bone contact with the lateral vertebral body wall by tightening the bone screws. The anterior screws are inserted after temporary fixation of a targeting device and opening of the cortex. Because of the heart shape of the vertebral body, the anterior screws are usually 5 mm shorter than the posterior screws. The fixation of the constraint plate and

screw implant is completed with the insertion of a locking screw that locks the polyaxial mechanism of the posterior screws (**Figure 8**).

Wound Closure
The retractor is moved, and the gap in the diaphragm is sutured thoracoscopically wherever necessary (**Figure 9**). We recommend that every incision in the attachment longer than 2 cm be sutured thoracoscopically to ensure that a hernia does not occur. The thoracic cavity is irrigated, blood clots are removed, and a chest tube is inserted with the end placed in the costodiaphragmatic recess. The lung is reinflated under thoracoscopic view. The portals are closed, first with adaptive sutures of the muscle layer and subcutaneous tissue, followed by an intracutaneous running bioabsorbable suture of the skin. The chest tube is connected to a chest drainage device with a water-sealed chamber. A radiographic check with the image amplifier is performed in both planes in the operating room before the sterile drapes and instruments are removed.

———————————————■

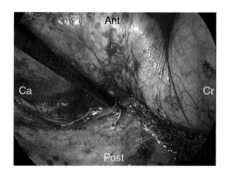

Figure 9 The diaphragm is sutured closed. Ant = anterior, Ca = caudal, Cr = cranial, Post = posterior.

Postoperative Regimen

The patient is intubated while still in the operating room. Ventilation is recommended only for patients with a higher risk of lung failure, such as patients with a posttraumatic lung contusion, chronic pulmonary dysfunction, a long surgical time or high blood loss, and a low body temperature. The patient is kept in the intensive care unit overnight. On the morning of the first postoperative day, the thoracic drain is clamped and a radiograph of the chest is obtained. If the lung has expanded fully, the chest tube is removed, and the patient is transferred out of intensive care. Postoperative radiographs and CT scans are performed on the second postoperative day (**Figure 10**).

Beginning on the first postoperative day, the patient is mobilized without a corset, avoiding torsion and kyphosis. The patient is instructed to perform intensive breathing exercises. Physical therapy is started during the first week, including standing and walking, so the patient can gradually resume activities of daily living. Sports activities and heavy load bearing are prohibited for the first 3 months. The patient is usually discharged after 5 to 6 days and usually continues physical therapy in a rehabilitation center.

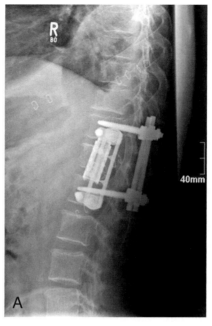
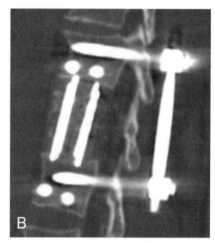

Figure 10 Postoperative images of the spine obtained after posterior and anterior reduction, stabilization, and decompression. Lateral radiograph (**A**) and two-dimensional sagittal CT reconstruction (**B**) show the spinal profile restored and the anterior column reconstructed by use of a distractible vertebral body replacement device.

Avoiding Pitfalls and Complications

Given the direct proximity of vital structures, the potential for complications with spine surgery is high. Compared with the thoracic spine, surgery at the level of the thoracolumbar junction carries less risk of neurologic complications because the spinal cord tapers at this level and the spinal canal is relatively wide. Even more attention must be paid to the anteriorly situated vessels, however. At the level of the thoracic spine, the spinal cord and greater vessels are at risk. Injury to these vessels represents a life-threatening complication that must be treated by immediate thoracophrenotomy with extensive exposure, mobilization, and tying of the vessels.

Injury to the spleen or thoracic duct also has been reported. This is best avoided by careful use of instruments and meticulous surgical technique. The thoracic duct usually is located close to the anterior circumference of the vertebral column and therefore can be avoided by staying close to the bony surface of the vertebra.

Overall, no evidence exists of a higher rate of complications with thoracoscopic spinal procedures after the surgeon has mastered the learning curve of the thoracoscopic technique. Attending bioskill laboratories and workshops and observing a spine surgeon experienced in thoracoscopic spine surgery are recommended ways of developing skill with the thoracoscopic procedure.

▌ Bibliography

Beisse R: Endoscopic surgery on the thoracolumbar junction of the spine. *Eur Spine J* 2006;15(6):687-704.

Beisse R: Video-assisted techniques in the management of thoracolumbar fractures. *Orthop Clin North Am* 2007;38(3): 419-429.

Beisse R, Mückley T, Schmidt MH, Hauschild M, Bühren V: Surgical technique and results of endoscopic anterior spinal canal decompression. *J Neurosurg Spine* 2005;2(2):128-136.

Beisse R, Potulski M, Beger J, Bühren V: Development and clinical application of a thoracoscopy implantable plate frame for treatment of thoracolumbar fractures and instabilities. *Orthopade* 2002;31(4):413-422.

Beisse R, Potulski M, Temme C, Bühren V: Endoscopically controlled division of the diaphragm: A minimally invasive approach to ventral management of thoracolumbar fractures of the spine. *Unfallchirurg* 1998;101(8):619-627.

Faciszewski T, Winter RB, Lonstein JE, Denis F, Johnson L: The surgical and medical perioperative complications of anterior spinal fusion surgery in the thoracic and lumbar spine in adults: A review of 1223 procedures. *Spine (Phila Pa 1976)* 1995;20(14):1592-1599.

Han PP, Kenny K, Dickman CA: Thoracoscopic approaches to the thoracic spine: Experience with 241 surgical procedures. *Neurosurgery* 2002;51(5, Suppl)S88-S95.

Kim DH, Jahng TA, Balabhadra RS, Potulski M, Beisse R: Thoracoscopic transdiaphragmatic approach to thoracolumbar junction fractures. *Spine J* 2004;4(3):317-328.

Knop C, Blauth M, Bastian L, Lange U, Kesting J, Tscherne H: Fractures of the thoracolumbar spine: Late results of posterior instrumentation and its consequences. *Unfallchirurg* 1997;100(8):630-639.

Mack MJ, Regan JJ, Bobechko WP, Acuff TE: Application of thoracoscopy for diseases of the spine. *Ann Thorac Surg* 1993; 56(3):736-738.

Magerl F, Aebi M, Gertzbein SD, Harms J, Nazarian S: A comprehensive classification of thoracic and lumbar injuries. *Eur Spine J* 1994;3(4):184-201.

McAfee PC, Regan JR, Zdeblick T, et al: The incidence of complications in endoscopic anterior thoracolumbar spinal reconstructive surgery: A prospective multicenter study comprising the first 100 consecutive cases. *Spine (Phila Pa 1976)* 1995;20(14):1624-1632.

Merkel P, Hauck S, Zentz F, Bühren V, Beisse R: Spinal column injuries in sport: Treatment strategies and clinical results. *Unfallchirurg* 2008;111(9):711-718.

Rosenthal D, Dickman CA: Thoracoscopic microsurgical excision of herniated thoracic discs. *J Neurosurg* 1998;89(2): 224-235.

Rosenthal D, Rosenthal R, de Simone A: Removal of a protruded thoracic disc using microsurgical endoscopy: A new technique. *Spine (Phila Pa 1976)* 1994;19(9):1087-1091.

Coding

CPT Codes		Corresponding ICD-9 Codes	
22556	Arthrodesis, anterior interbody technique, including minimal discectomy to prepare interspace (other than for decompression); thoracic	721.2 722.51 737.39	721.41 733.13 805.2
22558	Arthrodesis, anterior interbody technique, including minimal discectomy to prepare interspace (other than for decompression); lumbar	567.31 721.42 722.52	721.3 722.51 733.13
22842	Posterior segmental instrumentation (eg, pedicle fixation, dual rods with multiple hooks and sublaminar wires); 3 to 6 vertebral segments (List separately in addition to code for primary procedure)	342.1 342.90 343.0	342.9 343 343.1
22843	Posterior segmental instrumentation (eg, pedicle fixation, dual rods with multiple hooks and sublaminar wires); 7 to 12 vertebral segments (List separately in addition to code for primary procedure)	170.2 342.9 343	342.1 342.90 343.0
22844	Posterior segmental instrumentation (eg, pedicle fixation, dual rods with multiple hooks and sublaminar wires); 13 or more vertebral segments (List separately in addition to code for primary procedure)	170.2 342.9 343	342.1 342.90 343.0
22845	Anterior instrumentation; 2 to 3 vertebral segments (List separately in addition to code for primary procedure)	170.2 342.9 343	342.1 342.90 343.0
22846	Anterior instrumentation; 4 to 7 vertebral segments (List separately in addition to code for primary procedure)	170.2 342.9 343	342.1 342.90 343.0
22847	Anterior instrumentation; 8 or more vertebral segments (List separately in addition to code for primary procedure)	170.2 342.9 343	342.1 342.90 343.0
63085	Vertebral corpectomy (vertebral body resection), partial or complete, transthoracic approach with decompression of spinal cord and/or nerve root(s); thoracic, single segment	170.2 806.20 806.22	721.41 806.21 806.23
63086	Vertebral corpectomy (vertebral body resection), partial or complete, transthoracic approach with decompression of spinal cord and/or nerve root(s); thoracic, each additional segment (List separately in addition to code for primary procedure)	170.2 722.72 806.21	721.41 806.20 806.22
63087	Vertebral corpectomy (vertebral body resection), partial or complete, combined thoracolumbar approach with decompression of spinal cord, cauda equina or nerve root(s), lower thoracic or lumbar; single segment	170.2 721.41 722.72	567.31 721.42 722.73
63088	Vertebral corpectomy (vertebral body resection), partial or complete, combined thoracolumbar approach with decompression of spinal cord, cauda equina or nerve root(s), lower thoracic or lumbar; each additional segment (List separately in addition to code for primary procedure)	170.2 721.42 722.73	567.31 722.72 805.4

CPT copyright © 2010 by the American Medical Association. All rights reserved.

Chapter 34
Open Transthoracic Corpectomy/Fusion

S. Tim Yoon, MD, PhD
James A. Sanfilippo, MD

Indications

The open transthoracic approach to the thoracic spine allows surgical exposure of the anterior aspect of the spinal column. This approach was developed in the late 19th century for the treatment of spinal tuberculosis, or Pott disease. Current indications for this approach include infection (osteomyelitis and diskitis), primary or metastatic tumors, burst fractures associated with trauma, or large disk herniations that extend behind the vertebral body, when complete anterior decompression is required. The approach also is used to reconstruct anterior column defects and to improve correction and the fusion rate in deformity surgery.

Contraindications

Although the open thoracic approach can be performed safely, it also can be associated with significant morbidity.

The effect on the pulmonary system must always be carefully considered. In the perioperative period, open thoracotomy and the lung deflation or retraction that is necessary for exposing the spine are stressors on the pulmonary system. Therefore, careful evaluation of the patient's pulmonary status is required preoperatively. Studies have documented significant reduction in pulmonary function after thoracotomy for deformity surgery. Therefore, severe pulmonary compromise is a contraindication for open thoracotomy. The great vessels often lie close to the surgical area of the spine, and the segmental vessels that flow from them need to be controlled during the procedure. For this reason, prior surgery on the approach side must be considered carefully, and, when ligating the segmental vessels, consideration must be given to the blood supply of the spinal cord. Patients must be carefully chosen for this technique.

Alternative Treatments

Open transthoracic corpectomy and fusion can be highly effective in treating tumors, fractures, herniated disks, and various other spinal pathologies, but it is only one of many treatment options that should be considered for these spinal diseases. The decision to perform an open thoracic corpectomy should take into account patient comorbidities, lesion type, and the surgeon's experience. For instance, in a patient with poor pulmonary function, a posterior or posterolateral approach corpectomy, such as costotransversectomy or transpedicular techniques, may be preferred, to reduce the risk of pulmonary complications. Combined anterior and posterior approaches are also frequently used, especially with multilevel corpectomies. The location and size of the lesion also may impact the choice of open versus less invasive thoracic approaches. Less invasive transthoracic approaches include video-assisted thoracoscopy and mini-open thoracotomy using extreme lateral approach techniques. The surgeon's expertise also affects the choice of approach, as not all surgeons are equally adept at all approaches. Ultimately, the decision whether to use transthoracic corpectomy and fusion or an alterna-

Dr. Yoon or an immediate family member is a member of a speakers' bureau or has made paid presentations on behalf of Stryker and Biomet; serves as a paid consultant to or is an employee of Abbott; and has received research or institutional support from AO Spine, Medtronic Sofamor Danek, Nuvasive, Johnson & Johnson, Smith & Nephew, and Biomet. Neither Dr. Sanfilippo nor any immediate family member has received anything of value from or owns stock in a commercial company or institution related directly or indirectly to the subject of this chapter.

Table 1 Results of Open Transthoracic Corpectomy and Fusion

Author(s) (Year)	Number of Patients	Procedure or Approach	Mean Patient Age in Years (Range)	Mean Follow-up (Range)	Diagnosis	Results
Cotler et al (1985)	37	Anterior transthoracic or lumbar	NA	1 year minimum	Tumor, infection	21 patients with incomplete neurologic deficits improved; 10 recovered completely 25 of 27 patients (80%) followed for at least 1 year had solid fusions. 1 pseudarthrosis 1 delayed fusion 2 deaths in immediate postoperative period 3 deaths in first 6 weeks
Hosono et al (1995)	37	Anterior only	53.7 (10-80)	26.2 months	Metastatic tumor	84 patients had cervical, thoracic, or lumbar surgery 94% had pain relief 81% had motor improvement
Shehadi et al (2007)	47	Anterior	53 (35-84)	13 months median	Metastatic tumor	87 patients underwent various surgical treatments, including 47 anterior-only approaches. Significant improvement in pain and neurologic scores 11% had major complications
Street et al (2007)	24	Anterior, anterior and posterior, posterior	NA	NA	Metastatic tumor	VAS improvement 3.3 ECOG improvement 0.5
Lu et al (2010)	46	Anterior thoracic or lumbar	50.6 ± 16	NA	Osteomyelitis, metastasis, trauma	20 patients anterior only; 26 anterior and posterior. Mean ASIA score improvement 0.26 and 0.24, respectively. Complications rate 32% and 41%, respectively

NA = not available; VAS = visual analog scale; ECOG = Eastern Cooperative Oncology Group score; ASIA = American Spinal Injury Association.

tive approach should be made on a case-by-case basis to ensure that the approach used best fits the disease, patient, and surgeon.

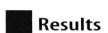

Results

Results specific to open transthoracic corpectomy and fusion are difficult to report because this technique is used for a multitude of different diagnostic indications, including tumor, fracture, osteomyelitis, disk herniation, and os-

sified posterior longitudinal ligament. Studies typically report on cohorts with a mix of diagnoses and a combination of anterior-only, anterior and posterior, and posterior-only corpectomies. In addition, no widely accepted criteria for "success" exist, making comparisons among studies even more difficult. A few of the more recent publications that include significant numbers of anterior transthoracic corpectomy cases are included in **Table 1**.

Technique

Preoperative Imaging and Considerations

Before performing an open transthoracic corpectomy, appropriate images should be obtained to help the surgeon fully understand the surgical anatomy, the character of the lesion in need of decompression, and the anatomy and number of the involved vertebra. Plain radiographs that include the cervicothoracic junction and the thoracolumbar junction are necessary to accurately identify the vertebral

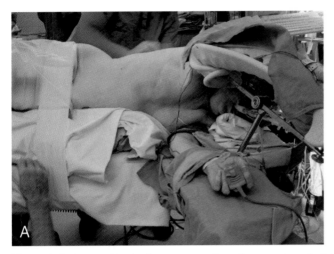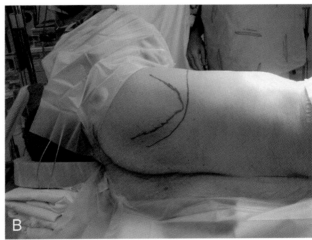

Figure 1 Patient positioning for open transthoracic corpectomy. **A,** Anterior view of a patient in the lateral decubitus position. The head is well supported, as are both arms, which are angled slightly superiorly to provide better access. Beanbags are useful to secure the patient. **B,** Posterior view of the patient in the lateral decubitus position. Note that the scapula and ribs are marked.

level. The surgical level should be identified preoperatively by counting levels both caudally, from the cervicothoracic junction, and cranially, from the thoracolumbar junction. Advanced imaging is essential when planning the procedure. CT is helpful in characterizing the bony anatomy and allows the surgeon to evaluate the bony destruction or compression present with tumor or infection. MRI is better at displaying soft-tissue properties and spinal cord compression.

Once the nature of the lesion and the patient's anatomy have been identified, the surgeon must choose the appropriate side on which to perform the approach. Typically, open thoracotomy and corpectomy is performed through a lateral thoracotomy. Therefore, it is important to determine the side of the approach based on the location and the extent of the lesion to be removed and the history of previous thoracic surgery. Generally, this means using a thoracotomy ipsilateral to the lesion; ie, a tumor extending from the left side of the vertebral body should be removed via a left-side approach. Less commonly, upper thoracic lesions may need to be addressed. In such cases, a direct anterior approach via a sternotomy or

manubriectomy may be required to provide better access and avoid the scapula. When planning surgery in the upper thoracic spine, the surgeon must remember that the heart and aortic arch lie along the ventral and left side of the vertebral bodies and can obstruct the spinal exposure. Therefore, a right-side approach may be easier at these levels. In the lower thoracic spine, the position of the liver makes an approach from the right more challenging, so a left-side approach, when possible, may be more appropriate. Also, if the lesion is not predominantly on one side, a left-side approach may be preferred because generally it is easier to mobilize the thoracic aorta than the vena cava, and the aorta is more durable than the vena cava.

Setup and Patient Positioning

The patient is placed on a standard radiolucent operating table, initially in the supine position. A decision should be made as to whether standard intubation or double-lumen intubation is to be used. At the lower thoracic levels, double-lumen intubation is usually not necessary, and the lung can be kept out of the surgical field with malleable retractors. If the midthoracic or

upper thoracic level is to be approached, double-lumen intubation is preferred because it allows single-lung ventilation, which permits optimal visualization of the surgical area. Double-lumen intubation requires greater skill on the part of the anesthesia team than does single-lumen intubation, and it requires a longer preparation time before surgery. Following successful intubation, a Foley catheter is placed to monitor urinary output during the surgery. The patient is then turned to the lateral decubitus position, with the side of the approach facing up (**Figure 1**, *A*). An axillary roll, such as an intravenous bag or rolled towel, is placed under the axilla. The hips are flexed 20° to 30° to take the stretch off the psoas muscle, and the knees are flexed 45° to 60°. A pillow is placed under the down knee to protect the peroneal nerve, and another is placed between the legs for comfort. The patient is then secured into position with a beanbag, tape, and/or belts such that the patient is secure even if repositioning of the operating table is required intraoperatively. The upper arm can be secured with special arm braces or simply supported with pillows between the arms. Care must be taken to ensure that the hardware used to maintain positioning does not interfere with the surgical field, the use of retraction, or the use of intraoperative imaging modalities. Better exposure of the spine can be obtained by bending the thoracic area to spread the up ribs. This is done by jackknifing, or "breaking," the bed. An additional bump can be placed under the thoracic region to help open the rib cage on the approach side (**Figure 1**, *B*). Once the table is jackknifed, the restraints must be checked once more and resecured as necessary.

Intraoperative imaging is then used to identify the appropriate surgical level. A C-arm is brought in to obtain perfect lateral imaging of the thoracic spine. The levels are counted up from the thoracolumbar junction and again down from the cervicothoracic junction and compared with the preoperative imaging and numbering. Another approach is to use an AP view to count the ribs from the T12 level and proceed cranially. A mark should be placed on the skin over the level of the lesion and another mark over the rib at that level (**Figure 1**, *B*). The patient is then prepared and draped in the usual sterile fashion.

The surgeon must remember that the spinal cord is relatively immobile and is sensitive to manipulation at the thoracic level. Intraoperative neural monitoring should be considered when spinal cord decompression or deformity correction is planned. A set of prepositioning and postpositioning somatosensory- and motor-evoked potentials can be helpful to determine position-related neural insults.

The Approach

The rib chosen for resection should be one or two levels proximal to the vertebra that needs to be exposed. A lateral spine radiograph can be helpful in the planning phase. As described earlier, a lateral fluorographic image can simplify the decision of where to locate the skin incision. During surgery, the ribs can be palpated and counted,

beginning with the 12th rib and proceeding cranially. The skin is incised over the appropriate rib, and the dissection is carried through the latissimus dorsi and serratus anterior muscles, both of which are innervated proximally. Subperiosteal dissection of the rib is performed with electrocautery and special rib dissectors. Typically, the rib is resected anteriorly to the anterior axillary line and posteriorly to the angle of the rib. Care should be taken with the neurovascular structures that run along the caudal interior surface of the rib. The parietal pleura is identified and incised, using great care to avoid damaging the underlying lung. A rib spreader can be used to gain additional space between the ribs. The ipsilateral lung can be pushed out of the way with malleable retractors or deflated to provide exposure of the spine when double-lumen intubation is used. The spine and overlying parietal pleura can now be visualized. A radiopaque marker is placed at the surgical level, and fluoroscopy again is used to reconfirm the surgical level.

The overlying pleura is incised and swept off the spine. The spine appears as a series of peaks and troughs, with the intervertebral disks corresponding to the peaks and the vertebral bodies corresponding to the troughs. The segmental vessels are identified over the vertebral body to be removed. Nutrient vessels to the spinal cord have their collateralization at the level of the foramen; therefore, these segmental vessels should be ligated at the midvertebral body to reduce the chances of compromising the blood supply to the spinal cord. One method of testing for vascular compromise of the spinal cord is to temporarily clamp the segmental vessels and then analyze the effect this has as measured by intraoperative monitoring.

The entire vertebral body must be exposed. This requires excision of the appropriate rib head or heads. Knowledge of the rib anatomy is important

because the rib articulates with the vertebra of the same number as well as the cranially adjacent vertebral body. It may be necessary to excise the rib head of the same numbered rib and the rib head of the caudally numbered rib. For example, to fully visualize the 7th vertebral body, the heads of the 7th and 8th ribs may need to be removed to gain full exposure of the transverse process, the pedicle, and the intervertebral disk above and below the body.

The Corpectomy

Before beginning the corpectomy, the surgeon must know the boundaries of the vertebra to be removed. First, the lateral and anterior boundaries are identified. This is accomplished safely by identifying the pedicle. A small curet is used to carefully dissect and identify the pedicle. Then a Penfield 4 elevator can be placed on the inferior margin of the pedicle to identify the neural foramen. When necessary, a burr can be used to drill away the lateral pedicle and thin the medial pedicle wall. A Kerrison rongeur can then be used to safely remove the remaining pedicle. With the pedicle removed, the lateral aspect of the spinal canal can be identified. A Penfield or Woodson probe can be used, if necessary, to further delineate the posterior vertebral body and posterior longitudinal ligament (PLL). Finding the cranial and caudal margins of the vertebral body consists of finding the intervertebral disks. A standard diskectomy can be performed, leaving the posterior anulus intact to protect the spinal canal.

The actual removal of the vertebral body can be accomplished in a variety of ways. A large malleable retractor is placed to protect the great vessels next to the spine. If the bone is to be used for future grafting, a series of rongeurs, curets, and osteotomes can be used. If bone graft is not a concern, a burr also can be used to quickly remove the vertebral body. Typically, it is safest to leave a thin posterior rim of

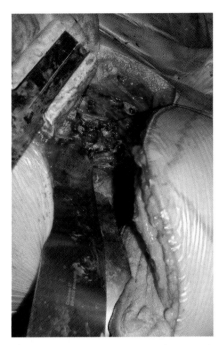

Figure 2 Intraoperative photograph shows rib retractors positioned superior to inferior and malleable retractors placed anterior to the spine to protect the large vessels and lung. The patient's head is to the right.

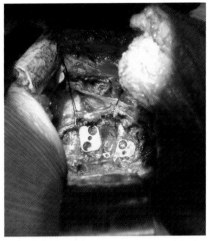

Figure 3 Intraoperative photograph shows staples placed in the lateral vertebra above and below the corpectomy defect. A small portion of a titanium mesh cage is visible at the corpectomy defect. The patient's head is to the right.

bone intact during the initial corpectomy; this rim of bone is removed carefully later in the corpectomy process. A thin rim of anterior bone often is left attached to the anterior longitudinal ligament to contain graft material and provide protection to the great vessels. Bony removal is carried across the midline and to the contralateral cortex of the vertebral body. Finally, the thin shell of posterior bone, which was left during the initial corpectomy, can be removed using a series of curets and reverse curets, collapsing the posterior wall of the body into the space created during the corpectomy. When a complete spinal canal decompression is desired, the contralateral pedicle should be identified, to ensure that the decompression has been carried adequately to the contralateral side. At this point, the PLL is encountered. If the PLL is not involved in the compressive pathology, it can be left intact. If it is involved, it can be removed at this time (**Figure 2**).

Reconstruction and Fusion

After the corpectomy is completed, the dual goals of mechanical reconstruction and fusion should be considered. Historically, structural bone graft combined with cancellous bone graft served this purpose. Rib harvested during the thoracotomy provides convenient material. The rib can be used as struts that are wedged into the corpectomy defect or morcellized and used as corticocancellous nonstructural bone graft. When more robust structural bone is desired, however, fibula autograft or allograft can be used, often in combination with the rib graft. Humeral or femoral shafts also are robust structural grafts. Using bone for structural graft has several advantages: it can be impacted into position relatively easily, it allows better radiographic imaging, and it permits direct fusion between host bone and structural graft.

Recently, cages made of synthetic materials such as titanium mesh (**Figure 3**), polyetheretherketone and expandable cages have been gaining popularity. These devices have several advantages: they are usually designed to prevent migration, and the expand-

able cages can simplify graft sizing and fitting. Disadvantages include their higher cost and the fact that bulky devices can occupy potential bone fusion bed and hinder visualization on radiographic and CT imaging.

The nonstructural graft material often is the rib graft. In cases not involving tumor or infection, the corpectomy bone can be used. These sources usually provide a generous amount of high-quality graft material. When local graft is insufficient, however, iliac crest bone or synthetics can be used.

When interbody fusion is not necessary, the surgeon may choose to use bone cement for structural support instead of bone or cages. The advantages of cement are that it is very cost effective, it fills in irregular surfaces, it is easy to use, and it provides immediate axial support and some rotational control when used with rebars. Before injecting the cement, the preferred technique is to use K-wires or staples that enter the end plate and occupy some of the corpectomy defect. Then, the cement is injected using a 60-mL Toomey syringe. It is important to remember that the cement will expand slightly while hardening, and care must be taken to prevent expansion into the spinal canal (**Figure 4**).

Additional stability can be achieved with instrumentation systems. Anterior-only instrumentation can be used with single-level corpectomy procedures, as long as good bone quality is present. Additional posterior instrumentation may be required in multilevel corpectomy, a highly unstable spine (three-column injury), or a spine with poor bone quality.

Wound Closure

After placement of the necessary implants, fluoroscopy is again used to visualize the corpectomy site and hardware. Copious irrigation is used, and any bleeding is controlled with thrombostatic agents and bipolar cautery. The lung is allowed to reinflate. Through an incision placed two or

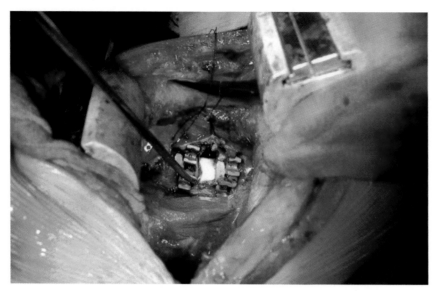

Figure 4 Intraoperative photograph shows cement in the corpectomy defect, covering the titanium mesh cage. Screws have been placed through the lateral vertebral body staples. The patient's head is to the right.

three levels caudal to the corpectomy incision, a chest tube is inserted and secured to the skin with suture. This allows for postoperative fluid drainage, manages potential air leaks, and prevents the development of postoperative pneumothorax. The rib spreader is removed, and the pleura is repaired, if possible, with small-gauge absorbable suture. Large sutures are used to approximate the ribs. The intercostal tissues are reapproximated and closed with absorbable suture. The skin is closed in standard fashion. A postoperative radiograph is taken to visualize the hardware and ensure proper lung reinflation.

Postoperative Regimen

Early mobilization is desirable. Dangling the legs over the side of the bed or sitting in a chair the day after the surgery is recommended if the patient is medically stable. Deep vein thrombosis prevention with sequential com-

pression devices should be used until the patient is discharged or highly mobile. The patient is asked to walk progressively more each day after surgery.

The chest tube should be set to a suction of –20 cm of water. Chest tube output should be monitored, and the tube should be removed at the earliest moment based on the institution's protocol. Although the patient can walk with the chest tube in place, it can hamper the patient's mobilization, as it can be uncomfortable and care must be taken to avoid accidental removal of the tube. Surgical reconstruction should be performed in a manner that allows ambulation and light physical activities postoperatively. Brace wear is not always necessary; however, in patients in whom rigid fixation is not accomplished, a brace should be used.

Periodic radiographic follow-up in the outpatient setting is required until solid arthrodesis is achieved. In cases of tumor, long-term surveillance imaging may be necessary. In cases of infection, long-term antibiotics should be given, with the involvement of an infectious disease specialist. The

erythrocyte sedimentation rate and C-reactive protein level should be monitored until they have normalized.

Avoiding Pitfalls and Complications

During the preoperative phase, understanding the proper indications and contraindications for the procedure is fundamental to avoiding pitfalls. The surgeon should consider alternatives to an open thoracotomy in patients with severe pulmonary compromise. Extubation may be difficult after open thoracotomy in these patients, and even after extubation, pulmonary function may worsen. Another contraindication is a history of previous thoracotomy. In these patients, exposure can be more difficult, and there is a higher risk of postoperative pleural effusions.

During surgery, multiple technical issues should be considered. Determining the best rib at which to perform the thoracotomy is important. A useful rule of thumb is to choose a site one or two ribs higher than the corpectomy level, but a lateral view (radiograph or intraoperative fluoroscopic visualization) can take away the guesswork and provide a more consistent entry site to the chest. The incision itself can significantly affect postoperative pain. One common mistake is to make a much larger incision than is necessary. Often, a relatively modest incision that is directly lateral to the corpectomy area is sufficient, and this will result in less postoperative pain than a larger incision. After entry into the chest cavity, it is important to identify and protect the large vessels. Vascular injury is rare, but when it occurs, it can be devastating. Typically, a malleable retractor is placed between the spine and the large vessels. It is preferable to perform the diskectomy above and below the ver-

Deformity Correction

Standard staple placement often does not allow significant active scoliosis correction at the time of implantation. With a flexible deformity, however, some correction of the scoliosis is often achieved merely with positioning of the patient on the operating table. Additional correction can sometimes be achieved using manual maneuvers at the time of staple placement to maximize the angular correction at each level. External manipulation of the rib cage and/or application of a gentle downward force on the segment of interest using a blunt pushing instrument can facilitate safe instrumentation in a more corrected position. This maneuver is difficult, however, and often yields less correction than desired. If these manual maneuvers are used, they should be performed both during the creation of pilot holes using the trial and during staple implantation.

When ligament tethers are used, these manual maneuvers usually are not required to correct the deformity. Sequential compression across vertebral body screws or anchors and tensioning of the ligament at each level achieves the desired segmental correction in a powerful yet controlled fashion.

Wound Closure

Standard closure of the chest is performed after reinflation of the lung and suctioning of excess air from the chest cavity. A small (20-French) chest tube can be placed at one of the incision sites and may be removed 1 to 3 days postoperatively as needed. Dissolvable sutures and Dermabond (Ethicon, Somerville, NJ) are used to close the skin.

Postoperative Regimen

The patient is mobilized as tolerated beginning on postoperative day 1 and is discharged home in 3 to 5 days. Activity is restricted for the first 6 weeks; walking is the most appropriate physical therapy. Significant bending, lifting, and twisting from a standing position should be avoided. Between 6 and 12 weeks, the activity restrictions are gradually lifted, with return to full activity allowed by 12 weeks. No brace is required.

As a growth modulation procedure, fusionless scoliosis surgery involving anterior vertebral stapling or ligament tethering seeks to not only actively correct the scoliosis during surgery but also achieve additional passive deformity correction with growth over time. For this reason, the passive correction of deformity should be monitored radiographically at 6-month intervals until the end of adolescent growth (approximately Risser stage 4).

Avoiding Pitfalls and Complications

The success of fusionless scoliosis surgery essentially depends on three factors: patient selection, implant type, and procedure execution. Appropriate patient selection requires a thorough understanding of idiopathic scoliosis in the skeletally immature patient and of the available methods used to accurately assess the risk of progression to a surgical curve. Patient selection should include consideration of implant type, as stapling seems to be less effective in curves of greater magnitude, especially in curves greater than 35°. A successful fusionless scoliosis procedure requires experience with endoscopic and open anterior spinal procedures and familiarity with available implants and their limitations. The surgeon should have sufficient experience to ensure safe and accurate placement of devices at all indicated levels of the spine and allow maximization of both active and passive correction of the deformity.

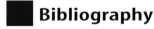

Bibliography

Akyuz E, Braun JT, Brown NA, Bachus KN: Static versus dynamic loading in the mechanical modulation of vertebral growth. *Spine (Phila Pa 1976)* 2006;31(25):E952-E958.

Betz RR, D'Andrea LP, Mulcahey MJ, Chafetz RS: Vertebral body stapling procedure for the treatment of scoliosis in the growing child. *Clin Orthop Relat Res* 2005;(434):55-60.

Betz RR, Kim J, D'Andrea LP, Mulcahey MJ, Balsara RK, Clements DH: An innovative technique of vertebral body stapling for the treatment of patients with adolescent idiopathic scoliosis: A feasibility, safety, and utility study. *Spine (Phila Pa 1976)* 2003;28(20):S255-S265.

Betz RR, Ranade A, Samdani AF, et al: Vertebral body stapling: A fusionless treatment option for a growing child with moderate idiopathic scoliosis. *Spine (Phila Pa 1976)* 2010;35(2):169-176.

Braun JT, Akyuz E, Ogilvie JW: The use of animal models in fusionless scoliosis investigations. *Spine (Phila Pa 1976)* 2005;30(17 Suppl):S35-S45.

Braun JT, Akyuz E, Ogilvie JW, Bachus KN: The efficacy and integrity of shape memory alloy staples and bone anchors with ligament tethers in the fusionless treatment of experimental scoliosis. *J Bone Joint Surg Am* 2005;87(9):2038-2051.

Braun JT, Hines JL, Akyuz E, Vallera C, Ogilvie JW: Relative versus absolute modulation of growth in the fusionless treatment of experimental scoliosis. *Spine (Phila Pa 1976)* 2006;31(16):1776-1782.

Braun JT, Lavelle WF, Ogilvie JW: The impact of genetics research on adolescent idiopathic scoliosis, in Newton PO, O'Brien MF, Shufflebarger HL, Betz RR, Dickson RA, Harms J, eds: *Idiopathic Scoliosis: The Harms Study Group Treatment Guide.* New York, NY, Thieme, 2010, pp 408-415.

Braun JT, Ogilvie JW, Akyuz E, Brodke DS, Bachus KN: Fusionless scoliosis correction using a shape memory alloy staple in the anterior thoracic spine of the immature goat. *Spine (Phila Pa 1976)* 2004;29(18):1980-1989.

Crawford CH III, Lenke LG: Growth modulation by means of anterior tethering resulting in progressive correction of juvenile idiopathic scoliosis: A case report. *J Bone Joint Surg Am* 2010;92(1):202-209.

Lonstein JE, Carlson JM: The prediction of curve progression in untreated idiopathic scoliosis during growth. *J Bone Joint Surg Am* 1984;66(7):1061-1071.

Newton PO, Faro FD, Farnsworth CL, et al: Multilevel spinal growth modulation with an anterolateral flexible tether in an immature bovine model. *Spine (Phila Pa 1976)* 2005;30(23):2608-2613.

Sanders JO, Khoury JG, Kishan S, et al: Predicting scoliosis progression from skeletal maturity: A simplified classification during adolescence. *J Bone Joint Surg Am* 2008;90(3):540-553.

Wall EJ, Bylski-Austrow DI, Kolata RJ, Crawford AH: Endoscopic mechanical spinal hemiepiphysiodesis modifies spine growth. *Spine (Phila Pa 1976)* 2005;30(10):1148-1153.

Coding

CPT Codes		Corresponding ICD-9 Codes	
20999	Unlisted procedure, musculoskeletal system, general	737.30 737.32 737.39 737.41 754.2	737.31 737.34 737.40 737.43
21899	Unlisted procedure, neck or thorax	737.30 737.32 737.39 737.41 754.2	737.31 737.34 737.40 737.43
22899	Unlisted procedure, spine	737.30 737.32 737.39 737.41 754.2	737.31 737.34 737.40 737.43

Chapter 37
Rib Anchors in Distraction-Based Growing Spine Implants

Wudbhav N. Sankar, MD
David L. Skaggs, MD

Indications

Using ribs instead of the spine as anchors has many potential advantages in distraction-based growing rods. Rib attachments may preserve motion. Ribs are attached to the spine via the costotransverse and costovertebral joints, and these joints permit a minimal amount of gliding motion. In contrast, traditional growing rods with spine anchors permit little motion of the vertebrae within the construct. As with any diarthrodial joint, prolonged immobilization can lead to spontaneous fusion. When converting growing rods to a final fusion construct, surgeons commonly discover spontaneous fusion of most, if not all, of the vertebrae within the construct. The use of ribs as anchor points could permit motion between vertebrae, thereby preventing or delaying spontaneous fusion; this technique, however, is too new to have tested this theory. Using ribs as anchors also avoids surgery on the spine, thereby preserving virgin tissue for future spine surgeries. In the pediatric patient, even minimal amounts of spinal dissection can lead to spontaneous fusion. Fu-

sion in the upper thoracic spine (T1 through T3) in young children has been shown to be particularly harmful to long-term pulmonary function; consequently, avoiding fusion in this region may be a particular benefit of this technique.

The indications for using ribs as anchors in growing spine systems are evolving. Based on the advantages noted above, the argument may be made to use rib attachments in children younger than 5 years of age, because they would be expected to have growing implants for at least 5 years and are at high risk for spontaneous fusion. Another indication is a preexisting fusion of the midthoracic spine (congenital or from previous surgery), in which additional fusion in the upper thoracic spine should be minimized. In cases of previous infection of growing implants, the ribs provide an area of new, uninfected tissue. Rib anchors also allow the surgeon to avoid sites of previous bony surgery, such as laminectomy. In addition to certain cases of early-onset scoliosis, one of the main indications for rib anchors is thoracic insufficiency syndrome from multiply fused ribs or

chest-wall restriction. In these cases, the primary culprit is the chest wall, not the spine, and it therefore makes sense to focus treatment on the ribs and chest by using rib anchors to achieve thoracic expansion.

Contraindications

Rib attachments tend to function poorly in cases of kyphosis because the ribs tend to pull backward over time as the spine falls forward. Upper thoracic kyphosis in particular is poorly controlled with rib attachments. In such cases, we prefer to use traditional growing rods, bent into kyphosis and attached cranially to the region of kyphosis, if possible. Another important contraindication is the patient or family who cannot tolerate repeated surgical procedures, for either medical or social reasons.

Dr. Skaggs or an immediate family member serves as a board member, owner, officer, or committee member of the Pediatric Orthopaedic Society of North America and the Scoliosis Research Society, is a member of a speakers' bureau or has made paid presentations on behalf of Medtronic Sofamor Danek and Stryker, serves as a paid consultant to or is an employee of Medtronic Sofamor Danek and Stryker, and has received research or institutional support from Medtronic Sofamor Danek. Neither Dr. Sankar nor any immediate family member has received anything of value from or owns stock in a commercial company or institution related directly or indirectly to the subject of this chapter.

Alternative Treatments

The use of traditional spine hooks on ribs is considered off-label by the US Food and Drug Administration (FDA); the decision to use off-label applications of spine implants in pediatric patients belongs to the physician. The use of spine hooks on ribs is increasingly becoming accepted; at least 6 of 22 orthopaedic surgeons serving as faculty at the 1st International Congress on Early Onset Scoliosis and Growing Spine in Madrid, Spain (November 2007) had used this technique in their practices.

A new expandable metal growing rod known as the Vertical Expandable Prosthetic Titanium Rib (VEPTR) (Synthes, West Chester, PA) is now available under the FDA humanitarian device exemption for the treatment of thoracic insufficiency syndrome in skeletally immature patients whose diagnoses fall into certain specific categories (**Figure 1**). These categories include flail chest syndrome; rib fusion and scoliosis; and hypoplastic thorax syndrome, including Jeune syndrome, achondroplasia, Jarcho-Levin syndrome, and Ellis–van Creveld syndrome; and progressive scoliosis of congenital or neurogenic origin without rib anomaly. The VEPTR device should not be used under the following conditions: inadequate strength of bone (ribs/spine) for attachment of the device, the absence of proximal and distal ribs for attachment of the device, absent diaphragmatic function, inadequate soft tissue for coverage of the device, age beyond skeletal maturity for uses of the device, age younger than 6 months,

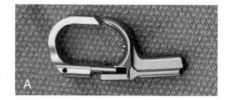
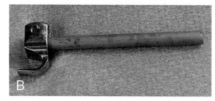

Figure 1 Examples of different rib anchors. **A,** A Vertical Expandable Prosthetic Titanium Rib (VEPTR) cradle (Synthes Spine, West Chester, PA). **B,** A standard spine hook. (Courtesy of Children's Orthopaedic Center, Los Angeles, CA.)

Table 1 Results With the Vertical Expandable Prosthetic Titanium Rib (VEPTR)

Authors (Year)	Number of Patients	Procedure	Patient Population	Mean Patient Age in Years (Range)
Campbell and Hell-Vocke (2003)	21	VEPTR, expansion thoracostomy	Congenital scoliosis with fused ribs	3.3 (0.3-8.4)
Campbell et al (unpublished data, 2005)*	16	VEPTR, expansion thoracostomy	Progressive EOS without fused ribs or congenital scoliosis	4.5 (1.4-9.5)
Emans et al (2005)	31	VEPTR, expansion thoracostomy	Thoracic insufficiency syndrome, fused ribs	4.2 (0.6-12.3)
Campbell et al (2007)	14	VEPTR, midthoracic thoracostomy	Cervical tilt‡, fused ribs, congenital scoliosis	4.4 (1.8-12.5)
Sankar et al (2010)	36	VEPTR vs rib-to-spine hybrid vs standard dual growing rods	EOS	4.8 (1.4-9.5)

NR = not reported; EOS = early-onset scoliosis.
*Campbell RM Jr, Smith MD, Mangos JA, et al: The treatment of thoracic insufficiency syndrome associated with progressive earlyonset scoliosis by opening wedge thoracostomy. *Presented at the 40th Annual Meeting of the Scoliosis Research Society.* Miami, FL, Oct. 27-30, 2005.
†A normal Cobb angle measures 0°. Any measurement >10° is indicative of scoliosis.
‡Normal cervical tilt is 0° (ie, no tilt).

known allergy to any of the device materials, and infection at the surgical site.

Patients with kyphosis are better treated with traditional growing rods with spinal anchors. Specialized devices and conventional spine hooks on ribs are both, in principle, growing implants with rib anchors, and they therefore can be used for similar indications. One practical advantage of using traditional spine implants on ribs rather than specialized devices is that no customized or unique equipment is needed because hooks that fit ribs are readily available on all spine implant systems. In addition, there is no need for institutional or research approval. If a rib-to-rib construct is planned (usually in conjunction with an opening thoracostomy), specialized device cradles provide a better distal attachment point than conventional spine hooks.

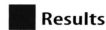

Results

The use of conventional spine hooks as rib anchors in growing spine systems is in its infancy, and therefore few data exist in the literature regarding their use. A multicenter trial currently is underway that is evaluating the safety and efficacy of these implants as rib anchors for spinal deformity. A few studies do exist describing the use of specialized devices for congenital or exotic scoliosis and for patients with thoracic insufficiency syndrome (Table 1). For the most part, such specialized devices have been shown to be effective in controlling curve severity

in these challenging patients. Depending on the series, curve correction in this heterogeneous patient population has been reported to be between 12° and 38°. In addition, serial lengthenings every 6 months have been shown to result in 7 to 12 mm of growth per year, depending on the series. In most cases, pulmonary status improved in these patients after treatment with the specialized devices.

Regardless of the type of implant, the complication rate often is high in growing spine surgery because of limited fixation and the need for repeated surgeries. A recent study by Sankar and associates compared the complication rates among VEPTR, rib-to-spine hybrid devices, and standard dual growing rods in a series of 36 children with early-onset scoliosis. Although the results did not reach

Table 1 (continued)

Mean Follow-up in Years (Range)	Results	Complications/Adverse Events
4.2 (1.8-6.2)	7.1%/year growth on concavity 6.4%/year growth on convexity Longitudinal growth of spine similar to that in normal children	NR
4.2 (2.0-8.8)	Mean Cobb angle[†] improved from 77° to 39° at final follow-up Postoperatively, 13/16 patients had stable respiratory function 2 patients improved, and 1 regressed	10/16 patients (62%) had a total of 19 complications including anchor migration (11), infection (3), and skin slough (2). Six additional patients developed junctional kyphosis above the VEPTR and 3 had progression of the lumbar curve below the construct.
2.6 (0.5-5.4)	Mean Cobb angle[†] improved from 55° to 43° at final follow-up Mean growth after the initial procedure was 1.2 ± 0.9 cm/year	8/31 patients had migration of anchors. Two cases of brachial plexus palsy or thoracic outlet syndrome and 2 deep infections were reported.
3.2 (2-5.8)	Mean cervical tilt[‡] improved from 28.8° to 22.9° at final follow-up Head and trunk decompensation and space available for lung improved in all patients	9/14 patients (64%) had at least 1 complication, including migration of anchors (8), S hook fracture (2), deep infection (4), and brachioplexopathy (1).
4.3 (2-9.8)	Complication rate of 2.3/patient in dual growing rods, 2.4/patient in VEPTR, but only 0.9/patient in hybrid rib-to-spine constructs	26/36 patients (72%) had at least 1 major complication. 72 unplanned surgeries were performed, including 51 revisions of instrumentation and 18 irrigation and débridements for infection.

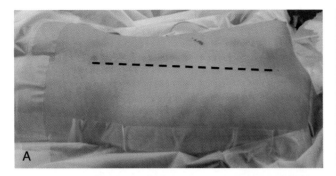

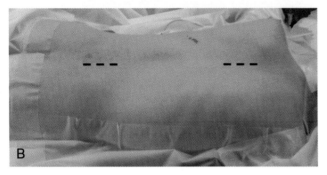

Figure 2 Dashed lines indicate the incisions that can be used to insert rib anchors and their connecting rods through a midline approach. A long midline incision (**A**) or two separate incisions (**B**) can be used. The latter choice necessitates submuscular tunneling to pass the implants.

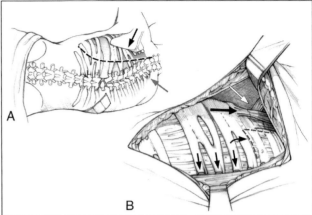

Figure 3 Illustrations show the lateral approach for inserting rib anchors. **A,** A J-shaped incision (broken line) is made starting halfway between the medial edge of the scapula (black arrow) and the posterior spinal processes of T1-T2 (gray arrow). **B,** Exposure should show the common insertion of the middle and posterior scalene muscle (thick black arrow). The neurovascular bundle (white arrow) lies immediately anterior to this. The safe zone for superior rib anchor insertion is posterior to the scalene muscle and on the second rib or lower (curved black arrow). The paraspinal muscles are reflected from lateral to medial by cautery up to the tips of the transverse processes (small black arrows). (Reproduced with permission from Campbell RM Jr: Opening wedge thoracostomy and titanium rib implant in the treatment of congenital scoliosis, in Tolo VT, Skaggs DL, eds: *Masters Techniques in Orthopaedic Surgery: Pediatrics*. Philadelphia, PA, Lippincott, Williams & Wilkins, 2008, pp 455-472.)

statistical significance, a strong trend toward a lower complication rate in the hybrid rib-to-spine group (86%) was evident, compared with patients with the specialized device (237%) or standard dual growing rods with spine-to-spine anchors (230%). The three groups were similar in terms of preoperative Cobb angle, kyphosis, age, and body mass index, and these factors did not seem to influence the complication rate.

Technique

Setup/Exposure

For conventional spine hooks on ribs, we generally position our patients prone, as in any typical spine fusion, taking care to pad all bony prominences. High-quality neurologic monitoring is essential when performing this surgery and must include both the upper and lower extremities. The approach is usually made through a midline skin incision because it is likely that this same incision will be used for the final spine fusion in the future. Depending on the specifics of the surgery, a long midline incision or separate incisions at the top and bottom of the construct can be made (**Figure 2**). After dissection through the subcutaneous tissues, a flap superficial to the paraspinal muscles is elevated laterally past the transverse processes. These are generally palpable as a point of resistance through the muscles. If any question exists, fluoroscopic imaging over a needle placed into bone clarifies the location. A combination of muscle splitting and cautery should bring the surgeon quickly to the ribs with minimal blood loss.

An alternative approach, which some surgeons find useful in cases of multiple fused ribs in which an opening thoracostomy is planned, is the lateral approach (although we still use the prone position, through a midline incision, for such patients). In this alternative approach, the patient is placed in the lateral decubitus position and prepared and draped from the top of the shoulders to the top of the pelvis. A curvilinear J incision is made, starting halfway between the medial edge of the scapula and the posterior spinous processes of T1-T2 (**Figure 3**). The incision is carried distally and swung laterally across the tenth rib. Cautery is used to transect the muscle layers in line with the skin incision down to the level of the ribs, and an anterior flap is elevated up to the costochondral junction. The paraspinal muscles are then elevated from lateral to medial up to the tips of the transverse processes.

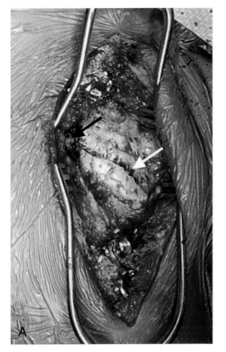 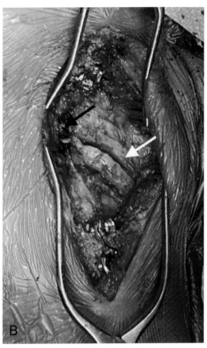

Figure 4 Intraoperative photographs taken prethoracostomy (**A**) and postthoracostomy (**B**). The interval for performing the thoracostomy is the groove between the two central fused ribs (white arrows). A Kerrison rongeur is used for the thoracostomy, which extends from the costochondral junction (not visualized) to the tips of the transverse processes (black arrows). (Courtesy of Children's Orthopaedic Center, Los Angeles, CA.)

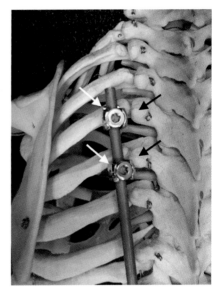

Figure 5 Model of the thoracic chamber. White arrows show correct placement of rib anchors, just lateral to the tips of the transverse processes (black arrows). (Courtesy of Children's Orthopaedic Center, Los Angeles, CA.)

For most cases of congenital or early-onset scoliosis treated with rib anchors, we have found it uncommon that a formal thoracotomy is required. In the treatment of scoliosis, thoracotomies have been shown to disrupt pulmonary function. Any tissue lysis between ribs cannot help but leave scar tissue, which is less mobile and functional than virgin intercostal muscle. In the absence of multiple rib fusions, the use of distraction-based rib implants is quite effective in opening up all rib spaces in a harmonious fashion.

In those few cases of congenital scoliosis with multiple rib fusions and stiff chest walls, an opening-wedge thoracostomy is indicated. The interval for performing the thoracostomy is the groove between the two central fused ribs. Usually the ribs are separate anteriorly, so the thoracostomy is started at the costochondral junction. The thoracostomy is performed using a combination of cautery to lyse muscle and fibrous adhesions and a Kerrison rongeur to osteotomize the rib fusion (**Figure 4**). The underlying pleura is protected using a Penfield elevator, which is inserted under the rib mass. The thoracostomy is carried medially to the tips of the transverse processes. A lamina spreader or rib distractor is then used to widen the thoracostomy until a minimum of two rib thicknesses of space has been achieved.

Instruments/Equipment/ Implants/ Required

When using traditional spine implants as rib anchors, little in the way of specialized equipment is necessary because hooks that fit around ribs are readily available in all spine implant systems. Standard hook inserters or partial rods can be used to place the rib anchors, and conventional spinal rods and connectors can be used to assemble the "growing" construct. For placement of specialized devices, specific instrumentation provided by the manufacturer is required for implantation.

Procedure

For standard spine hooks, care should be taken to ensure that the dissection on top of the rib is immediately adjacent to the transverse process only (**Figure 5**). Hooks tend to slide down the rib if soft tissues are dissected too laterally. In addition, the implants exert the most control on the spine when they are adjacent to the transverse process, as opposed to a more lateral placement. In the latter situation, the ribs tend to move cranially in a bucket-handle fashion, without influencing the spine. A 5-mm transverse incision is made with cautery just distal to the neurovascular bundle (again, just lateral to the transverse process). Ideally, the periosteum is preserved around the rib, to allow the rib to hypertrophy in response to stress. A Freer elevator is then used to

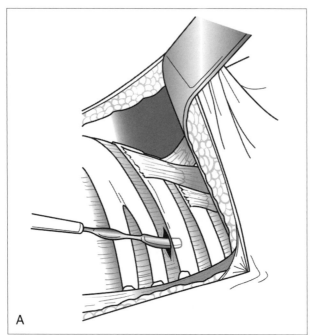
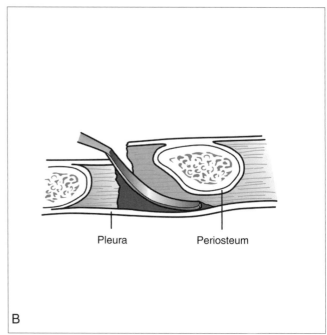

Figure 6 Drawings show dissection required before placing a conventional spine hook. **A,** A Freer elevator is used to dissect soft tissue anterior to the rib. **B,** Cross-sectional view demonstrates the appropriate tissue plane for dissection. (Adapted with permission from Campbell RM Jr: Opening wedge thoracostomy and the titanium rib implant in the treatment of congenital scoliosis with fused ribs, in Tolo VT, Skaggs DL, eds: *Masters Techniques in Orthopaedic Surgery: Pediatrics.* Philadelphia, PA, Lippincott, Williams & Wilkins, 2008, p 464.)

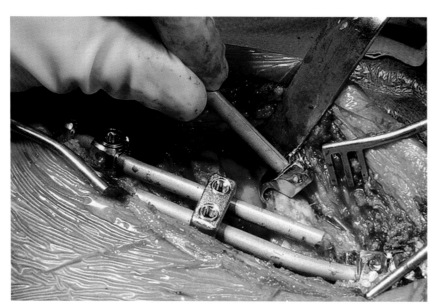

Figure 7 Intraoperative photograph demonstrates how a conventional upgoing spine hook is placed under the rib. (Courtesy of Children's Orthopaedic Center, Los Angeles, CA.)

dissect the soft tissue anterior to the rib, aiming to exploit the plane between the periosteum and the pleura (**Figure 6**). A conventional upgoing spinal hook is then placed into this interval using a standard hook inserter or a partial rod (**Figure 7**). The neurovascular bundle under each rib is not at risk during hardware placement (**Figure 8**). As we have become more comfortable with this technique over the years, we often now do no preliminary dissection about the rib and simply push the hook into place. In this technique, the hook is placed in a hook holder facing anteriorly and is then pushed anteriorly with the leading edge of the hook against the inferior edge of the rib. The hook is then rotated to face cranially as the leading edge of the hook passes against the anterior surface of the rib, and is pushed cranially to set the rib deeply in the hook. Usually a second upgoing hook is placed around an adjacent rib as well, to share the load. There is no need for a downgoing hook, because distractive forces keep the rib engaged in the hook, and a properly sized hook extends a bit cranially to the rib. If a specialized device cradle is being used, a similar insertion technique is performed, except that it often is safer to be subperiosteal with the rib dissec-

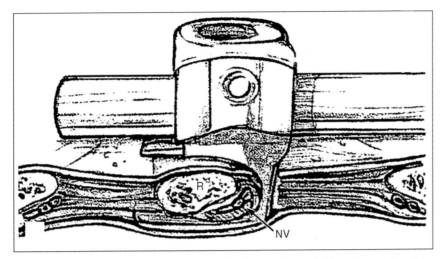

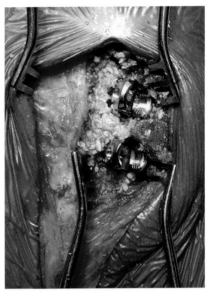

Figure 8 Cross-sectional drawing of a lumbar hook engaging a rib. Note the position of the rib (R) and neurovascular bundle (NV) in relation to the hook. The exact location of the neurovascular bundle within or outside of the hook is not important. (Adapted with permission from Skaggs DL, Buchowski JM, Sponseller P: Temporary distraction rods in the correction of severe scoliosis, in Tolo VT, Skaggs DL, eds: *Masters Techniques in Orthopaedic Surgery: Pediatrics*. Philadelphia, PA, Lippincott, Williams & Wilkins, 2008, pp 473-484.)

Figure 10 Intraoperative photograph depicts pedicle screws at two levels, which often are used for the distal anchor point. Allograft usually is placed before the rods to maximize bony contact. (Courtesy of Children's Orthopaedic Center, Los Angeles, CA.)

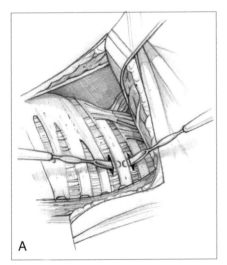

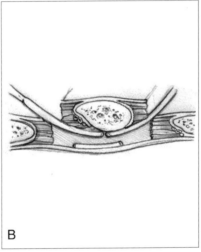

Figure 9 Drawings demonstrate creation of a soft-tissue tunnel for placement of the device cradle. **A,** A Freer elevator is used in both a superior and inferior direction subperiosteally around the rib to create a channel for the device cradle. **B,** Cross-sectional drawing shows the appropriate tissue plane for dissection. (Reproduced with permission from Campbell RM Jr: Opening wedge thoracostomy and the titanium rib implant in the treatment of congenital scoliosis with fused ribs, in Tolo VT, Skaggs DL, eds: *Masters Techniques in Orthopaedics Surgery: Pediatrics*. Philadelphia, PA, Lippincott, Williams & Wilkins, 2008, p 464.)

tion. A Freer elevator is then used in both a superior and inferior direction around the rib (or ribs, if one rib is too thin) to create a channel (**Figure 9**). The rib cradle cap is inserted into the superior end of the channel and the rib cradle is inserted into the inferior end of the channel. These two devices are aligned and connected with the cradle cap lock.

After proximal fixation, attention is turned to the distal anchor point. Through either the same or a separate midline incision, the lamina of the in-

tended vertebrae is subperiosteally dissected. Either single-level fixation with a downgoing supralaminar hook or two-level fixation with pedicle screws may be used. The theoretical advantage of a single-level hook construct is that no fusion is intended, and there is a certain amount of "slop" that may translate into motion and a lower risk of spontaneous fusion. The disadvantage of using a single hook is that it often migrates posteriorly over time, leading to either a bump that is concerning to the parents, or migration through the lamina and need for revision. During dissection, the interspinous ligament must be preserved or future distraction may lead to progressive kyphosis of the distal segment. When pedicle screws are used, they always should be placed in at least two adjacent levels, because "plowing" of the implants over time could injure nerve roots along the inferior border of the pedicle (**Figure 10**). If a two-level distal anchor point is chosen, the facet joint between the levels is then destroyed

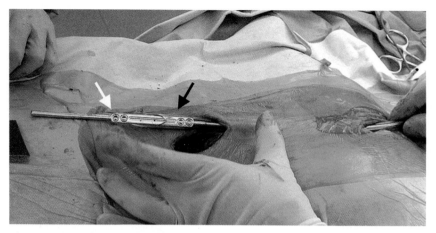

Figure 11 Intraoperative photograph demonstrates the two-incision approach. (The patient's head is to the right.) Spreading with a tonsil clamp (not shown) helps create a submuscular tunnel, and a chest tube (black arrow) can be used to safely shuttle the rod and connector (white arrow) between the two incisions. (Courtesy of Children's Orthopaedic Center, Los Angeles, CA.)

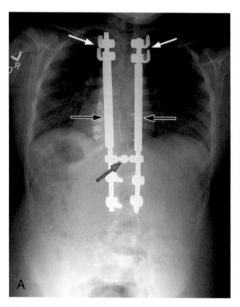
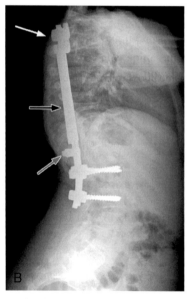

Figure 12 Postoperative PA (**A**) and lateral (**B**) radiographs after placement of dual growing rods with proximal rib anchors (white arrows). The locations of the growing rod connectors (black arrows) and the cross link (gray arrows) are indicated. (Courtesy of Children's Orthopaedic Center, Los Angeles, CA.)

with a narrow rongeur, and corticocancellous crushed allograft is placed in the joint. The exposed bone is decorticated and bone graft usually is placed before the rod is placed, to maximize bony contact.

If a single longitudinal incision was used, the separate upper and lower rods can be connected with either a traditional longitudinal growing rod connector or a side-to-side connector with the rods overlapping. If using a side-to-side connector, the surgeon should not rely on only one connector for the whole system because it could fail over time, perhaps as a result of bending moments. Specialized devices are connected by sliding the rib

sleeve (attached to the superior cradle) over the hybrid rod (attached to the lamina hook or pedicle screws). Regardless of the specific type of implant, the surgeon should account for the initial distraction maneuver during instrumentation when selecting the appropriate length of the rods. If two separate incisions were used for the exposure, a soft-tissue tunnel should be made between the two anchor sites for passage of the rods using a tonsil clamp. We shuttle the rods through a chest tube by inserting one end of the rod into the chest tube and safely passing the tube from one anchor to the other in a submuscular fashion (**Figure 11**).

This technique can be used with single or dual rods. Although unilateral rods are less invasive, they have fewer anchor points to share load. Balancing the curve can be problematic with single rods, both acutely, and even more over time. Like the traditional growing rod experience, we generally prefer dual rods because they seem more stable and less prone to loss of fixation. In addition, bilateral rods make balancing the spine easier, especially over time, and confer the ability to preferentially distract one side more than the other. As part of our dual-rod construct, we generally include a cross link (**Figure 12**).

When an opening wedge thoracostomy has been performed, a second rib-to-rib specialized device can be used laterally to assist in deformity correction and to reduce the load on the more medial rib-to-spine device (**Figure 13**). In such cases, the superior cradle should be placed around the same ribs that are encircled by the medial hybrid device, and the inferior cradle should be placed on a stable rib no lower than the tenth rib, because ribs 11 and 12 are floating.

Wound Closure

Prior to closure, the upper anchor site should be filled with warm saline, and the anesthesiologist should be asked

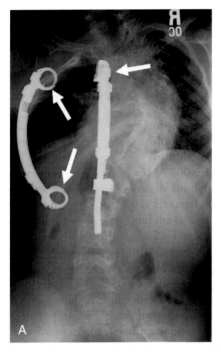

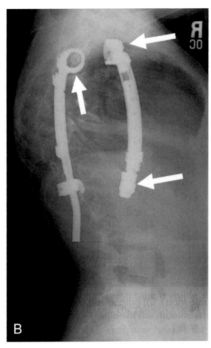

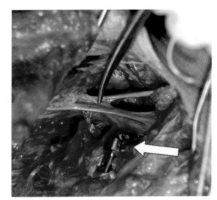

Figure 14 Cadaveric dissection demonstrates the brachial plexus (at the top of the tonsil clamp) draping over the first rib. The arrow indicates a VEPTR cradle on the first rib; rib anchors on the first rib alone should be avoided. (Courtesy of Children's Orthopaedic Center, Los Angeles, CA.)

Figure 13 Postoperative PA (**A**) and lateral (**B**) radiographs after opening thoracostomy and placement of the VEPTR device. The arrows indicate the rib anchors. (Courtesy of Children's Orthopaedic Center, Los Angeles, CA.)

to perform a Valsalva maneuver to look for a pleural leak. If bubbles are seen, a hemovac or chest tube should be placed into the pleural space for a few days. The wound is then closed in a layered fashion, using 1-0 braided absorbable suture for the musculocutaneous flap, a 2-0 suture for the dermis, and a running 3-0 monofilament absorbable suture for the final subcuticular layer. Compared with traditional growing spine implants, rib anchors tend to have good soft-tissue coverage, because they are located deep to the rhomboids and trapezius in a valley between the more prominent spine and scapula. As a result, raising local muscle flaps usually is not necessary. Incisions are dressed with adhesive skin closures, gauze, and occlusive dressings. For subsequent lengthenings, we seal the wound with skin glue after the final subcuticular layer and avoid using dressings to prevent unnecessary

"dressing trauma" to our young patients.

Postoperative Regimen

Diet is advanced as tolerated. Physical therapy is begun on the first postoperative day. If an arthrodesis has been performed at the distal anchor site, a thoracolumbosacral orthosis is used for 3 months. This orthosis helps to slow down young patients during the initial postoperative period and permits fusion at the distal anchor site. Patients are cleared for physical education and sports at the 3-month postoperative visit. Lengthenings usually are planned for every 6 months after the initial implantation.

Avoiding Pitfalls and Complications

The use of rib anchors is relatively straightforward, but several pearls should be kept in mind when performing the technique. As mentioned previously, it is important to keep the rib dissection and the hook as close to the transverse process as possible to prevent the hook from sliding laterally. If a supralaminar hook is used for the distal anchor, the interspinous ligament must be preserved to minimize the risk of distal kyphosis. Unlike spinal anchors, the hook-rib articulation is mobile, and plowing of the hook through the rib is likely to occur over time. In single-rod constructs with one hook on one rib, this complication can occur over a period of months to years. In contrast, we are not aware of any cases in which a spinal hook plowed through a rib when multiple hooks were used (on multiple ribs) or in cases of dual-rod constructs. If plowing occurs, however, it is easily remedied because the rib grows back, often with more—and stronger— bone than before, and the same rib can be used again.

A unique risk of using ribs as anchor points in distraction-based growing instrumentation is the possibility of neurologic injury to the upper extremity. An ongoing multicenter prospective study from the VEPTR study group found that neurologic injury to the upper extremity was six times more frequent than to the lower extremity. Thus, it is imperative that high-quality neuromonitoring be used for both the upper and lower extremities. One suspected mechanism for upper extremity injury is direct pressure of the first rib on the brachial plexus (**Figure 14**). To minimize this risk, the surgeon should avoid placing an anchor on the first rib (unless it is fused to other ribs). Another mechanism of upper extremity neurologic injury is direct impingement of the superior tip of the scapula into the brachial plexus, as the scapula is elevated off the chest wall. This mechanism is easily avoided, because there is no reason to elevate the scapula unless a thoracostomy is being performed, as is the case in most of these surgeries.

————————■

■ Bibliography

Campbell RM Jr, Adcox BM, Smith MD, et al: The effect of mid-thoracic VEPTR opening wedge thoracostomy on cervical tilt associated with congenital thoracic scoliosis in patients with thoracic insufficiency syndrome. *Spine* 2007;32:2171-2177.

Campbell RM Jr, Hell-Vocke AK: Growth of the thoracic spine in congenital scoliosis after expansion thoracoplasty. *J Bone Joint Surg Am* 2003;85:409-420.

Campbell RM Jr, Smith MD, Mayes TC, et al: The characteristics of thoracic insufficiency syndrome associated with fused ribs and congenital scoliosis. *J Bone Joint Surg Am* 2003;85:399-408.

Emans JB, Caubet JF, Ordonez CL, Lee EY, Ciarlo M: The treatment of spine and chest wall deformities with fused ribs by expansion thoracostomy and insertion of vertical expandable prosthetic titanium rib: Growth of thoracic spine and improvement of lung volumes. *Spine* 2005;30:S58-S68.

Karol LA, Johnston C, Mladenov K, Schochet P, Walters P, Browne RH: Pulmonary function following early thoracic fusion in non-neuromuscular scoliosis. *J Bone Joint Surg Am* 2008;90:1272-1281.

Newton PO, Perry A, Bastrom TP, et al: Predictors of change in postoperative pulmonary function in adolescent idiopathic scoliosis: A prospective study of 254 patients. *Spine* 2007;32:1875-1882.

Sankar WN, Acevedo DC, Skaggs DL: Comparison of complications among growing spinal implants. *Spine (Phila Pa 1976)* 2010;35:2091-2096.

Thompson GH, Akbarnia BA, Campbell RM Jr: Growing rod techniques in early-onset scoliosis. *J Pediatr Orthop* 2007;27:354-361.

Wilson TA, Rehder K, Krayer S, Hoffman EA, Whitney CG, Rodarte JR: Geometry and respiratory displacement of human ribs. *J Appl Physiol* 1987;62:1872-1877.

Coding

CPT Codes		Corresponding ICD-9 Codes	
22840	Posterior non-segmental instrumentation (eg, Harrington rod technique, pedicle fixation across one interspace, atlantoaxial transarticular screw fixation, sublaminar wiring at C1, facet screw fixation) (List separately in addition to code for primary procedure)	170.2 737.30 737.40	722.52 737.39 738.4
22842	Posterior segmental instrumentation (eg, pedicle fixation, dual rods with multiple hooks and sublaminar wires); 3 to 6 vertebral segments (List separately in addition to code for primary procedure)	722.52 737.39 738.4	737.30 737.40 756.11
22843	Posterior segmental instrumentation (eg, pedicle fixation, dual rods with multiple hooks and sublaminar wires); 7 to 12 vertebral segments (List separately in addition to code for primary procedure)	170.2 737.30 737.40	722.52 737.39 738.4
22844	Posterior segmental instrumentation (eg, pedicle fixation, dual rods with multiple hooks and sublaminar wires); 13 or more vertebral segments (List separately in addition to code for primary procedure)	170.2	737.30
22849	Reinsertion of spinal fixation device	737.30 737.40	737.39
32900	Resection of ribs, extrapleural, all stages	737.30 737.40	737.39

CPT copyright © 2010 by the American Medical Association. All rights reserved.

Chapter 38

Posterior Fixation of Thoracolumbar Burst Fractures

Darrel S. Brodke, MD
Justin Bundy, MD

■ Indications

Fractures of the thoracolumbar spine (T11 through L2) are common because of the area's anatomic location at the junction of the broadly kyphotic and relatively fixed thoracic spine and the more mobile and lordotic lumbar spine. Other anatomic changes, such as facet orientation, also play key roles in focusing the energy of a traumatic injury on this transitional region. Burst fractures in this zone account for up to 20% of major spine fractures. Although the treatment options for these fractures have changed over time, the goals of restoring stability, correcting deformity, and decompressing neural elements have remained constant.

Burst fractures result from an axial loading force, often accompanied by some flexion loading, and can be successfully treated nonsurgically. Surgical stabilization is warranted, however, when the fracture pattern results in significant loss of stability and deformity or when damage has occurred to the neurologic structures housed within the spinal canal. Management of burst fractures begins with a proper physical examination, a complete neurologic assessment, a review of the pertinent radiographic studies, and correct classification of the injury. When surgery is indicated, the posterior approach permits decompression with reduction of the fracture fragments, which can be accomplished directly via posterior decompression or indirectly using ligamentotaxis. This is followed by fixation of the unstable spine, usually using pedicle screw/rod instrumentation.

Although many thoracolumbar burst fractures are stable and can be treated in a thoracolumbosacral orthosis (TLSO), certain features of an injury may lead to a diagnosis of unstable fracture, which is best treated with surgery. The most unstable of all burst fractures have posterior column disruption, leading to dislocation at the injury level or, at the least, loss of the posterior tension band, which is important for long-term stability (Figure 1). Progressive kyphosis and an increased risk of long-term pain and deformity may result if the unstable fracture is not stabilized. Neurologic injury usually indicates instability, and surgical decompression and stabilization should be undertaken. For burst fractures without posterior column disruption or neurologic injury, other signs of instability may be used to determine treatment, although controversy exists about the relevance of these signs. Anterior column failure with kyphosis greater than 20° to 30°

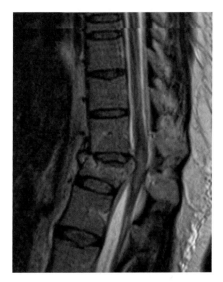

Figure 1 Preoperative sagittal MRI of a patient with an incomplete spinal cord injury demonstrates a large retropulsed fragment of bone from a burst fracture compressing the spinal cord. Note the injury to the posterior ligamentous complex.

Dr. Brodke or an immediate family member serves as a board member, owner, officer, or committee member of the Cervical Spine Research Society and the North American Spine Society; has received royalties from DePuy and Amedica; serves as a paid consultant to or is an employee of DePuy, Medtronic Sofamor Danek, Amedica, and DFine; has received research or institutional support from DePuy, Medtronic Sofamor Danek, Pfizer, Biomet, Zimmer, and Stryker; and owns stock or stock options in Amedica and Syndicom. Neither Dr. Bundy nor any immediate family member has received anything of value from or owns stock in a commercial company or institution related directly or indirectly to the subject of this chapter.

or progression of kyphosis after bracing and mobilization suggests instability, and surgical stabilization may be considered. Other indicators include anterior vertebral body collapse greater than 50% and canal compromise more than 50%; in isolation, however, these findings may not indicate surgical treatment.

Contraindications

In neurologically intact patients with stable burst fractures (<20° of kyphosis, <50% of vertebral body height loss, <50% of canal compromise), nonsurgical management with TLSO bracing is successful. Care must be taken to ensure that no disruption in the posterior ligamentous complex is present, as stated previously. This is best evaluated by imaging and typically is indicated by splaying or widening of the interspinous space, diastasis of the facet joints, or facet perch/subluxation. If doubt remains, MRI, which can show ligamentous disruption, may be used. Standing radiographs with the patient in a brace also may provide useful information.

Surgical fixation may be contraindicated for critically ill trauma patients and should be coordinated with experienced trauma surgeons. Although treatment of impending pulmonary demise may be aided by stabilization of the spine to allow mobilization, once pulmonary decline is in progress, the patient may be at great risk in the operating room. Other relative contraindications include anticoagulation treatment, a Morel-Lavallée lesion overlying the approach, hemodynamic instability, and head injury with high intracranial pressures. The importance of the team approach to surgical decision making and timing cannot be overemphasized.

Alternative Treatments

In patients with large retropulsed fragments of bone causing compression on the spinal cord or thecal sac and subsequent incomplete neurologic injury, anterior decompression has been used with excellent results. Although some authors warn that excess bleeding occurs in acute fractures treated anteriorly, others believe that the benefit of direct decompression of retropulsed fragments in a cord-injured patient and reconstruction of the anterior and middle column of the spine warrant such treatment. A large deformity (kyphosis >30°) with anterior comminution may be especially difficult to reduce from a posterior approach and may be best treated by direct anterior reduction, especially if surgical intervention is delayed more than 3 or 4 days. This approach can be combined with posterior instrumentation as an initial step or after the anterior surgery has been completed.

Results

The long-term results of posterior fixation for burst fractures show excellent fusion rates and improvements in neurologic grade when incomplete injury is present (**Table 1**). Posterior fixation can be divided into two categories: short-segment fixation and long-segment constructs, bypassing the injured segment by two or more levels. Shorter fixation can lead to loss of stability or reduction, whereas longer fixation requires fusion of more segments of the spine. Both techniques have been used with great frequency and, within defined indications, both stabilize burst fractures and prevent progressive deformity with excellent fusion rates. An alternative to longer fixation that may provide more stability than short-segment fixation (one

above and one below) is the placement of screws at the level of the fracture. This has been used with reported success and few complications.

Technique

Setup/Exposure

Setup begins with correct fracture classification and a complete neurologic assessment. Plain radiographs; CT with axial, coronal, and sagittal reformations; and possibly MRI are used to classify and evaluate injury morphology. Thorough assessment of the entire spine should be undertaken to exclude other adjacent and nonadjacent spine fractures. Perioperative cord perfusion should be optimized with a mean arterial pressure greater than 85 mm Hg, particularly in neurologically compromised patients. Intraoperative spinal cord monitoring should be used in patients with some or full distal neurologic function. Baseline motor- and somatosensory-evoked potential recordings should be obtained before positioning for comparison. The patient is then carefully rolled prone onto an operating room table with a spine frame or onto gel rolls. The operating room table should be radiolucent, to accommodate intraoperative fluoroscopy and localizing radiographs.

A standard posterior midline incision is made, centered over the fracture, and the paraspinal muscles and fascia are released from the spinous process and lamina from one or two segments above the injury to one or two segments below. The interspinous ligament is maintained if possible, but a defect may be noted from the traumatic insult. Deep retractors are placed with care to avoid the facet capsule until a verifying radiograph is obtained. The exposure is completed once the level is verified by dissecting out laterally to expose the transverse processes and removing soft tissue from the bone for complete exposure and landmark identification.

Table 1 Results of Thoracolumbar Burst Fracture Fixation

Authors (Year)	Number of Patients	Procedure(s)	Mean Patient Age in Years (Range)	Mean Follow-up (Range)	Fusion rate	Results
McLain et al (1993)	19	Short-segment posterior	29 (15-58)	15 months (4-28)	56%	>5° postoperative deformity in 10 of 16
Danisa et al (1995)	6 / 16 / 27	Combined / Anterior / Posterior	36.8 (13-63) / 35 (19-62) / 37.7 (19-75)	27 months (6-54)	100% / 100% / 100%	No statistical differences between techniques in neurologic recovery or maintenance of kyphosis at final follow-up
Been and Bouma (1999)	27 / 19	Combined / Posterior	26.8 / 33.7	7 years / 4.5 years	100% / 100%	No statistical difference in neurologic recovery or long-term kyphosis. Early >5° loss with posterior technique
Shen et al (2001)	47 / 33	Nonsurgical / Short-segment posterior	47 (19-64) / 42 (20-64)	24 months	100%	No functional or radiographic differences at 2 years
Yue et al (2002)	32	Posterior two segments above and below	41.3 (21-76)	22 months	100%	Sagittal alignment improved 62.2%. Gardner kyphotic angle* improved 33.3%. Good to excellent results reported
Wood et al (2003)	22 / 25	Nonsurgical / Short-segment posterior	18-66	44 months (24-118)	96%	No statistically significant difference in sagittal plane, VAS, or return to work. Significant increase in cost and complications in surgery group

NR = not reported; VAS = visual analog scale.
*The Gardner kyphotic angle is formed by lines drawn on the lower end plate of the fractured vertebra and the upper end plates of the adjacent vertebra.

Instruments/Equipment/Implants Required

A short- or long-segment construct can be selected, depending on fracture morphology, bone quality, and the location of injury. A variety of instrumentation systems are available, and the surgeon should be familiar enough with them to identify which one will best counteract the pattern of injury. In general, hook-rod constructs require longer moment arms over more instrumented segments and are used less often than pedicle screws. Sublaminar wiring rarely is used in trauma patients, because of the inherent risk to the already compromised cord. Segmentally placed pedicle screws are used most often because they provide three-column fixation, which increases construct stiffness and may reduce the level of fused segments (**Figure 2**). Screw insertion is relatively safe in the low thoracic and lumbar spine; difficulty increases higher in the thoracic region.

Procedure

Once adequate exposure is obtained, decompression can be accomplished through a full laminectomy or a unilateral laminotomy, for decompression of the neural elements and to allow access for impaction of the posterior vertebral body fragment if necessary (**Figure 3**). We prefer internal fixation with pedicle screws because they provide rigid, three-column segmental fixation. We usually place the instrumentation and reduce the spine before assessing and further reducing the intracranial fragment, because the ligamentotaxis may accomplish all that is required. This can be assessed once the fracture is re-

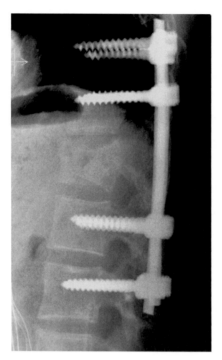

Figure 2 Postoperative lateral radiograph shows reduction of a burst fracture and restoration of overall sagittal alignment using a pedicle screw construct.

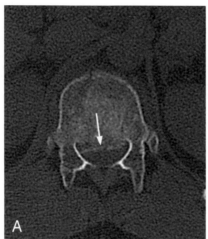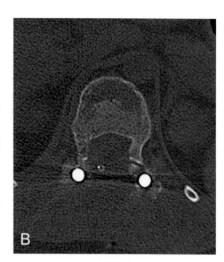

Figure 3 Axial CT scans of a patient with a burst fracture at T12. **A,** Preoperative scan shows a sizeable retropulsed fragment (arrow) occupying a large volume of the spinal canal. **B,** Postoperative scan shows the laminectomy defect and reduction of the fragment, which was performed using a posterior approach only.

duced and stabilized. In the lumbar spine, the standard anatomic landmark for the junction of the middle of the transverse process with the facet is used for placement of the screws. In the thoracic spine, the pedicles are identified by observing the relationship among the transverse process, the facet joints, and the pars interarticularis, depending on the level. The T12 pedicle tends to be in line with the transverse process and placement is initiated down the axis of the transverse process. At T11, the pedicle is in line with the cranial end of the transverse process, slightly more medial than T12. At T10 and above, the pedicle is entered at the junction of the lateral third of the facet and the cranial edge of the transverse process.

The entrance of the pedicle is decorticated and a curved pedicle probe is introduced with a slight curve aiming laterally (**Figure 4,** *A* through *C*). The probe is advanced 15 to 20 mm deep in this fashion (**Figure 4,** *D*). The probe is then removed, rotated so that the curve is aimed medially, and advanced to approximately 40 mm deep (**Figure 4,** *E*).

Once the screw track is created, a small ball-tipped probe can be used to evaluate the track (**Figure 5**). It should reveal no medial or lateral breach; if necessary, fluoroscopy also can be used to evaluate the placement and length of the pedicle screw. The track is then undertapped and reprobed, and the screw can then be placed. We typically use 5.5- to 6-mm–diameter screws with a length of 40 to 45 mm in the low thoracic and upper lumbar spine, and we usually place a screw 5 mm shorter on the left side because of the risk of penetration of and injury to the aorta (**Figure 6**). We often determine screw diameter and length preoperatively by studying the CT scan.

The spine typically is instrumented two levels above and two levels below the injured segment. Depending on the injury pattern, the injured level itself may be instrumented, which can reduce the need to instrument more than one level above and below the

injured segment. The length of the construct is based on the amount of comminution, the spread of the fragments, and the amount of sagittal plane reduction needed. Once all screws are placed, a rod is placed (either slightly lordotic or straight) and the screws are reduced to the rod. Generally, monoaxial screws allow more controlled and successful fracture reduction. Gentle distraction, usually less than 1 cm, can assist with ligamentotaxis but should be used with care to avoid overdistracting injured facets or increasing kyphotic deformity.

If hooks are placed in the thoracic spine instead of screws, we recommend a claw construct with a downgoing laminar hook and upgoing pedicle hook at offset levels to avoid placing multiple intracanal implants at the same level. In hook stabilization, it is standard to stabilize three levels above the fracture rather than two.

Fusion and Wound Closure

The wound is irrigated copiously, and final decortication of the posterior elements and transverse processes is

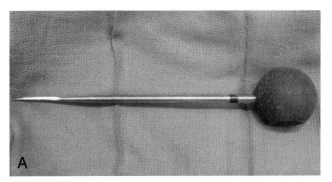

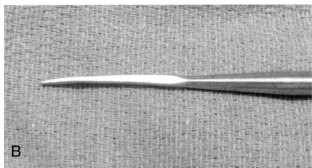

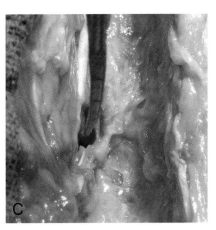

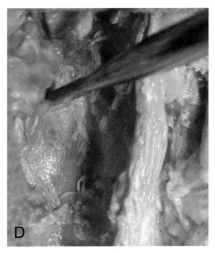

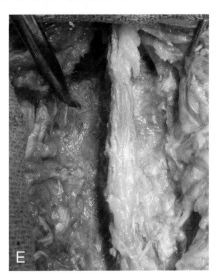

Figure 4 A curved pedicle probe is frequently used for placement of thoracic pedicle screws. **A,** Photograph of the probe. **B,** Close-up of the curved tip. Intraoperative photographs show the use of the pedicle probe. **C,** The probe is ready to be placed, with the curve aimed laterally. **D,** The probe is advanced 15 mm into the pedicle with the curve still aimed laterally. **E,** The probe is then aimed medially and advanced farther, to a 40-mm depth.

done using a burr or gauge. Autograft, harvested from the iliac crest, is the standard fusion material, although local autograft mixed with allograft chips or other bone-graft extenders may be substituted. The graft material is placed around the screws, rods, and lateral gutters. A deep drain may be placed near the instrumentation. The fascia is then closed, using interrupted bioabsorbable sutures. The subcutaneous tissue is closed with smaller interrupted bioabsorbable sutures, and the skin is closed with either a running bioabsorbable subcuticular stitch or interrupted nylon stitches.

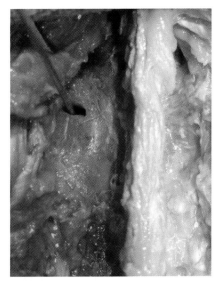

Figure 5 Intraoperative photograph shows a small ball-tipped probe placed down the pedicle track to palpate the walls of the pedicle.

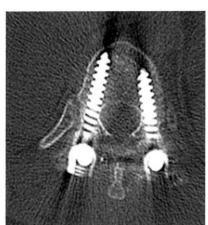

Figure 6 Postoperative axial CT scan of a patient who sustained a burst fracture shows a shorter screw on the patient's left side, with proper pedicle placement to avoid iatrogenic injury.

Postoperative Regimen

Pain management encompasses multiple modalities, including scheduled long- and short-acting narcotics, acetaminophen, muscle relaxants, antiseizure medications, and cyclooxygenase-2 (COX-2) inhibitors. Depending on the type of injuries, we try to mobilize patients as quickly as possible. Immediate sitting up in bed and, if possible, ambulation are encouraged. All patients receive mechanical deep vein thrombosis prophylaxis, usually compression stockings and foot pumps. If patients are unable to ambulate, they are started on low-molecular-weight heparin after 24 to 36 hours. If a drain was placed, it typically is removed on postoperative day 2, depending on output. A fitted TLSO is ordered for patients to wear for 3 months when out of bed. Benefits are related directly to compliance, and bracing can serve as a reminder of injury, limiting activity until solid fusion is achieved.

Avoiding Pitfalls and Complications

Potential complications associated with posterior fixation of thoracolumbar fractures include instrumentation failure, pseudarthrosis, loss of correction, and infection. More devastating complications include neurologic injury and even intraoperative mortality. Understanding the biomechanics of the fracture pattern is critical in selecting the appropriate fusion levels and in deciding whether to include anterior column support. Careful reduction of any bone fragments causing loss of neurologic function must be included in the procedure (**Figure 7**). Finally, a thorough understanding of vertebral and pedicle anatomy and adherence to fixation principles can help surgeons avoid the complications previously reported.

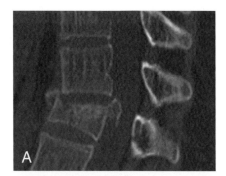
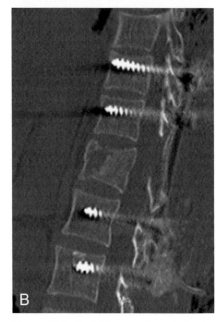

Figure 7 Sagittal CT scans of a patient who sustained a burst fracture. **A,** Preoperative scan. **B,** Postoperative scan shows complete reduction of the compressive fragment using posterior pedicle screw fixation two segments above and below the injured level.

Bibliography

Been HD, Bouma GJ: Comparison of two types of surgery for thoraco-lumbar burst fractures: Combined anterior and posterior stabilisation vs. posterior instrumentation only. *Acta Neurochir (Wien)* 1999;141(4):349-357.

Danisa OA, Shaffrey CI, Jane JA, et al: Surgical approaches for the correction of unstable thoracolumbar burst fractures: A retrospective analysis of treatment outcomes. *J Neurosurg* 1995;83(6):977-983.

Katonis P, Christoforakis J, Kontakis G, et al: Complications and problems related to pedicle screw fixation of the spine. *Clin Orthop Relat Res* 2003;(411):86-94.

McLain RF, Sparling E, Benson DR: Early failure of short-segment pedicle instrumentation for thoracolumbar fractures: A preliminary report. *J Bone Joint Surg Am* 1993;75(2):162-167.

Parker JW, Lane JR, Karaikovic EE, Gaines RW: Successful short-segment instrumentation and fusion for thoracolumbar spine fractures: A consecutive 41/2-year series. *Spine (Phila Pa 1976)* 2000;25(9):1157-1170.

Sasso RC, Cotler HB: Posterior instrumentation and fusion for unstable fractures and fracture-dislocations of the thoracic and lumbar spine: A comparative study of three fixation devices in 70 patients. *Spine (Phila Pa 1976)* 1993;18(4):450-460.

Shen WJ, Liu TJ, Shen YS: Nonoperative treatment versus posterior fixation for thoracolumbar junction burst fractures without neurologic deficit. *Spine (Phila Pa 1976)* 2001;26(9):1038-1045.

Sjostrom L, Karlstrom G, Pech P, Rauschning W: Indirect spinal canal decompression in burst fractures treated with pedicle screw instrumentation. *Spine (Phila Pa 1976)* 1996;21(1):113-123.

Vaccaro AR, Lehman RA Jr, Hurlbert RJ, et al: A new classification of thoracolumbar injuries: The importance of injury morphology, the integrity of the posterior ligamentous complex, and neurologic status. *Spine (Phila Pa 1976)* 2005; 30(20):2325-2333.

Wood KB, Bohn D, Mehbod A: Anterior versus posterior treatment of stable thoracolumbar burst fractures without neurologic deficit: A prospective, randomized study. *J Spinal Disord Tech* 2005;18(suppl):S15-S23.

Wood K, Buttermann G, Mehbod A, et al: Operative compared with nonoperative treatment of a thoracolumbar burst fracture without neurological deficit: A prospective, randomized study. *J Bone Joint Surg Am* 2003;85-A(5):773-781.

Yue JJ, Sossan A, Selgrath C, et al: The treatment of unstable thoracic spine fractures with transpedicular screw instrumentation: A 3-year consecutive series. *Spine (Phila Pa 1976)* 2002;27(24):2782-2787.

Coding

CPT Codes		Corresponding ICD-9 Codes	
20937	Autograft for spine surgery only (includes harvesting the graft); morselized (through separate skin or fascial incision) (List separately in addition to code for primary procedure)	170.2 733.13	724.6 733.81
22612	Arthrodesis, posterior or posterolateral technique, single level; lumbar (with or without lateral transverse technique)	170.2 721.42 722.10	721.3 722.0 737.39
22614	Arthrodesis, posterior or posterolateral technique, single level; each additional vertebral segment (List separately in addition to code for primary procedure)	170.2 722.52 737.39	722.10 724.02 738.4
22842	Posterior segmental instrumentation (eg, pedicle fixation, dual rods with multiple hooks and sublaminar wires); 3 to 6 vertebral segments (List separately in addition to code for primary procedure)	342.1 342.90	342.9 343

Chapter 39

Treatment of Fractures and Dislocations at the Spinopelvic Junction

Thomas A. Schildhauer, MD, PhD
Carlo Bellabarba, MD
M. L. Chip Routt, Jr, MD
Jens R. Chapman, MD

■ Indications

The posterior pelvic ring and lower lumbar spine form a complex transition zone consisting of an interwoven array of osseous and ligamentous structures. These structures are subject to a wide constellation of musculoskeletal and neurologic injuries and associated internal organ system injuries. Injury mechanisms range from high-energy trauma to trivial injuries that may cause insufficiency fractures. Factors that favor surgical intervention for such injuries include high-grade disruption of the mechanical integrity of the posterior osteoligamentous junction, the presence of neurologic injury, a need for patient mobilization, and failure of nonsurgical care because of persistent pain or progressive deformity. The treatment chosen should be appropriate for the patient's physiologic circumstances, provide the best possible environment for nerve regeneration in cases of neural injury, and facilitate early mobilization after restoration of functional alignment. Predicting stability following injuries to the posterior pelvic ring and lumbosacral junction can be daunting because of the variability of the trauma, the infrequent incidence of such injuries in areas outside of major trauma centers, and a multitude of patient-related confounding factors. Frank dislocations and the presence of predominantly ligamentous injuries are sound indications for surgical care because of the predictably poor outcomes of nonsurgical treatment.

Unacceptable fracture malalignment is another appropriate surgical indication for open reduction and internal fixation because closed or percutaneous fixation techniques usually are limited in their capacity for fracture reduction. Of course, open fractures of the lumbopelvic junction, which can be hidden in the form of disruptions of the rectal and/or the vaginal vault, are clear indications for timely surgical débridement and reconstruction. The posterior integument covering the lumbopelvic junction is a critical element when considering treatment. Generally unique to this region, severe closed but extensile fasciocutaneous degloving of the lumbodorsal fascia from the underlying muscle structures, referred to as the Morel-Lavallée lesion, poses an additional important clinical variable. Ideally, the treatment of multiply injured patients restores a stable lumbopelvic junction, which expedites mobilization efforts. The timing of such an intervention and the type of surgery chosen have to be individualized to suit the specific patient. Patients with compromised lumbosacral

Dr. Bellabarba or an immediate family member is a member of a speakers' bureau or has made paid presentations on behalf of Smith & Nephew and has received research or institutional support from Synthes, AO Spine, and DePuy. Dr. Chapman or an immediate family member serves as a board member, owner, officer, or committee member of the North American Spine Society, AO Spine International, AO Spine North America, and the American Cervical Spine Research Society; is a member of a speakers' bureau or has made paid presentations on behalf of Medtronic Sofamor Danek and Synthes USA; serves as a paid consultant to or is an employee of Synthes USA; serves as an unpaid consultant to DePuy, Stryker, Alseres Pharmaceuticals, and Paradigm Spine; has received research or institutional support from DePuy, Medtronic Sofamor Danek, Synthes, Stryker, and the Hansjoerg Wyss Foundation; and has received nonincome support (such as equipment or services), commercially derived honoraria, or other non–research-related funding (such as paid travel) from Synthes, Stryker, and Medtronic Sofamor Danek. Neither of the following authors nor any immediate family member has received anything of value from or owns stock in a commercial company or institution related directly or indirectly to the subject of this chapter: Dr. Schildhauer and Dr. Routt.

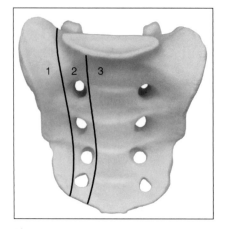

Figure 1 The Denis classification system divides the sacrum into three zones. Zone 1 injuries are lateral to the neuroforamina in their most medial excursion and rarely are associated with neurologic injuries, mainly in the form of L5 lesions. Zone 2 injuries run through the neuroforamina in their most medial fracture and have a percentage of associated L5 or S1 root injuries. Zone 3 injuries are defined as any fracture that runs through the spinal canal. They are associated with lower sacral plexus injuries and are associated with cauda equina injuries in more than 50% of cases. Bilateral vertical sacral fractures usually are type 3 injuries. Upon closer inspection, these injuries usually will feature an interconnecting transverse fracture extension, creating the so-called "sacral-U" fracture variants.

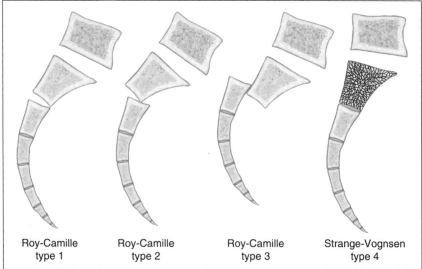

Roy-Camille type 1	Roy-Camille type 2	Roy-Camille type 3	Strange-Vognsen type 4

Figure 2 The Roy-Camille and Strange-Vognsen subdivision of transverse Denis zone 3 fractures by fracture pattern. Type 1 injuries feature kyphotic deformity but no translation. Type 2 injuries are characterized by kyphosis and translation, in contrast to type 3 injuries, in which the rostral segment is dislocated into hyperextension. Strange-Vognsen added a type 4, indicating comminution of the upper sacral body. (Courtesy of Jens R. Chapman, MD, Seattle, WA.)

roots due to impingement of neural elements appear to benefit from surgical intervention within 2 weeks. Patients who cannot mobilize because of disproportionate pain despite some form of brace or protected weight-bearing status may manifest functional instability of the lumbopelvic junction and deserve reevaluation for surgical stabilization.

The most relevant sacral fracture classification, proposed by Denis and associates, classifies fractures according to the location of the fracture relative to the spinal canal and neuroforamina, which also influences the likelihood of neurologic injuries and patient outcomes (**Figure 1**). Denis zone 3 injuries, which involve the sacral canal, are rarely longitudinally oriented fractures, however; they are most commonly complex sacral fracture patterns that include transversely or obliquely oriented components with associated displacement in the sagittal plane. To properly reflect these injury patterns, Roy-Camille and associates and Strange-Vognsen have developed a subclassification of the Denis zone 3 fractures (**Figure 2**).

Lumbopelvic fixation is indicated in injuries to the lumbosacral junction that produce multidirectional instability. These primarily occur under two circumstances. In the first, a vertical sacral fracture, which constitutes the posterior pelvic ring injury, extends rostrally into or medial to the S1 superior facet, thereby disarticulating the L5-S1 facet from the stable sacral fracture fragment (**Figure 3**). In the second circumstance, the multiplanar sacral fracture mentioned previously, comprised of bilateral longitudinal fractures and a transverse fracture component, separates the upper central sacrum and the remainder of the spine from the peripheral sacrum and attached pelvis. The result of this fracture pattern and its variants is dissoci-ation of the lumbar spine from the pelvic ring and functional lumbosacral instability. These injuries frequently are associated with neurologic deficits ranging from lower extremity monoradiculopathies to complete cauda equina deficits. Attempts at surgical decompression of the compromised neural elements, however, would lead to further instability of the lumbosacral junction.

Lumbopelvic fixation also is indicated in posterior pelvic ring injuries associated with severe osteoporosis or bony comminution or in sacral fractures with concomitant posterior ilium fractures, which may preclude any other standard posterior pelvic ring osteosynthesis technique such as iliosacral screw or transiliac plate osteosynthesis. Other reasons for considering lumbopelvic fixation as a salvage procedure to stabilize the lumbosacral junction include secondary displacement after standard osteosynthesis techniques of the posterior pelvic ring, pseudarthrosis, and bony defects after tumor and infection.

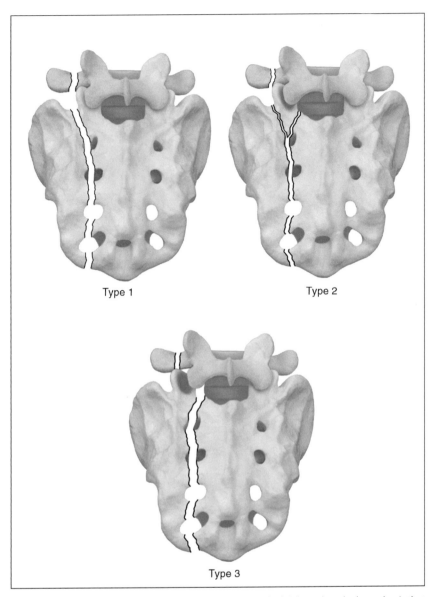

Type 1

Type 2

Type 3

Figure 3 The Isler classification of lumbosacral injuries, which is based on the hypothesis that longitudinally oriented fractures extending medial to or within the S1 superior facet result in lumbosacral instability, whereas fractures that extend lateral to the S1 superior facet do not. Type 1 injuries are lateral to the L5-S1 facet; type 2 injuries are through the facet; type 3 injuries exit medial to the facet. (Courtesy of Jens R. Chapman, MD, Seattle, WA.)

Contraindications

As noted above, the major challenge in managing injuries to this area is the difficulty of predicting stability in the face of numerous surrounding factors. Multiply injured patients may benefit from the optimization of systemic vital organ functions before undergoing

open and invasive lumbopelvic surgery. Patients with posterior degloving (Morel-Lavallée) lesions pose a particularly complex treatment challenge because of their increased risk of infection and need for repeat soft-tissue procedures. Clearly, indiscriminately aggressive surgical intervention can lead to a harrowing escalation of treat-

ment needs, with a high potential for unsatisfactory outcomes. Delays in surgery, however, can lead to soft-tissue breakdown, predispose to thromboembolism or pulmonary decompensation, and adversely affect the chances of neurologic recovery. Most nondisplaced or minimally displaced fractures without malalignment of adjacent articulations will not require surgical stabilization.

Alternative Treatments

The basic decision-making tree traditionally differentiates between nonsurgical and surgical treatment. Nonsurgical options can range from simple activity restrictions (restricted weight bearing, a wheelchair with reclining back) to more burdensome forms of care that last for weeks to months, such as unilateral or bilateral hip spica braces or prolonged recumbent skeletal traction with measures to protect against thromboembolic and cardiopulmonary complications. Surgical treatment ranges from percutaneous external devices, such as anterior half-pin fixators serving as temporizing or supplemental devices, to separate posterior ring stabilization efforts or resuscitation clamps that assist resuscitation by closing down the expanded volume of a traumatically disrupted pelvis. A useful but simple decision-making tool that can be used to assess the stability of a lumbosacral injury intended for nonsurgical care is the ability of the patient to mobilize without disproportionate pain. Patients with instability usually will not tolerate mobilization efforts, even with the help of orthotic devices.

Table 1 Results of Surgical Sacral Fracture Fixation

Authors (Year)	Number of Patients	Procedure	Mean Patient Age in Years (Range)	Mean Follow-up in Months (Range)	Results
Schildhauer et al (1998)	34	Triangular lumbopelvic fixation	35 (19-72)	19 (8-52)	91% uneventful healing 12% complications
Nork et al (2001)	13	Sacroiliac screw fixation	39 (21-60)	14 (7-48)	100% screw safety No loss of reduction 78% neurologic recovery No improvement of preoperative kyphotic deformity
Bellabarba et al (2006)	18	Segmental lumbopelvic fixation	32 (15-59)	25 (7-37)	No loss of fixation 83% neurologic improvement rate 16% wound infection
Tötterman et al (2006)	32	Not standardized surgery	33 (16-57)	17 (12-30)	91% sensory impairment 63% gait impairment 59% bowel/bladder/sexual impairment Late impairment associated with injury severity and associated injuries but not fracture characteristics
Tötterman et al (2007)	31	Not standardized surgery	35 (19-63)	17 (12-30)	33% return to work 65% functional independence High degree of poor outcomes with neurologic injury, sexual dysfunction, bowel and bladder control issues
Gardner et al (2009)	68	Percutaneous sacroiliac screws	39 (9-72)	NR	71% intraosseous screw placement 29% juxtaforaminal No neurologic or vascular deterioration

NR = not reported.

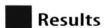

Results

The variety of injury types and magnitude, the lack of consistently applied injury and outcome classification systems, and a relatively low incidence of fractures and dislocations at the junction of the lumbosacral spine and pelvis have precluded comparative studies to evaluate various treatment algorithms. **Table 1** summarizes the results of various published studies that have investigated clinical outcomes after the surgical treatment of sacral fractures. In our experience, surgical decompression and lumbopelvic fixation for sacral fracture-

dislocations with spinopelvic dissociation and cauda equina deficits (Roy-Camille types 2 through 4) resulted in fracture healing in all patients without secondary loss of reduction. Average sacral kyphosis improved from 43° to 21°, and 83% had full or partial recovery of bowel and bladder deficits. Wound infection occurred in 16% of patients, two thirds of whom originally had been diagnosed with traumatic closed soft-tissue degloving lesions. Surgical re-exploration was required in 11% of patients because of seroma/pseudomeningocele formation. At the latest follow-up examination, 31% of patients had at least one broken longitudinal rod between the

lowest lumbar and most rostral iliac screw. Because of the lack of a sacroiliac (SI) joint arthrodesis and the resulting likelihood of eventual fatigue failure of the rods between the iliac and lumbar screws, this was interpreted as an incidental finding in the absence of referable clinical symptoms, such as pain with weight bearing or external hip rotation, and in the absence of radiographic signs of loss of fracture reduction. Conversely, in patients without rod failure, bridging callus of the posterolateral arthrodesis mass to the ilium could be identified on follow-up radiographs.

Tötterman and associates assessed the outcomes of patients with sacral fractures using validated outcomes scores and found a clear correlation between poor outcomes and loss of sexual function, loss of bowel and bladder control, and neurologic injuries. Again, these studies underscore the importance of identifying injuries and providing the best possible environment for neurologic recovery by systematic assessment and comprehensive neural element decompression and sacral reconstruction, as well as the seamless incorporation of rehabilitation measures in patients with neurologic injuries.

Positive results for iliosacral screw fixation in the treatment of sacral fractures have recently been published by Gardner and associates, who observed 100% acceptable screw placement without neurologic complications in 106 consecutively placed screws over a 21-month period. Nork and associates found that, for sacral fracture patterns that result specifically in spinopelvic instability, iliosacral screw fixation provided a reliable, minimally invasive approach to the stabilization of less severely displaced sacral U-type fractures, specifically those in which the safe zone for iliosacral screw fixation was sufficient and in which kyphocorrection was not deemed to be an essential component of treatment. They noted no screw-related complications, neurologic or otherwise. In two separate reports, Bellabarba and associates reviewed the results for and complications associated with segmental spinopelvic fixation from the lower lumbar spine to the ilium in severely displaced and comminuted sacral fractures with cauda equina syndrome. They noted a 25% rate of wound complications, including a 16% rate of infection, that were severe enough to require reoperation. No neurologic complications were identified, nor were any long-term wound or infectious issues. Reliable fracture healing in acceptable alignment was universally achieved in each of these extremely severe sacral fractures, with

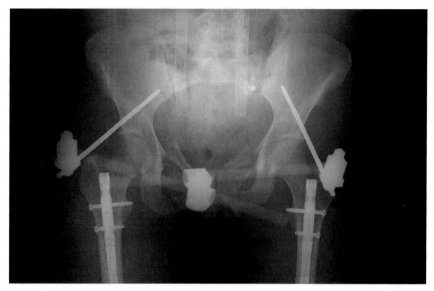

Figure 4 AP radiograph illustrates an anterior half-pin external fixator construct, which can provide temporary anterior ring reduction and aid in resuscitation efforts for pelvic ring bleeding. In general, external fixator constructs have limited biomechanical stabilization properties and commonly are limited in their durability because of pin-tract infections. (Courtesy of Jens R. Chapman, MD, Seattle, WA.)

more than 80% of patients experiencing substantial neurologic improvement.

Techniques

The surgical treatment of sacral fractures and posterior pelvic ring trauma is performed as early as possible after the emergent needs of vital organ systems have been met and the patient has been deemed physiologically stable for sacral reconstructive surgery, ideally within 2 weeks of the injury. Emergent surgical intervention is recommended only in patients with (1) open fractures; (2) lumbodorsal, presacral soft-tissue compromise caused by displaced fracture fragments; and (3) a deteriorating neurologic examination.

In patients with open fractures, appropriate wound débridement should be performed as soon as the hemodynamic condition is stable. Rectal involvement usually requires early loop colostomy, preferably of the transverse

colon, followed by a distal colonic wash-out. Soft-tissue contusions and Morel-Lavallée lesions have to be addressed; nonviable tissues require early and sometimes repetitive débridement. Degloved soft-tissue pockets require thorough débridement along with dead-space eradication and drainage techniques. Planned serial wash-outs and vacuum drainage techniques have shown promise in the management of these complex conditions.

Most commonly, a clinically relevant anterior pelvic ring disruption is first reconstructed as anatomically as possible to promote indirect reduction of the posterior pelvic ring and provide at least partial pelvic stability. Anterior pelvic stabilization can consist of anterior external pelvic fixation with pins in the iliac crest or anterior inferior iliac spine (**Figure 4**), plating of the symphysis, or antegrade and retrograde superior pubic ramus screw fixation. Upon completion of this part of the pelvic ring reconstruction, the posterior pelvic ring and lumbosacral junction injury can be

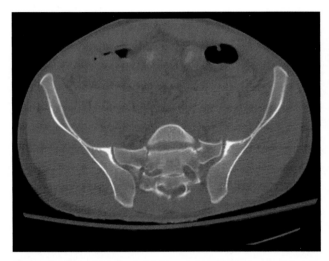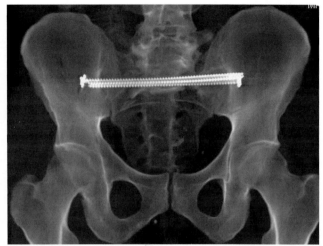

Figure 5 **A,** Preoperative axial CT scan shows a Denis zone 3 Roy-Camille type 1 injury. **B,** Postoperative AP pelvic view with bilaterally placed iliosacral screws, both anchored in the S1 segment. (Courtesy of Jens R. Chapman, MD, Seattle, WA.)

addressed as needed with the patient in the supine or even the prone position as deemed necessary.

Percutaneous Iliosacral Screw Fixation

Percutaneous iliosacral screws (**Figure 5**) have revolutionized the treatment options for posterior pelvic ring injuries because they are soft-tissue friendly and offer meaningful stabilization for most cases. Knowledge of the intricacies of the technique and its limitations is important for safe screw placement. Postoperatively, patients need to undergo a period of protected weight bearing to avoid overloading the construct.

This technique requires a good understanding of posterior pelvic ring anatomy and careful study of specific patient anatomic factors. In particular, patients with transitional vertebral anatomy may not be suitable for this technique because of the inconsistent visualization in such patients of important radiographic landmarks during intraoperative fluoroscopy. Some authors have suggested using CT guidance for iliosacral screw fixation, but this technique has failed to gain popularity because of logistic concerns in managing polytraumatized patients and the protracted operating

times when intraoperative manipulation is required.

Percutaneous iliosacral screw placement is performed with the patient supine on a radiolucent table, such as a Jackson table (Mizuho OSI, Oakland, CA), with a C-arm positioned to allow straight AP and pelvic inlet and outlet views. A true lateral sacral view and iliac and obturator oblique views also can be helpful. The best possible closed fracture reduction should be performed before actual surgical intervention. This can be done in several ways: with skeletal traction, anterior pelvic ring external fixation, internal fixation of the anterior pelvic ring, or manipulation of Schanz pins inserted into several pelvic ring structures suitable for pin placement. Closed reduction attempts have been reported to be much more successful if performed within 48 hours of injury. This likely is because of the increasing intestinal obstruction and soft-tissue contractions caused by an increasingly consolidating fracture hematoma. After the patient is appropriately prepared and draped, an incision between the greater trochanter and gluteus medius tuberosity is performed to allow access to a suitable starting point. Blunt dissection to the outer iliac crest with

an instrument such as a cannulated trocar is followed by creation of a bony starting point. A guidewire—usually long and terminally threaded—is then advanced incrementally into the first sacral segment or other desired target locations. The placement of this wire is checked using multiplanar fluoroscopy, usually with pelvic inlet and outlet views. The choice of implant can greatly influence the success of this form of fixation. For example, terminally threaded devices are suitable for achieving fracture compression in simple vertical fractures without foraminal involvement, whereas fully threaded screws placed as noncompressive transfixation screws usually are preferable for comminuted fracture patterns. Dual screws can be important for more displaced fractures or in cases of osteopenia. This procedure is technically demanding and therefore generally is performed by an orthopaedic trauma surgery specialist.

External Fixation

External fixation of the pelvic ring has maintained a role in the emergent management of unstable pelvic ring fractures and can provide adjuvant stability to posterior pelvic ring disruptions. Usually, single-pin fixation is achieved through the anterior infe-

pelvic ring injury is not stabilized and if the iliac screws do not have a strong purchase within the cancellous bone of the ilium (eg, in osteoporosis or when only short and thin iliac screws are available). In these situations, it is important to initially stabilize the anterior pelvic ring injury with a "dynamic" osteosynthesis, such as a superior pubic ramus screw, and then perform posterior sacral fracture reduction and fixation. If the posterior reduction and triangular osteosynthesis is performed first, without having a perfect anterior ring reduction, then a secondary anterior pelvic ring reduction and osteosynthesis becomes difficult to achieve because of problems in overcoming the much stronger posterior ring fixation. This may result in malreduction or early loosening and failure of the anterior pelvic ring fixation.

Overdistraction of an injured unstable L5-S1 facet joint also is a concern when performing lumbopelvic fixation techniques, especially when performing a distraction maneuver for sacral fracture reduction. The surgeon should therefore actively search for an

injury to the L5-S1 facet preoperatively on the CT scans. If such an injury is present and if distraction forces are applied along the longitudinal connecting rod of the lumbopelvic fixation for vertical reduction of the sacral fracture, this reduction maneuver should be followed by horizontal fixation with an iliosacral screw. The distraction force over the injured L5-S1 facet should be released subsequently, and the appropriate alignment of the L5-S1 junction should be restored prior to final tightening of the lumbopelvic implants.

Lumbopelvic fixation is primarily effective as a bridging osteosynthesis stabilizing a reduced fracture and not as a "distracting" osteosynthesis. Overdistraction at the lumbopelvic junction also can occur when the bony facet is intact but the joint capsule is disrupted, which may happen due to injury or iatrogenically when L5 pedicle screws are positioned. Tilting at the L5-S1 junction resulting from overdistraction should be differentiated from tilting resulting from insufficient reduction of the injured hemipelvis. In the latter case, the sa-

cral ala may engage on an uninjured or nondisplaced L5 transverse process.

Distraction along a longitudinal connecting rod of the lumbopelvic fixation construct may result in displacement of the fracture laterally and posteriorly along the vector of the rod, if it is contoured only in one plane. We prebend the longitudinal rod in an S shape in the frontal as well as in the sagittal plane. Rotating the rod within the L5 pedicle screw and the iliac screw during reduction maneuvers may then help to close down the fracture site. The lumbopelvic fixation should never be finalized before performing the horizontal fixation with the iliosacral screw. It should instead be a simultaneous procedure, using the longitudinal connecting rod for vertical reduction, followed by horizontal fixation with the iliosacral screw and then finalization of the lumbopelvic fixation with correction of any distraction at the lumbosacral junction.

Bibliography

Bellabarba C, Schildhauer TA, Vaccaro AR, Chapman JR: Complications associated with surgical stabilization of high-grade sacral fracture dislocations with spino-pelvic instability. *Spine (Phila Pa 1976)* 2006;31(11, Suppl)S80-S88, discussion S104.

Denis F, Davis S, Comfort T: Sacral fractures: An important problem. Retrospective analysis of 236 cases. *Clin Orthop Relat Res* 1988;227:67-81.

Gardner MJ, Farrell ED, Nork SE, Segina DN, Routt ML Jr: Percutaneous placement of iliosacral screws without electrodiagnostic monitoring. *J Trauma* 2009;66(5):1411-1415.

Isler B: Lumbosacral lesions associated with pelvic ring injuries. *J Orthop Trauma* 1990;4(1):1-6.

Klineberg E, McHenry T, Bellabarba C, Wagner T, Chapman JR: Sacral insufficiency fractures caudal to instrumented posterior lumbosacral arthrodesis. *Spine (Phila Pa 1976)* 2008;33(16):1806-1811.

Kothbauer K, Schmid UD, Seiler RW, Eisner W: Intraoperative motor and sensory monitoring of the cauda equina. *Neurosurgery* 1994;34(4):702-707.

Krappinger D, Larndorfer R, Struve P, Rosenberger R, Arora R, Blauth M: Minimally invasive transiliac plate osteosynthesis for type C injuries of the pelvic ring: A clinical and radiological follow-up. *J Orthop Trauma* 2007;21(9):595-602.

Kuklo TR, Potter BK, Ludwig SC, et al: Radiographic measurement techniques for sacral fractures consensus statement of the Spine Trauma Study Group. *Spine (Phila Pa 1976)* 2006;31(9):1047-1055.

Lindahl J, Hirvensalo E, Böstman O, Santavirta S: Failure of reduction with an external fixator in the management of injuries of the pelvic ring: Long-term evaluation of 110 patients. *J Bone Joint Surg Br* 1999;81(6):955-962.

Nork SE, Jones CB, Harding SP, Mirza SK, Routt ML Jr: Percutaneous stabilization of U-shaped sacral fractures using iliosacral screws: Technique and early results. *J Orthop Trauma* 2001;15(4):238-246.

Pohlemann T, Angst M, Schneider E, Ganz R, Tscherne H: Fixation of transforaminal sacrum fractures: A biomechanical study. *J Orthop Trauma* 1993;7(2):107-117.

Reilly MC, Zinar DM, Matta JM: Neurologic injuries in pelvic ring fractures. *Clin Orthop Relat Res* 1996;329(329):28-36.

Routt ML Jr , Nork SE, Mills WJ: Percutaneous fixation of pelvic ring disruptions. *Clin Orthop Relat Res* 2000;375:15-29.

Roy-Camille R, Saillant G, Gagna G, Mazel C: Transverse fracture of the upper sacrum: Suicidal jumper's fracture. *Spine (Phila Pa 1976)* 1985;10(9):838-845.

Schildhauer TA, Bellabarba C, Nork SE, Barei DP, Routt ML Jr, Chapman JR: Decompression and lumbopelvic fixation for sacral fracture-dislocations with spino-pelvic dissociation. *J Orthop Trauma* 2006;20(7):447-457.

Schildhauer TA, Josten C, Muhr G: Triangular osteosynthesis of vertically unstable sacrum fractures: A new concept allowing early weight-bearing. *J Orthop Trauma* 1998;12(5):307-314.

Schildhauer TA, Ledoux WR, Chapman JR, Henley MB, Tencer AF, Routt ML Jr : Triangular osteosynthesis and iliosacral screw fixation for unstable sacral fractures: A cadaveric and biomechanical evaluation under cyclic loads. *J Orthop Trauma* 2003;17(1):22-31.

Schildhauer TA, McCulloch P, Chapman JR, Mann FA: Anatomic and radiographic considerations for placement of transiliac screws in lumbopelvic fixations. *J Spinal Disord Tech* 2002;15(3):199-205.

Strange-Vognsen HH, Lebech A: An unusual type of fracture in the upper sacrum. *J Orthop Trauma* 1991;5(2):200-203.

Tötterman A, Glott T, Madsen JE, Røise O: Unstable sacral fractures: Associated injuries and morbidity at 1 year. *Spine (Phila Pa 1976)* 2006;31(18):E628-E635.

Tötterman A, Glott T, Søberg HL, Madsen JE, Røise O: Pelvic trauma with displaced sacral fractures: Functional outcome at one year. *Spine (Phila Pa 1976)* 2007;32(13):1437-1443.

Chapter 40
Anterior Approaches to the Lumbar Spine

Salvador A. Brau, MD, FACS

■ Indications

Anterior approaches to the lumbar spine have been used for decades, but in the early 1990s they became much more prevalent because of the introduction of threaded cages and bone dowels for anterior lumbar interbody fusion (ALIF). The use of these cages declined in the late 1990s but was followed by the introduction of artificial disks that require an anterior approach for deployment. Today, interest in artificial disks is not as strong, but new devices for stand-alone fusion have been introduced that also require an anterior approach.

Originally, these approaches were considered to be highly risky because of the potential for injury to the iliac vessels and the superior hypogastric plexus. Since descriptions of the mini-open lateral approach and the mini-open anterior approach were published in 2000, however, hundreds of general and vascular surgeons have been trained in these techniques, resulting in a much reduced incidence of complications. These new approaches are muscle sparing, are undertaken via the retroperitoneal route, and can be performed quickly and safely, giving the spine surgeon excel-

lent exposure of the entire disk space. Thus the old "shark-bite," anterolateral incision and the traditional left "paramedian" incision have been abandoned in many spine surgery centers where these newer approaches have become the standard. More importantly, the need for revision surgery has become more common, and these mini-open approaches disrupt the retroperitoneal tissues far less than the older incisions, facilitating an easier return to either adjacent levels or to the same level for revisions.

Spine surgeons should, therefore, avail themselves of a well-trained "access surgeon" if they have a significant number of patients who require an anterior approach. Unfortunately, no formal training programs exist that teach general or vascular surgery residents and fellows how to perform these procedures. Postgraduate courses and preceptorships sponsored by several device manufacturers and postgraduate institutions can help train practicing general and vascular surgeons interested in access to the lumbar spine, however. Once the access surgeon is trained properly, he or she needs to become familiar with the needs of spinal surgeons and the devices they use to determine the best approach for any particular instrumentation. Once ap-

propriate experience has been gained, the access surgeon can become a valuable resource to the spine surgeon in helping to design specific anterior approach plans for patients with difficult approach issues, such as those found in adjacent-level degeneration, revision of a previously instrumented level, and prior retroperitoneal surgery. Access surgeons also are able to handle any complications, such as iliac vein laceration or iliac artery thrombosis, that may arise during the original surgery. Their presence can ensure that no delay will occur in the recognition and treatment of such problems—a delay that could lead to catastrophic outcomes.

The indications for an anterior approach are dictated by the spine surgeon.

——————■

■ Contraindications

Only relative contraindications exist for the anterior lumbar approach. In general, the presence of several comorbidities in the same patient, such as diabetes, hypertension, heart disease, pulmonary disease, and obesity, should prompt a consult to the access surgeon, who can then determine if the risks of the anterior lumbar approach are justifiable. The following types of patients have a significantly increased risk of complications and

Dr. Brau or an immediate family member is a member of a speakers' bureau or has made paid presentations on behalf of Abbott and serves as a paid consultant to or is an employee of Blackstone Medical, Medtronic Sofamor Danek, Synthes, and Gore Medical.

should be evaluated thoroughly by the access surgeon before undergoing any anterior lumbar surgery: patients who have had prior retroperitoneal surgery such as a radical hysterectomy or a prostatectomy with lymph node dissection, laparoscopic hernia repairs, ureteral surgery, or vascular reconstruction of the aorta or iliac vessels (whether open or endovascular); those who have undergone radiation to the pelvis or retroperitoneum; and those with severe vascular occlusive disease or aneurysms. Calcification of the iliac vessels and aorta in itself is not a contraindication to anterior lumbar surgery; however, the access surgeon should educate patients with this condition about the increased risk of arterial thrombosis and should encourage the spine surgeon to have an alternative plan in case full anterior exposure cannot be obtained, so that the proper devices are available that can be deployed from a more anterolateral direction.

Alternative Treatments

Although some devices, such as artificial disks, stand-alone fusion cages, and anterior plates, need to be deployed through a full anterior exposure so they can be aligned at the midline of the vertebral body, certain alternative devices can be implanted into the disk space from a more anterolateral or direct lateral direction. The mini-open anterolateral approach, the anterolateral transpsoatic approach (ALPA), the anterolateral retroperitoneal approach (ARPA), and the extreme lateral approach all can be used to deploy devices that do not require alignment with the midline, including nucleus replacement devices, femoral ring allografts, and lateral cages.

Results

The results following ALIF and arthroplasty using the mini-open anterior approach have been remarkably good, with approach complications remaining very low. A very large unpublished series of 2,020 approaches in 2,013 patients reported an incidence of 0.29% for arterial injury and of 1.1% for venous injury. Only 5 patients in that series (0.24%) had any significant sequelae arising from these complications. The incidence of retrograde ejaculation in the male patients of the series was 0%. Thus, the anterior approach can be done with significantly reduced approach risks and may produce better results for the spinal procedure, whether it is arthrodesis or arthroplasty.

Technique

Setup/Exposure

The access surgeon and the spine surgeon should discuss the planned procedure well in advance and become well aware of each other's needs. The access surgeon, in particular, needs to know which level needs exposure and which device will be used. The overall medical status of the patient; the patient's age, body mass index, and sex; the presence or absence of pedal pulses; and the history of any prior retroperitoneal surgery are important to convey to the access surgeon. The AP and lateral radiographs and CT or MRI scans of the spine should be evaluated by the access surgeon to see whether any calcifications of the vessels, osteophytes, scoliosis or rotation of the spine, or aberrant locations of the iliac vessels in relation to the target level are present.

The patient is placed in the supine position on a radiolucent table with an inflatable bag under the lumbar re-

gion. Inflation of the bag permits extension of the spine at the time of diskectomy and graft placement, if needed.

A pulse oximeter placed on the first or second toe of the patient's left foot will provide an early warning for left iliac artery thrombosis should blood oxygen saturation levels not return to baseline levels after removal of the retractors, especially at L4-5. The saturation levels should be noted at the beginning of the operation as a baseline measurement. Upon placement of the retractors, especially at L4-5, saturation levels can fall to 0 in as many as 80% of patients. Should this happen, the spine surgeon has only 45 to 50 minutes to complete the spinal procedure. If more time is needed, the retractors should be released for a few cardiac cycles to allow the saturation to return to baseline levels. The retractors can then be reapplied, but the spine surgeon then has only 30 minutes to complete the procedure. If necessary, this maneuver can be repeated every 30 minutes. If the saturation does not return to baseline levels and remains 8 to 10 points below baseline, then further vascular investigation is necessary to determine the source of the deficit. The patient can be evaluated in the operating room by measuring segmental pressures and using an intraoperative arteriogram and then treated as necessary via the same incision or through a femoral endovascular approach. Removing the patient from the operating room, especially to go to the radiology department for angiography, will result in unnecessary delays in treatment, which could then give rise to further complications, such as a compartment syndrome.

A nasogastric or orogastric tube is placed once the patient is under anesthesia. The tube is removed at the end of the procedure. Complete muscle relaxation is necessary throughout the procedure.

Instruments/Equipment/ Implants Required

No special instruments are required to perform this approach to the lumbar spine. It is preferable, however, to use a table-held retractor with reverse-lipped anterior lumbar surgery (ALS) retractor blades that can be deployed once the exposure is completed. These retractors act as a lever to provide adequate exposure through a small incision. They also are radiolucent, so they do not interfere with fluoroscopic visualization of the posterior end plates. The use of sharp-tip retractor blades, such as a Hohmann, or Steinmann pins is discouraged because of the potential for vessel injury when deploying or removing them, especially when less experienced surgeons are involved.

Procedure

The access surgeon stands on the left of the patient and the assistant on the right. Transverse incisions are used for single-level approaches, and vertical or slightly oblique incisions are used for multiple-level access. This incision needs to be localized depending on the angle of L5-S1 and on the relationship of L4-5 to the iliac crest as seen on a lateral plain radiograph. The relationship of L4-5 to the iliac crest allows the surgeon to place the incision precisely by palpating the iliac crest and then moving the incision site caudally or cranially, depending on that relationship. Proper placement of this small incision is crucial in placing the working sleeves, templates, and inserters at the proper angle parallel to the vertebral end plates. Fluoroscopy should be used during incision placement when the access surgeon has not had sufficient experience to place the incision accurately after looking at the static films.

The incision is begun at the midline and is carried transversely to the lateral edge of the rectus muscle. For two-level exposure, the incision should be more oblique, starting mid-

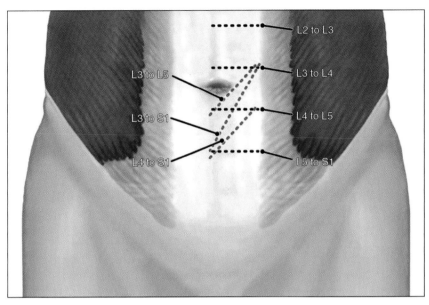

Figure 1 Drawing indicates the approximate location of the incision, depending on target level(s) to be exposed, for the anterior lumbar approach. The red and black dashed lines indicate the location of the incision. (Courtesy of Salvador Brau, MD, Los Angeles, CA.)

line at the level of the lower disk and ending at the level of the upper disk at the lateral edge of the left rectus muscle. For three levels, the obliquity increases. The incision may be vertical at the midline but never paramedian (**Figure 1**).

The incision is carried to the anterior rectus sheath, and then the rectus fascia is incised from 1 cm to the right of the midline to the edge of the rectus laterally. The anterior rectus sheath is elevated anteriorly away from the muscle belly for a distance of 4 to 6 cm both superiorly and inferiorly to allow for full mobilization of the rectus muscle. This is an important step in keeping this muscle from becoming an obstacle when the right-sided retractor is deployed. Medial, lateral, and posterior dissection of the muscle is then performed, taking great care to avoid injury to the inferior epigastric vessels. The rectus muscle is now easily retracted both medially and laterally (**Figure 2**). The lateral dissection of the rectus muscle is performed only in single-level cases and does not result in rectus muscle paresis. In approaches involving two or more levels,

lateral dissection of this muscle is not necessary because the incision is larger and the lateral aspect of the posterior rectus sheath can be accessed and incised with ease while retracting the muscle laterally from the midline.

In single-level cases, with the rectus muscle initially retracted medially, the posterior sheath is incised until the peritoneum is seen shining through. The edges should be grasped with a hemostat and the sheath dissected carefully from the peritoneum and incised as far inferiorly and superiorly as possible. The peritoneum is carefully pushed posteriorly at the edge of the fascial incision, and a plane is slowly developed between the peritoneum and the undersurface of the internal oblique and transversus muscles and fascia. This leads the surgeon into the retroperitoneal space (**Figures 3** and **4**).

Careful blunt-finger dissection is continued posteriorly, and then medial pushing is initiated to elevate the peritoneum away from the psoas muscle. The genitofemoral nerve can be identified easily over the psoas. The ureter usually can be identified as the

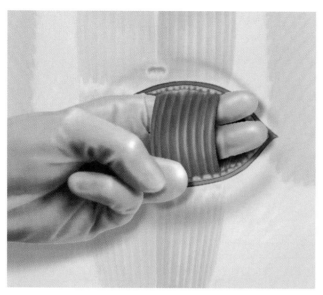

Figure 2 Drawing depicts mobilization of the left rectus muscle for the single-level approach. The patient's head is at the top. (Courtesy of Salvador Brau, MD, Los Angeles, CA.)

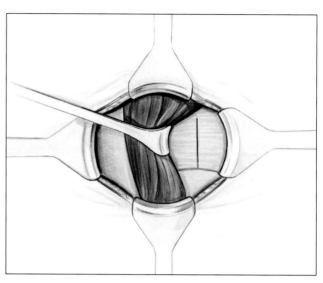

Figure 3 Drawing shows the incision on the posterior rectus sheath. The incision should be as lateral as possible. The patient's head is at the top. (Courtesy of Salvador Brau, MD, Los Angeles, CA.)

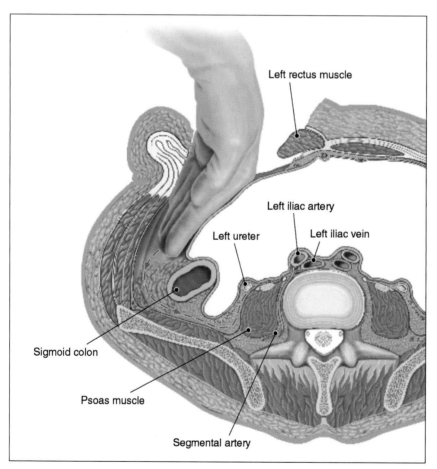

Figure 4 Drawing demonstrates how the surgeon's hand carefully pushes the peritoneum posteriorly at the edge of the fascial incision, developing a plane to elevate the peritoneum and its contents away from the retroperitoneal structures. (Courtesy of Salvador Brau, MD, Los Angeles, CA.)

peritoneum is lifted away from the psoas. Both of these structures should be preserved from injury.

Once the psoas is identified, a Harrington retractor is used to keep the peritoneal contents out of the way and allow further dissection. A Balfour retractor is then inserted to keep the incision open in the craniocaudal plane. A dry lap sponge tucked above the upper blade of the retractor is helpful in keeping retroperitoneal fat from creeping down and obscuring the field (**Figure 5**).

For operations on L4-5, or for operations that combine L4-5 with either L3-4 or L5-S1, the iliolumbar vein(s) must be ligated and cut. The entire lengths of the common and external iliac arteries are exposed, and they are mobilized as far distally as possible. This is extremely important in preventing stretch to the artery when retracted to the right. The incidence of left iliac artery thrombosis can be reduced by this maneuver. Careful blunt dissection then is started along the lateral edge of the artery to expose the left common iliac vein just underneath it. The dissection is continued posteriorly to identify the iliolumbar

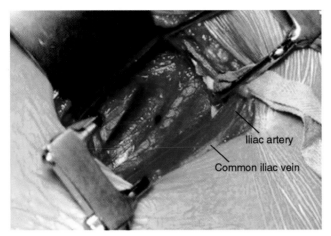

Figure 5 Intraoperative photograph demonstrates the initial visualization of the iliac vessels following elevation of the peritoneum. The patient's head is at the diagonal top right.

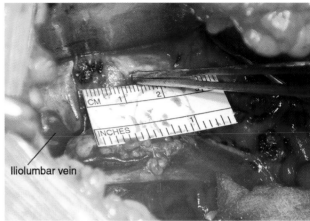

Figure 6 Intraoperative photograph shows identification of the iliolumbar vein. The patient's head is to the right. The forceps point to the middle of the L4-5 disk. The most common location of the iliolumbar vein is 1.5 cm caudal to this disk.

vein(s), which crosses the body of L5 and dives into the left paraspinous area (**Figure 6**). Ligation should be performed in place before transection and not too close to the junction with the iliac vein itself to avoid injuring the wall of the vein. For any operation that involves L4-5, these maneuvers are imperative to avoid avulsion of this vein.

The left iliac vein and artery now can be mobilized away from the spine using gentle, peanut-sponge dissection. In most patients, the vein "peels" away easily from the anterior surface of the spine (**Figure 7**). In some patients, however, an intense inflammatory reaction occurs in the plane between the vein and the anterior longitudinal ligament, especially when osteophytes are present; in such cases, the dissection can be quite difficult and tedious.

All of the vascular structures are thus swept from left to right, allowing adequate visualization of the disk involved. Once this part of the exposure has been completed, the Balfour and Harrington retractors are removed.

The table-held retractor then is set up. The surgeon's left hand reenters the retroperitoneal space with the rectus now moved laterally, and the fin-

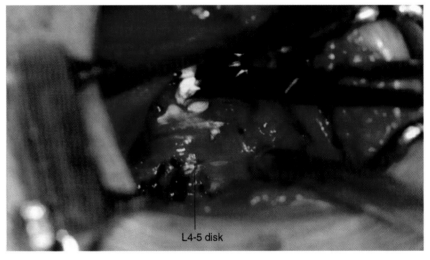

Figure 7 Intraoperative photograph depicts blunt dissection with a peanut sponge toward the right side of the disk space at L4-5. The patient's head is to the right.

gers find their way to the right side of the spine, following the planes previously dissected. A reverse-lipped, radiolucent 1-in blade of appropriate length is placed onto the right side of the spine using the finger(s) as a guide (**Figure 8, A**). This blade then is attached to the table-held retractor system and pushed to the right to elevate the vascular structures and expose the anterior surface of the spine (**Figure 8, B**). The reverse lip keeps the blade anchored to the edge of the spine, prevents it from slipping anteri-

orly once tension is applied, and allows for leverage, thus making a small incision possible.

A second blade is placed on the left side of the spine and attached to the table-held system to complete the exposure (**Figure 8, C**). Commonly, additional retractor blades need to be placed superiorly or inferiorly to complete the exposure (**Figure 9**). With these blades well anchored to the lateral wall of the vertebral column, the spinal surgeon and assistant can work on the disk with relative confidence

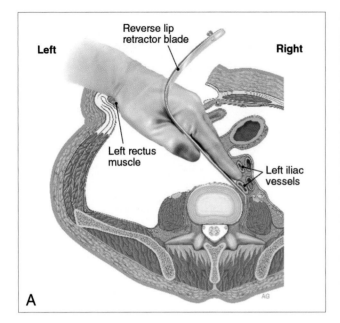

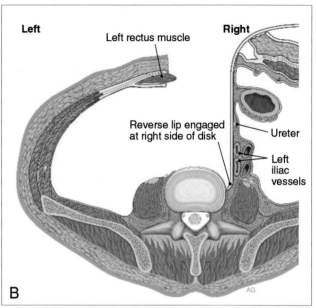

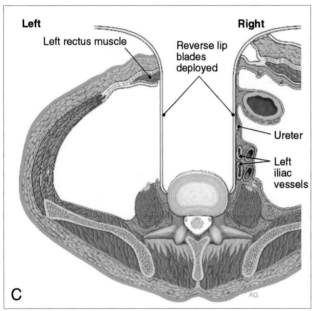

Figure 8 Drawings demonstrate the elevation of the vascular structures and exposure of the anterior surface of the spine for the anterior lumbar approach. **A,** Digital dissection under the vessels, with the surgeon's hand guiding the retractor blade toward the right side of the disk space. **B,** A reverse-lip blade is deployed on the right side, protecting the vessels and nerve plexus. **C,** Both reverse-lip blades are deployed. (Courtesy of Salvador Brau, MD, Los Angeles, CA.)

that the vessels will not slip around the retractors and become exposed to injury.

For operations on L5-S1, exposure usually lies between the iliac vessels below the aortic bifurcation. Blunt dissection is started anterior and medial to the left iliac artery toward the promontory. The L5-S1 disk is palpated, and dissection is carried out toward it until the middle sacral vessels become apparent. At this point, the superior hypogastric plexus can be seen in most patients, running with the peritoneum, much as the ureter does, as it is elevated away from the promontory (**Figures 10,** *A* and *B*). Once the peritoneum is thus elevated and the middle sacral vessels are identified clearly, it becomes easy to continue pushing the peritoneum and the nerve fibers to the right, protecting the fibers from possible injury. It is very important to look for this sympathetic plexus and for the approach surgeon to become familiar with its location if injury is to be avoided. The middle sacral vessels can then be cauterized with bipolar cautery or clipped and transected to further expose the disk space. The left iliac vein sometimes needs to be widely mobilized to allow adequate exposure. This vein is seen deep to the artery and can be swept further to the left with a peanut sponge to expose that side of the disk (**Figure 10,** *C*).

Chapter 43

Anterior Lumbar Corpectomy

Paul T. Rubery, Jr, MD

■ Indications

Anterior lumbar corpectomy involves surgical resection of nearly the entire vertebral body through an anterior approach to the spine. This allows broad decompression of the neural elements and can result in substantial mobility of the lumbar spine. Typically, the surgeon will perform a reconstruction involving a load-bearing implant and, frequently, a rigid stabilizing device.

The most common indication for corpectomy is symptomatic compression of the conus medullaris or cauda equina by bone or other material encroaching from the anterior direction. Lumbar burst fractures and pathologic burst fractures related to metastatic disease or vertebral osteomyelitis are the most common sources of such compression (**Figures 1** and **2**).

Lumbar corpectomy also is useful in the correction and reconstruction of posttraumatic kyphosis (malunited burst fracture) and in the correction of rigid coronal decompensation, as is seen in patients with severe scoliosis and congenital scoliosis due to hemivertebrae.

——————————■

■ Contraindications

Contraindications to anterior lumbar corpectomy are relative contraindications. Patients with previous retroperitoneal surgery, extensive intra-abdominal surgery, disorders of the great vessels, or a history of extensive external-beam radiotherapy to the retroperitoneum are relatively contraindicated because the surgical exposure of the spine may prove risky or impossible. Anterior corpectomy usually requires mobilization of the great vessels and can involve substantial hemorrhage. Consequently, patients whose overall medical condition is tenuous may be managed more safely with other approaches. Anterior corpectomy in the upper lumbar spine generally requires thoracoabdominal exposure, and patients who have marginal pulmonary function may not tolerate thoracotomy or sectioning of the hemidiaphragm.

——————————■

■ Alternative Treatments

Lumbar vertebral body removal and neural element decompression can also be accomplished through posterior approaches. Both posterolateral decompression and transpedicular decompression can be used to relieve impingement on the neural tissues from anteriorly based pathology. The thoracic techniques described in chapters 26 and 28 as well as modifications of the lumbar techniques described in chapter 46 can be adapted to this purpose. Posterior lumbar osteotomies, which are reviewed in chapter 61, are an excellent alternative for correcting both fixed coronal and sagittal plane imbalance.

——————————■

■ Results

Anterior lumbar corpectomy is used for the management of diverse pathologies, including fractures, tumors, and infections of the lumbar vertebrae. Understandably, the results of the procedure will vary according to the underlying disease state. Most recent reports are retrospective reviews of prospective clinical series (**Table 1**).

When used for the treatment of fracture, this technique is very successful. Canal obstruction by fracture

Dr. Rubery or an immediate family member has received royalties from LAGeT LLC, serves as an unpaid consultant to Kensey Nash has received research or institutional support from the Musculoskeletal Transplant Foundation and the National Institutes of Health (NIAMS & NICHD), and owns stock or stock options in Johnson & Johnson.

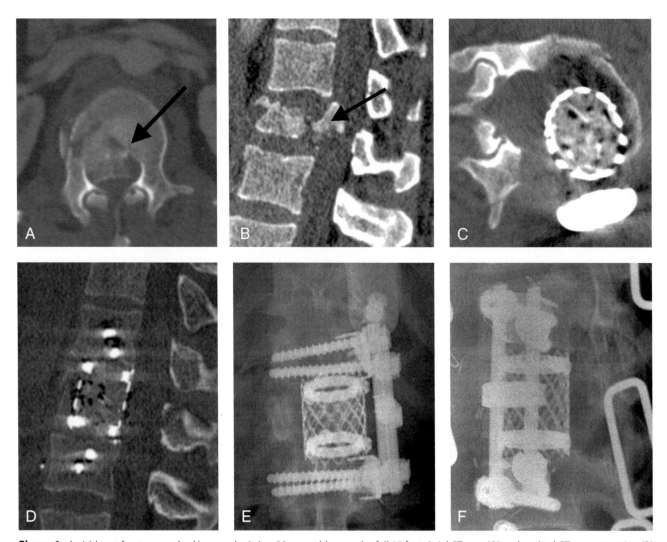

Figure 1 An L1 burst fracture resulted in paraplegia in a 38-year-old man who fell 15 feet. Axial CT scan (**A**) and sagittal CT reconstruction (**B**) demonstrate the burst fracture (arrows). Postoperative axial CT scan (**C**) and sagittal CT reconstruction (**D**) show the correction after an anterior L1 corpectomy and placement of a titanium cage and anterior screw-rod fixation device. Note the thorough decompression of the canal. Plain AP (**E**) and PA (**F**) radiographs show the instrumentation and the restoration of normal spinal alignment.

fragments is effectively relieved; typical preoperative canal compromise of 50% usually is relieved completely. Patients with incomplete neurologic deficit generally improve by one Frankel grade after surgery. Kyphosis correction is excellent, with typical residual kyphosis of less than 10°, and is well maintained at follow-up. Fusion rates are high (93% to 100%), and pain at follow-up is minimal or nonexistent in more than 90% of patients.

Results in tumor and infection surgeries are slightly harder to assess be-cause there are fewer patients, and such patients tend to have more systemic illnesses impacting their care. Many either require additional posterior reconstruction to address the pathology or undergo reconstruction with nonfusion techniques using polymethylmethacrylate (PMMA) after tumor resection. In small series, however, the rate of successful resolution of infection is extremely high, even when titanium cages are used anteriorly for the reconstruction. The fusion rate in infection (generally treated with anterior and posterior ap-proaches) is close to 100% in small series, and neurologic improvement in patients with incomplete deficits is common. Among tumor patients, pain relief is excellent. Neurologic improvement rates in patients with incomplete deficits are 20% to 40%, and improvement of one Frankel grade can be expected. Fusion rates in tumor patients often are not assessed, likely because of the high mortality of these patients in the postoperative period and the use of techniques using PMMA rather than biologic reconstruction.

the muscle. The ilioinguinal and genitofemoral nerves can be injured or irritated by self-retaining retractors resting on the surface of the psoas.

Major vascular injury is less common with a multidisciplinary surgical team. In my experience, intraoperative vessel injuries occur when the exposure is not quite adequate and the spine team attempts to compensate through vigorous retraction. It is important to ensure adequate access before allowing the exposure surgeon to leave the operating room. Cautery should be avoided on the L5-S1 disk and the sacral promontory to prevent injury to the sympathetic plexus.

Neural decompression proceeds more quickly, efficiently, safely, and thoroughly if the pedicle osteotomy technique is used to identify the dural sac before beginning decompression. Caution must be exercised when using the high-speed burr on posterior cortical bone, especially in fractures and on the contralateral side of the spine. The diamond burr, although less aggressive, is much less likely to snag or tear the dura and underlying nerve roots.

Vertebral bone quality can compromise reconstruction. If the bone is poor, subsidence of the strut is frequent. Using struts with a larger cross-sectional area can mitigate this tendency. Anterior spinal fixation devices often require bicortical purchase by the anchoring screws or bolts. Failure to achieve bicortical purchase can markedly compromise the construct. The vertebral diameter can be measured on preoperative CT scans to estimate anchor length. The vertebral diameter should be measured within the corpectomy defect. Finally, when creating the pathway for the anchors, a tap should be used to feel capture of the opposite cortex, and the path then should be rechecked for accuracy and length with a pedicle "feeler" probe.

Retroperitoneal seroma or lymphocele is a relatively rare complication. Controlling sites of lymphatic leak is a component of preventing this problem. My colleagues and I have a heightened awareness that the increasing use of BMP-2, particularly in off-label applications in the lumbar spine, correlates with increasing incidence of this problem. Anecdotal reports exist of recalcitrant lymphoceles requiring long-term indwelling percutaneous drains and even additional surgery. To date, there are no studies confirming causation by BMP-2.

The direct anterior incision carries the risk of incisional hernia, and the anterolateral incision occasionally results in denervation of a portion of the abdominal wall. This creates a patulous and occasionally uncomfortable abdominal wall on the side of the approach. This condition is not a hernia and cannot be repaired with additional surgery.

Bibliography

Bianchi C, Ballard JL, Abou-Zamzam AM, Teruya TH, Abu-Assal ML: Anterior retroperitoneal lumbosacral spine exposure: Operative technique and results. *Ann Vasc Surg* 2003;17:137-142.

Brodke DS, Gollogly S, Bachus KN, Mohr RA, Nguyen BK: Anterior thoracolumbar instrumentation: Stiffness and load sharing characteristics of plate and rod systems. *Spine* 2003;28:1794-1801.

D'Aliberti G, Talamonti G, Villa F, et al: Anterior approach to thoracic and lumbar spine lesions: Results in 145 consecutive cases. *J Neurosurg Spine* 2008;9:466-482.

Faro FD, White KK, Ahn JS, et al: Biomechanical analysis of anterior instrumentation for lumbar corpectomy. *Spine* 2003; 28:E468-E471.

Gumbs AA, Shah RV, Yue JJ, Sumpio B: The open anterior paramedian retroperitoneal approach for spine procedures. *Arch Surg* 2005;140:339-343.

Holman PJ, Suki D, McCutcheon I, Wolinsky JP, Rhines LD, Gokaslan ZL: Surgical management of metastatic disease of the lumbar spine: Experience with 139 patients. *J Neurosurg Spine* 2005;2:550-563.

Kaneda K, Taneichi H, Abumi K, Hashimoto T, Satoh S, Fujiya M: Anterior decompression and stabilization with the Kaneda device for thoracolumbar burst fractures associated with neurological deficits. *J Bone Joint Surg Am* 1997;79: 69-83.

Kirkpatrick JS: Thoracolumbar fracture management: Anterior approach. *J Am Acad Orthop Surg* 2003;11:355-363.

Korovessis P, Petsinis G, Koureas G, Iliopoulos P, Zacharatos S: Anterior surgery with insertion of titanium mesh cage and posterior instrumented fusion performed sequentially on the same day under one anesthesia for septic spondylitis of thoracolumbar spine: Is the use of titanium mesh cages safe? *Spine* 2006;31:1014-1019.

McDonnell MF, Glassman SD, Dimar JR II, Puno RM, Johnson JR: Perioperative complications of anterior procedures on the spine. *J Bone Joint Surg Am* 1996;78:839-847.

McDonough PW, Davis R, Tribus C, Zdeblick TA: The management of acute thoracolumbar burst fractures with anterior corpectomy and Z-plate fixation. *Spine* 2004;29:1901-1908.

Coding

CPT Codes		Corresponding ICD-9 Codes	
22558	Arthrodesis, anterior interbody technique, including minimal discectomy to prepare interspace (other than for decompression); lumbar	567.31 721.42 722.52	721.3 722.51 733.13
22845	Anterior instrumentation; 2 to 3 vertebral segments (List separately in addition to code for primary procedure)	170.2 342.9 343	342.1 342.90 343.0
22846	Anterior instrumentation; 4 to 7 vertebral segments (List separately in addition to code for primary procedure)	170.2 342.9 343	342.1 342.90 343.0
63087	Vertebral corpectomy (vertebral body resection), partial or complete, combined thoracolumbar approach with decompression of spinal cord, cauda equina or nerve root(s), lower thoracic or lumbar; single segment	170.2 721.41 722.72	567.31 721.42 722.73
63088	Vertebral corpectomy (vertebral body resection), partial or complete, combined thoracolumbar approach with decompression of spinal cord, cauda equina or nerve root(s), lower thoracic or lumbar; each additional segment (List separately in addition to code for primary procedure)	170.2 721.41 722.72	567.31 721.42 722.73
63090	Vertebral corpectomy (vertebral body resection), partial or complete, transperitoneal or retroperitoneal approach with decompression of spinal cord, cauda equina or nerve root(s), lower thoracic, lumbar, or sacral; single segment	170.2 806.4 806.6	567.31 806.5
63091	Vertebral corpectomy (vertebral body resection), partial or complete, transperitoneal or retroperitoneal approach with decompression of spinal cord, cauda equina or nerve root(s), lower thoracic, lumbar, or sacral; each additional segment (List separately in addition to code for primary procedure)	170.2 806.4 806.6	567.31 806.5

Chapter 47

Unilateral Partial Laminotomy (Laminaplasty) for Bilateral Decompression

Paul H. Young, MD
Jason P. Young, MD

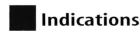

Indications

The indications for unilateral partial laminotomy (laminaplasty) are similar to those for standard lumbar decompression. Patients with degenerative lumbar spinal stenosis and predominant leg pain in whom nonsurgical therapy has failed are good surgical candidates. An ideal candidate for laminaplasty is a thin patient with leg pain and radiographic evidence of central canal, subarticular, and/or foraminal stenosis. Patients who require a bilateral decompression are best suited because subarticular and foraminal decompression contralateral to the partial laminotomy is readily accomplished.

Contraindications

Patients with grade II or higher spondylolisthesis require decompression with fusion and generally are not candidates for laminaplasty alone. Patients with a significant component of congenital spinal stenosis also are

poor candidates for partial laminotomy because neural compression in this setting is nonsegmental in the spinal canal and complete laminectomies usually are required to relieve the stenosis.

Alternative Treatments

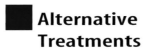

The classic treatment of symptomatic lumbar spinal stenosis is a wide decompression via a bilateral paraspinal exposure. Although this technique creates maximal exposure for bilateral decompression, morbidity is associated with the dissection of the muscle and stabilizing interspinous/supraspinous ligaments. Unilateral partial laminotomy for bilateral decompression (laminaplasty) is a less invasive technique that allows effective bilateral decompression while limiting superficial exposure to one side.

Patients with grade I degenerative spondylolisthesis are potential candidates for laminaplasty, especially those who cannot tolerate a more ex-

tensive fusion procedure. Patients with grade I degenerative spondylolisthesis and a collapsed disk with minimal segmental motion may be ideally suited for laminaplasty.

Results

The effectiveness of partial laminotomy (laminaplasty) in enlarging the cross-sectional areas of the spinal canal and foramen has been confirmed in cadaveric and clinical studies using postoperative CT. Clinical outcomes following lumbar laminaplasty compare favorably to other decompressive techniques, with successful outcomes in 87% to 93% of patients (**Table 1**).

Technique
Setup/Exposure
Following intubation, the patient is placed prone on a Wilson frame, which is positioned to widen the interlaminar spaces for easier entry. A freely hanging abdomen is essential for reducing excessive epidural bleeding. Neuromuscular paralytics are avoided during surgery to allow the surgeon to monitor twitching in case

Neither of the following authors nor any immediate family member has received anything of value from or owns stock in a commercial company or institution related directly or indirectly to the subject of this chapter: Dr. Paul H. Young and Dr. Jason P. Young.

Table 1 Results of Unilateral Partial Laminotomy for Bilateral Decompression

Authors (Year)	Number of Patients	Type of Treatment	Mean Patent Age in Years (Range)	Mean Follow-up (Range)	Results
Spetzger et al (1997)	29	Microdecompression	61 (NR)	18 months (NR)	88% good or excellent
Weiner et al (1999)	30	Microdecompression	64 (NR)	9 months (NR)	87% fair or very good
Iguchi et al (2000)	151	Decompression	70 (43-76)	13 years (10-17)	35% excellent 22% good
Costa et al (2007)	374	Unilateral laminotomy	72 (39-82)	36 months (NR)	90% improvement
Weiner et al (2007)	27	Unilateral decompression	62 (37-83)	29 months (20-48)	21 satisfied 6 unsatisfied
Sasai et al (2008)	48	Unilateral microdecompression	69 (47-84)	46 months (24-71)	57% very satisfied 26% fairly satisfied
Orpen et al (2010)	100	Microdecompression	65 (43-79)	3 years (2-5)	Instability in 4

NR = not reported.

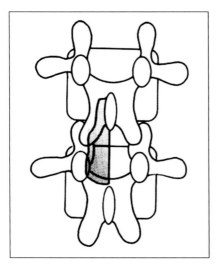

Figure 1 Drawing depicts a left-side unilateral partial laminotomy, in which half of the cranial and the top of the caudal lamina, the entire ligamentum flavum to the interspinous ligament medially, and the medial part of the facet joint laterally are removed (shaded area).

of excessive thecal sac and/or nerve root retraction.

The iliac crest provides the superficial landmark for localizing the lower lumbar levels. Generally, the lateral iliac crest is at the same level as the L4-5 interspace.

The operating position of the surgeon depends on the side of the pathology. For central, paracentral, and subarticular stenosis alone, the surgeon stands on the side of the greater pathology, and the partial laminotomy is performed on that side. For foraminal zone stenosis, the surgeon stands contralateral to the stenosis, and the partial laminotomy is performed on the side contralateral to the pathology. In cases of bilateral symptoms, a left-sided approach is preferred for a right-handed surgeon.

The incision is placed in relation to the interspinous spaces. At L4-L5, central canal stenosis usually is just cranial to the L4-5 interspinous space. At succeedingly higher levels, the area of stenosis is progressively more cranial in relation to the interspinous space.

A 2.5-cm midline incision usually is adequate for a single-level decompression. A curvilinear incision is made in the thoracolumbar fascia just off the midline. The paraspinal muscles are then subperiosteally dissected. This dissection is carried laterally to the facet joint, taking care to avoid violating the facet capsule. A McCulloch retractor is then placed, with the hook positioned against the interspinous ligaments, and the blade portion of the retractor retracting the paraspinal muscles over the facet joint. The cranial and caudal pars, half of the caudal and cranial laminae, the inferior aspect of the interspinous ligament medially, and the middle of the facet joint laterally should be easily visible after the exposure (**Figure 1**). The operating microscope is brought in at this stage.

Procedure

IPSILATERAL CENTRAL DECOMPRESSION (PARTIAL LAMINOTOMY)

The lower half of the cranial lamina is removed using a side-cutting high-speed burr. Beginning medially near the base of the spinous process and proceeding laterally to the base of the inferior articular facet, the lamina is resected to the underlying ligamentum flavum (**Figure 2**, *A*). Care is taken to preserve 5 to 10 mm of the pars interarticularis to prevent postoperative instability. As the resection reaches half of the cranial lamina, the protective ligamentum flavum thins and terminates, with visualization of the epidural fat and dura. A similar laminotomy is then performed at the upper edge of the caudal lamina, again proceeding from the base of the spinous process laterally (**Figure 2, B**). The ipsilateral ligamentum flavum is then removed to unroof the ipsilateral spinal canal (**Figure 2, C**).

CONTRALATERAL CENTRAL DECOMPRESSION

To perform the contralateral central decompression, the microscope is turned laterally and/or the table is tilted away from the surgeon. The line of vision should extend underneath the interspinous ligament across the midline (**Figure 3, A and B**). A blunt probe is used to separate the dura from the overlying ligamentum flavum. The contralateral cranial and caudal laminae are then undercut, beginning at the base of the spinous processes and proceeding laterally within the canal (**Figure 3, C**). In a stepwise fashion, the contralateral cranial and caudal laminae are burred away, followed by resection of the intervening ligamentum flavum. This successive resection is carried laterally until the contralateral traversing root pedicle is visualized, indicating that the lateral recess has been reached (**Figure 3, D**). A probe is passed cranial and caudal in the central canal to confirm adequate decompression.

CONTRALATERAL SUBARTICULAR DECOMPRESSION

The lateral attachments of the ligamentum flavum to the medial facet joint capsule (subarticular stenosis) are removed using a high-speed burr or a rongeur. The medial tip of the superior articular process is similarly resected. To complete the subarticular decompression, a burr is used to res-

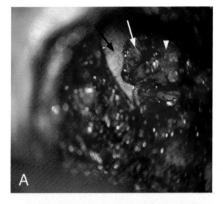
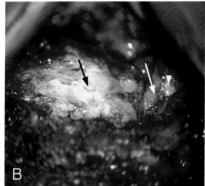
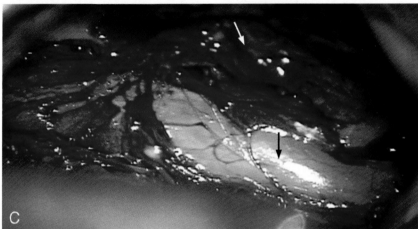

Figure 2 Intraoperative photographs demonstrate ipsilateral central decompression (partial laminotomy). The patient's head is to the left. **A**, Removal of half of the cranial lamina (black arrow) to the exposed ligamentum flavum (white arrowhead) and epidural space (white arrow). **B**, Removal of the top of the caudal lamina (white arrowhead), with exposed epidural space (white arrow/black arrow) and length of ligamentum flavum. **C**, The exposed thecal sac (black arrow) following removal of the ipsilateral ligamentum flavum (white arrow).

culpture the remaining bone and create a smooth transition between the lamina and the pedicle. Adequate contralateral subarticular decompression is verified when the traversing nerve root is inspected with a nerve hook.

CONTRALATERAL FORAMINAL DECOMPRESSION

After adequate decompression of the contralateral central and subarticular zones, a good view of the traversing root foramen is achieved. Any bone and/or soft tissue impinging on the traversing root foramen can be resected easily with a burr or a rongeur as the root passes from medial to lateral along the inferior aspect of the pedicle (**Figure 4, A and B**). To visual-

ize the inferior aspect of the exiting nerve root within the foramen and allow palpation of the pedicle, portions of the cranial lamina and the inferior facet are removed in a stepwise fashion (**Figure 4, C**). At the conclusion of the contralateral foraminal decompression, a blunt probe should be able to follow the exiting and traversing nerve roots into the extraforaminal zone. A final inspection of the contralateral decompression should reveal adequate resculpting of the contralateral spinal column (**Figure 5, A**).

IPSILATERAL SUBARTICULAR DECOMPRESSION

The microscope is redirected ipsilaterally. The ipsilateral subarticular decompression is started by removing the medial aspect of the hypertrophied inferior articular process with a burr or a rongeur. The medial border of the traversing root pedicle is revealed by following the cranial edge of the caudal lamina laterally. The traversing root can then be identified, and the hypertrophic medial tip of the superior facet can be resected safely by progressing cranially along the medial edge of the pedicle. The partial medial facetectomy is performed in a manner that removes more deep bone than superficial bone (to minimize facet disruption). Care is taken to preserve at least half of the facet joint to maintain stability. Adequate ipsilateral subarticular decompression is achieved when the medial facet is flush with the ipsilateral pedicle and the traversing nerve root passes freely into its foramen (**Figure 5**, *B*).

IPSILATERAL FORAMINAL DECOMPRESSION

Ipsilateral foraminal decompression is performed using the intertransverse approach. The paraspinal muscles are stripped further laterally to the transverse processes. The pars and the caudal facet joint are clearly identified (**Figure 6**, *A*). The tip of the superior facet is resected slightly. The intertransverse ligaments and associated soft tissue are then detached medially using a curet, and the nerve root is visualized. The foraminotomy is then continued from lateral to the pars into the canal. After adequate decompression, a probe should pass readily from inside the canal into the extraforaminal zone, and the tip of the probe can be visualized from the intertransverse interval (**Figure 6**, *B*).

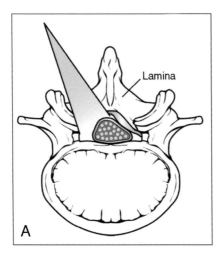
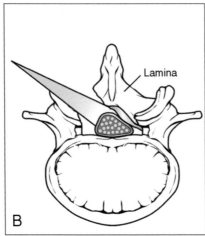
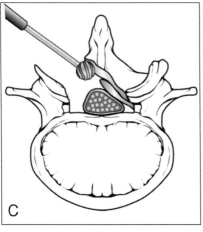
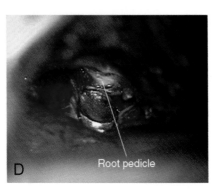

Figure 3 Images depict contralateral central decompression. Drawings depict the ipsilateral angle of vision (**A**) and the change in the angle of vision across the midline to the undersurfaces of the contralateral lamina and underlying ligamentum flavum (**B**). **C,** Drawing demonstrates the undercutting of the contralateral laminae. **D,** Intraoperative photograph of the contralateral traversing root pedicle following undercutting of the lamina. The patient's head is to the left.

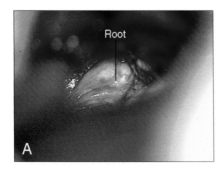
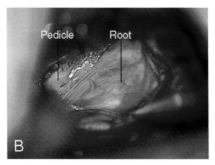
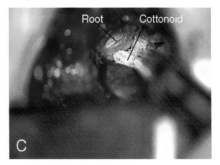

Figure 4 Intraoperative photographs demonstrate contralateral foraminal decompression. The patient's head is to the left. **A,** The contralateral traversing root following decompression. **B,** The contralateral traversing root following decompression at a higher magnification. **C,** The contralateral exiting root following decompression. Note the cottonoid used for hemostasis of the contralateral epidural space.

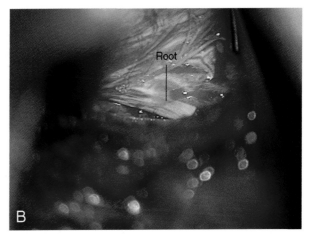

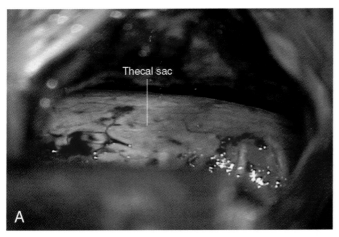

Figure 5 Intraoperative photographs across the thecal sac show contralateral subarticular decompression. The patient's head is to the left. **A,** A final inspection of the contralateral decompression should reveal adequate resculpturing of the contralateral spinal column. **B,** Inspection of the ipsilateral traversing root following foraminotomy.

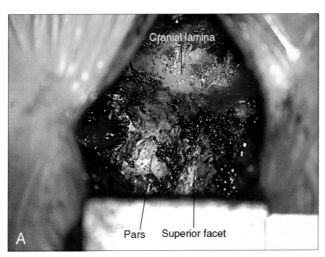

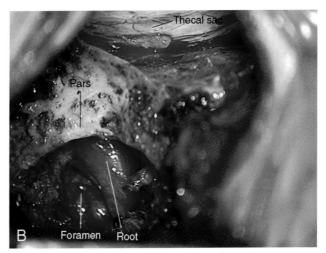

Figure 6 Intraoperative photographs demonstrate ipsilateral foraminal decompression. The patient's head is to the left. **A,** The relationships of the cranial lamina, the pars, and the superior facet. **B,** The ipsilateral exiting nerve root inside the foramen and the relationship of the exiting root and foramen to the lateral pars.

Wound Closure

Prior to closure, the decompression is verified to ensure that the exiting and traversing nerve roots pass freely into their respective foramina, bilaterally (**Figure 7**). The resected bony surfaces also are inspected to ensure that no sharp edges or oozing surfaces exist. The paraspinal muscles are injected with 0.5% bupivacaine for postoperative analgesia and to allow the muscles to reoppose the bone. The wound is irrigated with antibiotic solution and closed routinely in layers.

■ Postoperative Regimen

Patients generally are discharged the same day. They are instructed to begin ambulating immediately without restrictions. Prolonged sitting and strenuous lifting are avoided for a few weeks, whereupon an exercise therapy regimen is initiated.

■ Avoiding Pitfalls and Complications

The most common complication during lumbar laminaplasty is an inadver-

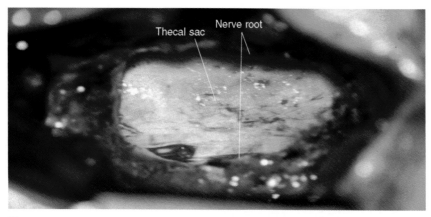

Figure 7 Intraoperative photograph shows verification of the bilateral thecal sac and nerve root decompression before closure. The patient's head is to the left.

tent dural tear. When a dural tear is encountered, a watertight repair generally should be attempted. Other potential complications include neurologic injury and epidural hematoma. Neurologic injury can be prevented by careful attention to the anatomic location of the nerve roots at all times during the procedure. Prior to aggressive bone/soft-tissue resection, the nerve root should be identified clearly. Although little epidural bleeding is encountered during central canal decompression, venous bleeding is common in the lateral zone.

Bibliography

Costa F, Sassi M, Cardia A, Ortolina A, De Santis A, Luccarell G, Fornari M: Degenerative lumbar spinal stenosis: Analysis of results in a series of 374 patients treated with unilateral laminotomy for bilateral microdecompression. *J Neurosurg Spine* 2007;7(6):579-586.

Gunzburg R, Keller TS, Szpalski M, Vandeputte K, Spratt KF: A prospective study on CT scan outcomes after conservative decompression surgery for lumbar spinal stenosis. *J Spinal Disord Tech* 2003;16(3):261-267.

Iguchi T, Kurihara A, Nakayama J, Sato K, Kurosaka M, Yamasaki K: Minimum 10-year outcome of decompressive laminectomy for degenerative lumbar spinal stenosis. *Spine (Phila Pa 1976)* 2000;25(14):1754-1759.

Kleeman TJ, Hiscoe AC, Berg EE: Patient outcomes after minimally destabilizing lumbar stenosis decompression: The "Port-Hole" technique. *Spine (Phila Pa 1976)* 2000;25(7):865-870.

McCulloch JA, Young PH: *Essentials of Spinal Microsurgery*. Philadelphia, PA, Lippincott-Raven, 1998.

Oertel MF, Ryang YM, Korinth MC, Gilsbach JM, Rohde V: Long-term results of microsurgical treatment of lumbar spinal stenosis by unilateral laminotomy for bilateral decompression. *Neurosurgery* 2006;59(6):1264-1270.

Orpen NM, Corner JA, Shetty RR, Marshall R: Micro-decompression for lumbar spinal stenosis: The early outcome using a modified surgical technique. *J Bone Joint Surg Br* 2010;92(4):550-554.

Patond KR, Kakodia SC: Interlaminar decompression in lumbar canal stenosis. *Neurol India* 1999;47(4):286-289.

Poletti CE: Central lumbar stenosis caused by ligamentum flavum: Unilateral laminotomy for bilateral ligamentectomy. Preliminary report of two cases. *Neurosurgery* 1995;37(2):343-347.

Postacchini F, Cinotti G, Perugia D, Gumina S: The surgical treatment of central lumbar stenosis: Multiple laminotomy compared with total laminectomy. *J Bone Joint Surg Br* 1993;75(3):386-392.

Sasai K, Umeda M, Maruyama T, Wakabayashi E, Iida H: Microsurgical bilateral decompression via a unilateral approach for lumbar spinal canal stenosis including degenerative spondylolisthesis. *J Neurosurg Spine* 2008;9(6):554-559.

Schillberg B, Nyström B: Quality of life before and after microsurgical decompression in lumbar spinal stenosis. *J Spinal Disord* 2000:13(3):237-241.

Spetzger U, Bertalanffy H, Naujokat C, von Keyserlingk DG, Gilsbach JM: Unilateral laminotomy for bilateral decompression of lumbar spinal stenosis: Part I. Anatomical and surgical considerations. *Acta Neurochir (Wien)* 1997;139(5):392-396.

Spetzger U, Bertalanffy H, Reinges MH, Gilsbach JM: Unilateral laminotomy for bilateral decompression of lumbar spinal stenosis. Part II: Clinical experiences. *Acta Neurochir (Wien)* 1997;139(5)397-403.

Thomas NW, Rea GL, Pikul BK, Mervis LJ, Irsik R, McGregor JM: Quantitative outcome and radiographic comparisons between laminectomy and laminotomy in the treatment of acquired lumbar stenosis. *Neurosurgery* 1997;41(3)567-574.

Weiner BK, McCulloch JA: Microdecompression without fusion for radiculopathy associated with lytic spondylolisthesis. *J Neurosurg* 1996;85(4):582-585.

Weiner BK, Patel NM, Walker MA: Outcomes of decompression for lumbar spinal canal stenosis based upon preoperative radiographic severity. *J Orthop Surg Res* 2007;2:3.

Weiner BK, Walker M, Brower RS, McCulloch JA: Microdecompression for lumbar spinal canal stenosis. *Spine (Phila Pa 1976)* 1999;24(21):2268-2272.

Williams RW, McCulloch JA, Young PH: *Microsurgery of the Lumbar Spine.* Rockville, MA, Aspen, 1990.

Coding

CPT Codes		Corresponding ICD-9 Codes	
63050	Laminoplasty, cervical, with decompression of the spinal cord, two or more vertebral segments	721.1 723.0	722.71 724.00
63051	Laminoplasty, cervical, with decompression of the spinal cord, two or more vertebral segments; with reconstruction of the posterior bony elements (including the application of bridging bone graft and non-segmental fixation devices (eg, wire, suture, mini-plates), when performed)	721.1 723.0	722.711 724.00

CPT copyright © 2010 by the American Medical Association. All rights reserved.

Chapter 48

Posterior Pedicle Screw Fixation With Posterolateral Fusion

Steven S. Lee, MD

Indications

The evolution of transpedicular spine instrumentation systems has allowed surgeons to change and improve their approaches to a variety of spinal disorders. Increased biomechanical stability has increased the ability of surgeons to maintain or restore the spine to normal alignment. Education, training, and increased experience have reduced the complications associated with the use of posterior pedicle screws. Fixed-angle screws and plates have developed into various polyaxial screw and rod systems. The rods themselves now include the option of being rigid or dynamic. Finally, unique screw-head locking mechanisms of some instrumentation systems have their own reported advantages.

Pedicle screws are commonly used in the treatment of a wide variety of spinal conditions. Acquired and congenital lumbar spondylolisthesis are two of the more accepted indications for these transpedicular screws. Trauma, tumor, iatrogenic instability (eg, after wide decompression), deformity correction, and degenerative disk disease are other common indications for posterior pedicle screw fixation with posterior fusion.

Screws have been used with both traditional open and newer minimally invasive approaches. Surgeons have placed posterior pedicle screws to augment lumbar interbody fusions. This has been done either with or without a posterior fusion.

Although the current use of pedicle screws encompasses a wide variety of diagnoses, most of the published literature presents techniques and results associated with spondylolisthesis. This may stem from similar inclusion and exclusion criteria that would allow for comparisons among the different study populations. This chapter focuses on the use of lumbar pedicle screws associated with an open posterior spinal fusion.

Contraindications

The main contraindication to using pedicle screws pertains to the anatomy of the pedicle and/or vertebral body. A screw may not be able to obtain proper fixation into the pedicle. The pedicle may be too small to accommodate the diameter of even the smallest screws (**Figure 1**). Traumatic fractures that involve the pedicle may not permit stable fixation. Iatrogenic fractures

through the pedicle also may occur intraoperatively during nerve decompression or screw insertion and can lead to loss of fixation. Poor bone quality due to tumors or osteoporosis also may preclude the use of pedicle screws at various levels. Many of these factors can be assessed preoperatively with thoughtful evaluation and planning to avoid unforeseen technical problems.

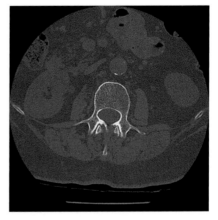

Figure 1 Axial CT scan of the lumbar spine through the level of the pedicle demonstrates a right pedicle that is considerably smaller than the left. Consideration of pedicle size and anatomy is a prerequisite for safe and adequate fixation with pedicle screws.

Alternative Treatments

When pedicle screws cannot be placed or loss of fixation has occurred intraoperatively, the initial option is to proceed with a standard noninstrumented posterior fusion for the original level(s) planned.

Other options can be considered if rigid fixation is imperative. If spinal decompression is not performed and the lamina is intact, a hybrid construct can be used, with modular laminar hooks attached via a rod to an intact pedicle screw. Alternatively, the surgeon can obtain stability with an additional level of screw fixation cranial or caudal to the insufficient pedicle. Finally, certain situations may allow preservation of stability with unilateral screw fixation, thus avoiding the unplanned addition of more surgical levels.

Polymethylmethacrylate has been used in osteoporotic bone to improve screw fixation. It can be injected into the screw tract immediately before final screw insertion. Care must be taken to ensure that no cortical breach or pedicle fracture has occurred that would allow the cement to extrude into the spinal canal.

Results

Results for the use of this technique in degenerative spondylolisthesis have been very favorable. Radiographic posterolateral fusion rates and clinical success rates have ranged from 41% to 100% (**Table 1**). Interestingly, several studies have shown that good clinical outcomes can be obtained even without a solid fusion. Unfortunately, the results for discogenic back pain have not been as favorable. Although the posterolateral fusion rates remain high, similar clinical success has not been attained without disk removal

and interbody stabilization. More recent studies on lumbar fusion have looked at outcomes with posterior lumbar interbody fusions or transforaminal interbody fusions rather than posterolateral fusions alone. Various bone-graft substitutes and biologic agents have been developed and used to increase fusion rates and lower the morbidity associated with autologous iliac crest bone grafting. Few studies have been performed to determine the most effective of these materials and techniques for use in posterolateral fusion. The development of adjacent-segment disease still remains problematic after any lumbar fusion technique. Symptomatic adjacent-segment disease is reported in 12% to 18% of patients during follow-up ranging from 4 to 12 years. Whether this is from increased biomechanical stress at the nonfused segment or the natural progression of degenerative disk changes at the adjacent disks remains a subject of considerable controversy.

Technique

Setup/Exposure
The patient is positioned prone on a well-padded Jackson spine table. The abdomen should be hanging free to prevent congestion of the venous plexus surrounding the spinal cord. The arms are positioned to protect the brachial plexus. The eyes and face are positioned with great care to prevent iatrogenic injury.

A standard midline incision is centered over the surgical levels. Sharp dissection is made through the skin and subcutaneous tissue until the lumbar fascia is identified. The appropriate levels are identified after palpation and identification of the spinous processes.

Bilateral subperiosteal dissection of the paraspinal muscles is performed to expose the spinous process, interlaminar space, and lamina laterally to the

facet joints (**Figure 2**, *A*). The facet joint capsule of the level to be fused can then be stripped from medial to lateral. The dissection is then taken ventrally, following the contour of the superior articulating facet. The transverse process can then be palpated, and its broad surface is exposed laterally to its edge (**Figure 2**, *B*).

The surgeon should be aware of the segmental lumbar blood vessels that supply the paraspinal musculature. Brisk bleeding from these small arteries may be encountered in the area lateral to the facet as the transverse process is being exposed. Careful dissection also is imperative during exposure of the superior transverse process. This adjacent facet joint capsule is to be preserved because this joint is not to be incorporated into the fusion (**Figure 2**, *C*).

After the exposure is completed, self-retaining retractors can be placed for the subsequent steps of the procedure. These retractors should be released intermittently to prevent ischemic muscle injury. The lateral gutters over the exposed transverse processes can be packed with gauze for added hemostasis. Spinal decompression can be performed before or after placement of the pedicle screws.

If no decompression is needed, the initial dissection may need to extend only just lateral to the facets so that the proper pedicle screw entry point can be identified. Because a posterior fusion can be performed across the remaining lamina, spinous processes, and facet joints, the full exposure of the transverse processes may be unnecessary, thus sparing further paraspinal muscle injury and trauma.

Instruments/Equipment/ Implants Required
Proper radiographic imaging is required for the safe placement of pedicle screws. C-arm fluoroscopy can identify the relevant bony anatomy and help ensure proper positioning of the screws (**Figure 3**).

Table 1 Results of Posterior Spinal Fusion

Author(s) (Year)	Diagnosis	Number of Patients*/ Procedure	Mean Patient Age in Years (Range)	Mean Follow-up (Range)	Fusion Rate*	Clinical Results
Lorenz et al (1991)	"Degenerative conditions"	a: 39; Inst PSF, ICBG b: 29; Noninst PSF, ICBG	a: 40 (22-53) b: 36 (22-53)	a: 31 mo (18-45) b: 26 mo (18-40)	a: 100% b: 41.4%	Inst had significantly higher fusion rates and better clinical outcomes.
Zdeblick (1993)	Isthmic and degenerative spondylolisthesis Degenerative disease Degenerative scoliosis Pseudarthrosis	a: 51; Noninst PSF, ICBG b: 35; Semi-rigid PSF, ICBG c: 37; Inst PSF, ICBG	a: 55 (26-80) b: 43 (27-75) c: 39 (20-74)	16 mo (9-28)	a: 65% b: 77% c: 95%	a: 71% G/E b: 89% G/E c: 95% G/E Inst fusion groups had better overall results.
Fischgrund et al (1997)	Degenerative spndylolisthesis	a: 33; Noninst PSF, ICBG b: 35; Inst PSF, ICBG	a: 66 (52-80) b: 69 (53-86)	28 mo (24-36)	a: 45% b: 82%	a: 85% G/E b: 76% G/E NSD
Thomsen et al (1997)	Isthmic spondylolisthesis Primary degeneration Degeneration after prior surgery	a: 64; Noninst PSF, ICBG b: 62; Inst PSF, ICBG	a: 43.5 (20-66) b: 46 (20-67)	24 mo	a: 85% b: 68%	a: 74% global satisfaction b: 82% global satisfaction NSD
France et al (1999)	Degenerative disease Failed back surgery syndrome Isthmic and degenerative spondylolisthesis	a: 34; Noninst PSF, ICBG b: 37; Inst PSF, ICBG	a: 43 (19-76) b: 43 (23-73)	a: 40 mo (12-65) b: 40 mo (12-71)	a: 64% b: 76%	a: 56% G/E b: 57% G/E NSD
Fritzell et al (2002)	Degenerative disease	a: 68; Noninst PSF, ICBG b: 62; Inst PSF, ICBG c: 71; Interbody fusion with Inst PSF, ICBG	a: 44 (25-62) b: 43 (25-65) c: 42 (28-59)	24 mo	a: 72% b: 87% c: 91%	a: 41% G/E b: 50% G/E c: 46% G/E NSD
Weiner and Walker (2003)	Degenerative disease Degenerative spondylolisthesis	a: 27; Noninst PSF, ICBG b: 32; Noninst PSF, ICBG with autologous growth factor	a: 56 (31-80) b: 61 (32-84)	24 mo	a: 91% b: 62%	Autologous growth factor showed inferior fusion rates. No clinical outcome data reported.
Kornblum et al (2004)	Degenerative spondylolisthesis	a: 22 with solid fusion after Noninst PSF, ICBG b: 25 with pseudarthrosis after Noninst PSF, ICBG	a: 73 b: 72	7 years + 8 months (5-14 years)	a: 100% b: 0%	a: 86% G/E b: 56% G/E Solid fusion group had significantly better long-term outcomes.
Dimar et al (2006)	Degenerative disease	a: 45; Inst PSF, ICBG b: 53; Inst PSF, rhBMP-2 and CRM	a: 52.7 b: 50.9	24 mo	a: 73.3% b: 90.6%	Both groups showed significant clinical improvement. NSD
Glassman et al (2007)	Degenerative disease Spondylolisthesis Degenerative scoliosis Postdiskectomy instability Pseudarthrosis Adjacent-level disease	a: 35; Inst PSF, ICBG b: 48; single-level Inst PSF, rhBMP-2 c: 27; multilevel Inst PSF, rhBMP-2 d: 16; revision Inst PSF, rhBMP-2	60 (27-84)	27 mo (24-38)	a: 88.6% b: 95.8% c: 100% d: 75%	Quality of fusion with commercially available rhBMP-2 equivalent to ICBG for PSF. No clinical outcome data reported.
Vaccaro et al (2008)	Degenerative spondylolisthesis	a: 19; Noninst PSF, OP-1 (rhBMP-7) putty b: 7; Noninst PSF, ICBG	a: 63 (43-80) b: 67 (51-79)	4 years	a: 68.8% b: 50%	a: 73.7% successful b: 57.1% successful NSD

*The numbers of patients and fusion rates reported for these studies represent only those available at latest follow-up.

Inst = instrumented fusion; PSF = posterior spinal fusion; ICBG = iliac crest bone graft; Noninst = noninstrumented fusion; G/E = good and/or excellent clinical results; NSD = no significant difference between groups; rhBMP = recombinant human bone morphogenetic protein; CRM = compression-resistant matrix; OP = osteogenic protein.

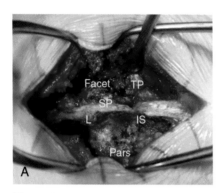
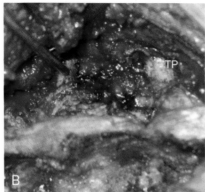
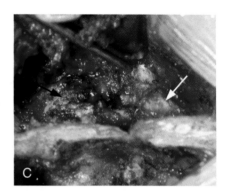

Figure 2 Intraoperative photographs demonstrate surgical exposure for posterior pedicle screw fixation with posterolateral fusion. The patient's head is to the right. **A,** Open exposure of the posterior lumbar spine. A standard midline approach has been made to expose the spinous processes, the lamina, the pars interarticularis, and the facet joints. **B,** The broad surfaces of the transverse processes are exposed to their tips laterally for proper preparation of the posterolateral fusion bed. **C,** Careful exposure at the superior joint level is important to keep the facet joint capsule intact because this joint will not be fused. Note that the normal facet joint capsule on the right (white arrow) remains intact, whereas the hypertrophic joint on the left (black arrow) has been fully exposed. IS = interlaminar space; L = lamina; SP = spinous process; TP = transverse process.

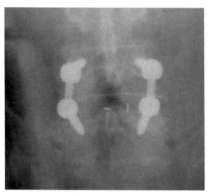

Figure 3 PA fluoroscopic view demonstrates the correct placement of the pedicle screws. The use of C-arm fluoroscopy during the procedure can help with the appropriate placement of pedicle screws.

The screws are available in a wide variety of diameters and lengths to accommodate almost any pedicle size and shape. The longitudinal rods come in precut lengths in a lordotic shape. Longer rods can be cut to custom length and contoured to fit the orientation of the screws and anatomy. Finally, cross-links can be used to bridge the bilateral rods to increase stability.

Procedure

The key component of the procedure is the identification of the starting point for pedicle screw insertion. Anatomic landmarks and fluoroscopic imaging are used together to ensure proper screw placement. The size of the pedicles increases gradually from L1 to L5. The medial angulation of the pedicle also increases, from approximately neutral at L1 to approximately 25° to 30° at L5.

The entry point can be estimated by finding the intersection of a line drawn vertically at the facet joint margin and a line drawn horizontally through the middle of the transverse process. A high-speed burr tip can then be used to decorticate this starting point (**Figure 4**, *A*). A sharp awl can be used in softer bone.

Alternatively, the pedicle entry points can be identified fluoroscopically, using a radiopaque marker. This can be very effective, especially in the smaller upper lumbar pedicles. The use of fluoroscopy also is beneficial in cases in which the normal anatomy is obscured by advanced degenerative changes at the facets or distorted by spinal deformity. An AP view shows a clear outline of the pedicles and a linear projection of the identification of the starting point. Once the marker is directly over the starting point, the burr tip can decorticate this position.

A blunt pedicle probe can then be started through the entry point (**Figure 4**, *B*). Prior to deeper insertion of the probe, the starting point and initial trajectory can be confirmed to be positioned appropriately by AP and lateral fluoroscopic projections. These views also can help to promote the proper angle of insertion and medialization of the eventual screw position. The probe can then be advanced gently to the appropriate depth into the vertebral body. If a lateral fluoroscopic view is taken with the probe fully inserted, it can be used to choose a screw with the corresponding length.

A ball-tipped feeler is then inserted into the tract and used to circumferentially palpate the bony tunnel (**Figure 4**, *C*). This is done to identify any breaches of the bony cortex along the screw tract. Any medial or inferior violation can affect the exiting nerve root. Superior or lateral breaks through the pedicle can affect the proximal nerve root. Anterior breaches through the vertebral body cortex risk injury to the anterior great vessels. If a cortical breach is suspected, the blunt pedicle probe can be redirected and repositioned.

The screw tract is then tapped the length of the pedicle. The feeler is used again to confirm intact bone. The screw is then inserted finally to the appropriate depth through the pedicle and into the vertebral body (**Figure 4**, *D*). The surgeon continues to direct the screws medially during insertion. The overlying muscle and soft tissue can sometimes change the path of the screw so that the tip can veer off its initial prepared tract. This may result in improper placement of the screw, leading to loss of fixation or even neurovascular injury. The "wall" of retracted tissue is a significant concern in patients who are obese or in revision surgical procedures where the soft tissue is less pliable. The tip of the screw should reach to the junction of the middle and anterior thirds of the vertebral body.

If difficulty is encountered in identifying the position of the pedicle, or if concern exists about the aberrant position of a screw, a laminotomy or extensive laminectomy can be performed for tactile palpation with instruments and/or visual confirmation of the anatomy. The fluoroscopy unit also can be angled directly along the plane of the pedicle to determine if the screw has cut out laterally outside the vertebral body or if it is not within the confines of the pedicle border. These situations occur more frequently in deformity cases.

Once the spinal decompression and screw placement have been completed, the transverse processes are re-exposed with retractors. The bone over the lateral pars, transverse processes, and facet joints is decorticated with a high-speed burr to expose healthy bleeding bony surfaces for the fusion bed. If no decompression was needed, the posterior lamina, spinous processes, and facet joints also may be decorticated. The bone graft of choice (autologous bone, bone-graft substitute, and/or biologic agents) is then placed across the fusion bed and in the

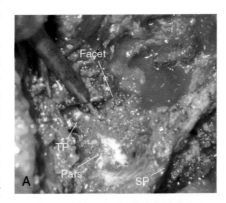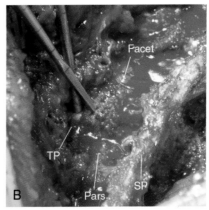
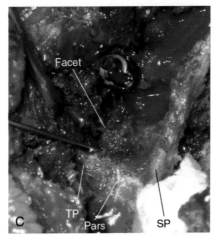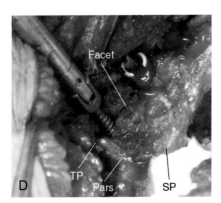

Figure 4 Intraoperative photographs demonstrate the sequence of pedicle screw insertion. The patient's head is to the upper right, diagonally. **A,** A high-speed burr tip can be used to decorticate the entry point for pedicle screw insertion. **B,** A pedicle probe is positioned at the entry point of the pedicle. The suction tip is in position at the midlevel of the transverse process, which is at the level of the pedicle. **C,** A ball-tipped feeler is used to circumferentially palpate the pedicle screw tract to ensure that no cortical disruption is present, which can lead to neurovascular injury or loss of fixation. **D,** Directing the screw medially during final placement is important to prevent the screw from veering off its initial prepared tract. SP = spinous process; TP = transverse process.

lateral gutters, spanning the levels to be fused.

The rods can then be connected to the screw heads. Compression or distraction across the screws can be performed after securing the most inferior or superior screw to the rod. Reduction of deformities also can be attempted through the screws and rods. Any of these manipulations should be done with great care so that the fixation and purchase of the screw into the bone are not compromised. This is especially pertinent in elderly patients, who are at risk for osteopenia

and osteoporosis. The instrumentation finally is secured after tightening of the screw locking mechanisms with the appropriate torque limiter.

Wound Closure

The lumbar fascia is closed in a watertight manner with interrupted sutures. It may be possible to reapproximate the paraspinal muscles with absorbable suture as a separate layer before closure of the fascia. The fascia also may be reattached to any remaining spinous processes at the upper and lower ends of the wound.

Subfascial and subcutaneous drains can be used. The subcutaneous tissue and skin are closed in a routine manner.

━━━━━■

Postoperative Regimen

Patients who have undergone routine posterior instrumented fusion performed for degenerative disorders and mild (lower than grade II) spondylolisthesis are allowed to be out of bed and ambulating with therapists on the first postoperative day. A simple abdominal binder often is used, mainly for comfort but also as a gentle reminder to limit initial lumbar motion such as bending and twisting. Patients who have had posterior fusion for trauma, tumor, or significant deformity or who have had multilevel procedures may require more rigid external support. This may involve the use of thoracolumbosacral braces or lumbosacral orthoses with thigh extensions for lumbosacral reconstructions.

Mechanical prophylaxis against deep vein thrombosis involves the combined use of sequential compression devices and lower extremity graded compression stockings. In high-risk patients with significant medical comorbidities, consideration is given to the addition of chemoprophylactic agents such as low-molecular-weight heparin.

The Foley catheter is removed when the patient is sufficiently ambulatory. Surgical drains usually are removed on the first or second postoperative day, depending on output.

Early pain control is helpful to allow patients to participate early in physical therapy and to promote a sense of recovery and well-being. Patient-controlled analgesia is used immediately after surgery along with appropriate oral analgesic agents.

During the first 6 weeks after surgery, patients are allowed to ambulate as tolerated, and walking is greatly encouraged. Heavy lifting (more than 15 lb) and repetitive lumbar bending or twisting motions are restricted. Some patients are allowed to work from home if their job duties are sedentary. Between 6 and 12 weeks, increased low-impact aerobic exercise and outpatient physical therapy is initiated. Return to light-duty work activities may be started at the same time. At approximately 6 to 9 months after surgery, patients with occupations requiring heavy labor may return to work activities. Some patients may not be allowed or able to return to their usual heavy manual labor occupation for up to a year. Between 4 months and 8 months, patients are allowed to return to moderate recreational activities.

━━━━━■

Avoiding Pitfalls and Complications

Preoperative preparation and planning are the most important factors in avoiding pitfalls and potential complications. Proper radiographic imaging should be reviewed so that the planned instrumentation can be anticipated in terms of screw size, length, and angles of insertion. If any concerns exist that specific bony anatomy is not readily appreciable on plain radiographs or MRI, a CT scan should be obtained.

In the elderly population, bone strength may be compromised by osteoporosis. A dual-energy x-ray absorptiometry scan can be reviewed to determine whether supplemental fixation with bone cement is needed to prevent screw failure.

Fluoroscopy can be quicker and more efficient than obtaining multiple intraoperative radiographs for pedicle screw placement. Multiple angled views can be obtained to help with proper screw insertion and placement. The intensifier can be angled along the path of the pedicle to determine the orientation of the implants. The intensifier should always be centered on the area of interest to prevent problems with parallax.

Two more recent technologies have gained interest among surgeons for use during instrumented spinal fusion procedures. First, electromyelographic readings during screw insertion can help to detect cortical violation by screws and thus reduce potential spinal nerve injury. Second, advances in computer navigation systems have resulted in improved screw placement. These technologies may be helpful in cases with complex anatomy. Their advantages still must be weighed against the increased cost, the longer surgical time, and the variability of results of the different available systems.

Improving exposure can help when screw insertion is difficult. A wider laminectomy or laminotomy can be performed to palpate and even visualize the borders of the pedicle of interest.

If a screw loses purchase or the screw is placed incorrectly, reinsertion in a new trajectory may be attempted if the pedicle is of adequate size and good bony purchase is obtained. Sometimes reinsertion is not possible, so the level may have to be skipped. In such cases, two options generally are available: the fusion could be extended so that the next pedicle can provide a fixation point, or unilateral screw fixation could be accepted by the surgeon.

Patients with postoperative radiculopathy and/or possible poor pedicle screw placement should undergo immediate evaluation with a CT scan (**Figure 5**). Plain radiographs may not adequately assess the actual position of a screw. If nerve root injury or irritation results from an improperly placed screw, the screw should be removed.

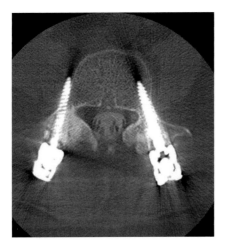

Figure 5 Axial CT scan shows the right-side screw (shown on the left) veering laterally outside the margin of the pedicle and vertebral body. Patients with unexplained postoperative radiculopathy after instrumentation or possible inadequate screw placement should be evaluated with a CT scan.

Long-term problems with pedicle screws include screw breakage, loosening and pull-out, and late kyphosis deformity. Careful attention to biomechanical principles and surgical technique can help to prevent these problems. Relying only on the strength of the pedicle screws without proper surgical preparation for bony fusion will lead to implant failure. Late kyphosis deformity and implant fatigue will occur with inadequate anterior column support. In such situations, the surgeon must consider surgical techniques other than just posterior instrumented spinal fusion.

Bibliography

Cheh G, Bridwell KH, Lenke LG, et al: Adjacent segment disease following lumbar/thoracolumbar fusion with pedicle screw instrumentation: A minimum 5-year follow-up. *Spine* 2007;32:2253-2257.

Dimar JR, Glassman SD, Burkus KJ, Carreon LY: Clinical outcomes and fusion success at 2 years of single-level instrumented posterolateral fusions with recombinant human bone morphogenetic protein-2/compression resistant matrix versus iliac crest bone graft. *Spine* 2006;31:2534-2539.

Fischgrund JS, Mackay M, Herkowitz HN, Brower R, Montgomery DM, Kurz LT: 1997 Volvo Award winner in clinical studies: Degenerative lumbar spondylolisthesis with spinal stenosis. A prospective, randomized study comparing decompressive laminectomy and arthrodesis with and without spinal instrumentation. *Spine* 1997;22:2807-2812.

France JC, Yaszemski MJ, Lauerman WC, et al: A randomized prospective study of posterolateral lumbar fusion: Outcomes with and without pedicle screw instrumentation. *Spine* 1999;24:553-560.

Fritzell P, Hägg O, Wessberg P, Nordwall A: Chronic low back pain and fusion: A comparison of three surgical techniques. A prospective multicenter randomized study from the Swedish Lumbar Spine Study Group. *Spine* 2002;27:1131-1141.

Ghiselli G, Wang JC, Bhatia NN, Hsu WK, Dawson EG: Adjacent segment degeneration in the lumbar spine. *J Bone Joint Surg Am* 2004;86:1497-1503.

Glassman SD, Carreon L, Djurasovic M, et al: Posterolateral lumbar spine fusion with INFUSE bone graft. *Spine J* 2007; 7:44-49.

Kornblum MB, Fischgrund JS, Herkowitz HN, Abraham DA, Berkower DL, Ditkoff JS: Degenerative lumbar spondylolisthesis with spinal stenosis: A prospective long-term study comparing fusion and pseudarthrosis. *Spine* 2004;29:726-733.

Lorenz M, Zindrick M, Schwaegler P, et al: A comparison of single-level fusions with and without hardware. *Spine* 1991; 16:S455-S458.

Park P, Garton HJ, Gala VC, Hoff JT, McGillicuddy JE: Adjacent segment disease after lumbar or lumbosacral fusion: Review of the literature. *Spine* 2004;29:1938-1944.

Thomsen K, Christensen FB, Eiskjaer SP, Hansen ES, Fruensgaard S, Bünger CE: 1997 Volvo Award winner in clinical studies: The effect of pedicle screw instrumentation on functional outcome and fusion rates in posterolateral lumbar spine fusion. A prospective, randomized clinical study. *Spine* 1997;22:2813-2822.

Vaccaro AR, Whang PG, Patel T, et al: The safety and efficacy of OP-1 (rhBMP-7) as a replacement for iliac crest autograft for posterolateral lumbar arthrodesis: Minimum 4-year follow-up of a pilot study. *Spine J* 2008;8:457-465.

Weiner BK, Walker M: Efficacy of autologous growth factors in lumbar intertransverse fusions. *Spine* 2003;28:1968-1971.

Zdeblick TA: A prospective, randomized study of lumbar fusion: Preliminary results. *Spine* 1993;18:983-991.

Coding

CPT Codes		Corresponding ICD-9 Codes	
22612	Arthrodesis, posterior or posterolateral technique, single level; lumbar (with or without lateral transverse technique)	170.2 721.42 722.10	170.3 722.0 737.39
22614	Arthrodesis, posterior or posterolateral technique, single level; each additional vertebral segment (List separately in addition to code for primary procedure)	170.2 721.42 722.10	170.3 722.0 737.39
22842	Posterior segmental instrumentation (eg, pedicle fixation, dual rods with multiple hooks and sublaminar wires); 3 to 6 vertebral segments (List separately in addition to code for primary procedure)	342.1 342.90 343.0	342.9 343
20936	Autograft for spine surgery only (includes harvesting the graft); local (eg, ribs, spinous process, or laminar fragments) obtained from same incision (List separately in addition to code for primary procedure)	170.2 733.13	724.6 737.30
63047	Laminectomy, facetectomy and foraminotomy (unilateral or bilateral with decompression of spinal cord, cauda equina and/or nerve root[s], [eg, spinal or lateral recess stenosis]), single vertebral segment; lumbar	722.73 724.02	722.83
63048	Laminectomy, facetectomy and foraminotomy (unilateral or bilateral with decompression of spinal cord, cauda equina and/or nerve root[s], [eg, spinal or lateral recess stenosis]), single vertebral segment; each additional segment, cervical, thoracic, or lumbar (List separately in addition to code for primary procedure)	722.73 724.02	722.83

No. 2-0 absorbable suture is used to close the subcutaneous layer. Adhesive skin closures can be used to appose the skin edges.

Postoperative Regimen

Postoperatively, patients are given oral pain medications and a patient-controlled analgesia device. The patient-controlled analgesia typically is weaned on postoperative day 2, and patients go home taking the oral pain medication. Stockings and sequential compression devices are used for deep vein thrombosis prophylaxis. Antibiotics are discontinued once all drains and the catheter have been removed. Typically, most patients go home on postoperative day 3. They are given a lumbosacral corset for comfort.

Patients are followed regularly. If they are doing well at the 3-month follow-up and no instrumentation failure is evident on radiographs, they are sent to physical therapy for range-of-motion and strengthening exercises as needed.

Avoiding Pitfalls and Complications

The key to successful placement of percutaneous pedicle screws is obtaining good images. It is worthwhile to take the time to obtain good images before preparation and draping.

Also, strict adherence to the guidelines for proper placement of the Jamshidi needle is important. If the imaging shows that the needle is too far medial or lateral, the surgeon should start over and repeat the process until the desired placement has been achieved. If the initial skin incision has been placed too far medial or lateral and the skin or soft tissues are interfering with the proper placement or trajectory of the needle, another incision should be made so that the needle can be placed optimally. Optimal placement of the needle should not be sacrificed for cosmesis.

Tapping or placing of the pedicle

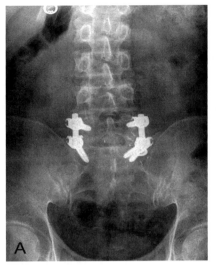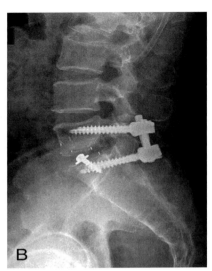

Figure 5 AP (**A**) and lateral (**B**) radiographs show the final placement of the percutaneous pedicle screws at L5-S1.

screw should be done with the C-arm in the lateral projection. Frequent images should be taken to ensure that the guidewire does not catch on the tap or the pedicle screw. This could drive the guidewire anteriorly and have disastrous consequences, because the great vessels lie anterior to the vertebral body. If the tap comes out during the tapping process, the C-arm should be brought back to the AP projection, the needle should be used to find the hole again, and the process should be repeated. Although strict adherence to protocol and attention to detail cannot prevent all complications, it can certainly reduce the incidence of unwanted complications.

Bibliography

Foley KT, Gupta SK, Justis JR, Sherman MC: Percutaneous pedicle screw fixation of the lumbar spine. *Neurosurg Focus* 2001;10(4):E10.

Kim DY, Lee SH, Chung SK, Lee HY: Comparison of multifidus muscle atrophy and trunk extension muscle strength: Percutaneous versus open pedicle screw fixation. *Spine (Phila Pa 1976)* 2005;30(1):123-129.

Lee SH, Choi WG, Lim SR, Kang HY, Shin SW: Minimally invasive anterior lumbar interbody fusion followed by percutaneous pedicle screw fixation for isthmic spondylolisthesis. *Spine J* 2004;4(6):644-649.

Schizas C, Kosmopoulos V: Percutaneous surgical treatment of chance fractures using cannulated pedicle screws: Report of two cases. *J Neurosurg Spine* 2007;7(1):71-74.

Schizas C, Michel J, Kosmopoulos V, Theumann N: Computer tomography assessment of pedicle screw insertion in percutaneous posterior transpedicular stabilization. *Eur Spine J* 2007;16(5):613-617.

Schwender JD, Holly LT, Rouben DP, Foley KT: Minimally invasive transforaminal lumbar interbody fusion (TLIF): Technical feasibility and initial results. *J Spinal Disord Tech* 2005;18(suppl):S1-S6.

Wiesner L, Kothe R, Schulitz KP, Rüther W: Clinical evaluation and computed tomography scan analysis of screw tracts after percutaneous insertion of pedicle screws in the lumbar spine. *Spine (Phila Pa 1976)* 2000;25(5):615-621.

Coding

CPT Codes		Corresponding ICD-9 Codes	
22558	Arthrodesis, anterior interbody technique, including minimal discectomy to prepare interspace (other than for decompression); lumbar	567.31 721.42 722.52	721.3 722.51 733.13
22585	Arthrodesis, anterior interbody technique, including minimal discectomy to prepare interspace (other than for decompression); each additional interspace (List separately in addition to code for primary procedure)	567.31 905.1 905.6	733.13 905.5
22845	Anterior instrumentation; 2 to 3 vertebral segments (List separately in addition to code for primary procedure)	170.2 342.1 342.9	342.90 343 343.0

CPT copyright © 2010 by the American Medical Association. All rights reserved.

Chapter 50

Posterior Lumbar Interbody Fusion

Hieu Ball, MD, MPH

Indications

Lumbar decompression and fusion procedures have been used to successfully treat degenerative conditions, instability, coronal and sagittal deformity (**Figure 1**), postlaminectomy syndrome, failed diskectomy, trauma, tumor, and infection. In cases in which lumbar decompression and arthrodesis are necessary to treat radicular and axial back pain, several surgical approach options are available. From a biomechanical standpoint, anterior column devices in conjunction with posterior instrumentation provide an optimally rigid construct that takes advantage of the 80% load-bearing anterior column and allows the fusion to heal under compression rather than tension alone, the latter of which occurs in posterior-only constructs.

In patients who have unfavorable anterior anatomy (eg, calcified aorta, abdominal obesity) or a prior treatment history (history of retroperitoneal surgery, radiation therapy, etc), a direct anterior approach to the lumbar spine may not be prudent clinically and in some cases not possible technically. In these difficult cases, the posterior lumbar interbody fusion (PLIF)

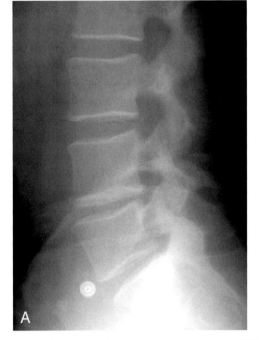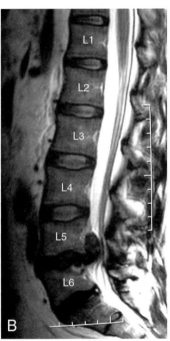

Figure 1 Lateral radiograph (**A**) shows lateral retrolisthesis of L4 on L5 and collapse of L5-6 in a patient with six lumbar vertebrae. **B,** Sagittal MRI of the same patient shows a large disk herniation at L4-5 and an annular tear noted at L5-6.

procedure allows for circumferential (360°) fusion from a posterior-only approach. Through this technique, the anterior column can be addressed, resulting in an increased surface area for fusion and greater stability with placement of an intervertebral structural device (eg, bone, polyetherether-ketone [PEEK], titanium) and bone graft or other osteoinductive agent. The advantages of PLIF include improved biomechanics (6 to 18 times greater stiffness than posterior screws alone) and improved local biologic conditions for the fusion surface area. Direct decompression of the lumbar neural anatomy can be performed in addition to stable instrumented arthrodesis with segmental fixation. The PLIF technique may be performed

Dr. Ball or an immediate family member serves as a board member, owner, officer, or committee member of the San Ramon Surgery Center and serves as a paid consultant to or is an employee of Medtronic Sofamor Danek and Synthes.

Table 1 Results of Posterior Lumbar Interbody Fusion

Authors (Year)	Number of Patients	Procedure	Mean Patient Age in Years (Range)	Mean Follow-Up in Months	Fusion Success Rate (%)
Suk et al (1997)	36	PLIF with pedicle screw fixation and posterolateral fusion	44.4	39.6	100
Agazzi et al (1999)	78	PLIF	47	28	90
Freeman et al (2000)	60	PLIF with instrumented posterolateral fusion	44 (19-69)	63.6	83
Brantigan et al (2000)	178	PLIF with pedicle screw placement	44	48	98.9
Okuda et al (2006)	251	PLIF	60	50	98.8

PLIF = posterior lumbar interbody fusion.

with or without transpedicular fixation, but stability, a reduced risk of implant migration, and higher rates of fusion are associated with PLIF used in conjunction with pedicle screw fixation. Improved sagittal balance also is attainable by a combination of a large anterior implant size inserted under distraction, followed by compression of the instrumentation using the PLIF cage as a pivot point to improve lordosis and enhance stability and local fusion conditions so that a local environment of fusion under compression is created.

Methods of performing PLIF include traditional open decompression and fusion techniques as well as minimally invasive methods with specialized retractor and rod-screw insertion systems that minimize soft-tissue trauma of the posterior paraspinal musculature.

Contraindications

Although patient selection is crucial in determining the success of any surgery, no strict contraindications exist for PLIF. In general, bone mineral density (BMD) must be considered in any instrumented procedure because low BMD may place patients at risk for graft malposition or migration and screw loosening unless the loads are distributed across multiple vertebrae. In patients with prior lumbar surgery, a higher risk for durotomy exists because the PLIF technique requires gentle retraction of the dura to allow access to the disk space and insertion of the interbody implant.

Alternative Treatments

In patients who have healthy facet joints and no instability on dynamic flexion and extension radiographs, motion-sparing technologies such as total disk replacement or dynamic posterior stabilization methods are possible options. With respect to circumferential fusion alternatives, the direct anterior, retroperitoneal approach allows for a complete diskectomy and fusion (anterior lumbar interbody fusion [ALIF]) with placement of a large structural fusion cage device. This method of anterior interbody graft/cage placement may be performed with anterior plating or in conjunction with posterior instrumentation. Another anterior column technique is direct lateral diskectomy and fusion via a retroperitoneal, transpsoas approach (extreme lateral interbody fusion [XLIF]/direct lateral interbody fusion [DLIF]). This technique may be performed through a traditional open iliolumbar incision or through a mini-open or minimally invasive incision when done in conjunction with special retractor systems and neuromonitoring methods to avoid injury to the genitofemoral nerve and lumbar plexus. This technique may be used in conjunction with lateral plating or posterior instrumentation methods.

Another posterior circumferential decompression and arthrodesis technique is transforaminal lumbar interbody fusion (TLIF). This technique is very similar to PLIF but carries the advantage of a more lateral approach, thus minimizing the dural retraction necessary for cage insertion. TLIF is detailed in chapter 51.

Transforaminal Lumbar Interbody Fusion

Stephen Timon, MD

Indications

Transforaminal lumbar interbody fusion (TLIF) is a reliable, cost-effective, and reproducible technique in the repertoire of the spinal surgeon. TLIF allows for a circumferential fusion, achieved through a single incision, without the morbidity and mortality of an anterior approach.

Although there are many options for treating degenerative disorders of the spine, TLIF has significant advantages over other modalities. In addition to the anterior fusion provided by TLIF, stability is achieved through pedicle screw fixation. Direct decompression of both central and foraminal stenosis is performed through a single posterior incision. Additionally, lateral recess and far lateral stenosis can be decompressed with the removal of the pars interarticularis and the inferior facet.

TLIF is indicated when nonsurgical treatment of low-grade spondylolisthesis, scoliosis, kyphosis, postlaminectomy degenerative disorders, or other degenerative conditions of the lumbar spine has failed.

Contraindications

Relative contraindications for TLIF include high-grade spondylolisthesis with loss of disk height, revision surgery with fixed anterior deformity, and severe fractures that would necessitate anterior corpectomy. In patients with axial back pain only, the use of fusion is controversial at this time. Severe osteoporosis is a contraindication to instrumented lumbar fusion, as is active infection.

Alternative Treatments

Many options exist for lumbar fusion within the armamentarium of the spinal surgeon. Excellent results have been reported for anterior lumbar interbody fusion (ALIF), posterior lumbar interbody fusion (PLIF), posterolateral lumbar fusion (PLF), and circumferential fusion. Emerging technologies, such as extreme lateral interbody fusion (XLIF) and disk arthroplasty, have produced favorable results as well.

Results

The long-term results of TLIF are excellent, especially for patients in whom TLIF is the primary procedure. Fusion rates have surpassed those reported for posterior-only surgery and are consistent with results from two-incision circumferential fusions (Table 1). Reported fusion rates for TLIF have been in the 89% to 94% range. Relief of neurologic symptoms has been reliable. Because the use of TLIF has become more widespread in the past 6 years, it is necessary to closely examine outcomes not only from a retrospective vantage point but also prospectively.

Techniques

Setup/Patient Positioning

TLIF is performed from a posterior approach. To safely expose the spine and the neural elements, the patient must be appropriately positioned. After informed consent is obtained, the patient is brought to the operating theater. General endotracheal intubation is usually required, as well as a Foley catheter. Vascular access is essential, including large-bore intravenous lines, arterial lines, and, in certain circumstances, central lines. Compressive stockings are placed on the lower extremities, and sequential

Dr. Timon or an immediate family member serves as a board member, owner, officer, or committee member of the Irving Coppell Surgical Hospital and the Pine Creek Medical Center; has received royalties from Seaspine; and serves as a paid consultant to or is an employee of Seaspine, Stryker, and Vertebron.

Table 1 Fusion and Outcome Data from Clinical Studies on Posterior TLIF

Authors (Year)	Number of Patients	Procedure or Approach	Mean Patient Age in Years (Range)	Mean Follow-up in Months (Range)	Fusion Success Rate (%)	Results
Lowe and Tahernia (2002)	40	TLIF	44.9 (24.1-69.2)	36 (30-42)	90	85% good or excellent results
Salehi et al (2004)	24	TLIF	42.6 (30-59)	16.9 (7.8-26)	91.7	Average hospital stay: 6.9 days 6 serious complications
Potter et al (2005)	100	TLIF	38 (18-72)	34 (24-61)	93	81% reported >50% reduction in symptoms 76% satisfied with results 20 minor complications
Hackenberg et al (2005)	52	TLIF	48.6 (19-69)	46 (36-64)	89	Significant reductions in VAS and ODI scores 4 (8%) serious complications
Lauber et al (2006)	39	TLIF	48.1 (17-80)	35.4 (24-78)	94.8	Significant improvement in pain and function scores Slip grade reduction:* Grade I: 18% to 13% Grade II: 33% to 15% 3 (7.6%) serious complications

TLIF = transforaminal lumbar interbody fusion, VAS = visual analog scale, ODI = Oswestry Disability Index.

*Slip grade reduction, Meyerding classification.

compression devices aid in the prevention of deep vein thrombosis.

Morbidly obese patients present a challenge. Blood pressure readings obtained with a cuff may not be accurate in these patients because the cuff may be too small or it may be misplaced on the upper arm. Placement of an arterial line may be necessary.

At this point, the patient is ready for positioning on the surgical table. Many options are available when choosing a table. The purpose of the table is to provide a safe, stable platform for the operation. Attention must be addressed to the patient's axillary area and the face (especially the eyes), as well as the lumbar spine. Significant pressure in the axillary region can lead to brachial plexus palsies. Neuromonitoring of the upper extremities, including somatosensory-

evoked potentials and motor-evoked potentials, can help identify early changes in the potentials of the nerves of the brachial plexus and thus notify the surgeon that repositioning is needed. The patient's face must be accessible. Positioning must allow easy access to the ventilation tubing and prevent kinking of the tube. Furthermore, care must be taken to ensure that no pressure is exerted on the eyes because this pressure has been postulated as a potential cause of postoperative blindness.

Finally, positioning of the patient must provide the surgeon adequate access to the lumbar spine. It is essential to minimize the amount of pressure on the patient's abdomen because this will indirectly reduce the blood in the epidural vessels and subsequently reduce the amount of blood loss. Addi-

tionally, the design of the table must allow the patient to be positioned with the appropriate amount of sagittal contour (kyphosis, lordosis, etc), and the table must be radiolucent to allow for appropriate imaging.

Instruments/Equipment/Implants Required

As in all spinal procedures, the implants and instruments used vary. Many types of implants, constructed of a variety of substances, can be used for TLIF. TLIF implants often are composed of allograft bone, titanium, and now, most commonly, polyetheretherketone (PEEK). Each type has its own advantages and disadvantages. For example, titanium is radiopaque, allograft bone can be brittle, and PEEK can deform. Materials are not the only factors that affect the nature of the implants. Size, curvature, lordosis, and availability to hold graft material all can play an important role in fusion.

Size is an important factor because only a limited amount of space is available for fusion along the end plates, and large grafts take up significant surface area that can instead be available for fusion. Small grafts may provide more surface area for fusion, have increased pressure per area measured, and lend themselves to more subsidence. Therefore, a compromise size is necessary. Curvature of the graft also is significant. Grafts range from straight to a curvature of greater than 50°. The more highly curved, or banana-shaped, grafts allow for a more anterior placement of the graft and, by increasing the distance from the anatomic fulcrum, can produce more lordosis per level; however, placement of such grafts can be more technically demanding. Lordosis produced by straight grafts is determined by the graft itself; a banana-shaped graft can produce a higher degree of lordosis. Finally, some implants have fenestrations that allow osteoinductive material to be placed within the graft, whereas other grafts have no fenestrations and provide anterior support only.

Procedure

The patient undergoing the procedure described in this section has a grade I spondylolisthesis at L4-L5 (**Figure 1**). After the lumbar spine has been adequately exposed out to the tips of the transverse process (**Figure 2**, *A* and *B*), retractors are inserted, and the levels are confirmed with a scout radiograph. Pedicle screws are generally placed in anticipation of the transforaminal lumbar interbody graft (**Figure 2**, *C* and *D*). Exposure of the disk space must be accomplished, usually through a generous laminectomy that exposes the thecal sac, the exiting nerve root, the traversing nerve root, the anulus fibrosus, and the facet joint (**Figure 2**, *E* through *F*). At this point, a dural retractor is inserted. With the

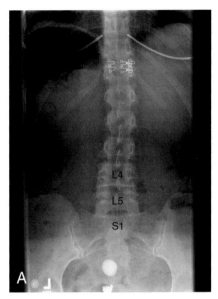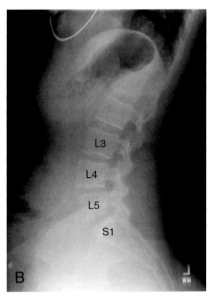

Figure 1 Preoperative PA (**A**) and lateral (**B**) radiographs of the lumbar spine in a 48-year-old woman with grade I L4-L5 spondylolisthesis.

nerve roots protected, the pars interarticularis is resected along with the inferior facet (**Figure 2**, *G* and *H*). This leaves the superior facet in direct visualization and allows a generous foraminotomy to be performed using a Kerrison rongeur. The remaining portions of the superior facet are removed while preserving the integrity of the pedicle. The disk is now adequately exposed, and the neural structures are well visualized (**Figure 2**, *I*).

After the appropriate level once again has been confirmed, an annulotomy is performed just superior and extending slightly medial to the pedicle. After the annulotomy is performed, removal of most of the nucleus pulposus is required. It is essential to provide as large a surface as possible for anterior fusion. Scrapers and pituitary rongeurs are used to remove as much disk material as possible. Curets, both straight and curved, are used to remove the cartilaginous end plates. Rasps are then used to roughen up the end-plate bone to bleeding bone, to provide an appropriate bed for fusion. Serial-sized trial grafts are inserted to determine the ap-

propriate sizing of the actual graft. At this point, the graft (TLIF cage) is inserted, generally under fluoroscopic guidance (**Figure 3**, *A* and *B*). The graft is then rotated with impactors into its final position (**Figure 3**, *C* and *D*). Local bone and/or fusion augmentors are placed posterior to the graft in the disk space. The graft is then locked into its final position by compressing the pedicle screws (**Figure 4**).

Wound Closure

After the cages have been implanted, the pedicle screws have been locked into position, and the appropriate decompression has been performed, but before the final graft material is inserted, the wound should be copiously irrigated. Significant debate has surrounded the use of antibiotic solutions, and, to date, no consensus opinion has been achieved. After the irrigation is complete, the fascia should be closed primarily if possible. The first layer is usually closed with heavy (No. 1-0 or 0) absorbable sutures to provide a watertight seal. In larger patients, No. 2-0 absorbable sutures can be used to close the suprafascial dead

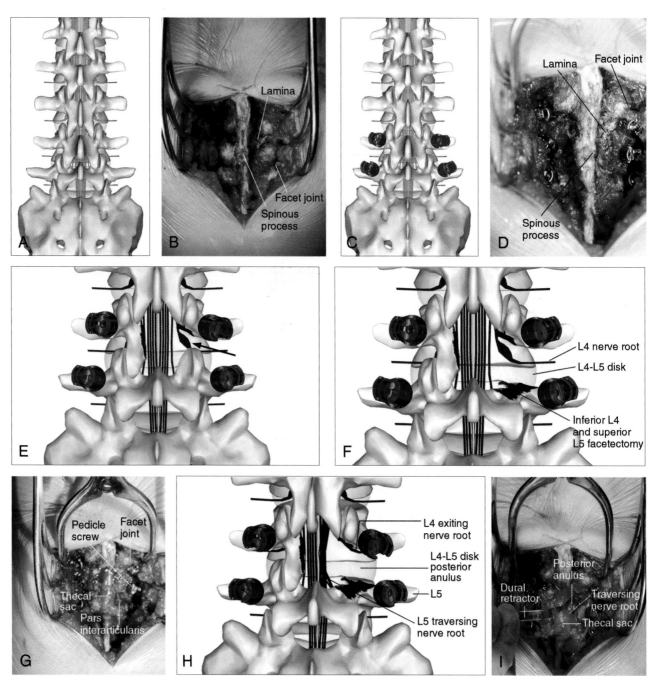

Figure 2 Transforaminal lumbar interbody fusion. **A,** Illustration of the posterior lumbar spine. **B,** Intraoperative photograph shows the same view of the lumbar spine after exposure has been accomplished. Note that the integrity of the facet joints has been preserved. **C,** Illustration of the lumbar spine shows pedicle screw placement at L4 and L5. **D,** Intraoperative photograph shows pedicle screw placement in a two-level TLIF. Illustrations show the lumbar spine after placement of the pedicle screws following laminectomy and unilateral removal of the pars interarticularis (arrow) (**E**) and after removal of the inferior facet and part of the superior facet (**F**). **G,** Intraoperative photograph shows the same area after generous laminectomy was performed following pedicle screw placement. **H,** Illustration shows the traversing L5 nerve root and the thecal sac retracted medially to expose the posterior anulus. **I,** Intraoperative photograph shows a dural retractor being used to expose the disk space while protecting the traversing nerve root.

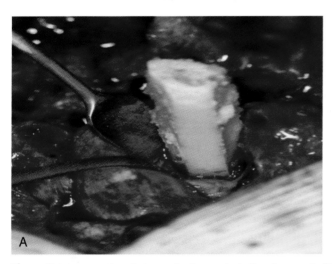
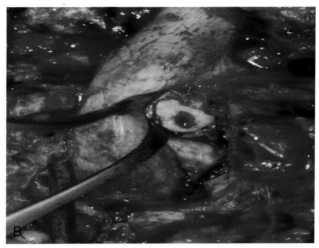

Figure 5 Intraoperative photographs demonstrate the placement of the graft. The patient's head is at the top. **A,** The fibula graft is placed in the transsacral channel. **B,** The fibula graft is seated in the sacrum and recessed 2 mm.

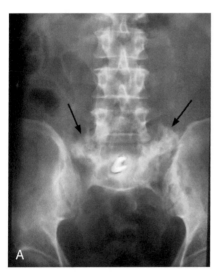
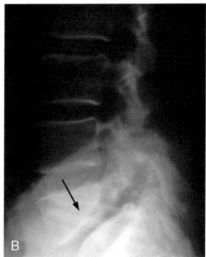

Figure 6 Postoperative radiographs demonstrate graft position. **A,** The posterolateral fusion mass (arrows) is seen on this AP view. **B,** The fibula graft (arrow) is seen on this lateral view.

Avoiding Pitfalls and Complications

Although the Bohlman technique for interbody fusion in the lumbosacral spine is a demanding surgical technique, it can be learned and its results are reproducible. Pitfalls and complications can be avoided by using the following guidelines. When placing the guide pin, it is important to avoid overzealous retraction of the dural sac because doing so can lead to neurologic problems. Protection of the thecal sac is critical when reaming the transsacral channel to avoid inadvertently tearing the dura. A poorly fashioned graft can require overly aggressive tamping, resulting in graft fracture during placement. To avoid this, precise graft carpentry is required. Even when deformity correction is avoided, L5 neurapraxias can occur. They are always transient and usually resolve in the first month after surgery.

Postoperative Regimen

Our postoperative treatment after lumbar spinal fusion surgery consists of a pain management program with multiple modalities, combined with immediate weight bearing as tolerated. Deep vein thrombosis prophylaxis includes compression stockings and mechanical compression devices. If a patient was on anticoagulation medication for prophylaxis or treatment of medical comorbidities preoperatively, we generally maintain it for 7 days postoperatively.

We do not use any external orthosis postoperatively.

■ Bibliography

Bartolozzi P, Sandri A, Cassini M, Ricci M: One-stage posterior decompression-stabilization and trans-sacral interbody fusion after partial reduction for severe L5-S1 spondylolisthesis. *Spine (Phila Pa 1976)* 2003;28:1135-1141.

Beutler WJ, Frederickson BE, Murtland A, Sweeney CA, Grant WD, Baker D: The natural history of spondylolysis and spondylolisthesis: 45-year followup evaluation. *Spine (Phila Pa 1976)* 2003;28:1027-1035.

Bohlman HH, Cook SS: One-stage decompression and posterolateral and interbody fusion for lumbosacral spondyloptosis through a posterior approach: Report of two cases. *J Bone Joint Surg Am* 1982;64:415-418.

Boxall D, Bradford DS, Winter RB, Moe JH: Management of severe spondylolisthesis in children and adolescents. *J Bone Joint Surg Am* 1979;61:479-495.

Goyton M, Ouellet J, Arlet V: Favorable outcome in the treatment of high grade L5-S1 spondylolytic spondylolisthesis with autogenous fibular strut grafting. *Spine J* 2006;6:153S-154S.

Hanson DS, Bridwell KH, Rhee JM, Lenke LG: Dowel fibular strut grafts for high-grade dysplastic isthmic spondylolisthesis. *Spine (Phila Pa 1976)* 2002;27:1982-1988.

Lamberg TS, Remes VM, Helenius IJ, et al: Long-term clinical, functional, and radiological outcomes 21 years after posterior or posterolateral fusion in childhood and adolescent isthmic spondylolisthesis. *Eur Spine J* 2005;14:639-644.

Meyerding H: Low backache and sciatica pain associated with spondylolisthesis and protruded intervertebral disc: Incidence, significance, and treatment. *J Bone Joint Surg Am* 1941;23:461-470.

Molinari RW, Bridwell KH, Lenke LG, Ungacta FF, Riew KD: Complications in the surgical treatment of pediatric high-grade isthmic dysplastic spondylolisthesis: A comparison of three surgical approaches. *Spine (Phila Pa 1976)* 1999;24:1701-1711.

Roca J, Ubierna MT, Cáceres E, Iborra M: One-stage decompression and posterolateral and interbody fusion for severe spondylolisthesis: An analysis of 14 patients. *Spine (Phila Pa 1976)* 1999;24:709-714.

Sasso RC, Shively KD, Reilly TM: Transvertebral transsacral strut grafting for high-grade isthmic spondylolisthesis L5-S1 with fibular allograft. *J Spinal Disord Tech* 2008;21:328-333.

Smith JA, Deviren V, Berven S, Kleinstueck F, Bradford DS: Clinical outcome of trans-sacral interbody fusion after partial reduction for high-grade L5-S1 spondylolisthesis. *Spine (Phila Pa 1976)* 2001;26:2227-2234.

Smith MD, Bohlman HH: Spondylolisthesis treated by a single-stage operation combining decompression with in situ posterolateral and anterior fusion: An analysis of eleven patients who had long-term follow-up. *J Bone Joint Surg Am* 1990;72:415-421.

Coding

CPT Codes		Corresponding ICD-9 Codes	
22612	Arthrodesis, posterior or posterolateral technique, single level; lumbar (with or without lateral transverse technique)	170.2 721.42 722.10	721.3 722.0 737.39
22614	Arthrodesis, posterior or posterolateral technique, single level; each additional vertebral segment (List separately in addition to code for primary procedure)	170.2 721.42 722.10	721.3 722.0 737.39
22842	Posterior segmental instrumentation (eg, pedicle fixation, dual rods with multiple hooks and sublaminar wires); 3 to 6 vertebral segments (List separately in addition to code for primary procedure)	342.1 342.90 343.0	342.9 343 343.1
22843	Posterior segmental instrumentation (eg, pedicle fixation, dual rods with multiple hooks and sublaminar wires); 7 to 12 vertebral segments (List separately in addition to code for primary procedure)	170.2 342.9 343	342.1 342.90 343.0

Chapter 56
Lateral Transpsoas Approach/Fusion

Shay Bess, MD
Jim A. Youssef, MD

■ Indications

The anterior vertebral column sustains approximately 80% of the spinal axial load. Vertebral interbody fusion provides a superior biomechanical environment for spinal arthrodesis compared with stand-alone instrumented posterior spinal fusion. When combined with posterior spinal implants, interbody fusion reduces the amount of unsupported cantilever load exposed to the posterior segmental implants, increasing the implant endurance limit. Aside from the biomechanical advantages provided by interbody fusion, posterior lumbar fusions that are supplemented with interbody fusion demonstrate greater arthrodesis rates than stand-alone posterior spinal fusion. Therefore, relative indications for lumbar interbody fusion include symptomatic degenerative disk disease with or without instability; recurrent disk herniation; degenerative spondylolisthesis; adjacent level stenosis; degenerative scoliosis;

existing pseudarthrosis; or patients at risk for pseudarthrosis, including patients with deficient posterior elements (eg, postlaminectomy) and patients with poor healing capacity (due to nicotine abuse, antiseizure medication use, diabetes, and other medical comorbidities). Other indications include revision surgery for failed previous interbody implants or failed lumbar total disk arthroplasty, and diskitis or osteomyelitis without active infection. Another benefit of interbody fusion is that the approach releases the anterior column, allowing the inserted structural device to restore lumbar lordosis, indirectly decompress the neural elements, and correct coronal plane deformities. Interbody fusion can be used for patients with flat back deformity, large and/or stiff lumbar scoliotic deformities, or lateral lumbar listhesis.

Techniques available for lumbar interbody spinal fusion include anterior lumbar interbody fusion (ALIF), posterior lumbar interbody fusion (PLIF), transforaminal lumbar inter-

body fusion (TLIF), and lateral transpsoas interbody fusion. The benefits of lateral transpsoas interbody fusion compared with traditional interbody fusion techniques include limited posterior paraspinal muscle dissection compared with PLIF or TLIF, minimal neural element retraction, avoidance of epidural scar dissection during revision spinal fusion for postlaminectomy surgery compared with PLIF and TLIF, decreased blood loss, decreased surgical time, reduced anterior abdominal dissection and vascular retraction compared with ALIF (especially for multilevel interbody fusion), and safer access to the retroperitoneal space and disk space in patients who have had prior open abdominal surgery compared with ALIF. Further advantages of this approach include indirect neural decompression and restoration of proper sagittal and coronal alignment. Additionally, the lateral approach allows for a more complete diskectomy and insertion of a larger structural interbody device than with PLIF and TLIF. Furthermore, preservation of the anterior and posterior longitudinal ligaments is accomplished via this technique (**Figure 1**).

The lateral transpsoas approach for fusion requires a comprehensive understanding of the relevant anatomy that will be encountered during the procedure. Relevant structures that

Dr. Bess or an immediate family member has received royalties from Pioneer, is a member of a speakers' bureau or has made paid presentations on behalf of Stryker and DePuy, serves as a paid consultant to or is an employee of NuVasive and Alphatec Spine, and has received research or institutional support from DePuy. Dr. Youssef or an immediate family member has received royalties from DePuy, NuVasive, Osprey, SeaSpine, and Aesculap/B. Braun; serves as a paid consultant to or is an employee of DePuy, NuVasive, Stryker, Aesculap/B. Braun, and SeaSpine; serves as an unpaid consultant to Stryker and DePuy; has received research or institutional support from DePuy, NuVasive, Stryker, Stryker BioTech, and Biosurface Engineering Technologies; and owns stock or stock options in Amedica and Vertiflex.

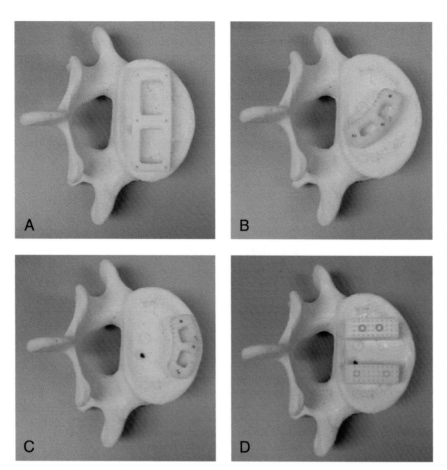

Figure 1 Illustration demonstrates the differences in structure and footprint among the lateral transpsoas interbody fusion (extreme lateral interbody fusion) device (**A**) TLIF interbody devices (**B** and **C**), and the PLIF interbody device (**D**).

accessible from a lateral approach because the disk space sits below the pelvis, which limits access to this level. Preoperative radiographs must be evaluated for iliac crest obstruction of the disk space planned for lateral access. If the disk space is obscured by the pelvis, or if interbody fusion is planned at L5-S1, alternative techniques for lumbar interbody fusion should be made. Additionally, if a right-sided approach is desired, the disk space at T12-L1 (and often the disk space at L1-2) will likely be obstructed by the liver, requiring either a left-sided approach or an alterative technique for interbody fusion. High-grade spondylolisthesis (≥grade III) is a relative contraindication because of the risk for implant misplacement. Severe osteoporosis (defined as a T score greater than –2.5) or systemic infection also are contraindications to performing this procedure. Furthermore, lateral access at the superior lumbar disk spaces (T12-L2) may be difficult in patients who have had prior bilateral renal surgery, previous retroperitoneal surgery, or radiation because of retroperitoneal scarring.

will be encountered include the psoas musculature, the lumbar plexus, the iliac vessels, and the peritoneum. Preoperative imaging studies, including MRI and CT, are paramount to preoperative planning. The anatomy of the lumbar plexus is worthy of review before undertaking this technique. The relative "safe zone" for entry into the disk space varies based on the surgical location. For example, the locations of the exiting nerve roots are more posterior at L1-2 as compared with L4-5, where these neural structures lie in a more anterior location. Anatomic studies indicate that at L4-5, the nerve trunk lies directly in the path of the initial guidewire at the center of the disk. During patient positioning, extension of the hip moves the nerves

more posteriorly, although positioning with the hips in flexion reduces psoas retraction and mitigates postoperative thigh pain with active hip flexion. Therefore, the use of intraoperative electromyographic (EMG) neuromonitoring is recommended when performing these procedures.

Contraindications

The lateral retroperitoneal approach is anatomically feasible from the T12-L1 disk space to the L4-5 disk space in the lumbar spine. The thoracic spine also is safely accessible up to T4 via a transthoracic lateral approach. The L5-S1 intervertebral disk space is not

Results

Published reports on lateral approach surgery have focused on techniques, whereas patient outcomes following the procedure largely have been limited to conference presentations (**Table 1**). Initial experience using the lateral approach in the United States reported no vascular or abdominal complications. In a presentation at the 12th International Meeting on Advanced Spinal Techniques, one author reported that approximately 3% of patients had temporary hip flexor weakness and one patient (0.07%) had a transient foot drop. The average hospital stay was 1 day. Subsequent presentations at North American Spine

Table 1 Early Clinical Results of Lateral Transpsoas Interbody Fusion

Authors (Year)	Indication	Number of Patients	Mean Age in Years (Range)	Mean Follow-up (Range)	Fusion Success Rate	Results
Diaz et al (2006)	Lumbar scoliosis	39	68 (58-80)	(1-3 years)	NR	No complications Postoperative improvement in VAS and ODI Reduction in scoliosis curve magnitude
Akbarnia et al (unpublished presentation, 2008)*	Lumbar scoliosis	13	60.5 (37-84)	9 months (2-28)	NR	Postoperative improvement in VAS and ODI Lumbar curve correction and restoration of lumbar lordosis 55% rate transient thigh pain and/or weakness
Rodgers et al (2008)	Morbidly obese patients with degenerative disk disease	43	54 (31-78)	NR	100% graded as Lenke 1 or 2 fusion	Postoperative VAS improvement 2 postoperative medical complications No visceral or vascular complications

NR = not reported; VAS = visual analog scale; ODI = Oswestry Disability Index.
*Akbarnia BA, Varma VV, Bess S, et al: Extreme lateral interbody fusion (XLIF) safely improves segmental and global deformity in large adult scoliosis: Preliminary results on 13 patients. Electronic poster presentation, International Meeting on Advanced Spinal Techniques (IMAST) 15th annual meeting, July 8-11, 2008, Hong Kong, China.

Society meetings describing use of the technique for lumbar scoliosis have reported reduction in the visual analog pain scale and improvement in the Oswestry Disability Index, approximately 55% lumbar curve correction, and restoration of lumbar lordosis in patients at up to 3-year follow-up. Finally, another group of authors concluded that the utility of the lateral approach also has been demonstrated in the morbidly obese population. Obviously, obese patients have more retroperitoneal fat than the normal population, enlarging the retroperitoneal space. Additionally, when placed in the lateral position, the pannus in obese patients pulls the abdominal contents away from the spine. Positioning the patient laterally allows easy access to the retroperitoneal space in the obese population, thereby facilitating access to the disk space (**Figure 2**).

Wright retrospectively reviewed 145 patients who underwent lateral transpsoas fusion. The study assessed the number of levels treated, the average blood loss, and the surgical time, along with the use of neuromonitoring technology. The average surgical time was 74 minutes, and the average blood loss was 88 mL. Retractor repositioning occurred 46% of the time as a result of nerve detection.

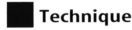

■ Technique

Setup

Preoperative planning using MRI, radiographs, and CT scans can help dictate the desired approach—left or right. The location of great vessels and exiting lumbar plexus, along with coronal and sagittal preoperative deformity, will help determine the safest approach to the desired levels. Once the approach side is determined, the patient is placed on a surgical table in the lateral decubitus position opposite the approach side. The surgical table must be radiolucent and be able to rotate and

flex/bend. The greater trochanter should be placed directly over the table break to facilitate retraction of the iliac crest. An axillary roll is placed, and the patient is secured to the surgical table at the axilla, the pelvis, and lower extremities (**Figure 3**) with cloth tape before table flexion. This technique helps prevent patient migration and facilitates retraction of the pelvis and correction of scoliosis. Appropriate hip flexion also limits the need for psoas retraction intraoperatively.

Once the patient is secured and the table is flexed, fluoroscopy is used to verify that the patient is in the true lateral position. The surgical table is then rotated as well as tilted to ensure an accurate view of the disk space is visualized on fluoroscopy in the AP and lateral planes. This visualization allows the surgeon to work parallel to the disk space and perpendicular to the floor. Correct disk space alignment on fluoroscopy is essential for patients who have scoliosis so that vertebral rotation is eliminated on the

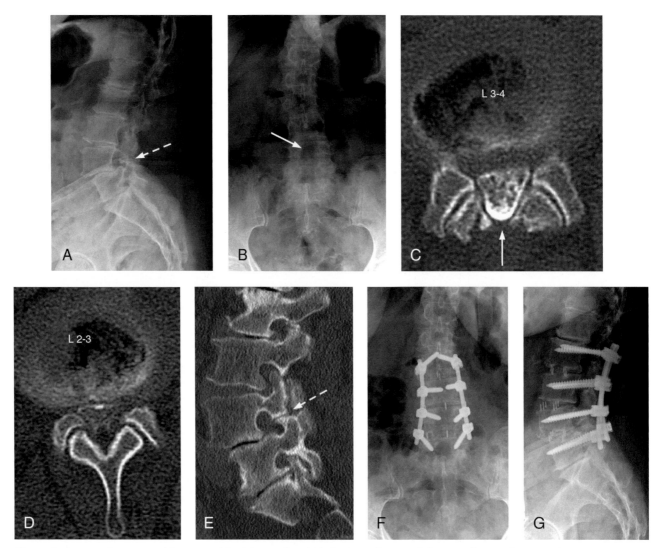

Figure 2 Images of a 75-year-old woman with a history of morbid obesity and type 1 diabetes mellitus. Following colectomy via anterior laparotomy, she presented with back and leg pain after remote L3-L5 decompression. Lateral (**A**) and AP (**B**) radiographs demonstrate L4 pars fracture (dashed arrow), complete L4 laminectomy (solid arrow), and grade I L4-5 spondylolisthesis. **C,** Axial CT myelogram demonstrates complete L4 laminectomy (arrow). **D,** CT scan demonstrates L4 pars defect and spinal stenosis. **E,** Sagittal CT scan demonstrates L4-5 spondylolisthesis and spinal stenosis at L2-3 and L3-4 (dashed arrow). AP (**F**) and lateral (**G**) radiographs 1 year following L2-3, L3-4, and L4-5 lateral transpsoas interbody fusion, L2 through L5 instrumented posterior spinal fusion, and L2-3 and L3-4 decompression.

images and safe lateral access to the disk space is ensured (**Figure 4**).

Instruments/Implants/ Equipment Required

Required instruments include sequentially larger diameter EMG guidance dilators, which are used to dilate the psoas muscle when approaching the desired disk space. A three-blade retractor with light source grooves in the retractor blades is used for appropriate disk visualization. Standard disk eval-

uation instruments, including Cobb elevators, pituitary rongeurs, endplate shavers, ring and cupped curets, and sequentially sized trial implants, are used to remove the disk. Final implants are device specific, but most are made of polyetheretherketone and are packed with bone graft material.

Exposure

The desired disk space is located on a lateral radiograph by intersecting two guidewires over the center of the disk

space, and the location is marked on the skin. The skin is prepared and draped in routine sterile fashion. A two-incision technique is advocated to approach the lateral disk space. The first incision is a counterincision made just lateral to the erector spinal muscles, approximately one fingerbreadth from the desired incision over the disk space. This counterincision is used to initially access and develop the retroperitoneal space so that a safe lateral approach to the disk space is ensured. The retroperitoneal space is developed via the initial counterincision, using blunt dissection with scissors and finger manipulation. Care is taken to avoid perforation of the peritoneal space when penetrating the thoracolumbar fascia to access the retroperitoneal space (**Figure 5**, *A*). Once the retroperitoneal space has been entered, an index finger is used to develop the retroperitoneal space and gently sweep and mobilize the peritoneum and viscera to further develop the retroperitoneal space. The psoas muscle, the transverse process, and the disk space are palpated; the finger is rotated and brought to the skin surface just beneath the region of the skin that was marked overlying the lateral disk space; and a second incision is made over the protecting finger (**Figure 5**, *B* and *C*). The fascia is penetrated, and a dilator is carried down to the psoas with the protection of the finger (**Figure 5**, *D*).

Once the psoas has been reached with the dilator, a transpsoas approach to the lateral disk space is performed using neurologic monitoring to avoid injury to the lumbar plexus, the dilator is secured to the disk space, and AP and lateral fluoroscopic images are obtained to confirm adequate positioning (**Figure 5**, *E*). Using fluoroscopic images, the dilator should be secured in the middle of the disk space on the lateral view and directly parallel to the disk space on the AP view. Using finger protection and neurologic monitoring, dilators of increasing diameter are sequentially passed through the lateral incision down to the lateral disk space. Once the largest dilator has been docked safely on the lateral aspect of the desired disk space, and no evidence is present of EMG irritation to any of the exiting nerve roots, then an illuminated multiblade retractor is positioned by sliding it over the largest dilator. This placement also is done using neuromonitoring on the retractor itself to ensure that the blades of the retractor do not cause any iatro-

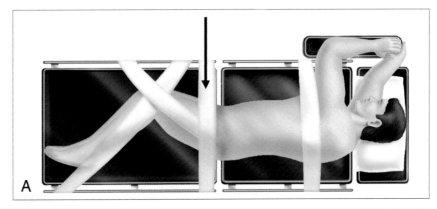

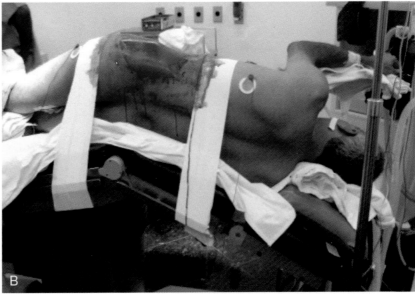

Figure 3 Positioning for lateral transpsoas interbody fusion. **A,** Illustration demonstrates overhead view of the patient on the surgical table. Note the location of the greater trochanter (arrow) at the level of the table break and the locations where the patient is secured to the table. **B,** Clinical photograph shows patient secured to the surgical table in preparation for lateral transpsoas interbody fusion. (Courtesy of Luis Pimenta, MD, São Paulo, Brazil.)

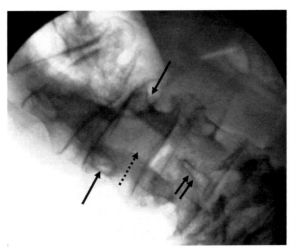

Figure 4 AP fluoroscopic image demonstrates alignment of the pedicles (solid arrows) to ensure no evidence of vertebral rotation. The spinous process also can be used to align the AP plane (double arrow); however, the pedicles are a more consistent landmark, especially in patients who have had a prior laminectomy (dashed arrow).

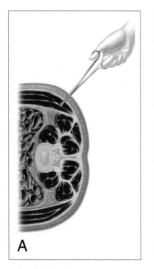
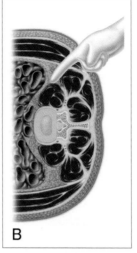
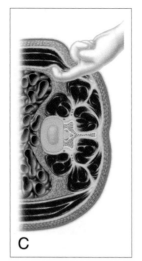
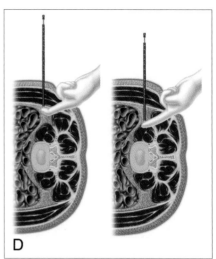

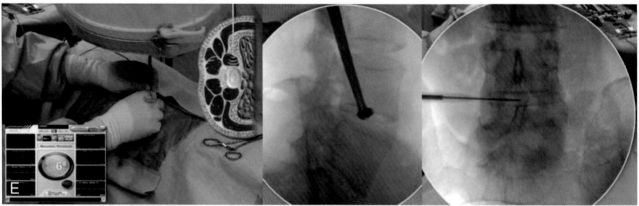

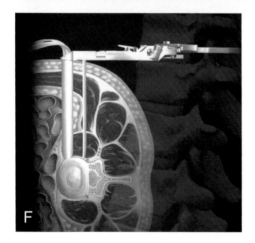

Figure 5 Retroperitoneal access and lateral transpsoas diskectomy. **A,** Blunt penetration of the thoracoabdominal fascia into the retroperitoneal space. Finger dissection into the retroperitoneal space (**B**) and undermining to the skin surface (**C**) in preparation for the direct lateral incision. **D,** The thoracolumbar fascia is penetrated (left), and a dilator is inserted down to the psoas with protection of a finger (right) from the counterincision to ensure safe dilator passage. **E,** Once the psoas is reached, the transpsoas approach proceeds, using neurologic monitoring to protect the lumbar plexus (left). Following transpsoas passage, the dilator is secured to the interspace, and lateral (middle) and AP (right) fluoroscopic images are obtained to confirm adequate positioning at the interspace. **F,** Dilators are used to develop the retroperitoneal space and transpsoas plane, and a retractor is placed to retract and protect the viscera and psoas.

genic nerve injury (**Figure 5**, *F*). The retractor is expanded gently and secured to the operating room table to prevent any migration during the procedure. Confirmation of retractor location using intraoperative biplanar fluoroscopy is required for execution

of the remainder of the procedure. Next, an intraoperative EMG wand is recommended to palpate the working space and stimulate the final retractor blade location as a final measure to protect against avoidable neurologic injury (**Figure 5**, *E*).

Procedure

Once the lateral retractor is in place and secured, the remainder of the psoas overlying the disk space is visualized through the retractor and is bluntly dissected and retracted off the disk space. Monopolar cauterization is not recommended because the zone of injury caused by monopolar cauterization may extend beyond the desired region and injure the lumbar plexus. If bleeding occurs during dissection, we recommend using bipolar cautery or topical hemostatic agents (eg, thrombin or gel foam). Once visualized and isolated, the lateral anulus is incised sharply, and the diskectomy is performed in routine fashion using a combination of curets and pituitary rongeurs. Curets are useful in removing the cartilaginous end plates from the respective superior and inferior vertebral bodies. Distraction across the interspace will be facilitated by releasing the contralateral anulus fibrosus using a curet or a tissue elevator. This release is performed using fluoroscopic imaging to prevent excessive penetration beyond the contralateral anulus.

After the diskectomy is completed, trial interbody implants are used to measure the disk space and confirm adequate fit and fill of the interbody device. Care is taken to avoid overdistraction of the disk space so that the vertebral end plates are not compromised and postoperative implant subsidence does not occur. The final structural interbody device is placed and final radiographs obtained. Ideally, the implant is centered in the disk space extending across the apophyseal ring (**Figure 6**, *A* and *B*). The end plates are prepared to punctate bleeding without aggressive end-plate violation. The interbody device can be filled with morcellized autograft, allograft, and/or bone-graft substitute. The use of bone morphogenetic protein in the interbody device has been described, but this represents an off-label use.

Wound Closure

After completing the procedure, hemostasis is confirmed to prevent postoperative psoas hematoma. The thoracolumbar fascia is closed meticulously to prevent a postoperative hernia. The

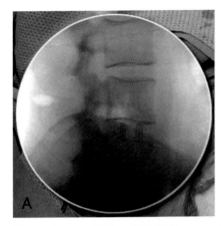 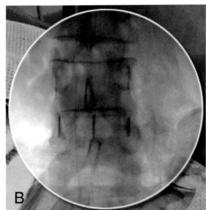

Figure 6 Lateral (**A**) and AP (**B**) fluoroscopic images of the final lateral interbody device placement. Ideally, the interbody device is placed in the center of the disk space, or just anterior to the center, and extends across the entire disk space. (Courtesy of NuVasive, San Diego, CA.)

deep dermis and skin are closed in layers. A drain is not routinely necessary.

Postoperative Regimen

Patients are encouraged to ambulate immediately after surgery as tolerated. If a staged procedure is performed in which a multilevel lateral interbody fusion is the initial procedure, patients are encouraged to ambulate during the time interval from the index surgery until the posterior instrumented fusion procedure is performed. To avoid a prolonged hospital stay, patients also may be discharged home after the initial interbody procedure and return for the second-stage posterior procedure at a later date. A postoperative orthosis should be considered on a case-by-case basis.

As with other spinal fusion procedures, bending, twisting, and lifting more than 25 lb is discouraged during the first 3 months postoperatively. Driving usually is permitted 6 to 8 weeks after surgery.

Avoiding Pitfalls and Complications

As indicated previously, a true lateral approach requires a proper knowledge of the pertinent anatomy and proper patient positioning. If the dissection sways anteriorly, the peritoneal contents and abdominal vascular structures are at risk. If the procedure strays too far posteriorly, the neural foramen and exiting nerve root are at risk. During the surgical dissection, it is highly recommended to use the two-incision technique. The two incisions are (1) a direct lateral incision overlying the desired lateral disk space and (2) a counterincision that is placed just lateral to the lateral border of the paraspinal musculature. The counterincision is used initially to develop the retroperitoneal space. Once the retroperitoneal space is developed, a finger is placed through the counterincision to guide the approach from the direct lateral incision to the lateral disk space. This process helps protect the viscera when approaching the lateral disk space. Real-time, dynamic, and discrete neurologic monitoring should be used to protect the lumbar plexus during the entire procedure. Preoperatively, the axial MRI/CT images should be inspected to ensure that the abdominal vessels do not abnormally overlie the lateral disk space and to analyze the neural structures at the surgical levels. Additionally, the surgeon should be certain that the pelvis does not prohibit access to the disk space, as described previously. Blunt dissection should be used whenever possible, avoiding monopolar cautery, to protect the viscera and the lumbar plexus. Patients also should be counseled that they may have transient thigh pain and/or numbness postoperatively due to the transpsoas approach. Hip flexion during intraoperative patient positioning may decrease the incidence of such postoperative symptoms. Adequate fluoroscopic visualization during the procedure and strict adherence to working directly lateral to the disk space will prevent end-plate perforation during diskectomy and implant insertion, especially in the presence of osteoporotic bone, and will prevent implant misplacement. End-plate preservation during diskectomy and implant insertion will reduce postoperative graft subsidence and maintenance of disk height restoration, restoration of lumbar lordosis, and scoliosis correction until arthrodesis occurs. Finally, patience and thoughtfulness during the procedure and adequate surgeon training are paramount for a successful procedure.

Bibliography

Bridwell KH: Load sharing principles: The role and use of anterior structural support in adult deformity. *Instr Course Lect* 1996;45:109-115.

Diaz R, Phillips F, Pimenta L, Guerrero L: XLIF for lumbar degenerative scoliosis: Outcomes of minimally invasive surgical treatment out to 3 years postoperatively. *North American Spine Society 21st Annual Meeting.* Poster presentation. Seattle, WA, September 26-30, 2006; *Spine J Meeting Abstracts* 2006;6(5):75S.

Ozgur BM, Aryan HE, Pimenta L, Taylor WR: Extreme lateral interbody fusion (XLIF): A novel surgical technique for anterior lumbar interbody fusion. *Spine J* 2006;6(4):435-443.

Rodgers W, Cox C, Gerber E: Extreme lateral interbody fusion (XLIF) in the morbidly obese. *North American Spine Society 23rd Annual Meeting.* Oral presentation. Toronto, Ontario, Canada, October 14-18, 2008; *Spine J Meeting Abstracts* 2008;8(5, suppl):112S.

Coding

CPT Codes		Corresponding ICD-9 Codes	
22558	Arthrodesis, anterior interbody technique, including minimal discectomy to prepare interspace (other than for decompression); lumbar	567.31 721.42 722.52	721.3 722.51 733.13
22845	Anterior instrumentation; 2 to 3 vertebral segments (List separately in addition to code for primary procedure)	170.2 342.9 343	342.1 342.90 343.0
22851	Application of intervertebral biomechanical device(s) (eg, synthetic cage(s), threaded bone dowel(s), methylmethacrylate) to vertebral defect or interspace (List separately in addition to code for primary procedure)	170.2 342.9 343	342.1 342.90 343.0
63090	Vertebral corpectomy (vertebral body resection), partial or complete, transperitoneal or retroperitoneal approach with decompression of spinal cord, cauda equina or nerve root(s), lower thoracic, lumbar, or sacral; single segment	170.2 806.4 806.6	567.31 806.5

CPT copyright © 2010 by the American Medical Association. All rights reserved.

Chapter 57
Percutaneous Transsacral Lumbar Interbody Fusion

Kasra Rowshan, MD
Nitin Bhatia, MD

Indications

Lumbar interbody fusion commonly is used to reduce instability and painful motion secondary to trauma, degenerative disease, iatrogenic instability, tumor, or infection. Interbody fusion has become increasingly popular because of its improved rates of fusion, restoration of disk and foraminal height, promotion of lordosis, and possibly improved functional outcome. Recently, less invasive surgical procedures have been advocated as options to prevent extensive paraspinal muscle dissection and resultant postoperative dysfunction. Continuous muscle retraction of longer than 1 hour has been associated with increased pain and disability postoperatively from local muscle necrosis and degeneration of neuromuscular junctions. Accordingly, procedures that reduce the amount of muscle dissection required to approach the spine may lower the morbidity and improve the outcome of associated surgical procedures.

Percutaneous transsacral lumbar interbody fusion is a minimally inva-sive method of interbody fusion that is designed specifically to address lumbosacral spine disease using the presacral space. The procedure recently was developed as a percutaneous alternative to anterior, posterior, and transforaminal lumbar interbody fusion (ALIF, PLIF, and TLIF, respectively) techniques. This technique uses the presacral space to access the L5-S1 disk space via percutaneous, image-guided instrumentation.

Indications for percutaneous transsacral lumbar interbody fusion are similar to those for traditional lumbar interbody fusion and include intractable low back pain secondary to degenerative disk disease with or without radicular symptoms; pseudarthrosis from a prior fusion; failed back surgery from an earlier diskectomy; or instability, including spondylolisthesis (grades I and II). Recent clinical studies have broadened the use to higher-grade spondylolisthesis, although in our experience, using the percutaneous transsacral lumbar interbody fusion technique in spondylolisthesis greater than grade II can pose difficulty because of the anatomic constraints of the lumbosacral junction.

Contraindications

Successful placement of the percutaneous transsacral lumbar interbody device requires adequate knowledge of anatomy to allow the trajectory of the screw to enter the S1 body, traverse the L5-S1 disk space, and end in the L5 body. Certain anatomic variants, such as abnormal sacral inclination or L5-S1 spondylolisthesis, may preclude the use of this device. Patients who have had previous retroperitoneal surgery, including spinal surgery, should not undergo this procedure because of the consequent scarring and altered anatomy, which can increase the risk of vascular or bowel injury. Other contraindications include coagulopathy, bowel disease (eg, Crohn disease, ulcerative colitis), pregnancy, severe lumbosacral scoliosis, sacral agenesis, severe spondylolisthesis, tumor, and trauma.

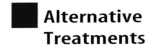

Alternative Treatments

Other variations of lumbosacral interbody fusion have been used for years

Dr. Bhatia or an immediate family member is a member of a speakers' bureau or has made paid presentations on behalf of Biomet, Stryker, and Alphatec Spine; serves as a paid consultant to or is an employee of Alphatec Spine, SeaSpine, and Biomet; and has received research or institutional support from Alphatec Spine and SeaSpine. Neither Dr. Rowshan nor any immediate family member has received anything of value from or owns stock in a commercial company or institution related directly or indirectly to the subject of this chapter.

Table 1 Outcomes of Percutaneous Presacral Lumbar Interbody Fusion

Authors (Year)	Number of Patients	Procedure or Approach	Mean Patient Age in Years (Range)	Mean Follow-up in Months (Range)	Fusion Success Rate	Results
Slosar et al (2001)	11	Percutaneous transsacral lumbar interbody fusion (4 patients also had posterior instrumentation)	50.3 (35-72)	22.7 (14-43)	100%, measured by CT scan at 6 months	Significant decrease in NRS and ODI, reduction in pain, and reduced morbidity at 1 year No noted complications Alternative to fibular strut graft for high-grade spondylolisthesis
Ledet et al (2005)	24 cadavers	Percutaneous transsacral lumbar interbody fusion in a cadaveric biomechanical study	N/A	N/A	N/A	Axial cage fixation showed increased stiffness and decreased ROM compared with intact spines Lateral and sagittal bending stiffness increased Extension and axial compression comparable to all other interbody devices
Asgarzadie et al (2007)	16	Percutaneous transsacral lumbar interbody fusion	NR	12	92%	26-point decrease between pre- and postoperative ODI 7-point decrease in VAS scores
Aryan et al (2008)	35	Percutaneous transsacral lumbar interbody fusion	54	17.5 (10-29)	91%	Average graft subsidence 1.6 mm, not correlated with outcome Local infection was noted complication Can be used as stand-alone or in combination with other fusion procedures
Stippler et al (2009)	36	Percutaneous transsacral lumbar interbody fusion and percutaneous pedicle screw placement	44 (20-61)	8 (3-20)	NR	40% reported resolution of pain 54% reported significant improvement of pain 3% symptoms worsened 3% symptoms unchanged

NRS = Numerical Rating Scale; ODI = Oswestry Disability Index; N/A = not applicable; ROM = range of motion; NR = not reported; VAS = visual analog pain scale.

with consistent outcomes. First used for Pott disease in 1906, ALIF has shown outstanding results. It is reported to have a fusion rate of more than 90%, a 91% rate of functional improvement, and a rate of significant pain relief greater than 84%. Similar fusion rates and functional outcomes are seen with PLIF and TLIF, although these variations have not been studied as extensively as ALIF. Newer methods of these classic interbody techniques have introduced reduced muscle dissection and minimally invasive approaches to the lumbar spine. Extreme lateral interbody fusion is not a useful technique at L5-S1 because of the difficulty in accessing the disk space created by the superimposed iliac wing.

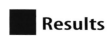

Results

Current literature suggests that percutaneous transsacral lumbar interbody fusion is a feasible, reproducible, and safe procedure with promising outcomes. Although short-term follow-up shows a high fusion rate with low revisions, long-term results have yet to be determined (**Table 1**). Although some authors suggest that the procedure can be used as a stand-alone procedure for L5-S1 interbody fusion, we feel that the procedure should be used in combination with minimally invasive or open posterior instrumentation techniques, such as pedicle screws or facet screws, because of the poor rotational stability in the stand-alone device. Biomechanical evaluations of axial cage fixation of L5-S1 have shown a significant increase in stiffness and reductions in range of motion relative to the intact state. Lateral and sagittal bending stiffness of the axial cage exceeded the other tested interbody devices in a cadaveric model.

Technique

Setup/Exposure

This technique uses a percutaneous fluoroscopically guided approach to S1 via the presacral space. The patient is placed prone on a Jackson table or other compatible radiolucent operating room table to allow for easy biplanar fluoroscopy. Optionally, a 20 French catheter is insufflated in the rectum with 10 mL of air for better visualization during subsequent fluoroscopy. The incision is located near the coccyx and the anus, and the buttocks can be retracted laterally and gently taped open to facilitate the procedure. The anus is then covered using occlusive dressings to isolate this contaminated region from the paracoccygeal surgical area. The area is washed and draped in a sterile manner.

The presacral space is composed of loosely organized connective tissue and is formed posteriorly by the parietal fascia covering the sacrum and anteriorly by the visceral fascia of the mesorectum. The rectum is surrounded by fat and defined posteriorly by the mesorectum fascial layer. MRI has shown the presacral space to measure 13 mm in males and 10.6 mm in females.

Sympathetic nerves arise at the L2-L3 level and form the preaortic plexus at the L4-5 disk space. They then connect with the hypogastric nerves at the sacral promontory. At this point, these nerves are 1 cm lateral to the midline and continue later-

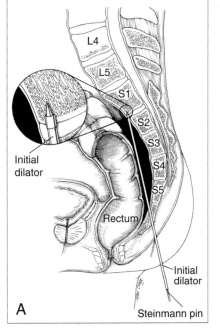
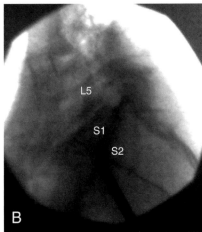

Figure 1 Percutaneous transsacral lumbar interbody fusion. **A,** Illustration demonstrates passage of the blunt dilator to the S1-2 level. **B,** Intraoperative lateral fluoroscopic image shows docking of the initial blunt dilator at the S1-2 level. (Part A is adapted from Eck JC, Hodges S, Humphreys SC: Minimally invasive lumbar spine fusion. *J Am Acad Orthop Surg* 2007 15:321-329.)

ally as they follow the internal iliac arteries. Parasympathetic fibers arise at S3-S4 in males and S2 through S4 in females and enter the pelvis laterally through the sacral foramen. Vascular structures in this region include the middle sacral artery and vein, which are located in the region of the sacral promontory more rostral than the working site S1-S2. The transverse sacral vein and midline sacral artery also are present; however, at this location they are small and have shown minimal bleeding risk. Hence, the risk to neurologic or vascular structures from this technique is minimal.

Instruments/Equipment/ Implants Required

The technique uses a percutaneous approach to the S1 presacral space. A Jackson table or equivalent radiolucent table is recommended. Surgical prepackaged systems should be on hand, consisting of 6-mm to 10-mm dilators, drills, exchange bushings,

and cannulas. Presacral implants of various lengths and diameters should be available for insertion. Bone grafting with autograft or allograft is optional.

Procedure

A 1.5-cm incision is made on the skin and underlying fascia, approximately 2 cm inferior to the right or left paracoccygeal notch, or just lateral to the coccyx. Blunt dissection is performed to ensure the fascia is opened appropriately. When the fascia is penetrated, a "pop" will be felt. Caution must be exercised during this maneuver to avoid plunging into the pelvis and causing injury to the adjacent structures, including the rectum.

Under fluoroscopic guidance, the blunt initial dilator is advanced slowly along the anterior midline of the sacrum to the inferior portion of the S1 body (**Figure 1**). Care must be taken to refrain from lifting the dilator from the anterior surface of the sacrum to prevent injury to the rectum or other retroperitoneal structures. Dilator advancement and placement is performed under frequent biplanar fluoroscopy to ensure that the dilator remains on the anterior surface of the sacrum and in the midline, away from the sacral foramen. The dilator trajectory and sacral starting point are created so that the cage can be advanced safely through S1 and into the L5 vertebral body. We use preoperative im-

aging studies to identify the ideal pin entry point and trajectory. All of our patients receive preoperative MRI scans of the sacrum to facilitate this planning (**Figure 2**). The goal is to pass through the middle of the L5-S1 disk space and end in the anterior aspect of the L5 vertebral body. In the AP plane, the pin should be midline.

After obtaining the ideal dilator location, the blunt central core is exchanged for a Steinmann pin, which is

then docked at the S1-S2 junction (**Figure 1**, *A*). Using a cannulated slap hammer, the blunt guide pin is tapped through the sacrum up to the level of the L5-S1 disk space. Frequent fluoroscopy is used to reconfirm the location. If the pin or dilator moves from the appropriate position, the procedure should be restarted, with the blunt dilator placed to ensure appropriate protection of the at-risk structures. A pin extension is attached to allow placement of a series of dilators that will dilate the presacral soft tissue and develop the bony working channel.

The first beveled 6-mm tubular dilator is advanced over the guide pin with the bevel placed ventrally. After contact with the anterior aspect of the sacrum, the dilator is rotated 180° to match the slope of the sacrum and driven with the slap hammer through the sacral cortex. The dilator is then removed, increasingly larger dilators are placed sequentially, and the steps are repeated. A thin-walled dilator sheath, which will function as the working corridor, is placed over the 10-mm dilator body (**Figure 3**, *A*). The dilator and guide pin are removed once the working corridor is placed.

Under frequent biplanar fluoroscopy, a 9-mm threaded reamer is advanced through the dilator sheath and into the sacrum to develop the osse-

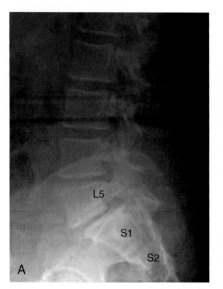

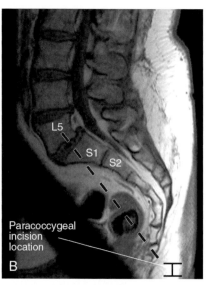

Figure 2 Preoperative imaging studies for percutaneous transsacral lumbar interbody fusion. **A,** Lateral radiograph. Note that the incision location and trajectory for the implant cannot be templated accurately on this image. **B,** Sagittal MRI. The paracoccygeal incision location is identified, and the implant trajectory (dashed line) can be templated preoperatively. This planning is especially important in patients with L5-S1 spondylolisthesis, as seen here.

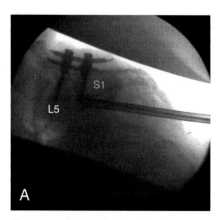

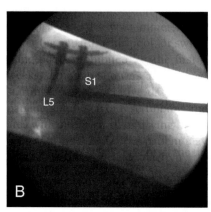

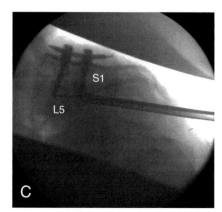

Figure 3 Fluoroscopic images demonstrate placement of the working corridor. **A,** Placement of the working corridor tube over the initial guide pin. **B,** Advancement of the initial reamer to the L5-S1 disk space. **C,** Advancement of the guide pin into the L5 vertebral body. Care must be taken to ensure that the proper trajectory is created, to allow containment of the implant within the S1 and L5 bodies.

Chapter 58

Pars Repair

Wellington K. Hsu, MD
Joseph K. Weistroffer, MD

Indications

Spondylolysis, which presents most commonly as a bone defect in the pars interarticularis, is widely believed to be caused by a stress fracture from repetitive loading. Although the prevalence of this condition in the general population has been reported to be between 3% and 6%, most cases are asymptomatic. In patients who are symptomatic, the most common symptom is low back pain, with or without radiation to the buttocks and posterior thighs. Hamstring tightness is a common finding, along with accentuation of the symptoms with hyperextension of the spine. Clinical presentation is common during the adolescent years and has an increased association with sporting activities such as gymnastics, weight lifting, and American football.

Although nonsurgical modalities, such as hyperextension bracing, restriction of sports activity, and rehabilitation therapy, are the mainstay of treatment, surgical treatment can be considered for patients in whom these modalities have failed after at least 6 months. Although lumbar fusion is sometimes indicated to prevent motion across a spinal segment, a successful direct pars interarticularis repair, which can retain normal physiologic spine biomechanics, can produce excellent results in the appropriate patient. For the adolescent or young adult patient with spondylolytic defects anywhere between L1 and L5, with an intact vertebral disk of normal height and minimal listhesis, a direct reconstruction of the pars has been shown to provide symptomatic relief. Furthermore, patients who experience a positive response to an infiltrative anesthetic injection into the pars defect have a high likelihood of improvement from surgical treatment (**Figure 1**).

Contraindications

Low-grade spondylolisthesis (grade I) is not an absolute contraindication to a pars repair, but the results and recommendations for these patients are controversial. Although some authors have reported using this procedure with success in adults who have spondylolistheses, others have opined that tensile forces across the pars defect from an existing slippage can lead to a reduced healing rate and poor clinical outcomes. Surgical repair of the pars is contraindicated in patients who have clinically significant degenerative disk disease or facet joint arthropathy. Furthermore, persistent pain that continues despite an anesthetic injection may demonstrate a different pain-generating source, such as the intervertebral disk. Because a direct pars repair would not address lower extremity symptoms from spinal stenosis, this procedure alone would fall short of expectations for patients with neurogenic claudication.

Alternative Treatments

For all symptomatic patients, continued activity modification, bracing, and other nonsurgical treatment modalities represent a reasonable approach even if symptoms persist past 6 months. In patients with significant spondylolysis or anterolisthesis of the spinal segment, a posterior lumbar spinal fusion can lead to excellent results. For patients with concomitant lower extremity symptoms, a decompressive laminotomy/laminectomy should be considered as an integral part of any surgical plan.

Dr. Hsu or an immediate family member serves as a paid consultant to or is an employee of Stryker and has received research or institutional support from Baxter Northwestern Alliance. Dr. Weistroffer or an immediate family member owns stock or stock options in Zimmer.

Results

The results of direct pars repair for spondylolysis generally have been promising, as demonstrated by healing rates and successful clinical outcomes. Although several techniques have been described, no long-term studies have compared constructs directly. Since its first description by Kakiuchi in 1997, the pedicle screw–laminar hook construct has gained popularity within the spine surgery community. Pars repairs tend to have better outcomes in younger patients (<40 years of age) and in those who have relatively normal disk pathology. Advanced degenerative changes have been shown to correlate with a poor outcome, whereas temporary symptom relief after a lidocaine injection into the pars portends a good prognosis. Most studies describe using iliac crest autograft as the biologic source of fusion; however, bone graft substitutes such as bone morphogenetic protein, allograft, and demineralized bone matrix also have been reported (Table 1).

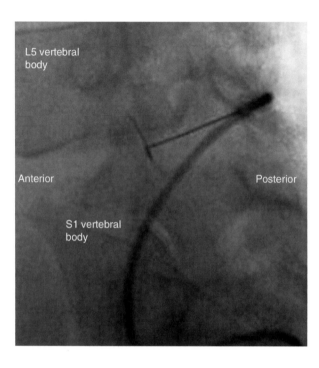

Figure 1 An oblique fluoroscopic image of a pars interarticularis injection with contrast medium along the posterior surface of the pars. Pain relief after pars infiltration can portend a good outcome from a direct pars repair.

Technique

Exposure

A standard posterior lumbar approach is used with the patient under general anesthesia in the prone position. A Wilson frame can be used to decompress the abdomen, allowing easier mechanical ventilation and reduced venous engorgement. The arms are abducted 75° to 85° on well-padded arm boards with the hands at the level of the head. The knees are flexed 20° to 30° to relieve stretch on the femoral nerve. Fluoroscopy may be used to localize the level of the incision before skin preparation with an antiseptic surgical solution.

Once the dermis is incised, the dissection is carried down to, but not into, the lumbodorsal fascia with elec-

Table 1 Results of Direct Pars Repair

Author(s) (Year)	Number of Patients	Procedure	Mean Patient Age in Years (Range)	Mean Follow-up in Months (Range)	Fusion Success Rate	Results
Bradford and Iza (1985)	22	Posterior wiring (Scott), autograft	24 (14-41)	(12-45)	90%	80% good to excellent
Kakiuchi (1997)	16	Pedicle screw-hook, ICBG	32 (12-60)	25 (24-28)	100%	81% excellent
Gillet and Petit (1999)	10	Pedicle screw–bent rod, ICBG	26 (16-48)	35 (7 to 63)	NR	70% good to excellent
Debnath et al (2007)	19	Buck technique (pars screw), ICBG	20 (15-34)	7 (4-10)	NR	82% excellent
Debusscher and Troussel (2007)	23	Pedicle screw–hook, allograft	34 (16-52)	59 (6-113)	91%	87% good to excellent

NR = not reported; ICBG = iliac crest bone graft.

trocautery. The lumbodorsal fascia is developed minimally with a Cobb elevator at the midline to assist in identifying it during closing at the end of surgery. Leaving the interspinous ligament intact at all levels, the dissection is carried in a subperiosteal fashion along the L5 spinous process (for an L5 pars repair) laterally to the lamina, taking care not to disrupt the facet capsule. The dissection need not expose the transverse process directly, although this structure should be palpable with a Penfield No. 4 or other probe to assist in placing the pedicle screw in the appropriate vertebral body. The pars interarticularis is then identified to confirm the bony defect and to establish the osseous anatomy necessary to ensure proper placement of the pedicle screw (**Figure 2**). The pars defect is thoroughly débrided of any fibrous or cartilaginous tissue, and the sclerotic bone margins are curettaged back to cancellous bleeding bone. Finally, the deep ligamentum flavum is released unilaterally from the undersurface of the inferior edge of the involved lamina with an up-angled Epstein curet. The curet should remain in contact with the undersurface of the lamina to prevent spinal canal violation.

Procedure

The pedicle screw is placed in the standard fashion with the starting point lateral to the facet joint and located by finding the intersection of the line axially bisecting the transverse process and the line created by the cranial extension of the lateral pars interarticularis arc (**Figure 2**). The posterior cortex is breached at this intersection with a pointed awl or oscillating burr. A pedicle finder tool is advanced through the pedicle and into the anterior half of the vertebral body in the appropriate orientation. A Holt probe is then used to ensure that the cortex of the pedicle and vertebral body are not violated. The posterior cortex can then be undertapped one

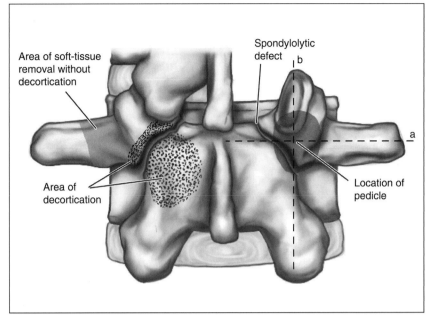

Figure 2 Drawing shows a posterior anatomic view of a lumbar vertebra with a pars interarticularis defect. The area shown is thoroughly curettaged of fibrous tissue to bleeding cancellous bone. The starting point of the pedicle screw is located by finding the intersection of the line axially bisecting the transverse process (a) and the line created by the cranial extension of the lateral pars interarticularis (b).

millimeter smaller than the anticipated pedicle screw diameter. After reexamination with a Holt probe to verify the integrity of the pedicle and measure the screw depth, the screw is placed along this track. For bilateral pars defects, the procedure is repeated for the contralateral pedicle. The placement of instrumentation can be performed under fluoroscopic assistance or with CT navigation.

Alternatively, a decompression of the traversing nerve root can be performed if subarticular stenosis and symptomatic radicular symptoms exist. The wound is irrigated copiously with sterile saline, and hemostasis is achieved with electrocautery, gel foam, and thrombin. A sublaminar hook is then secured under the affected lamina in the area prepared previously with the Epstein curet and attached loosely to the pedicle screw with an appropriate-length titanium rod (**Figure 3**). If necessary, a portion of the inferior articular facet can be

removed using an osteotome to facilitate laminar hook placement. Strips of autologous posterior iliac crest bone graft are then packed gently on top of the previously débrided pars defect, taking care not to introduce graft into the spinal canal or foramen. The use of other bone graft substitutes such as bone morphogenetic protein has been reported in the literature; however, this use remains off label and has not been studied in long-term clinical trials. Gentle compression is applied between the sublaminar hook and the pedicle screw after bone graft placement with the appropriate locking set screws tightened to the manufacturer's torque specifications (**Figure 4**).

Wound Closure

The wound is closed in a layered fashion with interrupted figure-of-8 stitches of No. 2 nonabsorbable braided sutures (over a suction drain if the surgeon chooses). The wound is reirrigated before interrupted deep

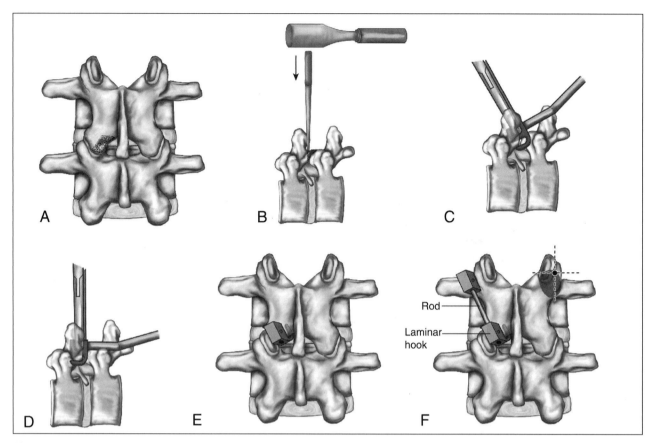

Figure 3 Drawings demonstrate sublaminar hook placement in the lumbar spine. After identification of the correct lamina (**A**), an osteotome is used to square off the leading edge to facilitate screw insertion (**B**). **C,** Using an appropriate inserter, the tip of the hook is used to locate the anterior surface of the lamina. **D,** The screw is positioned directly underneath the lamina, using a slight upward motion with the inserter, and secured with a hook holder. **E,** Final placement of the hook on the AP view should fall between the facet joint laterally and the spinous process medially. **F,** After pedicle screw placement, compression is placed across the screw-rod construct with set screws tightened to the manufacturer's specifications.

dermal buried stitches of 2-0 absorbable braided sutures are placed, followed by surgical staples or a subcuticular running stitch of 4-0 absorbable monofilament suture. Sterile tape strips, liquid adhesive, and petroleum gauze can be placed before a soft gauze dressing is applied.

Postoperative Regimen

The patient is placed in a custom-molded bivalve lumbosacral orthosis for 3 months with instructions for performing daily isometric core-

strengthening exercises. The dressing is kept in place for the first 3 days postoperatively and then changed at least once daily. The wound should be kept clean and dry, with immersion in water (eg, a bath, whirlpool, or swimming pool) prohibited for the first 4 weeks, although showers are allowed starting on postoperative day 3. The patient should avoid scrubbing the area with a washcloth or drying it vigorously with a towel. The patient may return to unrestricted activity 3 months postoperatively once weaned from the brace and after attaining full range of motion with good core muscle strength and tone.

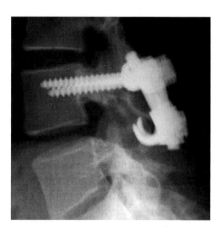

Figure 4 Plain lateral radiograph demonstrates the lumbar spine after successful pedicle screw–sublaminar hook placement at L4 for a spondylolytic defect. (Reproduced with permission from Bono CM: Low-back pain in athletes. *J Bone Joint Surg Am* 2004; 86(2):382-396.)

Avoiding Pitfalls and Complications

Selecting the proper instruments and instrumentation and taking care when performing the most delicate aspects of the procedure go a long way toward preventing the most common pitfalls and complications in pars repair. En-suring that the facet joint is not violated during the approach, the pars débridement, or the placement of the pedicle screw is important. Polyaxial pedicle screws should be used, and they should not be placed so deep that the motion of the head is restricted. The sublaminar hook should be placed in a configuration that maximizes the compression across the pars defect. Fi-nally, a sublaminar hook should be used that fits snugly onto the lamina. This will not only facilitate rod placement into a static device but also en-sure that the hook does not project too deeply into the neural canal.

———————■

Bibliography

Bono CM: Low-back pain in athletes. *J Bone Joint Surg Am* 2004;86-A(2):382-396.

Bradford DS, Iza J: Repair of the defect in spondylolysis or minimal degrees of spondylolisthesis by segmental wire fixation and bone grafting. *Spine (Phila Pa 1976)* 1985;10(7):673-679.

Buck JE: Direct repair of the defect in spondylolisthesis: Preliminary report. *J Bone Joint Surg Br* 1970;52(3):432-437.

Debnath UK, Freeman BJ, Gregory P, de la Harpe D, Kerslake RW, Webb JK: Clinical outcome and return to sport after the surgical treatment of spondylolysis in young athletes. *J Bone Joint Surg Br* 2003;85(2):244-249.

Debnath UK, Freeman BJ, Grevitt MP, Sithole J, Scammell BE, Webb JK: Clinical outcome of symptomatic unilateral stress injuries of the lumbar pars interarticularis. *Spine (Phila Pa 1976)* 2007;32(9):995-1000.

Debusscher F, Troussel S: Direct repair of defects in lumbar spondylolysis with a new pedicle screw hook fixation: Clinical, functional and Ct-assessed study. *Eur Spine J* 2007;16(10):1650-1658.

Gillet P, Petit M: Direct repair of spondylolysis without spondylolisthesis, using a rod-screw construct and bone grafting of the pars defect. *Spine (Phila Pa 1976)* 1999;24(12):1252-1256.

Jakob G: The operative treatment of the spondylolisthesis with compression screws (author's transl). *Arch Orthop Unfallchir* 1977;90(2):103-111.

Kakiuchi M: Repair of the defect in spondylolysis: Durable fixation with pedicle screws and laminar hooks. *J Bone Joint Surg Am* 1997;79(6):818-825.

Kimura M: My method of filing the lesion with spongy bone in spondylolysis and spondylolistesis. *Seikei Geka* 1968;19(4):285-296.

Roca J, Moretta D, Fuster S, Roca A: Direct repair of spondylolysis. *Clin Orthop Relat Res* 1989;246:86-91.

Ulibarri JA, Anderson PA, Escarcega T, Mann D, Noonan KJ: Biomechanical and clinical evaluation of a novel technique for surgical repair of spondylolysis in adolescents. *Spine (Phila Pa 1976)* 2006;31(18):2067-2072.

Coding

CPT Codes		Corresponding ICD-9 Codes	
63012	Laminectomy with removal of abnormal facets and/or pars inter-articularis with decompression of cauda equina and nerve roots for spondylolisthesis, lumbar (Gill type procedure)	738.4 756.12	756.11
22612	Arthrodesis, posterior or posterolateral technique, single level; lumbar (with or without lateral transverse technique)	170.2 721.42	721.3 722.0
22614	Arthrodesis, posterior or posterolateral technique, single level; each additional vertebral segment (List separately in addition to code for primary procedure)	170.2 722.52	722.10 724.02
22842	Posterior segmental instrumentation (eg, pedicle fixation, dual rods with multiple hooks and sublaminar wires); 3 to 6 vertebral segments (List separately in addition to code for primary procedure)	342.1 342.90	342.9 343

CPT copyright © 2010 by the American Medical Association. All rights reserved.

Chapter 59

Translaminar and Direct Facet Screw Placement

Isador H. Lieberman, MD, MBA, FRCSC

Indications

Despite the recent focus on the development of techniques to preserve spinal motion, spinal fusion will always be an important treatment for a variety of spinal pathologies. To stabilize the spine until a fusion consolidates, spine surgeons have used combinations of hooks, wires, screws, and rods. These implants have several disadvantages. They require an extensive soft-tissue dissection that can contribute to significant complications. To implant pedicle screws in a safe and anatomically correct position, the facet joint proximal to the segment to be fused needs to be exposed and may be damaged by the screw. These hardware constructs are expensive. Finally, these implants may form a bulky hardware mass that can be uncomfortable and could necessitate a subsequent operation to remove the implant.

Translaminar facet screw fixation (the translaminar approach developed by Magerl) or direct facet screw fixation (the direct facet pedicle screw approach developed by Boucher) could effectively address many of the issues identified above. These methods of fixation have been shown to be biomechanically equivalent to the more commonly used pedicle screw–rod constructs. In addition, these fixation techniques tend to be far less expensive, less invasive, and less bulky. The implants typically are off-the-shelf, readily available 4.5-mm cortical bone screws; however, proprietary sets and instruments are now available that allow percutaneous or computer-guided navigation insertion techniques.

Translaminar facet screw fixation and direct facet screw fixation can be used when single- or multiple-level fixation is needed to facilitate fusion in the setting of degenerative spine pathology in the presence of structurally intact facet joints. These methods may be used to supplement anterior interbody fusion with cages or structural allograft bone implants. The prerequisite for these fixation techniques is

that the anterior column is stable, meaning bone-on-bone disk degeneration or a stable interbody construct. Typically, single- or two-level constructs are easily performed. In rare cases, this technique can be used for three-level fixation. Some surgeons have used a unilateral facet fixation technique to supplement a contralateral pedicle screw construct. In all circumstances, appropriate bone fusion techniques must be used, including preparation of the bone-graft bed as well as the addition of the osteogenic, osteoconductive, and osteoinductive elements.

Contraindications

Translaminar facet screw fixation and direct facet screw fixation cannot be used in the presence of structurally compromised or missing facet joints. Other contraindications include significant deformity and isthmic spondylolysis or spondylolisthesis greater than grade I. In the presence of a degenerative spondylolisthesis higher than grade II, translaminar facet screws and direct facet screws may not be able to gain enough purchase across the subluxated joint to achieve adequate stability. Additional contraindications include deficient posterior elements (lamina and spinous process) for translaminar screws and

Dr. Lieberman or an immediate family member serves as a board member, owner, officer, or committee member of the Scoliosis Research Society, the Cleveland Clinic Foundation, and the Spine Arthroplasty Society; has received royalties from AxioMed, MAZOR Surgical Technologies, Merlot Orthopaedix, Stryker, Trans1, and CrossTrees; serves as a paid consultant to or is an employee of AxioMed, MAZOR Surgical Technologies, Merlot Orthopaedix, and CrossTrees; has received research or institutional support from AxioMed, MAZOR Surgical Technologies, Merlot Orthopaedix, Trans1, CrossTrees, Kyphon, Medtronic, Orthovita, Stryker, and DePuy; owns stock or stock options in AxioMed, MAZOR Surgical Technologies, Merlot Orthopaedix, and CrossTrees; and has received nonincome support (such as equipment or services), commercially derived honoraria, or other non–research-related funding (such as paid travel) from AxioMed, MAZOR Surgical Technologies, Merlot Orthopaedix, and CrossTrees.

Table 1 Biomechanical Studies

Authors (Year)	Testing Scenario	Conclusions
Rathonyi et al (1998)	Tested three-dimensional stability of intact spine, cage alone, translaminar screw alone, and cage and translaminar screw	Additional translaminar fixation significantly reduces motion in extension and axial rotation. Translaminar fixation alone better than cage alone
Ferrara et al (2003)	Tested the biomechanical effects of short-term and long-term cyclic loading on lumbar motion segments instrumented with either a pedicle screw or a transfacet pedicle screw construct	The stability provided by both transfacet pedicle screw fixation and traditional pedicle screw fixation was not compromised after repetitive cycling. Transfacet pedicle screw fixation appears equivalent biomechanically to traditional pedicle screw fixation.
Burton et al (2005)	Tested range of motion and stiffness with intact spine, cage alone, cage and facet screws, and cage and pedicle screws	Translaminar screw fixation was equivalent to bilateral pedicle fixation in all modes tested.

any situation in which the anterior column is deficient or unreconstructable. Relative contraindications include osteoporosis or an earlier surgery from which existing hardware or the presence of deformed anatomic structures may preclude safe implantation.

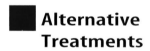

Alternative Treatments

The alternatives to translaminar facet screws and direct facet screws are the existing hook, wire, screw, and rod constructs. Depending on the spinal pathology and the extent of the reconstruction, multiple implants and combinations can be used.

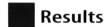

Results

The biomechanical characteristics and clinical results of translaminar facet screws and direct facet screws have been extensively investigated and reported in the literature. Studies reveal that these methods are biomechanically sound (**Table 1**), produce results comparable to other methods, provide a stable environment to facilitate fu-

sion, and result in good clinical outcomes (**Table 2**). These methods also have been shown to be safe and cost effective.

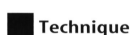

Technique

Patient Positioning
The patient is positioned prone on a typical spinal surgery frame to facilitate both the surgical exposure and any use of guidance or fluoroscopy. The preparation and draping is completed according to the surgeon's typical routine. Intraoperative fluoroscopy or plain radiographs are used to verify the surgical level and also may be used throughout the operation to assess the positioning of the screws.

Instruments/Equipment/ Implants Required
A drill and a screwdriver are the minimum equipment needed for the placement of the translaminar or direct facet screws. The implants typically are the commonly available 4.5-mm cortical bone screws. Several percutaneous guides and cannulae, reciprocating drills, fluoroscopic guides, robotic guides, and navigation systems are now available to help facilitate the implantation of the screws and increase the accuracy of placement,

but these advanced instruments are not absolutely necessary for the safe and effective use of the screws.

Surgical Technique
Implantation using an open exposure only is described here. Two trajectories are typically used: the direct facet pedicle screw approach (developed by Boucher and King) (**Figures 1** and **2**), and the translaminar approach (developed by Magerl) (**Figure 3**).

A traditional, less invasive open exposure to the surgical level is used. Through a small vertical midline incision, the spinous processes, laminae, and facet joints are exposed in a standard fashion. If decompression is needed, care should be taken to preserve the laminar arch and enough of the facet joints to accommodate the screws. Consideration may even be given to first implanting the screws and then proceeding with the decompression. Once exposed, the facet capsule is opened, and the joint surfaces are denuded of their cartilage. Bone graft of the surgeon's choice is then packed into the facet joint.

For the translaminar screw approach, a 3.2-mm drill bit is used to drill the base of the spinous process toward the facet joint between the cortices of the contralateral lamina, aiming to exit at the junction of the facet joint and the transverse process. This

Table 2 Clinical Studies Using Facet Fixation

Authors (Year)	Number of Patients	Mean Patient Age in Years (Range)	Mean Follow-up (Range)	Clinical Result	Fusion Rate	Complications
Jacobs et al (1989)	43	39	16 months Minimum 12 months	93% improvement	91%	No neurologic
Grob et al (1992)	72	49 (15-81)	24.4 months (12-47)	76% satisfied	94.5%	5 screw breakage 5 screws were not transfacet No neurologic
Benini and Magerl (1993)	166	NR	NR Case series, 1987-1991	NR	97.5%	NR
Reich et al (1993)	61	39 (16-65)	23 months (8-54)	93.4% excellent to good 6.6% unsatisfied	98.4%	No neurologic
Grob and Humke (1998)	173	53 (22-87)	58 months (42-71)	99 good 70 satisfactory 4 poor	94%	3% loosening 1 screw breakage 1 nerve irritation
Thalgott et al (2000)	46	46 (27-67)	33 months (24-42)	75.5% good or excellent	93.2%	No neurologic
Jang et al (2003)	18	NR	6 months (1-13)	100% excellent or good	NR	No malpositions or other complications
Yin et al (2004)	30	37 (29-61)	10 months (5-24)	97% anterior 98% posterior	100%	3.4% correction loss
Shim et al (2005)	20	54 (41-68)	19.5 months (10-28)	80% good to excellent 20% fair to poor	100%	10.8% lamina violation 15.4% screw malposition Articular process fracture at 1 level
Tuli et al (2005)	78 (38 pedicle screw, 40 translaminar)	44	12 weeks	Similar clinical outcome in the two groups	NR	10 complications in translaminar group 14 complications in pedicle screw group
Best and Sasso (2006)	43	NR	38 months (26-49)	VAS improved by average 4 points	95.3%	4.7% revision
Tuli et al (2007)	77 (37 pedicle screw, 40 translaminar)	44	3 years for translaminar 4 years for pedicle screw	33% revision rate for translaminar 27% revision rate for pedicle screw	18% nonunion for translaminar 3% nonunion for pedicle screw	5% adjacent-level degeneration for translaminar 14% adjacent-level degeneration for pedicle screw

NR = not reported; VAS = visual analog pain scale, range 0 to 10 (see Appendix).

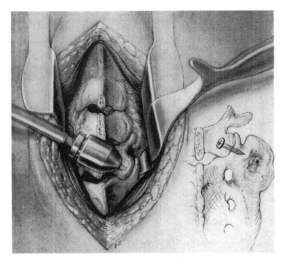

Figure 1 Illustrations demonstrate the King method of direct facet screw fixation.

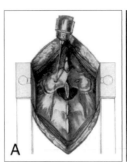
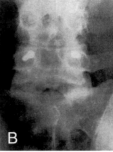
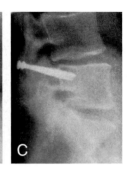

Figure 2 Images demonstrate the Boucher method of direct facet pedicle screw fixation. **A,** Illustration shows that all soft tissue has been removed out to and including the lateral articulations. The guide pin is withdrawn after penetrating the cortex of the ala. The obliquely placed screws avoid the nerve roots. AP (**B**) and lateral (**C**) radiographs demonstrate fusion between the fourth and fifth lumbar vertebrae. This placement of screws above the lumbosacral level seems to offer satisfactory stability and avoid root irritation. No external support is worn. (Reproduced with permission from Boucher HH: A method of spinal fusion. *J Bone Joint Surg Br* 1956;41(2):248-259.)

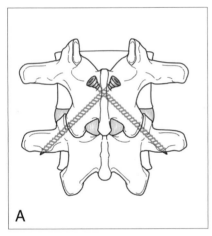
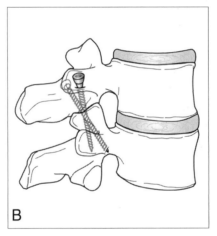

Figure 3 Drawings demonstrate the Magerl method of translaminar facet screw fixation. **A,** Posterior view shows the screws crossing through the spinous process. **B,** Lateral view shows the screws exiting at the junction of the facet joint and the transverse process.

drilling can be done through the midline incision or through a second stab opening with a guide tube (**Figure 4**). To place two screws through one spinous process without having the screws hit each other, one screw should be placed a bit more caudal and the other a bit more cranial (**Figure 3**). If the trajectory of the lamina is followed, the risk of penetrating the epidural space or injuring the dura or neural structures is negligible. After drilling with the 3.2-mm drill bit, a 4.5-mm tap is used to tap the hole. The length of the hole is then measured with a depth gauge. Finally, a 4.5-mm screw of the appropriate

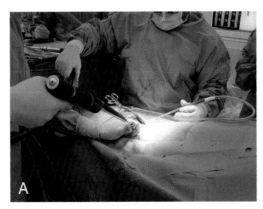
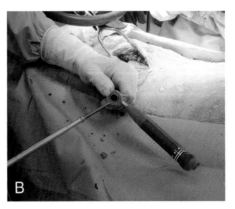
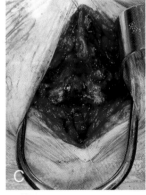

Figure 4 Intraoperative photographs demonstrate placement of translaminar facet screws. **A,** Drilling of the translaminar screw path through lamina and across facet joints. **B,** The insertion of a 4.5-mm cortical screw. **C,** The final position of the screws.

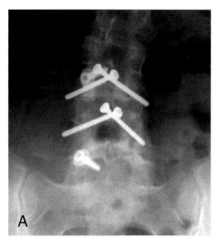

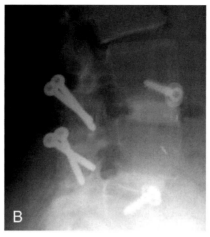

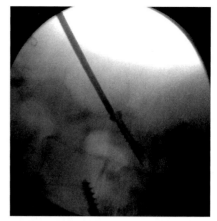

Figure 6 Fluoroscopic view shows percutaneous placement of facet screws.

Figure 5 AP (**A**) and lateral (**B**) radiographs show the proper placement of translaminar facet screws.

length is placed across the facet joint through the hole in the lamina (**Figures 4** and **5**). It is important to appreciate that the translaminar screw is not meant to be a lag screw; instead, it is intended as a stabilization and neutralization screw. As such, compressing the facet joint will result in facet fracture or spinous process fracture.

For the direct facet pedicle screw approach, the trajectory starts at the junction of the inferior facet and pars interarticularis of the vertebra above, aimed slightly laterally across the facet joint, and into the pedicle of the vertebra below (**Figures 1, 2, 6,** and **7**). The same drilling and tapping steps used for the translaminar screw approach apply in this approach. Direct facet screws may be applied as lag screws to compress the joint or as neutralization screws. Both uses require the appropriate joint preparation for fusion. If used as lag screws, overdrilling of the proximal hole is needed.

Translaminar facet screws are ideally suited for the L3-L4 and L4-L5 levels because of the anatomic relationships of the lamina and facet joints. At L5-S1, depending on the coronal orientation of the facet joints and the thinness of the lamina, direct facet screws may be easier to apply. Translaminar facet screws are pre-

cluded if the laminae are absent or if the facet surface area is compromised. Under these circumstances, direct facet pedicle screws are intuitively more appropriate.

Wound Closure

Wound closure depends on the method of application. If the screws

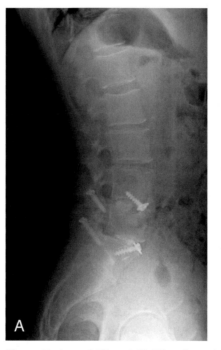

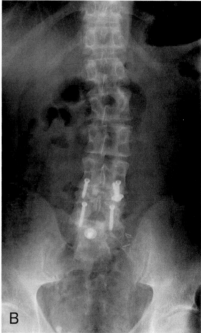

Figure 7 Lateral (**A**) and AP (**B**) radiographs show proper placement of percutaneous facet screws.

were implanted percutaneously, simple closure of the stab incisions is all that is required. If a greater exposure was needed to facilitate other surgical steps, such as a decompression, a typical layered closure of fascia and skin is performed.

———————■

Postoperative Regimen

Postoperative care following the use of translaminar facet screws or direct facet screws is no different than that ordered for any other fixation technique and tends to be specific to the pathology and surgeon preference. In general, because of the less invasive approach used during implantation, most patients recover sooner and are mobilized earlier than for other fixation techniques.

Avoiding Pitfalls and Complications

Although translaminar facet screw fixation and direct facet screw fixation are relatively simple techniques, as with all surgical procedures, complications are possible. A thorough appreciation of the relevant anatomy is critical before attempting to place these screws.

One potential complication is foraminal violation. The nerve root may be damaged or irritated by the drills or tools if the trajectory is not ideal or if the screw is malpositioned. In such a case, if the imaging studies show impingement on the nerve root, the screw should be removed and repositioned.

Another complication is inadequate decompression. The spine surgeon should never sacrifice a good decompression to preserve bone for fixation using translaminar or facet screws. If the amount of bone resected to achieve the desired decompression precludes the use of translaminar or direct facet screws, then alternate fixation techniques should be used.

Bibliography

Benini A, Magerl F: Selective decompression and translaminar articular facet screw fixation for lumbar canal stenosis and disc protrusion. *Br J Neurosurg* 1993;7(4):413-418.

Best NM, Sasso RC: Efficacy of translaminar facet screw fixation in circumferential interbody fusions as compared to pedicle screw fixation. *J Spinal Disord Tech* 2006;19(2):98-103.

Boucher HH: A method of spinal fusion. *J Bone Joint Surg Br* 1959;41-B(2):248-259.

Burton D, McIff T, Fox T, Lark R, Asher MA, Glattes RC: Biomechanical analysis of posterior fixation techniques in a 360 degrees arthrodesis model. *Spine (Phila Pa 1976)* 2005;30(24):2765-2771.

Ferrara LA, Secor JL, Jin BH, Wakefield A, Inceoglu S, Benzel EC: A biomechanical comparison of facet screw fixation and pedicle screw fixation: Effects of short-term and long-term repetitive cycling. *Spine (Phila Pa 1976)* 2003;28(12):1226-1234.

Grob D, Humke T: Translaminar screw fixation in the lumbar spine: Technique, indications, results. *Eur Spine J* 1998;7(3):178-186.

Grob D, Rubeli M, Scheier HJ, Dvorak J: Translaminar screw fixation of the lumbar spine. *Int Orthop* 1992;16(3):223-226.

Jacobs RR, Montesano PX, Jackson RP: Enhancement of lumbar spine fusion by use of translaminar facet joint screws. *Spine (Phila Pa 1976)* 1989;14(1):12-15.

Jang JS, Lee SH, Lim SR: Guide device for percutaneous placement of translaminar facet screws after anterior lumbar interbody fusion: Technical note. *J Neurosurg* 2003;98(1, Suppl):100-103.

King D: Internal fixation for lumbosacral fusion. *J Bone Joint Surg Am* 1948;30A(3):560-565.

Lieberman IH, Togawa D, Kayanja MM, et al: Bone-mounted miniature robotic guidance for pedicle screw and translaminar facet screw placement: Part I—Technical development and a test case result. *Neurosurgery* 2006;59(3):641-650.

Magerl FP: Stabilization of the lower thoracic and lumbar spine with external skeletal fixation. *Clin Orthop Relat Res* 1984;189:125-141.

Rathonyi GC, Oxland TR, Gerich U, Grassmann S, Nolte LP: The role of supplemental translaminar screws in anterior lumbar interbody fixation: A biomechanical study. *Eur Spine J* 1998;7(5):400-407.

Reich SM, Kuflik P, Neuwirth M: Translaminar facet screw fixation in lumbar spine fusion. *Spine (Phila Pa 1976)* 1993;18(4):444-449.

Shim CS, Lee SH, Jung B, Sivasabaapathi P, Park SH, Shin SW: Fluoroscopically assisted percutaneous translaminar facet screw fixation following anterior lumbar interbody fusion: Technical report. *Spine (Phila Pa 1976)* 2005;30(7):838-843.

Thalgott JS, Chin AK, Ameriks JA, et al: Minimally invasive 360 degrees instrumented lumbar fusion. *Eur Spine J* 2000;9(Suppl 1):S51-S56.

Togawa D, Kanyanja MM, Reinhardt MK, et al: Bone-mounted miniature robotic guidance for pedicle screw and translaminar facet screw placement: Part 2. Evaluation of system accuracy. *Neurosurgery* 2007;60(2 Suppl 1):ONS129-ONS139.

Tuli J, Tuli S, Eichler ME, Woodard EJ: A comparison of long-term outcomes of translaminar facet screw fixation and pedicle screw fixation: A prospective study. *J Neurosurg Spine* 2007;7(3):287-292.

Tuli SK, Eichler ME, Woodard EJ: Comparison of perioperative morbidity in translaminar facet versus pedicle screw fixation. *Orthopedics* 2005;28(8):773-778.

Yin QD, Zheng ZG, Cai JP: Pedicle screw fixation with translaminar facet joint screws for the treatment of thoracolumbar fracture. *Chin J Traumatol* 2004;7(6):354-357.

Coding

CPT Codes		Corresponding ICD-9 Codes	
22612	Arthrodesis, posterior or posterolateral technique, single level; lumbar (with or without lateral transverse technique)	170.2 721.42 722.10	721.3 722.0 737.39
22614	Arthrodesis, posterior or posterolateral technique, single level; each additional vertebral segment (List separately in addition to code for primary procedure)	170.2 722.52 737.39	722.10 724.02 738.4
22842	Posterior segmental instrumentation (eg, pedicle fixation, dual rods with multiple hooks and sublaminar wires); 3 to 6 vertebral segments (List separately in addition to code for primary procedure)	342.1 342.90 343.0	342.9 343 343.1
63047	Laminectomy, facetectomy and foraminotomy (unilateral or bilateral with decompression of spinal cord, cauda equina and/or nerve root[s], [eg, spinal or lateral recess stenosis]), single vertebral segment; lumbar	722.73 724.02	722.83
63048	Laminectomy, facetectomy and foraminotomy (unilateral or bilateral with decompression of spinal cord, cauda equina and/or nerve root[s], [eg, spinal or lateral recess stenosis]), single vertebral segment; each additional segment, cervical, thoracic, or lumbar (List separately in addition to code for primary procedure)	722.0 722.2 722.52	722.10 722.51 722.71
20930	Allograft for spine surgery only; morselized (List separately in addition to code for primary procedure)	170.2 733.13	724.6 733.81
20931	Allograft for spine surgery only; structural (List separately in addition to code for primary procedure)	170.2 733.13	724.6 733.81
20936	Autograft for spine surgery only (includes harvesting the graft); local (eg, ribs, spinous process, or laminar fragments) obtained from same incision (List separately in addition to code for primary procedure)	170.2 733.13	724.6 737.30

CPT copyright © 2010 by the American Medical Association. All rights reserved.

Chapter 60
Interspinous Spacers in the Lumbar Spine

Thomas Scioscia, MD
Adam C. Crowl, MD

◼ Indications

Patients with intermittent neurogenic claudication are common in a large spine practice. Standing upright is typically the most symptomatic position for these patients. Most patients describe symptomatic relief in a seated or flexed position, and many state that leaning over a shopping cart at the grocery store relieves their symptoms.

Interspinous spacers have been developed recently to treat patients with symptoms that are relieved by sitting or leaning over. It has been well demonstrated that flexion reduces the amount of stenosis by distracting the soft tissues (ligamentum flavum, posterior anulus, and facet capsule) and thereby opening the central spinal canal, lateral recess, and foramina. A correctly placed interspinous spacer mimics the flexed position at the implanted spinal segment, thus relieving the neurogenic claudication, which improves a patient's function.

Indications for interspinous technologies have been determined in a pivotal multicenter US Food and Drug Administration (FDA) study by Siddiqui and associates comparing a spacer implant technology with nonsurgical treatment. Currently, these indications include patients older than 50 years with classic neurogenic claudication symptoms of leg or buttock pain relieved by sitting. Instability should be limited to a stable grade I degenerative spondylolisthesis. Stenosis should be mild to moderate both clinically and on imaging studies to obtain the most dramatic results (**Figure 1**). The current recommendation is implantation for the treatment of one or two levels, but clinical success also has been achieved with three-level placement. These indications will change quickly as more companies develop implants. Studies are underway to prove efficacy in treating back pain from spondylosis and facet arthritis. Placement along with decompression may expand the indication to patients who do not get relief from sitting or who have a fixed neurologic deficit. Interspinous spacers offer an alternative to patients with stenosis who in the past were faced with a larger, more invasive surgery. In the future, we may see other clinical applications for these devices. Surgeons already are combining the technology with microdecompression to expand the indications and increase success rates. The theory behind the combination is to directly decompress the lateral recess and indirectly decompress the foramina while stiffening the segment. Treatment of spondylosis and facet arthritis also is being pursued. Interspinous devices and spinous process plates also are being explored to reduce segmental instability and motion to enhance the possibility of fusion through a minimally invasive approach.

———————◼

◼ Contraindications

An interspinous spacer is contraindicated in a patient with severe stenosis or a fixed neurologic defect. These conditions are better treated by direct decompression. Pain while sitting is a contraindication secondary to lack of efficacy in this patient population. Another contraindication is severe osteoporosis, because of the risk of spinous process fracture. Three-level surgery has not been studied extensively and at the current time cannot be recommended. Treatment of gross instability or scoliosis with a Cobb angle greater than 25° also will reduce efficacy. Ankylosis of the segment will make indirect decompression difficult because of the inability to distract the posterior

Dr. Scioscia or an immediate family member has received royalties from SeaSpine, is a member of a speakers' bureau or has made paid presentations on behalf of Kyphon and Medtronic Sofamor Danek, and serves as a paid consultant to or is an employee of DePuy. Dr. Crowl or an immediate family member serves as a paid consultant to or is an employee of Abbott and has received research or institutional support from Abbott and Biomet.

Table 1 Results of Clinical Studies of Interspinous Spacers

Authors (Year)	Number of Patients	Mean Patient Age in Years	Follow-up in Years	Success Rate
Zucherman et al (2005)	100	>50	2	73.1%
Kondrashov et al (2006)	18	67	4	78%
Anderson et al (2006)	42	>50	2	63.4%
Siddiqui et al (2007)	24	>50	1	54%

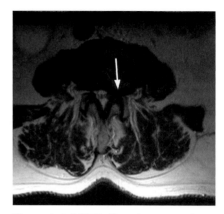

Figure 1 Axial MRI of L3-4 interspace shows mild to moderate left lateral recess stenosis (arrow). (Adapted with permission from Kyphon/Medtronic.)

structures. Previous laminectomy and isthmic spondylolisthesis at the affected level also are contraindications because of the lack of bony support for the implant. Treatment of the L5-S1 segment also may be difficult because of the lack of an S1 spinous process and supraspinous ligament.

Alternative Treatments

First-line treatment options for patients with intermittent neurogenic claudication remain nonsurgical. These include nonsteroidal anti-inflammatory drugs, activity modification, weight loss, and physical therapy. Epidural steroids can be helpful in calming down a flare of the disease and usually have some benefit. Those patients who do not improve may be candidates for surgical intervention.

Lumbar laminectomy is the most common surgical treatment of lumbar stenosis. Posterolateral fusion is added if the level has segmental instability. Interbody fusion also may add some benefit by increasing the fusion rate and reducing back pain. Unfortunately, these procedures carry the risk of infection, durotomy, iatrogenic nerve damage, radiculitis, nonunion, bone graft–site pain, hardware failure, misplacement of hardware, need for transfusion, adjacent-segment disease, and perioperative morbidity and mortality. This has led forward-thinking surgeons to consider interspinous spacers as a safer alternative.

Results

Biomechanical data supporting the use of interspinous spacers are substantial. Richards and associates showed in an MRI cadaver study that the canal area, subarticular diameter, and foraminal area all increased substantially after implantation (18%, 50%, and 25%, respectively). Siddiqui and associates had similar findings in an in vivo positional MRI study. Lindsey and associates showed that the implant favorably affected the disk by reducing nucleus and posterior anulus pressure without affecting the anterior anulus or adjacent-segment disks. Wiseman and associates found that facets also are unloaded by the device, reducing the mean force by 67% with no effect at adjacent facets. Lindsey and associates found that the only motion that was changed substantially was extension, and adjacent-segment kinematics were not affected.

Clinical results also support the use of interspinous spacers (**Table 1**). A large 2-year follow-up study showed results similar to those from laminectomy. A recent study by Kondrashov and associates studied patients at 4-year follow-up; 17 of 18 patients had improved function and showed improvement measured by the Oswestry Disability Index. One study looked specifically at the use of interspinous devices in patients with degenerative spondylolisthesis. This study showed significant improvements in those who received the device—63%, versus only 13% in those who underwent nonsurgical treatment.

Technique
Setup/Exposure

General anesthesia or local anesthesia with sedation can be used for the implantation of an interspinous spacer. The patient is positioned either in a flexed right lateral decubitis position or prone on a fully flexed Wilson frame. A 5- to 8-cm incision is made on the midline at the affected segment (**Figure 2**). The supraspinous ligament is spared by leaving a 1-cm cuff of soft tissue between the spinous processes (**Figure 3**). A Cobb elevator is then used to lift the paraspinal musculature off the sides of the spinous processes and the lamina. A self-retaining retractor of choice is placed to aid in visualization and exposure.

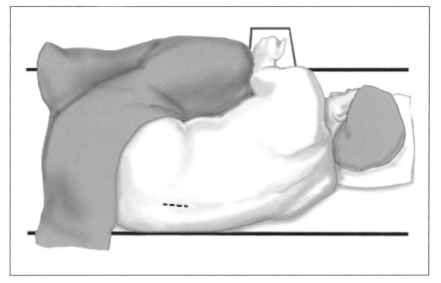

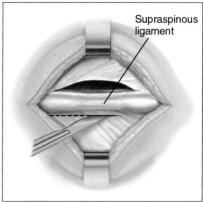

Figure 3 Illustration shows the sparing of the supraspinous ligament during the surgical approach. The patient's head is to the right. (Adapted with permission from Kyphon/Medtronic.)

Figure 2 Illustration demonstrates right lateral decubitus positioning for insertion of an interspinous device. The incision is indicated by the dashed line. (Adapted with permission from Kyphon/Medtronic.)

Instruments/Equipment/ Implants Required

Most interspinous devices are placed using only a few instruments and implants. A self-retaining retractor aids in visualization during preparation and insertion. The space for the interspinous device usually is opened using pointed dilators. The interspinous space is sized using a distractor. After distraction and sizing, the implant of choice is then implanted in the interspinous space, just posterior to the lamina and anterior to the supraspinous ligament.

Procedure

The interspinous ligament is pierced from the right side, with the small dilator as anterior as possible against the facets and lamina. The larger dilator is placed through the same hole and then the sizer is applied through the interspinous ligament between the spinous processes. The sizer is distracted using the amount of force equal to the grip used during a firm handshake. The tissue is held distracted for 30 seconds and then the sizer is regripped. The size of the implant is read off the sizer handle and

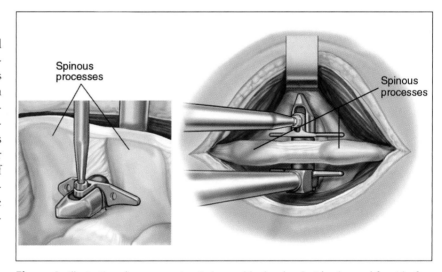

Figure 4 Illustration shows correct anterior positioning (against lamina and facets) of an interspinous device. The inset shows a lateral view. The patient's head is to the right. (Adapted with permission from Kyphon/Medtronic.)

then the implant is placed, staying as anterior as possible (**Figure 4**). The left wing is then placed and torqued to an audible "click." Preoperative and postoperative radiographs are used to verify correct placement of the spacer (**Figure 5**). A two-level procedure is performed similarly (**Figure 6**).

Wound Closure

The wound is irrigated and the fascia is closed with two running absorbable stitches approximating the fascia back to the supraspinous ligament. The skin is closed in the usual fashion, without the use of a drain.

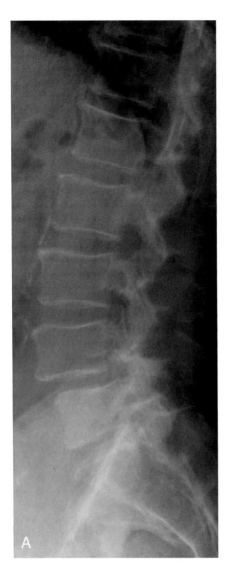
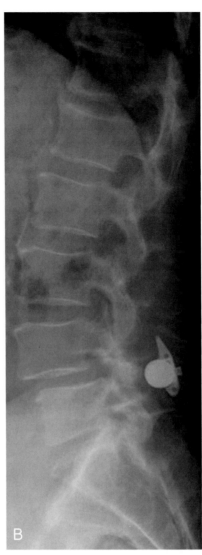

Figure 5 Lateral radiographs before (**A**) and after (**B**) implantation of an interspinous device at L4-5. (Reproduced with permission from Kyphon/Medtronic.)

Postoperative Regimen

The typical patient stays in the hospital less than 24 hours. Patients are advised to avoid excessive bending, twisting, or lifting during the first 6 weeks of treatment. A brace can be used to limit spinal motion if the patient has osteoporosis or if posterior placement of the device is inevitable because of anatomy. At 6 weeks after surgery, all bracing is discontinued and restrictions are lifted from patient activity.

Avoiding Pitfalls and Complications

The key to a successful outcome of placement of an interspinous device is proper patient selection. Although it is tempting to offer this procedure to elderly patients to improve their quality of life, the surgeon must not proceed unless the criteria for a successful surgery are met. Often the elderly have severe stenosis, back pain, osteoporosis, scoliosis, or preexisting medical conditions. When interspinous spacers are used to treat these conditions, a low success rate can be anticipated. Severe stenosis will not be relieved by indirect decompression, especially if the patient has neurologic deficit or sitting pain. Back pain may improve with these devices by unloading the facets, but relief may not be adequate. Osteoporosis could promote settling of the implant or fracture of the spinous process; both would lead to a clinical failure. Scoliosis may be so severe that foraminal stenosis may not be relieved or scoliosis may progress despite implantation. The severely debilitated patient may not regain the ability to walk because of physical decline. Selecting a patient with moderate stenosis who experiences complete relief with sitting is the best way to ensure success.

Technical pitfalls also are possible during the procedure. Implantation of the device too posterior could lead to supraspinous ligament failure and subsequent device migration. To avoid this complication, the implant should be placed adjacent to the facets. If the facets are hypertrophied (**Figure 7**), spurs can be trimmed or even broken off using rongeurs or dilators. Spinous process fracture can occur. Gentle and consistent force must be applied while using the sizer and during implantation of the implant. Erosion can render the implant ineffective. If the implant is oversized or an osteoporotic patient is not restricted in activity, settling can be seen early in the postoperative course.

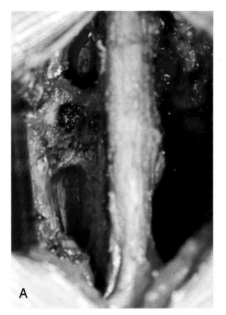 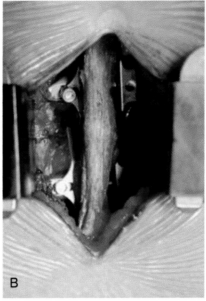

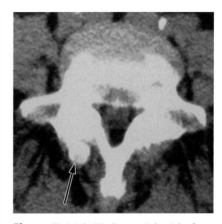

Figure 7 Axial CT shows right-side facet hypertrophy (arrow), which would impede anterior placement of an interspinous device. (Adapted with permission from Kyphon/Medtronic.)

Figure 6 Intraoperative photographs of a two-level procedure. **A,** Left microdecompression at L3 through L5 before implantation of two interspinous spacers. **B,** Correct placement of the spacers after microdecompression. (Reproduced with permission from Kyphon/Medtronic.)

Bibliography

Anderson PA, Tribus CB, Kitchel SH: Treatment of neurogenic claudication by interspinous decompression: Application of the X STOP device in patients with lumbar degenerative spondylolisthesis. *J Neurosurg Spine* 2006;4(6):463-471.

Booth KC, Bridwell KH, Eisenberg BA, Baldus CR, Lenke LG: Minimum 5-year results of degenerative spondylolisthesis treated with decompression and instrumented posterior fusion. *Spine (Phila Pa 1976)* 1999;24(16):1721-1727.

Bridwell KH, Sedgewick TA, O'Brien MF, Lenke LG, Baldus C: The role of fusion and instrumentation in the treatment of degenerative spondylolisthesis with spinal stenosis. *J Spinal Disord* 1993;6(6):461-472.

Hee HT, Castro FP Jr, Majd ME, Holt RT, Myers L: Anterior/posterior lumbar fusion versus transforaminal lumbar interbody fusion: Analysis of complications and predictive factors. *J Spinal Disord* 2001;14(6):533-540.

Herkowitz HN, Kurz LT: Degenerative lumbar spondylolisthesis with spinal stenosis: A prospective study comparing decompression with decompression and intertransverse process arthrodesis. *J Bone Joint Surg Am* 1991;73(6):802-808.

Kondrashov DG, Hannibal M, Hsu KY, Zucherman JF: Interspinous process decompression with the X-STOP device for lumbar spinal stenosis: A 4-year follow-up study. *J Spinal Disord Tech* 2006;19(5):323-327.

Lindsey DP, Swanson KE, Fuchs P, Hsu KY, Zucherman JF, Yerby SA: The effects of an interspinous implant on the kinematics of the instrumented and adjacent levels in the lumbar spine. *Spine (Phila Pa 1976)* 2003;28(19):2192-2197.

Richards JC, Majumdar S, Lindsey DP, Beaupré GS, Yerby SA: The treatment mechanism of an interspinous process implant for lumbar neurogenic intermittent claudication. *Spine (Phila Pa 1976)* 2005;30(7):744-749.

Siddiqui M, Karadimas E, Nicol M, Smith FW, Wardlaw D: Influence of X Stop on neural foramina and spinal canal area in spinal stenosis. *Spine (Phila Pa 1976)* 2006;31(25):2958-2962.

Siddiqui M, Smith FW, Wardlaw D: One-year results of X Stop interspinous implant for the treatment of lumbar spinal stenosis. *Spine (Phila Pa 1976)* 2007;32(12):1345-1348.

Weinstein JN, Lurie JD, Tosteson TD, et al: Surgical versus nonsurgical treatment for lumbar degenerative spondylolisthesis. *N Engl J Med* 2007;356(22):2257-2270.

Wiseman CM, Lindsey DP, Fredrick AD, Yerby SA: The effect of an interspinous process implant on facet loading during extension. *Spine (Phila Pa 1976)* 2005;30(8):903-907.

Zdeblick TA: A prospective, randomized study of lumbar fusion: Preliminary results. *Spine (Phila Pa 1976)* 1993;18(8): 983-991.

Zucherman JF, Hsu KY, Hartjen CA, et al: A multicenter, prospective, randomized trial evaluating the X STOP interspinous process decompression system for the treatment of neurogenic intermittent claudication: Two-year follow-up results. *Spine (Phila Pa 1976)* 2005;30(12):1351-1358.

Coding

CPT Codes		Corresponding ICD-9 Codes	
0171T	Insertion of posterior spinous process distraction device (including necessary removal of bone or ligament for insertion and imaging guidance), lumbar; single level	724.0 738.4 756.12	724.00 756.11
0172T	Insertion of posterior spinous process distraction device (including necessary removal of bone or ligament for insertion and imaging guidance), lumbar; each additional level (List separately in addition to code for primary procedure)	724.0 738.4 756.12	724.00 756.11

CPT copyright © 2010 by the American Medical Association. All rights reserved.

Indications

Sagittal deformity is a condition of spinal imbalance in which the patient is unable to maintain an upright posture in the sagittal plane (**Figure 1**). Of all spinal deformities in adults, fixed sagittal imbalance has the most negative impact on quality of life, producing both social and functional deficits. The ideal indication for a pedicle subtraction osteotomy (PSO) is sagittal deformity with a solid anterior column, from either previous fusion or ankylosing spondylitis (**Figures 2 and 3**). A PSO may be performed in a patient with open disk spaces, but a multilevel Smith-Petersen osteotomy with or without anterior fusion also should be considered. A PSO performed with open disk spaces leaves the proximal and distal aspects of the wedged vertebral body unattached to the hardware and therefore difficult to control. Furthermore, if a concomitant coronal imbalance of less than 6 cm exists, then an asymmetric PSO can be considered to address both the coronal and sagittal planes.

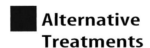

Contraindications

A PSO is a major surgical undertaking, and medical comorbidities must be considered as relative contraindications. The surgeon must be able to obtain fixation points proximal and distal to the planned osteotomy, so distorted anatomy and osteoporosis must be considered. The surgeon should be ready to abort the osteotomy should these fixation points not be obtainable, even if the decision is made intraoperatively. The rare patient who has severe fixed kyphoscoliosis with sagittal and coronal imbalance and shoulders parallel to the pelvis or tipping to the convex side of the deformity requires spinal shortening and translation that can best be achieved with a vertebral column resection.

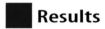

Alternative Treatments

The posterior osteotomy is only one of multiple techniques that surgeons should have in their armamentarium to treat the patient with spinal deformity. Combined anterior and posterior procedures and vertebral column resections have overlapping surgical indications with posterior osteotomies, but these procedures also have their own specific indications.

Results

A single-level PSO should provide approximately 30° of sagittal correction per level of osteotomy. (A PSO may be performed at more than one level if more correction is necessary.) The degree of correction per level can be improved by extending the anterior column or combining the osteotomy with a transforaminal lumbar interbody fusion at the suprajacent level. The amount of sagittal translation improvement also is dependent on the level of the osteotomy, with more correction obtained with a more distal osteotomy. Patient outcome parameters generally show high improvement in overall satisfaction and self-image but more moderate benefit in pain and functional measures (**Table 1**).

Dr. Tribus or an immediate family member serves as a board member, owner, officer, or committee member of the Medical Advisory Board and US Spine; has received royalties from Stryker and US Spine; is a member of a speakers' bureau or has made paid presentations on behalf of Stryker, Kyphon, and US Spine; serves as a paid consultant to or is an employee of US Spine and Stryker; has received research or institutional support from Medtronic; and owns stock or stock options in US Spine and ESM Technologies.

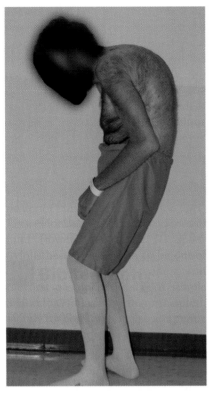

Figure 1 Clinical photograph of a patient with a severe fixed sagittal imbalance, which presents positional challenges that must be anticipated in the operating room.

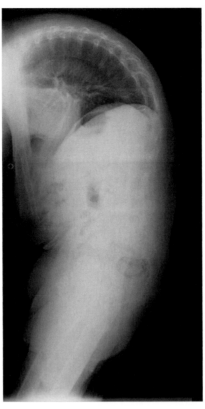

Figure 2 Lateral radiograph demonstrates severe ankylosing spondylitis that has created a devastating fixed sagittal imbalance.

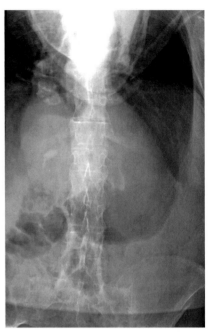

Figure 3 AP radiograph of a patient with ankylosing spondylolisthesis demonstrates both fused sacroiliac joints and a typical "bamboo spine."

Table 1 Results of Posterior Lumbar Pedicle Subtraction Osteotomy

Authors (Year)	Number of Patients	Mean Patient Age in Years (Range)	Mean Follow-up in Years (Range)	Fusion Success Rate	Average Correction (deg)	Results
Kim et al (2002)	45	34.6 (17-55)	3 (2-4)	No pseudarthroses	34	Improvement in activity, pain, psychosocial, and satisfaction scales
Murrey et al (2002)	59	47 (13-84)	4.5 (1-10)	No pseudarthroses	26.2	74.1% completely satisfied 18.5% relatively satisfied 7.5% not satisfied
Buchowski et al (2007)	108	54 (40-68)	(2-12)	NR	32	9 revisions for decompression
Kim et al (2007)	35	53.1	5.8 (5-7.6)	29% pseudarthrosis rate (8 of 35)	27	Satisfaction, 87% Improved image, 76% Improved function, 69% Improvement in pain, 66%
Chang et al (2008)	83	NR	Minimum 2-year follow-up	80/83 patients	42.2	Improved pain, self-image, and function on SRS scale

NR = not reported, SRS = Scoliosis Research Society.

▮ Technique

Setup/Exposure

The operation begins by addressing anesthesia concerns. In the patient who has a severe deformity, fibro-optic intubation, perhaps nasotracheal, should be considered to best obtain and protect the airway, particularly if the cervical spine is involved. The head must be well supported. When positioning the patient prone, the operating table must accommodate the patient, not vice versa. A preferred approach is to use a standard operating table with two separate four-post posterior frames split over the hinge of the table. Two pads are placed on the inferior portion of the cranial four-post frame to support the chest, and two pads are placed on the superior portion of the caudal frame to support the iliac crests and proximal thighs. The planned osteotomy is centered over the preflexed hinge (**Figure 4**). Once the osteotomy is performed, the table can be re-flexed, thus closing the osteotomy. The patient should be padded thoroughly. Neurologic monitoring should be considered for any osteotomy with planned angular correction of the spine, but its usefulness ultimately is dependent on the level of the osteotomy.

A standard posterior exposure is performed. Ideally, three levels of fixation above and below the planned osteotomy are exposed. Adding on to a previous fusion should be avoided unless junctional disease is present or additional levels are needed to improve the correction or provide necessary fixation points.

Instruments/Equipment/ Implants Required

A posterior osteotomy of the spine requires complete destabilization of the spine before realignment. Although laminar hooks and sublaminar wires may be used, three-dimensional control of the spine is best obtained by transpedicular fixation. Whether to

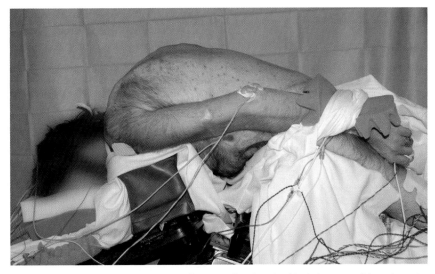

Figure 4 Photograph of a patient with severe fixed sagittal imbalance positioned on the operating table, which must accommodate the deformity. The table is flexed, with chest support and pelvic support on the two separate segments of the table.

use top-loading screws instead of a side-loading screw system depends on surgeon preference, but each option has relative advantages. Obtaining fixation both proximal and distal to the planned osteotomy before performing the osteotomy is of primary importance. Once the osteotomy is performed, the spine is highly unstable, and the spinal nerve is at risk for distraction injury. This lack of stability makes the placement of pedicle screws after the osteotomy is performed both challenging and dangerous, and if fixation is not attainable, the surgeon is left with an impossible reconstruction problem.

Procedure

PEDICLE SUBTRACTION OSTEOTOMY

After the exposure is completed, the osteotomy margins should be marked with a burr through the surface of the lateral fusion mass. Both sides should be marked clearly and in parallel. Asymmetric resection can result in coronal deformity, but it can be planned to correct a slight coronal imbalance. The area to be resected in the lateral fusion mass should be roughly centered about the pedicle and span from the proximal to the distal pars

interarticularis. Assuming that the pedicles to be resected are at L3, the resection would extend from the pars of L2 to the pars of L3. Thus, once the pedicle is resected and the osteotomy is closed, the L2 and L3 nerve roots would be exiting through one large foramen between the pedicles of L2 and L4.

Next, the laminectomy should be performed, before the formal resection of the lateral fusion mass. A wide laminectomy of L2, L3, and L4 accommodates the buckling thecal sac upon closure of the osteotomy. Should a dural tear be created during decompression, repair can be delayed until partial closure of the osteotomy. The redundancy created by shortening the posterior column creates ample dura, which can simplify the repair of even complicated tears. This technique can be particularly useful in patients with ankylosing spondylitis who may have dural atresia at the level of the lamina.

Performing the laminectomies early also allows access to the pedicles above and below the planned osteotomy. Instrumentation of these pedicles is particularly important and is greatly facilitated by performing the decompression first. The fixation

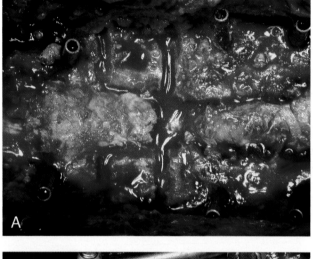

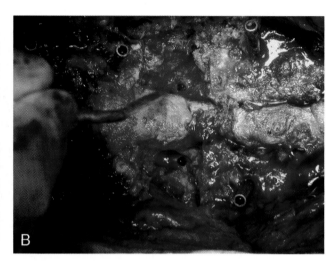

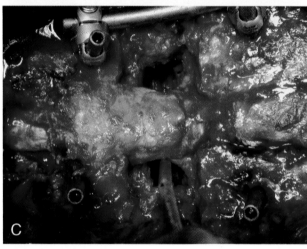

Figure 5 Intraoperative photographs demonstrate a pedicle subtraction osteotomy. The patient's head is, to the left. **A,** Fixation is obtained proximal and distal to the planned osteotomy. **B,** The lateral masses and pedicles are resected. **C,** Temporary rods may be placed to prevent premature closure of the osteotomy while the wedge resection of the vertebral body is being performed.

points, typically pedicle screws, should be established before completing the osteotomy, for two reasons. First, it is safer to place the hardware in a stable spine; once the osteotomy is completed, the spinal column may be grossly unstable, making work with mallets and pedicle finders potentially dangerous. Second, if fixation points cannot be established before the osteotomy is performed, the procedure can be aborted while spinal stability is still present (**Figure 5**, *A*). A radiograph taken at this point is useful to confirm screw placement.

Next, the lateral fusion mass is resected; a 5-mm burr or an osteotome may be used to define the borders. The surgeon should attempt to save the local bone graft because it can be quite

abundant and can obviate the need to obtain the graft for the fusion from the iliac crest. The resection isolates the posterior aspect of the pedicle. The neural elements are then retracted from the pedicle as the pedicle is resected (**Figure 5**, *B*). A burr may be used, working outward from inside the center of the pedicle. A rongeur can be a very safe alternative, providing good visualization and protection of the neural elements.

The resection continues anteriorly into the vertebral body. Bleeding can be brisk. Bipolar electrocautery can control the epidural bleeding, but the cancellous bone bleeding can be difficult to control. It is important to work efficiently and as a team, moving from side to side to pack the opposite side

with a hemostatic agent such as gel foam and thrombin. The surgeon should start the resection at the base of the pedicle, working anteriorly and medially. If pedicle screws were previously placed at the osteotomy site, the screw holes can be very useful landmarks for depth and point of focus for the apex of the resection. The combination of a burr and angled curets is used to join the resection at the midvertebral body. Suction can then be applied from one side while the surgeon continues to work from the other. The superior and inferior bone should be shaped as a wedge, angled posteriorly to align with the resection in the lateral fusion mass. The surgeon should not go through the cortex anteriorly. Although the cortex can be exposed, it also is feasible to leave approximately 1 cm of cancellous bone anteriorly. Then, closure of the osteotomy creates a greenstick fracture, which allows deformation and compression of the bone (**Figure 5,** *C*). Next, a reverse-angled curet is used to push the remaining posterior cortex of the vertebral body forward onto the area of vertebral resection, where it can be removed safely. A unilateral short rod can be placed, spanning the osteotomy to prevent it from closing prematurely. The lateral resection is thinned to the cortex, where it can be resected with a Kerrison rongeur. The segmental vessels can be injured during this step. An alternative approach is to use a bone tamp to bluntly greenstick the lateral cortex from the posterior and medial side. The tamp is progressively brought anterior to complete the greenstick fracture, allowing closure of the osteotomy.

An alternative to the described osteotomy for the patient with open disk spaces is the addition of an interbody fusion at the disk space above the pedicle resection. In this technique, the pedicle is resected in the fashion previously described, but the vertebral body resection is angled more proximally and includes the end plate and disk superiorly. The anterior apex of the resection is the junction of the middle and anterior thirds of the superior end plate. Allograft or a vertical cage can then be placed in the residual anterior disk space to provide a fulcrum for closure, and the osteotomy can be closed in the typical fashion (**Figures 6** and **7**).

If the patient has a concomitant moderate coronal deformity, an asymmetric wedge resection can be performed by resecting the greater amount of bone on the convexity. Thus, during careful closure of the osteotomy, the coronal deformity can be corrected. Three-dimensional resections add an additional plane of consideration. The surgeon can easily get

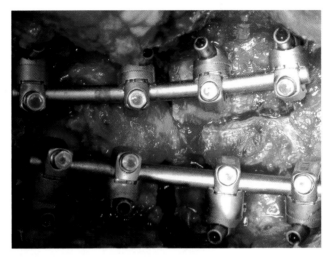

Figure 6 Intraoperative photograph demonstrates the final rods secured.

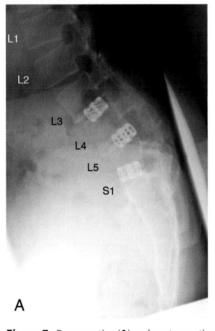
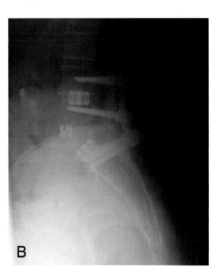

Figure 7 Preoperative (**A**) and postoperative (**B**) lateral radiographs of a patient with severe iatrogenic flatback. A pedicle subtraction osteotomy is combined with an instrumented transforaminal lumbar interbody fusion at L4-L5 which increases the degree of correction by maintaining anterior column height and allowing a broader posterior closure.

lost in the resection anatomy and the correction.

To close the osteotomy, the temporary rod must be loosened. It may be retained in place loosely to facilitate quick stabilization of the spine should the osteotomy site be rendered too unstable. The table is then re-flexed slowly while the surgeon directly inspects the osteotomy site and the neural elements. The re-flexing of the ta-

ble may be used to effect the closure. Alternatively, a spreading device can be placed in the osteotomy site or on the hardware, the table re-flexed while the surgeon holds the osteotomy open, and the distractor relaxed to close the osteotomy. Once the hardware is tightened, the table should be made flat to reduce pressure on the legs and chest. Intraoperative AP and lateral radiographs must be obtained to confirm spinal balance in both the coronal and sagittal planes after the fixation is secured and to ensure that no translation has occurred at the osteotomy site.

SMITH-PETERSEN OSTEOTOMY

The Smith-Petersen osteotomy provides approximately 10° of angular correction per level. It may be combined with an anterior release and fusion or performed as a stand-alone posterior approach. The resection is of the facet joint and/or lateral fusion mass and is combined with a laminectomy to prevent neural impingement during correction, as in the PSO. In contrast to the PSO, the pedicle is not resected, and the correction is obtained through the disk space. In the patient with a combined sagittal and coronal deformity with shoulder angulation tilted into the concavity, an anterior release followed by a posterior fusion with multilevel Smith-Petersen osteotomies can prove useful. It has been shown that the combined anterior and posterior approach with multiple Smith-Petersen osteotomies provides sagittal correction similar to a PSO with less blood loss, but it requires additional anterior exposure.

Wound Closure

Prior to closure, the wound should be irrigated, and a final check for foraminal patency should be performed. Closure of the osteotomy typically will create redundancy in the soft tissues and dead space in the depth of the wound. A standard side-to-side approximation of the fascial layer over a deep drain is followed by a layered closure of subcutaneous tissue and skin.

Postoperative Regimen

Given the magnitude of the surgical insult, the postoperative critical care management needs of the patient should be anticipated. Fluid resuscitation and evaluation is ongoing, with overnight intubation frequently necessary.

The effects of hip flexion and subsequent pelvic rotation on the fixation of the surgical construct must be considered, especially if the fixation extends to the pelvis. If the osteotomy is performed at L4, a thoracolumbosacral orthosis combined with a thigh cuff should be worn during all out-of-bed activities for 6 to 8 weeks. The patient is instructed to avoid flexion of the hip greater than 45°. Use of a bedpan is advocated when bone quality is in question. Alternatively, a tilt table may be used. The table assists the patient in rising to a standing position without flexing the hips. Once upright, the patient is free to walk around without a brace. This option requires a prolonged stay at a skilled nursing facility but has some advantages over home care because the patient gains independence by ambulating on a more regular basis.

Avoiding Pitfalls and Complications

In the patient with ankylosing spondylitis who has a fixed cervical spine, overcorrection via lumbar osteotomy can lead to great dissatisfaction because the patient's gaze will be above the horizontal. Undercorrection, especially when fusing short of the pelvis, will lead to recurrent kyphosis.

Early complications include atelectasis, pressure sores, deep vein thrombosis, wound hematoma, and ileus. Subacute and late complications include wound infection, loss of fixation, and nonunion. Neurologic complications should be evaluated aggressively. A new postoperative radiculopathy may be transient, but the surgeon must have a high index of suspicion that the neural elements may be trapped in the closure of the osteotomy site.

Bibliography

Bradford DS, Tribus CB: Current concepts and management of patients with fixed decompensated spinal deformity. *Clin Orthop Relat Res* 1994;306:64-72.

Bridwell KH: Decision making regarding Smith-Petersen vs. pedicle subtraction osteotomy vs. vertebral column resection for spinal deformity. *Spine (Phila Pa 1976)* 2006;31(19, suppl):S171-S178.

Bridwell KH, Lewis SJ, Lenke LG, Baldus C, Blanke K: Pedicle subtraction osteotomy for the treatment of fixed sagittal imbalance. *J Bone Joint Surg Am* 2003;85-A(3):454-463.

Buchowski JM, Bridwell KH, Lenke LG, et al: Neurologic complications of lumbar pedicle subtraction osteotomy: A 10-year assessment. *Spine (Phila Pa 1976)* 2007;32(20):2245-2252.

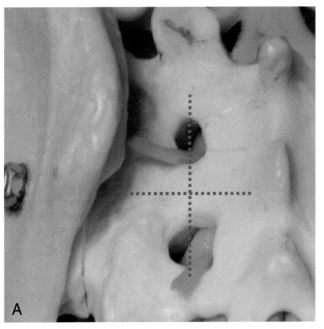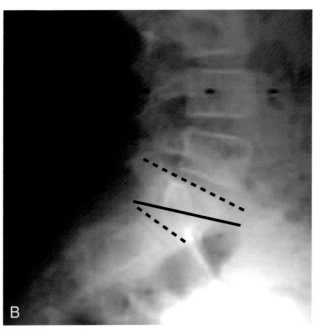

Figure 3 Zone 2 fixation. **A,** Pelvic model of the posterior S1 and S2 foramen. The S2-alar starting point is at the intersection of the dashed lines. **B,** Lateral radiograph of the lumbosacral spine. The dashed lines represent the superior S1 end plate and the S1-S2 physeal scar, and the solid line represents the lateral trajectory of an S2-alar screw toward the midpoint of the S1 vertebral body.

to be inserted and is then palpated again. Then the screw is inserted.

ZONE 2 FIXATION

Zone 2 fixation is not as strong as zone 1 fixation; nonetheless, several techniques for using various S2-type screws have been reported. One technique is to use an S2-alar screw. These screws may be used to augment S1 pedicle screw fixation. Again, bicortical fixation is necessary, and here, greater resistance to pullout forces is attained with laterally directed screw placement. These screws can, however, be prominent or tent the skin. The starting point for the S2-alar screw is slightly inferior to the lateral aspect of the first posterior foramen (centered between the first and second posterior foramen) (**Figure 3**, **A**). A burr is used to make a starting hole for screw insertion. Using fluoroscopic guidance, a straight pedicle developer is directed laterally and toward the midpoint of S1 (**Figure 3**, **B**). The awl is then removed, and the tract is assessed using a ball-tipped probe. The

length of the screw is marked on the probe and then measured, and the posterior cortex is undertapped using a tap at least 1 mm smaller than the diameter of the screw to be inserted. The screw is inserted under direct fluoroscopic visualization.

ZONE 3 FIXATION

Today, zone 3 fixation consists primarily of iliac screws. This technique offers the advantage of better pullout strength than the smooth intrailiac Galveston rods that were used primarily in the past. Screws also can be placed into sites of previously harvested grafts. Again, longer screws provide better resistance to flexion forces because they project farther anterior to the center of rotation. Furthermore, iliac screws may be removed after the lumbosacral fusion is solid—usually on an outpatient basis.

To insert the screws, the inner and outer ilium must be exposed at the level of the PSIS. The starting point is 1 cm proximal and 1 cm medial to the PSIS, and the trajectory is just supe-

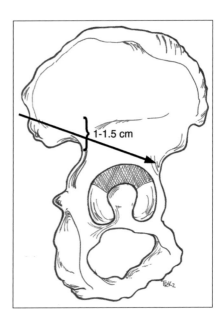

Figure 4 Zone 3 fixation. Drawing depicts the best iliac screw trajectory (arrow), capturing the strong bone just superior to the sciatic notch (within 1 to 1.5 cm).

rior to the sciatic notch (**Figure 4**). A curved pedicle developer (awl) is used to develop a channel for screw insertion, and the general trajectory is approximately 45° medial-lateral and

45° cranial-caudal. A ball-tipped probe is used to palpate the walls of the channel and to ensure complete intraosseous screw placement. Next, the length of the screw is marked on the probe and measured, and the starting point is undertapped. The iliac screw head must be recessed adequately to prevent prominent instrumentation. The screws are then connected with the longitudinal rod construct on the lumbar spine through connecting rods.

Wound Closure

The wound is closed in the standard fashion. Staples often are used in patients who have undergone multiple revisions.

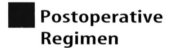

Postoperative Regimen

The standard postoperative regimen includes early ambulation and mobilization. A brace may be used, but its primary purpose is to slow the patient down and reduce forward flexion. Thigh extensions are not routinely used.

Avoiding Pitfalls and Complications

Complications following S1 screw fixation primarily involve a medially directed screw that breaches the medial cortex. This is best avoided by a thorough palpation of the screw tract, where four walls and a floor are palpated. Bicortical screws should be directed medially because a "straight-forward" trajectory at S1 may come in contact with the traversing L5 nerve root anterior to the sacral promontory.

For S2-alar screws, a complete understanding of sacral anatomy is necessary because a screw directed too far medially may come in contact with the traversing L5 nerve root anterior to the sacral promontory, and a screw directed too far laterally may violate the SI joint. Complications of iliac screw fixation include violation of and injury to the structures traversing the sciatic notch, acetabular violation, and instrumentation prominence. Again, as with all spine instrumentation techniques, a thorough understanding of spinal anatomy is mandatory, and postinstrumentation imaging is necessary to confirm well-placed instrumentation.

Pelvic instrumentation should be considered for patients with long fusions (L3 or higher); compromised bone quality as in osteoporosis; revision procedures; or significant lumbosacral kyphosis, as in a high-grade spondylolisthesis. Sacropelvic fixation serves as the construct "anchor" providing multiple fixation points anterior to the IAR and should be used to provide optimal stability.

Despite continued concerns, postoperative SI joint degeneration and other problems with the SI joint have not been identified with iliac fixation. Potential pelvic ring stress fractures are possible, however, and should be considered in the older patient when a significant change in symptoms occurs in the postoperative period.

Bibliography

Balderston RA, Winter RB, Moe JH, Bradford DS, Lonstein JE: Fusion to the sacrum for nonparalytic scoliosis in the adult. *Spine (Phila Pa 1976)* 1986;11(8):824-829.

Bridwell KH, Edwards CC II, Lenke LG: The pros and cons to saving the L5-S1 motion segment in a long scoliosis fusion construct. *Spine (Phila Pa 1976)* 2003;28(20):S234-S242.

Devlin VJ, Boachie-Adjei O, Bradford DS, Ogilvie JW, Transfeldt EE: Treatment of adult spinal deformity with fusion to the sacrum using CD instrumentation. *J Spinal Disord* 1991;4(1):1-14.

DeWald CJ, Vartabedian JE, Rodts MF, Hammerberg KW: Evaluation and management of high-grade spondylolisthesis in adults. *Spine (Phila Pa 1976)* 2005;30(6, suppl):S49-S59.

Eck KR, Bridwell KH, Ungacta FF, et al: Complications and results of long adult deformity fusions down to L4, L5, and the sacrum. *Spine (Phila Pa 1976)* 2001;26(9):E182-E192.

Edwards CC II, Bridwell KH, Patel A, Rinella AS, Berra A, Lenke LG: Long adult deformity fusions to L5 and the sacrum: A matched cohort analysis. *Spine (Phila Pa 1976)* 2004;29(18):1996-2005.

Emami A, Deviren V, Berven S, Smith JA, Hu SS, Bradford DS: Outcome and complications of long fusions to the sacrum in adult spine deformity: Luque-galveston, combined iliac and sacral screws, and sacral fixation. *Spine (Phila Pa 1976)* 2002;27(7):776-786.

Kostuik JP, Hall BB: Spinal fusions to the sacrum in adults with scoliosis. *Spine (Phila Pa 1976)* 1983;8(5):489-500.

Kostuik JP, Valdevit A, Chang HG, Kanzaki K: Biomechanical testing of the lumbosacral spine. *Spine (Phila Pa 1976)* 1998;23(16):1721-1728.

Kuklo TR, Bridwell KH, Lewis SJ, et al: Minimum 2-year analysis of sacropelvic fixation and L5-S1 fusion using S1 and iliac screws. *Spine (Phila Pa 1976)* 2001;26(18):1976-1983.

Lehman RA Jr, Kuklo TR, Belmont PJ Jr, Andersen RC, Polly DW Jr: Advantage of pedicle screw fixation directed into the apex of the sacral promontory over bicortical fixation: A biomechanical analysis. *Spine (Phila Pa 1976)* 2002;27(8):806-811.

McCord DH, Cunningham BW, Shono Y, Myers JJ, McAfee PC: Biomechanical analysis of lumbosacral fixation. *Spine (Phila Pa 1976)* 1992;17(8, suppl):S235-S243.

Neustadt JB, Shufflebarger HL, Cammisa FP: Spinal fusions to the pelvis augmented by Cotrel-DuBousset instrumentation for neuromuscular scoliosis. *J Pediatr Orthop* 1992;12(4):465-469.

Saer EH III, Winter RB, Lonstein JE: Long scoliosis fusion to the sacrum in adults with nonparalytic scoliosis: An improved method. *Spine (Phila Pa 1976)* 1990;15(7):650-653.

Smith SA, Abitbol JJ, Carlson GD, Anderson DR, Taggart KW, Garfin SR: The effects of depth of penetration, screw orientation, and bone density on sacral screw fixation. *Spine (Phila Pa 1976)* 1993;18(8):1006-1010.

Tsuchiya K, Bridwell KH, Kuklo TR, Lenke LG, Baldus C: Minimum 5-year analysis of L5-S1 fusion using sacropelvic fixation (bilateral S1 and iliac screws) for spinal deformity. *Spine (Phila Pa 1976)* 2006;31(3):303-308.

Weistroffer JK, Perra JH, Lonstein JE, et al: Complications in long fusions to the sacrum for adult scoliosis: Minimum five-year analysis of fifty patients. *Spine (Phila Pa 1976)* 2008;33(13):1478-1483.

Coding

CPT Codes		Corresponding ICD-9 Codes	
22630	Arthrodesis, posterior interbody technique, including laminectomy and/or discectomy to prepare interspace (other than for decompression), single interspace; lumbar	722.10 738.4 756.12	722.52 756.11 905.1
22632	Arthrodesis, posterior interbody technique, including laminectomy and/or discectomy to prepare interspace (other than for decompression), single interspace; each additional interspace (List separately in addition to code for primary procedure)	905.1 905.6	905.5 905.7
20660	Application of cranial tongs, caliper, or stereotactic frame, including removal (separate procedure)	805.0 805.02 805.04	805.01 805.03 805.06
20661	Application of halo, including removal; cranial	805.0 805.02 805.04	805.01 805.03 805.06
20662	Application of halo, including removal; pelvic	737.29 737.30	737.3 737.43
22840	Posterior non-segmental instrumentation (eg, Harrington rod technique, pedicle fixation across one interspace, atlantoaxial transarticular screw fixation, sublaminar wiring at C1, facet screw fixation) (List separately in addition to code for primary procedure)	170.2 342.9 343	342.1 342.90 343.0
22841	Internal spinal fixation by wiring of spinous processes (List separately in addition to code for primary procedure)	170.2 342.9 343	342.1 342.90 343.0
22842	Posterior segmental instrumentation (eg, pedicle fixation, dual rods with multiple hooks and sublaminar wires); 3 to 6 vertebral segments (List separately in addition to code for primary procedure)	342.1 342.90 343.0	342.9 343 343.1
22848	Pelvic fixation (attachment of caudal end of instrumentation to pelvic bony structures) other than sacrum (List separately in addition to code for primary procedure)	170.2 342.9 343	342.1 342.90 343.0

Chapter 64
Lumbar Scoliosis

Norman B. Chutkan, MD, FACS
John S. Clapp, MD

 Indications

Adult scoliosis has been defined as a curve in the coronal plane measuring greater than 10° in the skeletally mature patient. Multiple etiologies have been described for scoliosis, including primary (de novo) degenerative, progressive idiopathic, secondary adult (metabolic bone disease, tumor, limb-length inequality, and posttraumatic), and iatrogenic.

Consensus for surgical management of lumbar scoliosis has not been defined clearly in the literature to date. Our indications for surgical intervention in this patient population include progression of deformity resulting in spinal imbalance, a new onset or progression of a neurologic deficit, and intractable pain. These signs and symptoms often lead to a reduced quality of life and functional deterioration.

The most common clinical presentation is axial back pain, which can be accompanied by radiculopathy, neurogenic claudication, progressive neurologic deficit, and spinal imbalance. These findings also may exist in the absence of back pain. When considering surgical intervention, it is important to take into consideration the overall health of the patient, curve flexibility, bone quality, and the expectations of the patient (**Figure 1**).

Surgical management of patients with lumbar scoliosis can yield significant improvement in functional activity and pain relief. Posterior instrumentation is the mainstay of surgical correction. In selective patients with relatively flexible thoracolumbar or lumbar curves, anterior instrumentation may be considered; however, these patients tend to be the exception. Anterior column support with structural interbody grafting (anterior, posterior, or transforaminal lumbar interbody fusion) is associated with increased fusion rates and a lower incidence of hardware failure. Pelvic fixation is highly recommended in patients with long constructs that cross the lumbosacral junction (**Figure 2**).

Some patients with isolated radiculopathy may benefit from limited decompression. This may be considered in curves of less than 20° with less than 2 mm of lateral listhesis and radiographic evidence of autostabilization. Selective nerve root blocks are helpful in predicting successful outcomes in patients with primarily radicular symptoms.

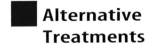

Contraindications

Surgical intervention in lumbar scoliosis is contraindicated in patients who are medically unable to tolerate major spine surgery. Other relative contraindications include severe osteoporosis, poor nutritional status, psychosocial disturbances, and unrealistic patient expectations. Caution should be exercised in patients with a history of chronic narcotic use and poor pain tolerance. Sedentary patients with low functional levels at baseline also should be considered with caution.

Alternative Treatments

A trial of nonsurgical therapy before surgery often is indicated in this patient population. Several options exist, including activity modification, nonsteroidal anti-inflammatory drugs,

Dr. Chutkan or an immediate family member serves as a board member, owner, officer, or committee member of the North American Spine Society and AO North America; has received royalties from Globus Medical; serves as a paid consultant to or is an employee of Globus Medical; and has received research or institutional support from Synthes. Neither Dr. Clapp nor any immediate family member has received anything of value from or owns stock in a commercial company or institution related directly or indirectly to the subject of this chapter.

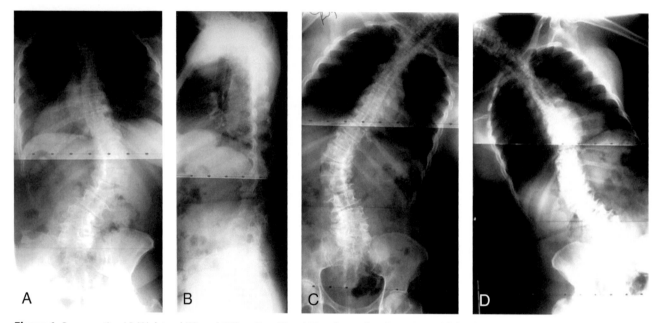

Figure 1 Preoperative AP (**A**), lateral (**B**), and AP bending (**C** and **D**) radiographs of a patient with lumbar scoliosis.

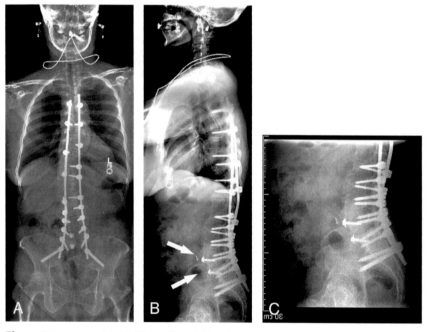

Figure 2 Postoperative AP (**A**) and lateral (**B**) radiographs and a focused lateral view of the lower lumbar spine (**C**) of the patient in Figure 1 show anterior structural grafts (arrows).

include pain relief and improvement in function and quality of life. Use of these modalities also can provide time for medical optimization before surgery, such as correction of nutritional deficiencies, treatment of osteopenia or osteoporosis, and increased stamina and cardiopulmonary reserve. Improvement of these factors can have a direct impact on postoperative recovery.

Results

Much of the literature concerning surgical management of adult lumbar scoliosis is retrospective (**Table 1**). Although surgical intervention has been shown to result in improvement in pain and function, there remains considerable concern for complications such as pseudarthrosis and adjacent-level degeneration. Improvement in outcome traditionally has been measured using many variable parameters, and evidence-based treatment is difficult given the many patient types and wide array of symptoms at presenta-

physical therapy, aqua therapy, and injections such as epidural steroid injections and selective nerve blocks. Fluoroscopically guided epidural steroid injections and selective nerve root blocks can be particularly helpful in

patients with isolated radiculopathy. Limited use of orthoses also may be beneficial. Patient education plays an important role in this process. The patient should be informed of the potential benefits of these therapies, which

tion. Overall, we believe that with proper patient selection and optimization before surgery, satisfactory outcomes can be achieved with surgical intervention.

———————■

Technique

Setup/Exposure

For an anterior approach for anterior column support of the lower lumbar/lumbosacral spine, the patient is placed supine on a radiolucent table and a muscle-sparing retroperitoneal approach is performed, usually by an access surgeon. For access to the thoracolumbar junction and the upper lumbar spine, a flank approach usually is undertaken. Recently, minimally invasive transpsoas approaches have been developed that allow placement of structural grafts above L5.

For the posterior procedure, the patient is placed prone on a spine frame, allowing the abdomen to hang free. A standard posterior approach is then performed. Hypotensive anesthesia with arterial monitoring can be useful in select patients for reduction of blood loss. Cell saver use also may be beneficial.

Instruments/Equipment/ Implants Required

Structural anterior column support can be achieved with allograft bone, metal cages, polyetheretherketone (PEEK) devices, or other implants (eg, carbon fiber). These may be placed via an anterior, lateral, or posterior technique. Pedicle screw fixation allows for correction of the deformity and increased fusion rates. Fluoroscopy and image guidance are useful in ensuring accurate placement of pedicle screws. Polyaxial screws can be helpful in reducing the load placed at the bone-screw interface in patients with significant deformity, particularly in the presence of osteoporosis.

Procedure

Once adequate posterior exposure is obtained, pedicle screws are placed in a standard fashion. Proximal and distal fixation of the construct is obtained, followed by sequential translation of the intervening vertebral bodies to correct the deformity. In lumbar curves, fusion to the thoracolumbar junction frequently is sufficient; however, care should be taken to avoid stopping at the apex of thoracic kyphosis. If concern for junctional kyphosis above the instrumentation is felt, then fusion to the proximal thoracic spine may be advisable. In patients with symptoms of radiculopathy and/or neurogenic claudication, laminectomies with decompression of the stenotic segments are performed. Facetectomies, particularly on the concave side of the curve, may be necessary to obtain adequate lateral recess and nerve root decompression. Facetectomies also may be necessary to increase flexibility for the correction of the curve and to allow access to the disk space. Patients with significant sagittal malalignment may require osteotomies for correction. The choice of osteotomy must be individualized to the specific patient.

Stopping the construct at L5 may be considered in patients with healthy-appearing lumbosacral disks and deep-seated L5 vertebrae (L5 vertebral body below the intercrestal line). In patients undergoing fusion to the sacrum, anterior column support at the lumbosacral junction increases fusion rates significantly and reduces the incidence of hardware failure. In long constructs, it is recommended that iliac screws be used for additional fixation. Placement of the iliac screws may be performed open, with exposure of the outer table of the ilium and visualization of the sciatic notch, or with the use of intraoperative fluoroscopy with oblique views of the iliac wings. Using a starting point on the inner table below the level of the top of the crest reduces the prominence of the iliac screws.

The choice of an anterior, lateral, or posterior approach for interbody grafting should be individualized to the specific patient. In patients with a history of prior abdominal surgery (particularly retroperitoneal procedures), a posterior approach may be more favorable. With male patients, it is important to discuss the associated risk of retrograde ejaculation. Structural interbody grafts (**Figure 2,** *C*) not only provide anterior column support but also may be used to aid correction. Posterior interbody grafting on the concavity of the curve is particularly useful in the restoration of disk space height. The decision whether to perform interbody grafting before or after posterior instrumentation may be individualized to the specific patient and the surgeon's preference. We typically perform anterior interbody grafting before posterior instrumentation; however, if posterior interbody grafts are used, they are generally placed after pedicle screw insertion. Focal compression and distraction also can be helpful in correcting segmental deformity; however, care should be taken to ensure that lumbar lordosis is not adversely affected, particularly with distraction.

The use of bone morphogenetic protein can be helpful in improving fusion rates, but in most cases this use is off-label. Spinal cord monitoring also is a useful adjunct, particularly electromyographic evaluation of the pedicle screws to confirm proper placement. The use of cross links can increase construct rigidity and is particularly helpful at the lumbosacral junction when combined with iliac screws (**Figure 3**).

In patients undergoing a limited decompression for isolated radiculopathy, care should be taken to avoid excessive bony resection. If it is necessary to remove more than 50% of the facet to achieve adequate decompression of the lateral recess, then consideration should be given to a concomitant segmental fusion. Minimally

Table 1 Results of Surgical Management for Adult Lumbar Scoliosis

Authors (Year)	Number of Patients/ Type of Study	Diagnosis	Mean Curve	Procedure or Approach	Staged
Swank et al (1981)	222/Retrospective	Idiopathic (160) Paralytic (44) Congenital (11) Miscellaneous (7)	80°	Anterior/posterior (multiple combinations)	Single stage, 174 (78%) Multiple stages, 48 (22%)
Grubb et al (1994)	53/Prospective cohort	Idiopathic (28) Degenerative (25)	58° idiopathic 28.6° degenerative	Anterior/posterior (multiple combinations)	50% 1 stage 50% ≥2 stages
Wu et al (2008)	26/Retrospective	Degenerative	16.5°	Instrumented PLIF	Single procedure in all cases
Kluba et al (2009)	26 surgical versus 29 nonsurgical/ Retrospective	Degenerative lumbar scoliosis	25° (range, 10°-66°)	Anterior/posterior (19) Posterior only (7)	Single procedure in all cases

PLIF = posterior lumbar interbody fusion.

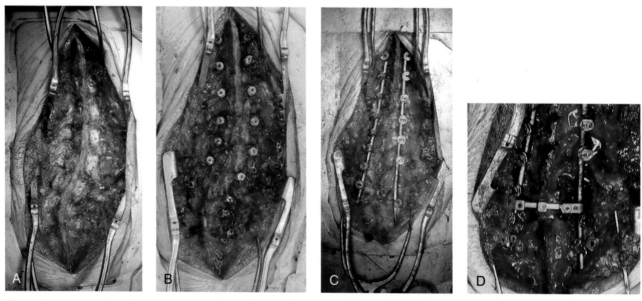

Figure 3 Intraoperative photographs of a patient with a significant scoliotic deformity show exposure (**A**), placement of pedicle screws (**B**), correction (**C**), and pelvic fixation with cross link (**D**).

Table 1 *(continued)*

Mean Patient Age in Years (Range)	Mean Follow-up (Range)	Complication Rate	Distal Extent of Fusion	Results
30.7	(3.4-4.3 years)	53% complication rate 11% pseudarthrosis 1.4% mortality rate	Increased incidence of pseudarthrosis with lower levels of fusion	68% free of pain Solid fusion 97%
40.9 (idiopathic) 63.3 (degenerative)	33 months	17.5% pseudarthrosis 36% revision rate in degenerative patients 25% revision rate in idiopathic patients	To sacrum: 67% (idiopathic) and 95% (degenerative)	Pain reduction 80% in idiopathic group, 70% in degenerative group Improved walking seen in both groups Improved sitting in idiopathic group Improved standing in degenerative group
64.2	3 years	19% adjacent segment degeneration, correlated with dissatisfied results	To sacrum: 7 of 26 (26%)	Oswestry Disability Index: 76.9% satisfied with surgical outcome
61.5 for surgical group	24 months minimum	11.5% pseudarthrosis 11.5% continued sciatica requiring additional decompression	Fusion ended before L5-S1 in all but 4 patients	Improved postoperative walking distance Reduced demand for analgesics

invasive decompression techniques are an attractive option but can be very demanding technically in the presence of significant deformity. Traditional laminectomies are associated with progression of the deformity (**Figure 4**) and eventual worsening of symptoms, and thus should be avoided if at all possible.

Wound Closure

Prior to closure, the wound is irrigated. The fascia is then closed using a 1-0 absorbable braided suture in an interrupted figure-of-8 pattern. A Jackson-Pratt drain is placed above the fascia, and 2-0 suture is used to close the subcutaneous layer. A deep drain also may be used when concern about poor patient hemostasis exists. Finally, staples are placed in the skin and a sterile dressing is applied before removal of the drapes.

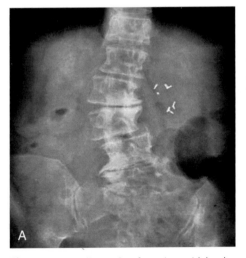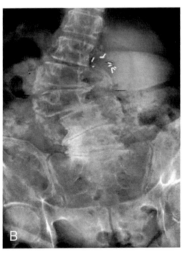

Figure 4 AP radiographs of a patient with lumbar scoliosis. Preoperative radiograph (**A**) and radiograph obtained following laminectomy (**B**) demonstrate progression of the deformity.

Postoperative Regimen

Monitoring in the intensive care unit may be necessary for patients with significant medical comorbidities or blood loss. Patients are mobilized as tolerated, typically mobilizing out of bed to a chair on postoperative day 1 and ambulating with assistance on postoperative day 2. Standard inpatient rehabilitation may be considered once the drain is discontinued and the

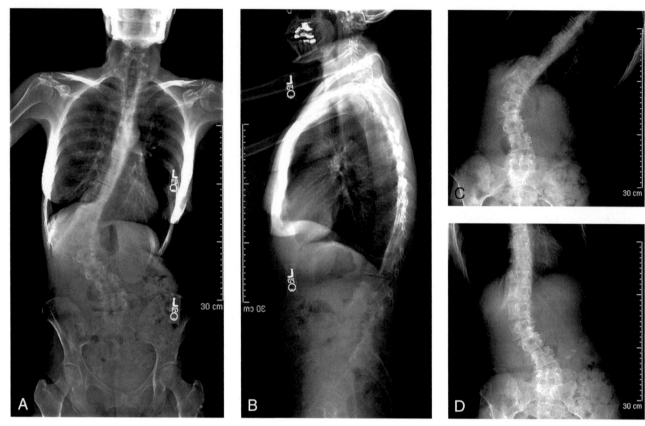

Figure 5 AP (**A**), lateral (**B**), and AP bending (**C** and **D**) radiographs of a patient with a significant scoliotic deformity.

wound appears to be healing adequately (usually 3 to 5 days after surgery).

———————————————■

Avoiding Pitfalls and Complications

Careful preoperative evaluation and planning are critical to reduce the risk of complications in this patient population. Patients should be medically optimized, with special attention given to correcting any nutritional abnormalities. A thorough review of imaging studies including full-length standing spine radiographs is mandatory (**Figure 5**). Sagittal alignment should be evaluated carefully, because postoperative sagittal malalignment

has been shown to correlate with poor outcomes. Every effort should be made to maintain or restore normal lumbar lordosis (**Figure 6, *A***). This may require a combination of anterior and posterior procedures and possibly osteotomies. Some osteotomies, particularly three-column osteotomies, can result in significant blood loss, and in some instances staged procedures may be necessary.

Patients undergoing long fusions to the sacrum are at significant risk for pseudarthrosis and implant failure even with anterior column support. The sacrum provides very poor bone for S1 screw fixation. Bicortical screw purchase or "tricortical" fixation at the sacral promontory may improve fixation. The addition of alar or S2 screws can be helpful, but they are limited in their ability to improve construct

strength. In most patients with long constructs, the use of pelvic fixation with iliac screws is recommended highly (**Figure 6, *B***).

Insertion of pedicle screws in patients with significant rotational deformity can be very challenging. Fluoroscopy and image guidance are both useful in determining correct screw orientation. Electromyographic testing of the screws may be used to detect any breaches of the medial pedicle wall. If any concern exists, then the pedicles should be inspected under direct visualization via a laminotomy.

Osteoporosis remains a challenge in many of these patients, most of whom are elderly. The use of cement to augment screw fixation can reduce the risk of fixation failure and screw pull-out. Augmentation of the vertebral body just superior to the instrumentation also may reduce the risk of adjacent segment fractures and kyphosis. It also is important not to neglect the medical management of osteoporosis in these patients.

Other complications such as infections, pneumonia, and urinary tract infections can be minimized with appropriate use of perioperative antibiotics, meticulous surgical technique, and early mobilization. Deep vein thrombosis prophylaxis also should be considered, particularly in patients who are slow to mobilize. Despite all these efforts, the complication rate for adult deformity surgery remains relatively high, and a frank and thorough discussion of possible adverse effects should be undertaken with each patient.

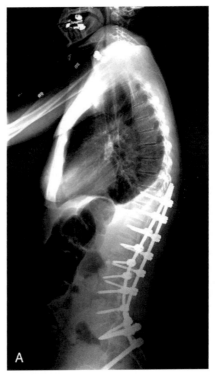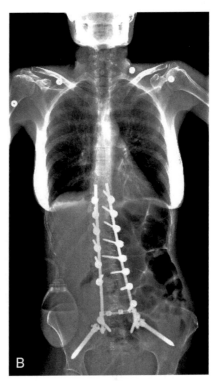

Figure 6 Postoperative lateral (**A**) and AP (**B**) radiographs of the patient in Figures 3 and 5.

Bibliography

Aebi M: The adult scoliosis. *Eur Spine J* 2005;14(10):925-948.

Anand N, Baron EM, Thaiyananthan G, Khalsa K, Goldstein TB: Minimally invasive multilevel percutaneous correction and fusion for adult lumbar degenerative scoliosis: A technique and feasibility study. *J Spinal Disord Tech* 2008;21(7): 459-467.

Anderson G, Albert T, Tannoury C: Adult scoliosis, in Spivak JM, Connolly PJ eds: *Orthopaedic Knowledge Update: Spine*, ed 3. Rosemont, IL, American Academy of Orthopaedic Surgeons, 2006, pp 331-338.

Deviren V, Patel VV, Metz LN, Berven SH, Hu SH, Bradford DS: Anterior arthrodesis with instrumentation for thoracolumbar scoliosis: Comparison of efficacy in adults and adolescents. *Spine (Phila Pa 1976)* 2008;33(11):1219-1223.

DeWald CJ, Stanley T: Instrumentation-related complications of multilevel fusions for adult spinal deformity patients over age 65: Surgical considerations and treatment options in patients with poor bone quality. *Spine (Phila Pa 1976)* 2006;31(19, Suppl)S144-S151.

Glassman SD, Carreon LY, Djurasovic M, et al: Lumbar fusion outcomes stratified by specific diagnostic indication. *Spine J* 2009;9(1):13-21.

Grubb SA, Lipscomb HJ: Diagnostic findings in painful adult scoliosis. *Spine (Phila Pa 1976)* 1992;17(5):518-527.

Grubb SA, Lipscomb HJ, Suh PB: Results of surgical treatment of painful adult scoliosis. *Spine (Phila Pa 1976)* 1994; 19(14):1619-1627.

Herron LD: Selective nerve root block in patient selection for lumbar surgery: Surgical results. *J Spinal Disord* 1989;2(2): 75-79.

Kim YB, Lenke LG, Kim YJ, Kim YW, Bridwell KH, Stobbs G: Surgical treatment of adult scoliosis: Is anterior apical release and fusion necessary for the lumbar curve? *Spine (Phila Pa 1976)* 2008;33(10):1125-1132.

Kluba T, Dikmenli G, Dietz K, Giehl JP, Niemeyer T: Comparison of surgical and conservative treatment for degenerative lumbar scoliosis. *Arch Orthop Trauma Surg* 2009;129(1):1-5.

Kostuik JP, Bentivoglio J: The incidence of low back pain in adult scoliosis. *Acta Orthop Belg* 1981;47(4-5):548-559.

Postacchini F: Surgical management of lumbar spinal stenosis. *Spine (Phila Pa 1976)* 1999;24(10):1043-1047.

Pritchett JW, Bortel DT: Degenerative symptomatic lumbar scoliosis. *Spine (Phila Pa 1976)* 1993;18(6):700-703.

Riew KD, Park JB, Cho YS, et al: Nerve root blocks in the treatment of lumbar radicular pain: A minimum five-year follow-up. *J Bone Joint Surg Am* 2006;88(8):1722-1725.

Swank S, Lonstein JE, Moe JH, Winter RB, Bradford DS: Surgical treatment of adult scoliosis: A review of two hundred and twenty-two cases. *J Bone Joint Surg Am* 1981;63(2):268-287.

Tribus CB: Degenerative lumbar scoliosis: Evaluation and management. *J Am Acad Orthop Surg* 2003;11(3):174-183.

Tsuchiya K, Bridwell KH, Kuklo TR, Lenke LG, Baldus C: Minimum 5-year analysis of L5-S1 fusion using sacropelvic fixation (bilateral S1 and iliac screws) for spinal deformity. *Spine (Phila Pa 1976)* 2006;31(3):303-308.

Watanabe K, Lenke LG, Bridwell KH, et al: Comparison of radiographic outcomes for the treatment of scoliotic curves greater than 100 degrees: Wires versus hooks versus screws. *Spine (Phila Pa 1976)* 2008;33(10):1084-1092.

Wu CH, Wong CB, Chen LH, Niu CC, Tsai TT, Chen WJ: Instrumented posterior lumbar interbody fusion for patients with degenerative lumbar scoliosis. *J Spinal Disord Tech* 2008;21(5):310-315.

Coding

CPT Codes		Corresponding ICD-9 Codes	
20937	Autograft for spine surgery only (includes harvesting the graft); morselized (through separate skin or fascial incision) (List separately in addition to code for primary procedure)	170.2 733.13 737.30	724.6 733.81
20938	Autograft for spine surgery only (includes harvesting the graft); structural, bicortical or tricortical (through separate skin or fascial incision) (List separately in addition to code for primary procedure)	170.2 733.13	724.6 733.81
22558	Arthrodesis, anterior interbody technique, including minimal discectomy to prepare interspace (other than for decompression); lumbar	567.31 721.42 722.52	721.3 722.51 733.13
22630	Arthrodesis, posterior interbody technique, including laminectomy and/or discectomy to prepare interspace (other than for decompression), single interspace; lumbar	722.10 738.4 756.12	722.52 756.11 905.1
22840	Posterior non-segmental instrumentation (eg, Harrington rod technique, pedicle fixation across one interspace, atlantoaxial transarticular screw fixation, sublaminar wiring at C1, facet screw fixation) (List separately in addition to code for primary procedure)	170.2 342.9 343	342.1 342.90 343.0
22842	Posterior segmental instrumentation (eg, pedicle fixation, dual rods with multiple hooks and sublaminar wires); 3 to 6 vertebral segments (List separately in addition to code for primary procedure)	342.1 342.90 343.0	342.9 343 343.1
22843	Posterior segmental instrumentation (eg, pedicle fixation, dual rods with multiple hooks and sublaminar wires); 7 to 12 vertebral segments (List separately in addition to code for primary procedure)	170.2 342.9 343	342.1 342.90 343.0
22844	Posterior segmental instrumentation (eg, pedicle fixation, dual rods with multiple hooks and sublaminar wires); 13 or more vertebral segments (List separately in addition to code for primary procedure)	170.2 342.9 343	342.1 342.90 343.0
22845	Anterior instrumentation; 2 to 3 vertebral segments (List separately in addition to code for primary procedure)	170.2 342.9 343	342.1 342.90 343.0
22846	Anterior instrumentation; 4 to 7 vertebral segments (List separately in addition to code for primary procedure)	170.2 342.9 343	342.1 342.90 343.0
22847	Anterior instrumentation; 8 or more vertebral segments (List separately in addition to code for primary procedure)	170.2 342.9 343	342.1 342.90 343.0
22848	Pelvic fixation (attachment of caudal end of instrumentation to pelvic bony structures) other than sacrum (List separately in addition to code for primary procedure)	170.2 342.9 343	342.1 342.90 343.0

CPT copyright © 2010 by the American Medical Association. All rights reserved.

Chapter 65
Pedicle-Based Posterior Dynamic Stabilization

Warren D. Yu, MD
Ehsan Tabaraee, MS, MD
Joseph R. O'Brien, MD

■ Indications

Spine fusion remains the standard surgical treatment of a wide range of painful spinal conditions, instabilities, and deformities. Patients undergoing arthrodesis are subject to several surgical morbidities, however, including approach-related morbidity, bone graft donor-site pain, pseudarthrosis, and adjacent-level degeneration. Nonfusion technologies have been developed with the goal of reducing arthrodesis-related morbidities. Implant types include total disk replacements, prosthetic nuclear implants, interspinous devices, pedicle-based dynamic stabilization, and facet replacements. Advantages of this class of devices include elimination of the need for bone graft, potentially reduced surgical morbidity, a theoretical decrease in adjacent-level disease, and avoidance of pseudarthrosis.

Several pedicle-based dynamic stabilization systems recently have been developed and are in various stages of

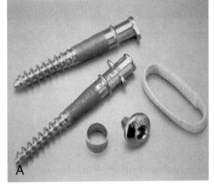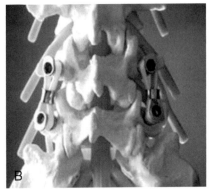

Figure 1 The Graf artificial ligament system. **A,** This system is composed of 5- to 7-mm titanium pedicle screws and looped 8-mm braided polyester bands. **B,** The Graf system in place. The bands are connected to the screws as compressive force is applied to the pedicle screws, to stabilize the surgical segment in lordosis. (Reproduced with permission from Kanayama M, Hashimoto T, Shigenobu K, Togawa D, Oha F: A minimum 10-year follow-up of posterior dynamic stabilization using Graf artificial ligament. *Spine (Phila Pa 1976)* 2007;32(18): 1992-1997.)

biomechanical and clinical evaluation. Posterior dynamic systems attempt to stabilize a spinal motion segment without requiring rigid spinal arthrodesis, theoretically reducing the risk of adjacent-level morbidity. Features common to this class of device include the use of pedicle fixation and

controlled motion at the index level. Variations in these devices occur predominantly in the differing biomechanics and materials of the interpedicular spacers that maintain motion at the index level. The Graf artificial ligament system (SEM, Montrouge, France) (**Figure 1**) and Dynesys dynamic stabilization system (Zimmer Spine, Minneapolis, MN) (**Figure 2**) have provided the longest clinical experience. Acceptable indications for the use of pedicle-based flexible rod stabilization devices are evolving constantly. In general, patients indicated for standard one- and

Dr. Yu or an immediate family member serves as a paid consultant to or is an employee of Zimmer and Kyphon and has received research or institutional support from Medtronic, Johnson & Johnson, and Stryker. Dr. O'Brien or an immediate family member is a member of a speakers' bureau or has made paid presentations on behalf of Stryker and DePuy; serves as a paid consultant to or is an employee of DePuy; and has received research or institutional support from DePuy and Stryker. Neither Dr. Tabaraee nor any immediate family member has received anything of value from or owns stock in a commercial company or institution related directly or indirectly to the subject of this chapter.

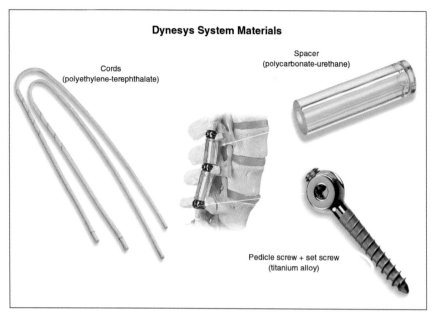

Dynesys System Materials

Cords
(polyethylene-terephthalate)

Spacer
(polycarbonate-urethane)

Pedicle screw + set screw
(titanium alloy)

Figure 2 The Dynesys dynamic stabilization system. The system includes a pedicle screw with a closed circular head. Through this head is threaded the polyethylene terephthalate (PET) cord, which limits flexion. The PET cord also is threaded through a polycarbonate-urethane (PCU) spacer that is placed between the pedicle screws. The spacer limits extension.

two-level instrumented fusions are potential candidates for pedicle-based dynamic stabilization. Common worldwide indications for pedicle-based dynamic stabilizations include grade 1 spondylolisthesis, spinal stenosis with moderate instability, recurring disk herniation, and degenerative disk disease with significant mechanical back pain. Before this surgical treatment is used, an appropriate course of nonsurgical treatment should have failed. Patients should have persistent mechanical and/or neurogenic symptoms, consistent with diagnostic imaging studies, requiring surgical decompression and stabilization.

Table 1 Results of the Graf Artificial Ligament System and the Dynesys Stabilization System

Authors (Year)	Study Type	Number of Patients	Approach	Mean Patient Age in Years (Range)
Graf system				
Hadlow et al (1998)	Retrospective review	53 (Graf) vs 30 (PLF)	Posterior	Graf: 42 PLF: 46
Hashimoto et al (2001)	Retrospective review	59	Posterior	61 (23-82)
Kanayama et al (2001)	Retrospective review	18 (Graf) vs 27 (PLF)	Posterior	Graf: 55 (32-73) PLF: 58 (28-79)
Rigby et al (2001)	Retrospective review	51	Posterior	41 (22-67)
Gardner and Pande (2002)	Retrospective review	40	Posterior	42 (17-60)
Madan and Boeree (2003)	Prospective randomized study	28 (Graf) versus 27 (ALIF)	Anterior (ALIF) Posterior (Graf)	NR

PLF = posterior lumbar fusion; JOA = Japanese Orthopaedic Association; VAS = visual analog scale; NR = not reported; ODI = Oswestry Disability Index; ALIF = anterior lumbar interbody fusion; LBP = low back pain.

Contraindications

Contraindications for pedicle-based dynamic stabilization include the general contraindications to spine surgery, such as acute trauma, active infection, systemic disease, or mental illness that would affect the patient's welfare or overall outcome. Relative contraindications include preoperative risk factors for the failure of standard spinal fusion such as obesity, smoking, multiple comorbidities, and medicolegal issues. In addition, malformations caused by scoliosis, severe spondylolisthesis, postlaminectomy destabilization, and multilevel disease (more than two levels) may need more rigid fixation than that provided by the flexible rod systems. In general, any pedicle-based device is unfavorable in patients with poor bone quality. The surgeon must be cautious when considering such surgery in patients with osteopenic, osteoporotic, or pathologic bone.

Alternative Treatments

Alternative treatments to pedicle-based dynamic stabilization include continued nonsurgical treatment, standard surgical fusion with rigid pedicle-based systems and bone grafting, and alternative posterior dynamic stabilization systems. Some nonsurgical options include weight loss, smoking cessation, abdominal strengthening, epidural injections, and pain management.

When used for isolated discogenic low back pain, decompression and fixation with rigid constructs has demonstrated higher fusion rates but not necessarily improved clinical outcome scores compared with uninstrumented fusions. Surgical fusion with rigid implants for stenosis and degenerative spondylolisthesis has demonstrated higher fusion rates and better clinical outcomes than uninstrumented fusion or decompression alone.

Other novel means of posterior dynamic stabilization include interspinous devices and facet replacements. Their effectiveness and indications are under investigation as an alternative to standard fusion.

Mean Follow-up in Years	Outcomes	Failure Rates	Conclusions
2.5	43% (Graf) vs 59% (PLF) good/excellent subjective relief	72% (Graf) vs 43% (PLF) by 2 years	Graf clinical outcomes worse at 1 year and higher reoperation rate at 2 years relative to fusion
3.4	Improved JOA and VAS scores at final follow-up significantly improved compared with preoperative values	NR	Effective for mild and early lumbar degenerative diseases with minimum flexion instability (<10°)
6	Graf had lower rate of adjacent-level degeneration radiographically and clinically	5.6% (Graf) vs 18.5% (PLF) reoperation rate for adjacent-level degeneration	Graf maintains mobility and sagittal alignment while decreasing adjacent-segment deterioration relative to fusion
4.25	Preop ODI 48 vs postop ODI 40 41% would have chosen not to have operation again	8%	Longer term results of this technique not encouraging
7	62% with excellent/good subjective scores 61% significant/total relief	23% had reoperations	Benefits of Graf ligamentoplasty are sustained in the longer term Revision rate high
2.1	93% (Graf ligamentoplasty) vs 78% (ALIF with cage) with satisfied results	0% (Graf) vs 4% (ALIF) reoperation	Graf results better than rigid fixation (ALIF with cage) in short term for patients with degenerative disk disease

Table 1 Results of the Graf Artificial Ligament System and the Dynesys Stabilization System *(continued)*

Authors (Year)	Study Type	Number of Patients	Approach	Mean Patient Age in Years (Range)
Graf system *(continued)*				
Kanayama et al (2005)	Prospective cohort	64	Posterior	66 (50-79)
Onda et al (2006)	Retrospective review	31	Posterior	61 (30-74)
Kanayama et al (2007)	Retrospective review	43	Posterior	58 (30-75)
Dynesys system				
Stoll et al (2002)	Multicenter prospective cohort	83	Posterior	58 (28-85)
Grob et al (2005)	Retrospective review	31	Posterior	50 (30-80)
Putzier et al (2005)	Retrospective review	35 (Dynesys + nucleotomy) vs 49 (nucleotomy alone)	Posterior	Dynesys 39 (23-58) Nucleotomy 36 (21-59)
Schnake et al (2006)	Prospective cohort	24	Posterior	71 (47-87)
Welch et al (2007)	Multicenter prospective cohort	101	Posterior	56 (27-79)
Bothmann et al (2008)	Prospective cohort	40	Posterior	NR
Ricart and Serwier (2008)	Prospective cohort	25	Posterior	71 (53-83)
Schaeren et al (2008)	Prospective cohort	19	Posterior	71 (47-87)
Würgler-Hauri et al (2008)	Prospective cohort	36	Posterior	58 (27-79)

PLF = posterior lumbar fusion; JOA = Japanese Orthopaedic Association; VAS = visual analog scale; NR = not reported; ODI = Oswestry Disability Index; ALIF = anterior lumbar interbody fusion; LBP = low back pain.

Mean Follow-up in Years	Outcomes	Failure Rates	Conclusions
5.6	VAS and sciatic symptoms significantly improved Flexion-extension motion average 4.7°	8% (5 of 64)	Procedure effective alternative to spinal fusion Degenerative slip not improved but motion maintained in 80% of patients
8.9	3.7 average decrease in VAS score 8.5 average increase in JOA score	6.5% (3 of original 46)	Provides stability and reduces symptoms of lumbar back pain and sciatica Viable alternative to rigid fusion
10	LBP and sciatica improved in degenerative spondylolisthesis and flexion instability Scoliosis and laterolisthesis associated with poor clinical outcome	7% reoperation	Beneficial for low-grade spondylolisthesis and flexion instability Limited use in scoliosis and laterolisthesis
3.2	Low back VAS improved 7.4 to 3.1 Leg VAS improved 6.9 to 2.4 ODI improved 54 to 23 Prolo Functional and Economic Scale scores also improved	16%	Safe and efficient in stabilizing spine Midterm results are highly comparable to fusion
2.8	Back VAS improved in 67% Leg VAS improved in 64% 50% had improved quality of life 68% would repeat procedure	19%	Reoperation rate relatively high No support for notion that semirigid fixation results in better patient outcomes than fusion
2.8	91% (Dynesys) vs 88% (nucleotomy alone) satisfied Minimal rate of disk degeneration observed in patients with Dynesys	0%	Dynesys use helps prevent progressive disk degeneration after nucleotomy for disk herniation
2.2	Significant reduction in leg VAS 87.5% satisfied and would undergo surgery again Radiographic implant failure high (17%) but none clinically significant	0%	Dynesys stabilization and decompression comparable to rigid fusions in elderly patients with spinal stenosis and degenerative spondylolisthesis
1	Leg VAS improved 80.3 to 25.5 Back VAS improved 54 to 29.4 ODI improved 55.6 to 26.3	10%	Early clinical outcomes promising Dynesys avoids greater tissue destruction and donor-site problems associated with fusion
1.3	73% had improvement on pain scores	27.5%	Better postop pain scores when done with nerve decompression Outcome data not superior to conventional rigid fixation
2.8	72% with very good results (defined by gains in clinical scores of >70%) 28% with good results (gains in clinical scores of 40% to 70%) No poor results	4%	Dynesys is acceptable alternative to fusion in degenerative spondylolisthesis at L4-L5 level
4.3	Overall satisfaction high and 95% would repeat procedure 47% with adjacent-level degeneration by 4 years	12% of original 25 revised	Excellent midterm results when used for spinal stenosis due to spondylolisthesis in elderly Results similar to instrumented fusion reported in literature Adjacent-level degeneration significant
1	73% excellent/good outcome on self-evaluation	19%	Outcomes for Dynesys stabilization after microdecompression do not reflect advantages compared with none or other stabilization systems High incidence of implant failure observed

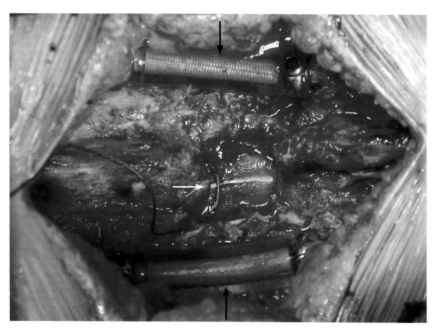

Figure 3 Intraoperative photograph depicts the standard midline exposure for the dynamic stabilization system implantation. The patient's head is to the right. Exposure is carried laterally to allow appropriate trajectory of the pedicle screw. The white arrow demonstrates the area of decompression. The black arrows depict the PET cords and PCU spacers.

Results

The Graf artificial ligament system and the Dynesys stabilization system are two implants with published short-term and midterm results. Table 1 summarizes clinical outcome studies of both systems. Other pedicle-based posterior dynamic stabilization devices include the Stabilimax (Applied Spine Technologies, Rocky Hill, CT), Isobar Dynamic Rod TTL (Scient'x USA, West Chester, PA), AccuFlex (Globus Medical, Audubon, PA), fulcrum-assisted soft stabilization (FASS), DSS Modular Stabilization (Paradigm Spine, New York, NY), Dynabolt (Vertiflex, San Clemente, CA), NFix II (Synthes, West Chester, PA), Axient (Innovative Spinal Technologies, Mansfield, MA), Potomac (K2M, Leesburg, VA), Cosmic (Ulrich Medical, Chesterfield, MO) and polyetheretherketone (PEEK) semirigid rod systems. Few clinical studies have been published about these devices. Biomechanical studies and case series have demonstrated that these devices show promise as alternatives to fusion with rigid pedicle screws systems, however.

Clinical trials have shown the pedicle-based flexible rod systems to be safe and effective. Average rates for revision and clinical outcome scores for back pain have been similar to those of standard fusion. Short-term and midterm radiographic and clinical data regarding decreased adjacent-level degeneration have been inconclusive, however. Overall, the clinical superiority of the pedicle-based posterior dynamic stabilization systems has yet to be proven definitively.

Technique

Setup/Exposure
The setup and positioning are similar to those used for standard posterior lumbar spine fusion. Prone or knee-chest positions are acceptable. The surgeon must take care to preserve the natural lordosis in the lumbar spine. Positioning with the abdomen hanging free will avoid pressure on the abdominal cavity that might result in excessive bleeding. Our preference is a Jackson table with standard chest, iliac crest, and thigh supports. The exposure is similar to that of standard posterior fusion. A midline incision is used, followed by dissection and lateral displacement of the paraspinal muscles (**Figure 3**). The goal of exposure is to reveal enough of the posterior column and in particular the transverse process for placement of pedicle-based screws. A caveat during this procedure is to use a greater than usual medial trajectory of the pedicle screws to avoid the index and superior facet joint and capsule, which require adequate lateral exposure of the transverse process. An alternative exposure uses the paramedian (Wiltse) approach. This exposure requires symmetric paramedian incisions located approximately 3 to 5 cm lateral to the midline, centered over the index level (**Figure 4**). Fluoroscopic localization often is helpful to determine the appropriate incision. The paraspinal muscles are divided below the posterior fascia. From L1 to L3, the division occurs between the multifidus and longissimus, and from L4 to S1, the division occurs between the iliocostalis and longissimus.

Decompression
Decompression is performed as necessary, depending on the pathology and clinical symptoms. A central decompression commonly is performed, followed by the necessary lateral recess and foraminal decompression (**Figure 3**). Because motion is preserved with this procedure, most implant manufacturers recommend preserving at least 50% of the facet joints to maintain adequate segmental stability.

Implants and Implant Insertion
A common feature in all pedicle-based posterior dynamic stabilization im-

Furthermore, histologic findings showed that CPC filled the screw threads and new bone formation occurred soon after surgery.

Coupler Connections

Pedicle screws augmented by coupler connections between bilateral screws have been studied. Single and double coupler groups were included in the testing. Both single and double coupler constructs improved pullout in the sagittal plane when compared with pedicle screws alone in cadaveric models with a BMD greater than 90 mg/mL. In cadaveric models with a BMD less than 90 mg/mL, however, the results were not significant.

Double Screws

The use of two small-diameter pedicle screws (double-screw fixation) implanted into a single pedicle also has been investigated. In a cadaveric biomechanical model, the pullout strength of the double-screw construct was not significantly different from that of single-screw fixation; however, stiffness and axial load to failure were increased significantly. The authors noted that, because of increased concern for pedicle breach, better adapted instrumentation is needed before this technique can be accepted widely.

Novel Screws

Expandable pedicle screws (EPS) also have been considered as an alternative treatment to pedicle fixation in osteoporotic bone. These screws are designed to expand within the vertebral body to improve purchase and screw-bone contact. Variations of these screw constructs include EPS systems that deploy fins into the surrounding bone, fenestrated outer screw sheaths that allow cement augmentation, and cannulated expandable pedicle screws augmented with cement. A review of the literature shows early promise for these novel screw designs.

Hydroxyapatite-Coated Screws

Hydroxyapatite (HA)-coated pedicle screws also have shown potential in the laboratory when compared with titanium-alone pedicle screws in osteoporotic bone. A study using osteoporotic beagle dog spines showed a statistically significant increase in mean resistance to pullout forces, up to 1.6 times that of titanium-alone screws. In addition, the HA-coated screws exhibited improved bony ingrowth as early as 10 days after surgery.

Concurrent Vertebroplasty Versus Balloon Kyphoplasty

An experimental cadaveric study investigated four techniques of pedicle screw fixation in osteoporotic bone: nonaugmented solid screws, perforated screws with vertebroplasty augmentation, solid screws with vertebroplasty augmentation, and solid screws with balloon kyphoplasty. The authors concluded that a perforated screw with vertebroplastic polymethyl methacrylate (PMMA) augmentation improved resistance to pullout and that balloon kyphoplasty was not superior to vertebroplasty in this application. Because of concerns over cement extravasation into the spinal canal, however, the American Academy of Orthopaedic Surgeons has recently released a strong recommendation against the use of vertebroplasty in osteoporotic spinal compression fractures.

Results

Many orthopaedic surgeons consider pedicle screw fixation to be the gold standard for fixation in the osteoporotic spine; however, this form of fixation is not without its concerns and complications. For this reason, industry and surgeons alike are constantly striving to develop more stable,

worry-free implants for this challenging patient population. Although many fixation and augmentation methods have shown promise in animal and biomechanical cadaveric testing (**Table 1**), few current, applicable clinical data exist. We recommend first attempting titanium pedicle screw fixation in these patients, with the understanding that the fixation may need to be augmented with laminar hooks or PMMA.

Technique

The senior author (J.J.A.) prefers to treat this difficult patient population with pedicle screw fixation. Despite being the most rigid form of fixation, pedicle screw fixation is not without its risks in the osteoporotic spine. As mentioned previously, a preoperative workup is essential in these patients. Preferably, this workup should be done by the patient's primary care physician or endocrinologist.

Instruments/Implants/ Equipment Required

The patient is positioned on a Jackson table. Standard instruments are used to perform a midline approach. We recommend neurophysiologic monitoring. Intraoperative fluoroscopy is used according to surgeon preference. Exposure can be achieved through many methods, which may include the use of rongeurs, curets, or Kerrison punches. A dural elevator, Woodson elevator, or Murphy probe can be used to palpate and localize the pedicles. The screw entry point is decorticated with a 5-mm ball-tipped high-speed burr. Pedicle screw holes are made with a pedicle probe or a No. 3-0 straight curet, and the pedicle walls are examined with a ball-tipped feeler. Fixation and closure depend on the particular implant and closure technique chosen by the surgeon.

Table 1 Results of Pedicle Screw Fixation in Osteoporotic Bone

Author(s) (Year)	Number of Patients	Mean Patient Age (Range)	Mean Follow-up (Range)	Fusion Success Rate	Results
Suzuki et al (2001)	33 (cadaver)	69 (46-89)	NA	NA	Pedicle screw vs pedicle screw augmented by single or double couplers. Pullout strength significantly increased with couplers in less osteoporotic bone but not significantly in severely osteoporotic spines.
Cook et al (2001)	21 with osteoporosis	49.8 (21-84)	35 mo (24-72)	86%	EPS system. 86% fusion in osteoporotic bone arm of study.
Taniwaki et al (2003)	14 (canine)	NA	4 wks	NA	Pedicle screws with CPC in osteoporotic bone vs pedicle screws alone in normal bone. Rigidity was similar and pullout strength greater in experimental group vs control.
Tan et al (2004)	24 (cadaver)	74.5 (48-90)	NA	NA	Pedicle screws augmented with laminar hooks, sublaminar wires, or CPC. All enhanced rigidity. CPC had less body translation.
Cook et al (2004)	21 (cadaver)	69.5 (45-84)	NA	NA	Pedicle screw fixation with and without PMMA. Increased pullout strength, stiffness, and energy to failure in the cemented expandable screw. Cemented conventional screw achieved pullout strength similar to noncemented expandable screw.
Hasegawa et al (2005)	2 (canine)	NA	10 days	NA	HA-coated screws vs pure titanium screws. Significantly increased pullout resistance with HA-coated screws. Histology showed new bone formation with HA coating and only fibrous tissue with titanium screws.
Takigawa et al (2007)	18 (cadaver)	82.7 (71-95)	NA	NA	NPS system with PMMA vs conventional screw. NPS showed significant increase in mechanical strength over conventional screw in pullout and cyclic load. No cement leakage into spinal canal or neuroforamina noted.
Jiang et al (2007)	72 (cadaver)	69.3 (61-79)	NA	NA	Double screw vs single screw. Increased stiffness and axial load to failure in double-screw pedicle screw fixation. All specimens were male and larger than average size. Further studies needed.
Fransen (2007)	3	81, 77, 74	7 mo	100%	Three case studies. Pedicle screw fixation with fenestrated screws that allow cement to be injected through implant. Author believes this provides additional stability.
Wan et al (2008)	6 (sheep)	NA	Group 1: 3 mo Group 2: 6 mo	NA	Osteoporotic femoral condyle fixation with EPS. Based on micro-CT and histology, EPS can increase stabilization as a result of bony ingrowth along the screws' expansive fissures.
Becker et al (2008)	5 (cadaver)	79.8 (72-89)	NA	NA	Nonaugmented solid screw vs perforated screw with vertebroplasty vs solid screw with vertebroplasty vs solid screw with balloon kyphoplasty. Vertebroplasty-augmented screws showed significantly higher pullout force than control.

NA = not applicable; CPC = calcium phosphate cement; EPS = expandable pedicle screws; NPS = novel pedicle screws; PMMA = polymethyl methacrylate; HA = hydroxyapatite.

Setup and Exposure

Setup and exposure do not vary from standard cases in which pedicle screws are used for fixation. After administration of general endotracheal anesthesia, the patient is placed prone on a Jackson table with appropriate padding over all bony prominences. Extra care is taken to handle osteoporotic patients gently during positioning, because pathologic fractures are much more likely to occur. Finally, as in any instrumented spine case, we recommend the use of neurophysiologic monitoring to mitigate neurologic damage and better ensure patient safety.

We have found that in most cases, standard, self-tapping pedicle screw systems are adequate for instrumentation of osteoporotic bone, but the surgeon should be prepared to augment standard fixation with larger-diameter screws, pedicle or laminar hooks, or PMMA. We prefer titanium implants to stainless steel because the elastic modulus of titanium is closer to that of bone. Having fluoroscopy and vertebroplasty equipment available also is recommended.

Standard exposure instruments are used to perform a midline approach to the spine, with exposure taken laterally to the tips of the transverse processes. Care should be taken to avoid fracture of the transverse processes because the surface area they provide for formation of a fusion bed is essential in the osteoporotic patient.

Procedure

Any decompressive portion of the procedure is performed using the surgeon's preferred technique, with care taken to preserve all excised bone to be used later as autograft material.

When decompression is complete, the identification of the pedicle screw entry points is performed using the described anatomic landmarks for the given level. If decompression has been performed at the level in question, the pedicle may be palpated directly with a dural elevator, Woodson elevator, or Murphy probe within the canal. Fluoroscopy also may be used according to surgeon preference. A 5-mm ball-tipped high-speed burr is used to decorticate the screw entry point. Then a pedicle probe or No. 3-0 straight curet is advanced carefully against resistance through the pedicle, using a "push-pull" technique to prevent plunging. Once the pedicle probe has been advanced through the isthmus of each pedicle, the screw holes are probed gently for cortical breaches with a ball-tipped feeler. Once each screw hole is confirmed to be sound, commercially available pedicle markers or disposable drill bits are placed in each hole in a different configuration on each side, and a lateral radiograph is obtained to identify any changes needed in trajectory or screw length.

Tapping is not recommended in osteoporotic bone because sharp taps are likely to create a false passage in soft bone and could lead to errant screw placement. Screws are placed in the standard fashion, ensuring that the screw with the largest possible diameter and greatest length is selected, to maximize screw-bone interface. Care is taken to evaluate the screw purchase at each level as the screw is advanced to detect poor purchase early. Transverse processes and any remaining laminar surfaces should then be decorticated with a high-speed burr, and bone graft should be placed over the desired fusion surface. Rods are placed in standard fashion, and final tightening is performed, taking care to use an anti-torque instrument to avoid placing undue stress on the pedicles. Fusions longer than two levels should be finished with cross connectors to further strengthen the construct.

If a pedicle is damaged during any portion of the procedure and concern arises over the ultimate integrity of the construct as a result, the surgeon must step back and carefully evaluate the options available. A well-placed screw that feels loose may be replaced with one of larger diameter. Before a screw is upsized, however, the pedicle walls should be palpated carefully to identify any obvious breach. Obtaining an imaging study to confirm screw location also is reasonable. Once the pedicle is confirmed to be intact, the larger screw may be placed.

If further investigation reveals that the pedicle is damaged significantly, consideration should be given to the use of laminar hooks at the level in question. In longer constructs with multiple other good fixation points, the surgeon may elect to leave the level uninstrumented on that side. Finally, in the rare case in which the quality of the bone is so poor that the screws seem to have wholly inadequate purchase, we recommend the use of PMMA augmentation. In this situation, vertebroplasty cannulas can be placed into the vertebral body through a prepared pedicle, and cement can be injected into the body under fluoroscopic guidance. Screws can then be replaced before the cement hardens, ensuring that the cement does not extrude into any pedicle of questionable integrity or, even more importantly, into the spinal canal.

Wound Closure

Closure is performed in the standard fashion. A drain may be placed if needed.

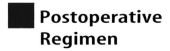

Postoperative Regimen

Patients with osteoporosis who undergo pedicle screw fixation should be braced appropriately for 3 months postoperatively. A custom molded rigid thoracolumbosacral orthosis is preferred. For constructs extending below L4, a unilateral leg extension is recommended. Electromagnetic bone stimulators may be prescribed to has-

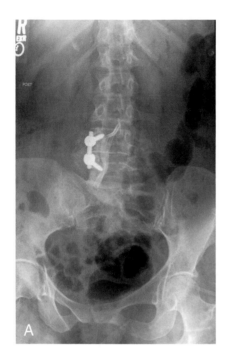
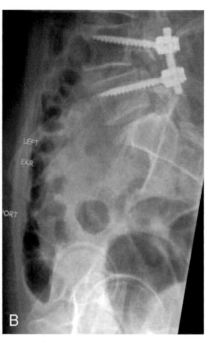

Figure 2 Postoperative AP (**A**) and lateral (**B**) radiographs of the lumbar spine of the patient shown in **Figure 1** confirm the placement of unilateral pedicle screws.

ten and ensure bony fusion. Postoperative physical therapy regimens should be advanced slowly to avoid undue stress on the construct. Radiographs are obtained at 6 weeks, 3 months, and 6 months and then every 3 months until fusion is solid (**Figure 2**).

Avoiding Pitfalls and Complications

Careful preoperative planning will help to avoid the most common pitfalls in the care of patients with an osteoporotic spine. The use of CT to evaluate pedicle size and morphology can ensure that the largest diameter, longest screws possible are used for optimal cortical bone purchase and maximal screw-bone interface. Knowledge of the severity of the osteoporosis can help the surgeon plan for cement augmentation and may lead to a decision to augment as part of the primary plan. Finally, the assessment of other risk factors, including corticosteroid use, tobacco use, diabetes, or other systemic illnesses, is of utmost importance.

Bibliography

American Academy of Orthopaedic Surgeons: *Clinical Practice Guideline on the Treatment of Symptomatic Osteoporotic Spinal Compression Fractures.* Rosemont, IL, American Academy of Orthopaedic Surgeons, September 2010. http://www.aaos.org/research/guidelines/SCFguideline.pdf.

Becker S, Chavanne A, Spitaler R, et al: Assessment of different screw augmentation techniques and screw designs in osteoporotic spines. *Eur Spine J* 2008;17(11):1462-1469.

Cook SD, Barbera J, Rubi M, Salkeld SL, Whitecloud TS III: Lumbosacral fixation using expandable pedicle screws: An alternative in reoperation and osteoporosis. *Spine J* 2001;1(2):109-114.

Cook SD, Salkeld SL, Stanley T, Faciane A, Miller SD: Biomechanical study of pedicle screw fixation in severely osteoporotic bone. *Spine J* 2004;4(4):402-408.

Fransen P: Increasing pedicle screw anchoring in the osteoporotic spine by cement injection through the implant: Technical note and report of three cases. *J Neurosurg Spine* 2007;7(3):366-369.

Hasegawa T, Inufusa A, Imai Y, Mikawa Y, Lim TH, An HS: Hydroxyapatite-coating of pedicle screws improves resistance against pull-out force in the osteoporotic canine lumbar spine model: A pilot study. *Spine J* 2005;5(3):239-243.

Hirano T, Hasegawa K, Washio T, Hara T, Takahashi H: Fracture risk during pedicle screw insertion in osteoporotic spine. *J Spinal Disord* 1998;11(6):493-497.

Jiang L, Arlet V, Beckman L, Steffen T: Double pedicle screw instrumentation in the osteoporotic spine: A biomechanical feasibility study. *J Spinal Disord Tech* 2007;20(6):430-435.

Kumano K, Hirabayashi S, Ogawa Y, Aota Y: Pedicle screws and bone mineral density. *Spine (Phila Pa 1976)* 1994;19(10): 1157-1161.

Shepard MF, Wang JC, Oshtory R, Yoo J, Kabo JM: Enhancement of pedicle screw fixation through washers. *Clin Orthop Relat Res* 2002;(395):249-254.

Suzuki T, Abe E, Okuyama K, Sato K: Improving the pullout strength of pedicle screws by screw coupling. *J Spinal Disord* 2001;14(5):399-403.

Takigawa T, Tanaka M, Konishi H, et al: Comparative biomechanical analysis of an improved novel pedicle screw with sheath and bone cement. *J Spinal Disord Tech* 2007;20(6):462-467.

Tan JS, Kwon BK, Dvorak MF, Fisher CG, Oxland TR: Pedicle screw motion in the osteoporotic spine after augmentation with laminar hooks, sublaminar wires, or calcium phosphate cement: A comparative analysis. *Spine (Phila Pa 1976)* 2004; 29(16):1723-1730.

Taniwaki Y, Takemasa R, Tani T, Mizobuchi H, Yamamoto H: Enhancement of pedicle screw stability using calcium phosphate cement in osteoporotic vertebrae: In vivo biomechanical study. *J Orthop Sci* 2003;8(3):408-414.

Vaccaro AR, Garfin SR: Pedicle screw fixation in the lumbar spine. *J Am Acad Orthop Surg* 1995;3(5):263-274.

Wan SY, Lei W, Wu ZX, et al: Micro-CT evaluation and histological analysis of screw-bone interface of expansive pedicle screw in osteoporotic sheep. *Chin J Traumatol* 2008;11(2):72-77.

Coding

CPT Codes		Corresponding ICD-9 Codes	
22520	Percutaneous vertebroplasty, one vertebral body, unilateral or bilateral injection; thoracic	733.0 733.01 733.09	733.00 733.02 733.13
22521	Percutaneous vertebroplasty, one vertebral body, unilateral or bilateral injection; lumbar	733.0 733.01 733.09	733.00 733.02 733.13
22522	Percutaneous vertebroplasty, one vertebral body, unilateral or bilateral injection; each additional thoracic or lumbar vertebral body (List separately in addition to code for primary procedure)	805.2	805.4
22523	Percutaneous vertebral augmentation, including cavity creation (fracture reduction and bone biopsy included when performed) using mechanical device, one vertebral body, unilateral or bilateral cannulation (eg, kyphoplasty); thoracic	733.13	805.2
22524	Percutaneous vertebral augmentation, including cavity creation (fracture reduction and bone biopsy included when performed) using mechanical device, one vertebral body, unilateral or bilateral cannulation (eg, kyphoplasty); lumbar	733.13	805.2
22525	Percutaneous vertebral augmentation, including cavity creation (fracture reduction and bone biopsy included when performed) using mechanical device, one vertebral body, unilateral or bilateral cannulation (eg, kyphoplasty); each additional thoracic or lumbar vertebral body (List separately in addition to code for primary procedure)	733.13 805.4	805.2

Coding *(continued)*

CPT Codes		Corresponding ICD-9 Codes	
22840	Posterior non-segmental instrumentation (eg, Harrington rod technique, pedicle fixation across one interspace, atlantoaxial transarticular screw fixation, sublaminar wiring at C1, facet screw fixation) (List separately in addition to code for primary procedure)	170.2 342.9 343	342.1 342.90 343.0
22841	Internal spinal fixation by wiring of spinous processes (List separately in addition to code for primary procedure)	170.2 342.9 343	342.1 342.90 343.0
22842	Posterior segmental instrumentation (eg, pedicle fixation, dual rods with multiple hooks and sublaminar wires); 3 to 6 vertebral segments (List separately in addition to code for primary procedure)	342.1 342.90 343.0	342.9 343 343.1
22843	Posterior segmental instrumentation (eg, pedicle fixation, dual rods with multiple hooks and sublaminar wires); 7 to 12 vertebral segments (List separately in addition to code for primary procedure)	170.2 342.9 343	342.1 342.90 343.0
22844	Posterior segmental instrumentation (eg, pedicle fixation, dual rods with multiple hooks and sublaminar wires); 13 or more vertebral segments (List separately in addition to code for primary procedure)	170.2 342.9 343	342.1 342.90 343.0
22845	Anterior instrumentation; 2 to 3 vertebral segments (List separately in addition to code for primary procedure)	170.2 342.9 343	342.1 342.90 343.0
22846	Anterior instrumentation; 4 to 7 vertebral segments (List separately in addition to code for primary procedure)	170.2 342.9 343	342.1 342.90 343.0
22847	Anterior instrumentation; 8 or more vertebral segments (List separately in addition to code for primary procedure)	170.2 342.9 343	342.1 342.90 343.0
22851	Application of intervertebral biomechanical device(s) (eg, synthetic cage(s), methylmethacrylate) to vertebral defect or interspace (List separately in addition to code for primary procedure)	170.2 342.9 343	342.1 342.90 343.0
72291	Radiological supervision and interpretation, percutaneous vertebroplasty, vertebral augmentation, or sacral augmentation (sacroplasty), including cavity creation, per vertebral body or sacrum; under fluoroscopic guidance	733.0 733.01 733.09 805.2	733.00 733.02 733.13 805.4
72292	Radiological supervision and interpretation, percutaneous vertebroplasty, vertebral augmentation, or sacral augmentation (sacroplasty), including cavity creation, per vertebral body or sacrum; under CT guidance	733.0 733.01 733.09 805.2	733.00 733.02 733.13 805.4

Chapter 68
Provocative Diskography in Spine Surgery

Eugene J. Carragee, MD

Indications

Provocative diskography is used to assess the possible contribution of an individual disk to an axial pain syndrome in a patient with severe disability. It is based on the theory that, absent other confounding factors, stimulating a symptomatic disk with a nuclear injection will be painful, whereas injecting a disk that normally is asymptomatic will not cause pain.

The use of provocative diskography in assessing patients with suspected discogenic pain is controversial. The test currently does not have a pathologic or imaging criterion standard (ie, gold standard) comparator to assess test validity. Therefore, the implications of a positive test are not scientifically clear. There has been no sensitivity or specificity analysis, but certain patient subgroups are generally accepted to be at higher risk for false-positive injections (**Table 1**). Professional societies and expert panels have published various guidelines and position papers regarding indications for the use of diskography inassessing possible discogenic pain (**Table 2**), all of which recommend careful consideration of patient selection factors when applying this test, if it is to be used at all.

Table 1 Subgroup Risks for False-Positive Diskography Injections

Subgroup	Risk Level	Means to Avoid Risk
Litigation	High	None
Psychologic distress	High	Pretest treatment or stabilization of psychologic problems, if possible
Multiple pain syndromes	High	Assess other pain syndromes for diagnosis type. Subjects with multiple pain syndromes who have vague diagnoses (eg, fibromyalgia, chronic myofascial pain syndrome, atypical chest or pelvic pain) likely are at greatest risk.
Analgesic/opioid dependency	Moderate	Avoid prolonged period without opioid/analgesic before diskography testing.
Previous disk surgery	Moderate	Patients who have had previous disk surgery are at moderate risk (25% to 55%) for pain with disk injection, whether they currently have pain or not.
Concurrent pelvic or spinal pathology (nondisk)	Moderate	No reliable method to exclude confounding pain nociception from nearby painful structures
Drug or alcohol addiction	Unclear	Not clear if previous drug or alcohol addiction confers an ongoing risk. Patients with ongoing drug and alcohol problems are poor candidates for diskography.

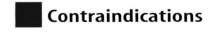

Contraindications

Several absolute contraindications to diskography have been established. As

Dr. Carragee or an immediate family member serves as a board member, owner, officer, or committee member of the North American Spine Society and the International Society for the Study of the Lumbar Spine; serves as a paid consultant to or is an employee of Orthokinematics, Intrinsic, BioAssetts, Simpirica, the Department of Justice, and the Department of Defense; has received research or institutional support from DePuy and AOSpine; and owns stock or stock options in Simpirica.

Table 2 Recommendations Regarding Provocative Diskography

Organization/Authors (Year)	Position	Caveats
American Pain Society Low Back Pain Guideline Panel/Chou et al (2009)	"In patients with chronic nonradicular low back pain, provocative discography is not recommended as a procedure for diagnosing discogenic low back pain (strong recommendation, moderate-quality evidence)."	"... even though positive pain responses with provocative discography are unlikely in healthy, asymptomatic patients without back pain, false-positive responses are common in persons without significant back pain but with somatization, other pain conditions, unresolved worker's compensation claims, or previous back surgery, and can occur even after incorporating low pressure threshold criteria."
Bone and Joint Decade 2000-2010 Task Force on Neck Pain and Its Associated Disorders/Nordin et al (2008)	Not recommended	"There is no evidence that pain reproduction on provocative disc injection identifies the injected disc as the cause of primary serious neck pain problems. There is weak evidence against provocative discography of the cervical spine in patients with neck pain. There is evidence (1 phase II study) that pain response to provocative discography cannot accurately distinguish between subjects with and without neck pain. There is no evidence that provocative cervical discography has clear utility in treating patients with neck pain (i.e., improves outcomes)."
American College of Occupational and Environmental Medicine (2008)	Not recommended for the evaluation of acute, subacute, or chronic low back pain.	None
COST B13 Working Group on Guidelines for Chronic Low Back Pain (European Guidelines)/Airaksinen et al (2006)	Not recommended for the evaluation of discogenic pain	There is moderate evidence that diskography is not a reliable procedure for the diagnosis of discogenic pain (level B).
International Spine Injection Society (ISIS)/Derby, Guyer, et al (2005)	Supports the use of diskography as a subjectively interpreted diagnostic test in select patients. "Discography is a test that is easily abused."	• Exercise caution when a positive pain response occurs (1) in a patient with psychologic distress; (2) with a high-pressure injection; (3) in a patient with a high opioid intake; (4) at the site of a previous diskectomy; (5) from multiple pain sources; or (6) in a patient with poor pain tolerance. • Pain that subsides quickly should be ignored. • All positive tests should be validated with a confirmatory pressurization.
North American Spine Society/ Guyer and Ohnmeiss (2003)	Supports the use of diskography in select situations	• Exercise caution in subjects with psychological factors influencing pain response. • Exercise caution in subjects with other pain sources in a common referred pain area. • Should not be used as a stand-alone test.

an invasive procedure, diskography is contraindicated in patients with serious and uncorrected platelet or coagulation disorders. Patients with suspected infection of the spine or surrounding structures should be excluded from this test. Finally, patients with allergies to the diskography dye must be assessed carefully to evaluate the risk of injection and whether pharmacologic prophylaxis is possible or reasonable.

Relative contraindications include the subgroups of patients unlikely to have meaningful results from disk injection. As noted in **Table 1**, these include patients with serious emotional distress, somatization tendencies, compensation disputes, multiple pain syndromes, and previous spinal surgery.

Finally, diskography, like any diagnostic test, should be considered only when the results will change the

prognosis or management of the disorder. For example, if spinal fusion will be performed whether the test is positive or negative, no reason exists to expose the patient to the discomfort, expense, and risk of the test. Conversely, a patient who is a poor surgical candidate because of medical illness or psychosocial factors will remain a poor candidate after the test regardless of the pain response to disk injection.

— ∎

Table 3 Results of Surgical Disk Operations Based on Diskography Results

Authors (Year)	Number of Patients	Selection Criteria	Procedure	Mean Patient Age in Years	Mean Follow-up in Years	Results
Madan et al (2002)	73	Consecutive cohort trial 32 screened with diskography 41 selected without diskography	Posterior lumbar interbody fusion	NR	2.4 (with diskography) 2.8 (without)	Outcomes not improved in the diskography screening group
Blumenthal et al (2005)	304	Single-level + lumbar diskography Highly selected cohort, excluded any psychosocial disorder	FDA trial of fusion versus Charité* disk replacement	40	2	Final ODI, 30-40 Final VAS, 30-40 70%-85% still taking opioid medications postoperatively; 50% working
Derby, Lettice, et al (2005)	17	Single level + lumbar diskography All with abnormal psychometric findings on SF-36 (MCS <40)	Anterior and posterior lumbar fusion	42.7	2	No significant improvement in PCS of SF-36 9 of 17 (55%) were worse on PCS
Carragee, Lincoln, et al (2006, *Spine*)	32	Single level + lumbar diskography Normal psychometric findings No compensation cases No other chronic pain processes	Anterior and posterior lumbar fusion	44	2	25%-30% high-grade results (VAS ≤2, ODI ≤15, return to work, no opioid medication) 40%-50% minimum acceptable results

NR = not reported, FDA = US Food and Drug Administration, ODI = Oswestry Disability Index, VAS = visual analog scale, SF-36 = Short-Form-36, MCS = Mental Component Summary, PCS = Physical Component Summary.

*Charité artificial disk, Depuy Spine, Raynham, MA.

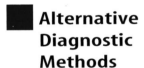

Alternative Diagnostic Methods

The best tool for diagnosing primary discogenic pain is a careful clinical history. The diagnosis is brought into serious question by the presence of such factors as multiple pain disorders, complex or chaotic social situations, a history of drug or alcohol abuse, inconsistent histories, litigation or compensation disputes in the absence of serious trauma, and psychiatric illness. The diagnosis of spinal pain from a single disk segment may be suggested by severe degenerative changes at that level on imaging studies. The presence of severe loss of disk height and modic changes around the end plates at a single level are imaging findings associated with high-grade relief of pain after surgical treatment. Conversely, normal or near-normal MRI findings indicate that the patient is less likely to have primary discogenic pain. Similarly, extensive deformity, gross instability, or severe spondylosis would suggest that discogenic pain is highly unlikely to be the primary pain generator.

Results

Most clinical series of diskography patients find that 70% to 90% of subjects have one or more disks that are painful when injected. It is unclear how many of these painful disk injections have discovered the primary cause of an axial pain syndrome. It also is unclear whether treatment options exist that have a high likelihood of relieving the axial pain syndrome by surgical or percutaneous techniques addressing the suspected disk.

The utility of diskography in determining outcomes of spinal surgery has been examined in a randomized clinical trial, which found it inferior to anesthetic disk injection. A meta-analysis was performed of the outcomes of spinal fusion in case and series reports of patients in whom diskography had and had not been used in patient selection. No advantage was found in outcomes when diskography-selected patients were compared with those selected for fusion on other clinical grounds.

In examining the outcomes of spinal fusion and other techniques for treating presumed discogenic pain, it appears that few studies in which diskography was used have followed rigorous outcomes determinations in multiple dimensions (pain, function, medication, and occupational status). Selected studies reporting these results are listed in **Table 3**. One study reported a best-case scenario, involving subjects with no known confounding factors to impede successful fusion outcome and positive single-level diskography. In this series, approximately 30% of these carefully selected patients had highly successful outcomes, and approximately 50% of participants achieved their minimum acceptable goals. Conversely, few patients (<10%) with single-level positive diskograms and significant psychologic comorbidities achieved even minimally successful outcomes.

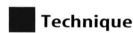

■ Technique

Setup/Exposure

ANESTHESIA AND POSITIONING

Provocative diskography requires the patient to be conscious and coherent enough to answer questions about the reproduction of pain. For that reason, it is essential to use adequate local anesthetic and as little general sedation as possible to keep the patient comfortable and yet avoid disorientation, uncooperative behavior, and somnolence. During debriefing after the procedure, the surgeon may ask procedure-related questions; consequently, the patient should be able to recollect the procedure if possible.

The back should be prepared and draped in a true sterile fashion. Careful positioning is important. The prone or lateral position is preferred by some diskographers. An oblique position also has been described, with the body at a 45° angle and rotated forward; this position may allow less movement during the procedure than the lateral position, because the patient is not balanced on the tip of the greater trochanter. The C-arm fluoroscope should then be positioned. Preliminarily tilting the x-ray beam cranially may achieve visualization of the disk space with the end plates appearing as a single line, facilitating optimal visualization of entry into the disk.

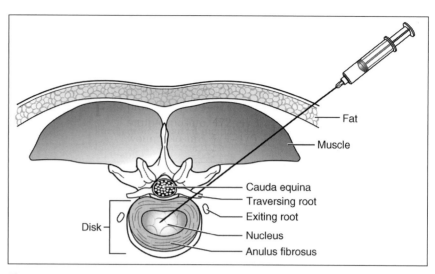

Figure 1 Drawing depicting needle placement for provocative diskography. The needles are inserted in an oblique extradural approach to enter the "safe zone" lateral to the facet and the traversing nerve root and posteromedial to the exiting nerve root. The annulus fibrosus is punctured, and the needle is placed in the center of the disk.

The C-arm may need to be tilted cranially to approximately 30° to 45° when approaching the lumbosacral junction.

ANTIBIOTICS

Some authors have advocated the use of a prophylactic broad-spectrum antibiotic such as cefazolin, clindamycin, or ciprofloxacin. Administration of the antibiotic can be intravenous, intradiskal, or a combination of the two. More recently, other authors have concluded that, when a double-needle technique is used, the risk of postdiskography diskitis is insufficient to justify the routine use of prophylactic antibiotics.

Instruments/Equipment Required

The procedure is performed with fluoroscopic guidance, and a high-resolution unit is preferred. A radiolucent table is required. The needles usually are between 22 and 25 gauge and 6 to 8 inches in length. Many clinicians use a double-needle technique, and the outer (stouter) needle can be curved gently to help placement at the L5-S1 level. Local anes-

thetic, antibiotic, and nonionic contrast are needed.

Procedure

Local anesthetic is infiltrated to the skin and sometimes the underlying musculature. Care should be taken to avoid the infiltration of local anesthetic as deep as the facet joint capsule or periosteum, because the anesthetic could spread to the foramen, epidural space, and margin of the disk, thus increasing the likelihood of a false-negative response from a generalized anesthetic effect.

The needles are inserted in an oblique extradural approach to enter the "safe zone" lateral to the facet and the traversing nerve root and posteromedial to the exiting nerve root (**Figures 1** through **3**). The needle should advance parallel to the end plate and pass just lateral to the superior articular process (SAP) yet medial to the exiting nerve root. The use of a curved distal needle tip, which can bend around the SAP yet allow positioning of the tip into the middle of the disk nucleus, has been advocated. The needles typically are placed on the side contralateral to the side on which the

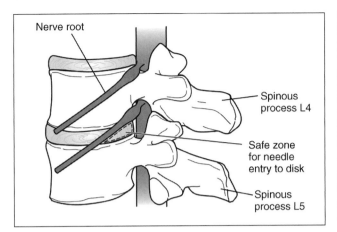

Figure 2 Drawing demonstrates the safe zone of needle entry into a disk. This anatomic "triangular working zone" avoids the exiting nerve root.

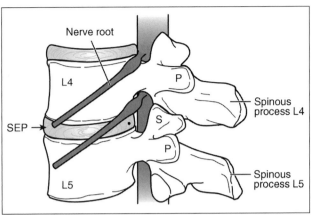

Figure 3 Proper positioning for L4-L5 diskogram. The superior articular process of L5 (S) is positioned midway in the superior end plate (SEP) of L5. Correct needle placement is shown by the black dot. P = pedicle of L4, L5.

pain is usually experienced. This is done to avoid confusing needle placement discomfort with injection pain; however, this thesis has been questioned by prospective analysis.

Placement of the needle in the center of the disk should be established by biplanar fluoroscopy or C-arm fluoroscopy, to be certain the injection will not extend into the anulus. Needles generally are placed in two or three consecutive levels. It is recommended that a low-osmolarity, nonionic contrast be used for diskography.

ASSESSMENT

The patient's response is reported with each injection into a disk. The patient should be comfortable and alert but remain unaware of the moment of injection, the level injected, and the amount injected. The most suspicious disk usually is injected last. After injection, pain response, injection pressure, and disk morphology need to be considered when assessing the diskogram.

Pain Response

As each level is injected, the patient should be questioned about whether pain is provoked. If so, the patient should be asked to compare this pain with the typical symptoms in terms of

quality and distribution. Pain responses are recorded at each level as: no pain, pressure alone, similar or exact pain (termed concordant), or dissimilar (discordant) pain. Pain usually is rated on a scale from 0 to 10. The patient should be observed for grimacing, distress, or other pain responses with injection.

Injection Pressure

The integrity of the disk can be determined by assessing the hydraulic pressure that the disk will hold with a defined injection volume. Pressure may dissipate rapidly or simply fail to increase in an incompetent disk secondary to leakage through the anulus or end plate. An intact disk/anulus and end-plate complex usually can hold pressure up to 90 mm Hg. It is essential to avoid pressures that are so high they produce false-positive results from end-plate deflection, facet distraction, or frank injury to the disk.

Disk Morphologic Characteristics

The contrast distribution within the disk, anulus, and peridiskal space may disperse into common patterns (cotton ball, lobular, irregular, fissured, ruptured) (Figures 4 and 5). The last two patterns, fissured and ruptured, contain fissures that extend

to or though the outer anulus. These patterns are presumed to be associated with the discogenic pain syndrome in some patients. The morphologic character of the disk can be further evaluated using CT after diskography; however, the utility of this additional test, which involves substantial radiation exposure, has not been demonstrated.

CRITERIA FOR A POSITIVE TEST

The basic criteria for a positive provocative diskogram are the reporting of "significant" pain upon injection (typically defined as ≥6 of 10 on a pain scale) and the reproduction of the patient's normal symptoms, not only in character but also in distribution. More recently, it has been proposed that disks can be classified on the basis of the pressure at which a significant pain response is recorded. Disks that produce a severe pain response at low pressures (<15 to 25 psi above opening values) have been termed "chemically sensitive" disks. Disks that produce a response at high pressures (>50 psi above opening values) have been termed "mechanically sensitive." Although avoiding high pressures is likely important, the utility of these low-pressure criteria has not been proven. Asymptomatic subjects have

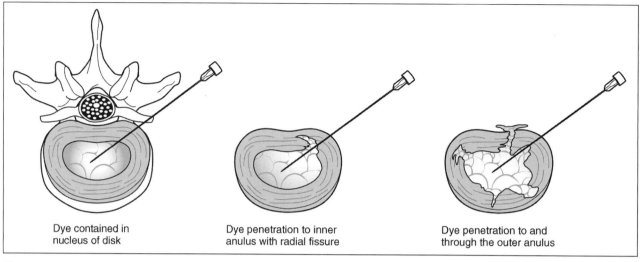

Figure 4 Common dye patterns with disk injection.

Diskogram type		Stage of disk degeneration
1. Cotton ball		No signs of degeneration. Soft white amorphous nucleus.
2. Lobular		Mature disk with nucleus starting to coalesce into fibrous lumps
3. Irregular		Degenerated disk with fissures and clefts in the nucleus and inner anulus
4. Fissured		Degenerated disk with radial fissure leading to the outer edge of the anulus
5. Ruptured		Disk has a complete radial fissure that allows injected fluid to escape. Can be in any state of degeneration.

Figure 5 Classification of disk degeneration patterns seen on diskography. (Adapted with permission from Adams MA, Dolan P, Hutton WC: The stages of disc degeneration as revealed by discograms. *J Bone Joint Surg Br* 1986;68:36-41.)

been found to have pain with relatively low-pressure injection.

Other criteria that sometimes are used to support a positive result include a "negative control" disk adjacent to a suspected symptomatic disk; an anular fissure to the outer anulus; physiologic measurements (eg, elevated heart rate with injection of the painful disk); exact pain reproduction only (ie, similar pain is not "positive"); or very intense pain only (≥7 of 10). Other authors have advocated challenging a positive diskography result with intradiskal anesthetic injection, followed by monitoring of pain relief and the ability to perform previously painful physical maneuvers. None of these criteria has been determined to establish the validity of a painful disk injection as a "true positive" finding for discogenic pain.

Postoperative Regimen

Patients usually are fit enough to leave the injection facility less than 1 hour after the procedure. If sedation is used, the patient should get a ride home and not drive for several hours. There are no specific activity restrictions after diskography. Patients should be cautioned regarding the signs and symptoms of infection but also counseled that this complication is very rare. Patients can bathe when comfortable enough.

Avoiding Pitfalls and Complications

Proper patient selection is the best strategy to avoid problems from this test. Many expert panels and organizations believe that this test has no value in the evaluation of axial pain syndromes. Clinicians who use the test must maintain a healthy skepticism about it, understand that the test may not be highly accurate, and avoid relying solely on the results of diskography without a general appreciation of the entire clinical situation. The most common pitfall is overconfidence in the results of diskography, resulting in a recommendation for invasive procedures that have little chance of success. Another pitfall is the use of diskography as a forensic test to evaluate a purported disk injury or the relative merits of a compensation claim. Clearly, this application of the test is not supported by any scientific medical evidence.

Finally, the surgeon must address the question of possible harm to the disk and the patient from diskographic needle puncture and injection. Patients with serious psychologic issues can experience exacerbation of their pain syndromes for many months after diskography, so diskography must be considered carefully in these patients. Furthermore, basic disk research has found that disk puncture in animal models can accelerate disk degeneration. Needle puncture in human cervical disks has been associated with rapid degenerative changes. Studies of experimental subjects undergoing diskography demonstrated progressive and clinically significant accelerated degeneration of punctured disks (with 22- and 25-gauge needles) compared with matched controls. The diskography subjects demonstrated greater disk height loss and disk signal loss and more disk herniations and end-plate reactive changes compared with controls. Furthermore, these changes were found predominantly on the side of the needle puncture and injection. Careful consideration of the risks and benefits of this currently poorly validated procedure is required.

Bibliography

Airaksinen O, Brox JI, Cedraschi C, et al: Chapter 4: European guidelines for the management of chronic nonspecific low back pain. *Eur Spine J* 2006;15(Suppl 2):S192-S300.

Hegmann KT, ed: *Occupational Medicine Practice Guidelines: Evaluation and Management of Common Health Problems and Functional Recovery in Workers*, ed 2. Elk Grove Village, IL, American College of Occupational and Environmental Medicine, 2008.

Blumenthal S, McAfee PC, Guyer RD, et al: A prospective, randomized, multicenter Food and Drug Administration investigational device exemptions study of lumbar total disc replacement with the CHARITE artificial disc versus lumbar fusion: Part I. Evaluation of clinical outcomes. *Spine (Phila Pa 1976)* 2005;30(14):1565-1575.

Carragee EJ, Alamin TF, Carragee JM: Low-pressure positive discography in subjects asymptomatic of significant low back pain illness. *Spine (Phila Pa 1976)* 2006;31(5):505-509.

Carragee EJ, Alamin TF, Miller J, Grafe M: Provocative discography in volunteer subjects with mild persistent low back pain. *Spine J* 2002;2(1):25-34.

Carragee EJ, Chen Y, Tanner CM, Truong T, Lau E, Brito JL: Provocative discography in patients after limited lumbar discectomy: A controlled, randomized study of pain response in symptomatic and asymptomatic subjects. *Spine (Phila Pa 1976)* 2000;25(23):3065-3071.

Carragee EJ, Lincoln T, Parmar VS, Alamin TF: A gold standard evaluation of the "discogenic pain" diagnosis as determined by provocative discography. *Spine (Phila Pa 1976)* 2006;31(18):2115-2123.

Carragee EJ, Tanner CM, Khurana S, et al: The rates of false-positive lumbar discography in select patients without low back symptoms. *Spine (Phila Pa 1976)* 2000;25(11):1373-1381.

Carragee EJ, Tanner CM, Yang B, Brito JL, Truong T: False-positive findings on lumbar discography: Reliability of subjective concordance assessment during provocative disc injection. *Spine (Phila Pa 1976)* 1999;24(23):2542-2547.

Chou R, Loeser JD, Owens DK, et al: Interventional therapies, surgery, and interdisciplinary rehabilitation for low back pain: an evidence-based clinical practice guideline from the American Pain Society. *Spine (Phila Pa 1976)* 2009;34(10):1066-1077.

Cohen SP, Larkin T, Fant GV, Oberfoell R, Stojanovic M: Does needle insertion site affect diskography results? A retrospective analysis. *Spine (Phila Pa 1976)* 2002;27(20):2279-2283.

Derby R, Guyer R, Lee SH, Seo KS, Chen Y: The rational use and limitations of provocative discography. *ISIS Scientific Newsletter* 2005;5:6-21.

Derby R, Howard MW, Grant JM, Lettice JJ, Van Peteghem PK, Ryan DP: The ability of pressure-controlled discography to predict surgical and nonsurgical outcomes. *Spine (Phila Pa 1976)* 1999;24(4):364-375.

Derby R, Lettice JJ, Kula TA, Lee SH, Seo KS, Kim BJ: Single-level lumbar fusion in chronic discogenic low-back pain: Psychological and emotional status as a predictor of outcome measured using the 36-item Short Form. *J Neurosurg Spine* 2005;3(4):255-261.

Guyer RD, Ohnmeiss DD, NASS: Lumbar discography. *Spine J* 2003;3(3, Suppl)11S-27S.

Madan S, Gundanna M, Harley JM, Boeree NR, Sampson M: Does provocative discography screening of discogenic back pain improve surgical outcome? *J Spinal Disord Tech* 2002;15(3):245-251.

Nordin M, Carragee EJ, Hogg-Johnson S, et al: Assessment of neck pain and its associated disorders: Results of the Bone and Joint Decade 2000-2010 Task Force on Neck Pain and Its Associated Disorders. *Spine (Phila Pa 1976)* 2008;33(4, Suppl)S101-S122.

Willems PC, Jacobs W, Duinkerke ES, De Kleuver M: Lumbar discography: Should we use prophylactic antibiotics? A study of 435 consecutive discograms and a systematic review of the literature. *J Spinal Disord Tech* 2004;17(3):243-247.

Coding

CPT Codes		Corresponding ICD-9 Codes	
72285	Discography, cervical or thoracic, radiological supervision and interpretation	723.0 724.1	723.1
72295	Discography, lumbar, radiological supervision and interpretation	724.2	724.02

Chapter 69

Computer-Assisted Spine Surgery

Choll W. Kim, MD, PhD
Ramin Raiszadeh, MD
William R. Taylor, MD
Steven R. Garfin, MD

Indications

Computer-assisted surgery (CAS), also referred to as computer-aided surgery, computer navigation, or surgical navigation, describes a closely related group of technologies that use preoperative or intraoperative images to localize surgical instruments in three-dimensional space in real time. Originally modified from intracranial frameless stereotaxy, CAS produces multiplanar views of instruments in relation to anatomy. Its advantages include reduced radiation exposure to the patient and the surgical team, increased accuracy, elimination of the need for cumbersome protective gowns, and clearance of the surgical field from the C-arm fluoroscope. In various surveys, surgeons indicated they were likely to use spinal navigation because of the reduced radiation exposure and elimination of the C-arm. The increased dependence on intraoperative fluoroscopy in spinal surgery presents a potentially significant occupational health hazard that could be mitigated in part by the use of navigation technology. In addition, elimination of the C-arm from the surgical field helps the surgeon avoid assuming uncomfortable positions to reach the surgical target and allows a second surgeon to assist from the opposite side. The use of CAS also reduces the need for uncomfortable lead gowns, providing additional ergonomic benefits (**Figure 1**).

Contraindications

Despite these advantages, the use of CAS in spine surgery has been limited. The main obstacles to the adoption of CAS among surgeons with little or no navigation experience appear to be the perceptions that it is not reliably accurate and is associated with a high frequency of intraoperative glitches, many of which appear to be related to software freezes and slowdowns that reduce the pace and tempo of the surgical procedure.

This suggests that a significant learning curve exists for effective use of CAS. During the learning curve period, extended setup times, intraoperative glitches, and wide variations in image stability erode user confidence. Significant improvements in software

Dr. Kim or an immediate family member serves as a board member, owner, officer, or committee member of the Society for Minimally Invasive Spine Surgery; has received royalties from Hydrocision; is a member of a speakers' bureau or has made paid presentations on behalf of Medtronic Sofamor Danek, Biomet, DePuy, Synthes, and Globus Medical; serves as a paid consultant to or is an employee of Medtronic, Synthes, and Globus Medical; has received research or institutional support from Medtronic Sofamor Danek, DePuy, Biomet, EBI, and Synthes; and owns stock or stock options in Hydrocision and Spinal Elements. Dr. Raiszadeh or an immediate family member serves as a paid consultant to or is an employee of Synthes and Sea-spine and has received nonincome support (such as equipment or services), commercially derived honoraria, or other non–research-related funding (such as paid travel) from Synthes and Sea-spine. Dr. Taylor or an immediate family member serves as a board member, owner, officer, or committee member of the Society for Minimally Invasive Spine Surgery, is a member of a speakers' bureau or has made paid presentations on behalf of Nuvasive, and serves as an unpaid consultant to Nuvasive. Dr. Garfin or an immediate family member serves as a board member, owner, officer, or committee member of the University of California San Diego, Spine Arthroplasty, the North American Spine Society, and the Orthopaedic Research Society; has received royalties from DePuy; is a member of a speakers' bureau or has made paid presentations on behalf of Biomet, Blackstone Medical, DePuy, Nuvasive, and Medtronic Sofamor Danek; serves as a paid consultant to or is an employee of DePuy, Kyphon, Nuvasive, Biomet, Blackstone Medical, Medtronic Sofamor Danek, Spinal Kinetics, Applied Spine, and Pioneer; has received research or institutional support from Abbott, Arthrocare, Biomet, DePuy, Kyphon, Lippincott, the National Institutes of Health (NIAMS & NICHD), Nuvasive, Stryker, Trimed, and the United Cerebral Palsy Research and Education Fund; and owns stock or stock options in Spinal Kinetics, AMS, and Pioneer.

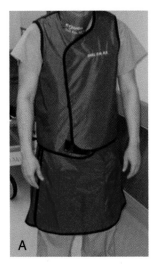 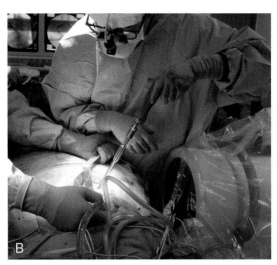

Figure 1 Ergonomic disadvantages of non-CAS procedures. **A,** When not using CAS, the surgeon should wear a full wraparound vest, skirt, thyroid shield, lead-lined protective glasses, and lead-lined gloves (not shown) for maximal protection against ionizing radiation. **B,** Encroachment of the C-arm into the surgical field often leads to awkward positions during key steps of the procedure, such as pedicle screw insertion. The proximity of the field generator also greatly increases the radiation dose effects.

and hardware technology to address these issues, combined with improved education and training programs using simplified techniques, will be needed for widespread adoption of this promising technology.

Results

The use of CAS during spine surgery, in particular instrumented lumbar fusions performed using minimally invasive surgery (MIS), has been shown to reduce radiation exposure to the surgical team and limit overall C-arm use. In experienced hands, pedicle screw insertion improves with the use of CAS (Table 1).

Table 1 Results of Computer-Assisted Spine Surgery

Authors (Year)	Number of Patients/ Specimens	Procedure or Approach	Parameter Measured	Results
Kalfas et al (1995)	30 patients 150 screws	Frameless stereotaxy pedicle screw insertion	Pedicle screw accuracy	149 of 150 screws inserted satisfactorily
Laine et al (2000)	100 patients	Randomized controlled trial of pedicle screw insertion: conventional insertion vs navigation	Rate of pedicle screw perforation	Perforation rate 13.4% in conventional group vs 4.6% in navigation group
Rampersaud et al (2000)	6 cadavers 96 screws	Pedicle screw insertion using fluoroscopy	Radiation exposure to surgeon	Dose rates 10 to 20 times greater than other procedures
Foley et al (2001)	12 pedicles	Pedicle screw insertion	Accuracy compared with real-time fluoroscopy	Close correlation between virtual image and real-time image Mean probe tip error 0.97 ± 0.40 mm Mean trajectory angle error 2.7° ± 0.6°
Kosmopoulos and Schizas (2007)	Meta-analysis 130 studies 37,337 screws	Thoracolumbar pedicle screw insertion	Accuracy of pedicle screw insertion	95.2% accuracy of navigated pedicle screw insertion 90.3% accuracy for non-navigated pedicle screw insertion
Sasso and Garrido (2007)	105 patients	L5-S1 instrumented fusion for spondylolisthesis	Surgical times	40-min reduction in surgical time using navigation
Kim et al (2008)	18 cadavers 10 patients	MIS TLIF using standard intraoperative FLUORO vs NAV	Radiation exposure to surgeon, surgical times	Increased fluoroscopy time (57.1 sec NAV group vs 147.2 sec FLUORO group) 12.4 mrem exposure for single-level MIS TLIF using FLUORO vs none with NAV No difference in overall surgery times

MIS TLIF = minimally invasive transforaminal lumbar interbody fusion, FLUORO = fluoroscopy, NAV = navigation-assisted fluoroscopy.

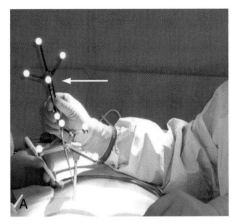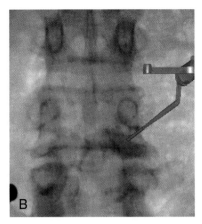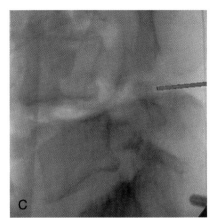

Figure 2 Use of the navigation probe to plan the incision and exposure in minimally invasive transforaminal interbody fusion (MIS TLIF). All images are captured in the navigation system at the beginning of the procedure, and the C-arm is taken out of the surgical field during surgery. The navigation computer stores all images as virtual images. Various navigation instruments can now be used with the virtual images, which are overlaid onto the image of the navigation tracking device. **A,** The navigation probe (arrow) is placed on the skin to plan the center of the incision and the trajectory of the approach. The patient reference tracker can be seen just below. **B,** AP fluoroscopic view depicts the tip of the probe docked lateral to the pedicles. **C,** Lateral fluoroscopic view shows the probe directly in line with the disk space. The tip can be extended by the navigation system to aid in alignment. The extension is shown in red.

Rampersaud and associates showed that MIS lumbar pedicle screw insertion can be associated with high levels of radiation exposure to the surgical team. Dose rates can be 10 to 20 times greater than nonspinal orthopaedic procedures. Kim and associates showed that using navigation during MIS transforaminal lumbar interbody fusion (TLIF) greatly reduces radiation exposure to the surgical team. Sasso and Garrido further showed that, in experienced hands, CAS reduces overall surgical time. Furthermore, the overall accuracy of pedicle screw insertion improves with CAS. Kosmopoulos and Schizas performed a meta-analysis of 130 studies and reported that the accuracy of navigated pedicle screw insertion was 95.2%, whereas nonnavigated pedicle screw accuracy was 90.3%.

Techniques

The use of CAS is most advantageous during MIS procedures that require significant real-time intraoperative fluoroscopy. The best-established MIS spinal fusion technique is TLIF. For the best results, the entire surgical team should be educated and trained in the use of CAS to minimize delays and intraoperative problems.

Instruments/Equipment Required

Because of the large number of additional instruments required to perform MIS procedures, combined with the additional instruments needed for CAS, it is useful to organize the instruments to be used in chronological order. These instruments include a CAS patient reference frame and set, an MIS retractor system, an MIS decompression tray, an MIS diskectomy tray, and an MIS pedicle screw system.

Image Acquisition

The patient reference tracker is placed into the posterior superior iliac spine using a 5-mm fluted pin (**Figure 2**, *A*). A standard 9-inch C-arm is fitted with the navigation tracker to allow image capture by the navigation computer. Multiple images of the lumbar spine are obtained and stored in the navigation system. During image acquisition, the surgical team can step away from the surgical field and behind lead shielding. No lead aprons are worn by the surgical team. Once the desired images are obtained, the C-arm is taken out of the surgical field. The navigation computer imports the fluoroscopic virtual images from the C-arm and relates them to the patient reference tracker, which in turn orients the navigation instruments and fluoroscopic images in three-dimensional space (**Figure 2**, *B* and *C*).

Surgical Technique for Navigation-Assisted TLIF

The navigation pointer is used to plan the incision (**Figure 2**, *B* and *C*). The entry point to a path directly in line with the disk space on the lateral image and down the lateral aspect of the facet joint on the AP image is marked (**Figure 2**, *C*). The skin and posterior fascia are incised, and blunt finger dissection is performed between the multifidus and longissimus muscles (**Figure 3**, *A*). A complete facetectomy and contralateral decompression are performed (**Figure 3**, *B* and *C*). Navigated, angled curets are used to perform a subtotal diskectomy from a

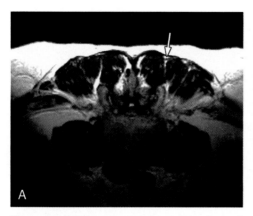
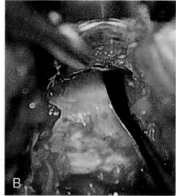
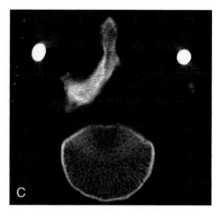

Figure 3 MIS TLIF using CAS. **A,** Axial MRI shows the intermuscular plane between the multifidus and longissimus muscles (arrow). Intraoperative photograph (**B**) and postoperative axial CT scan (**C**) demonstrate the facetectomy and decompression during the MIS TLIF technique.

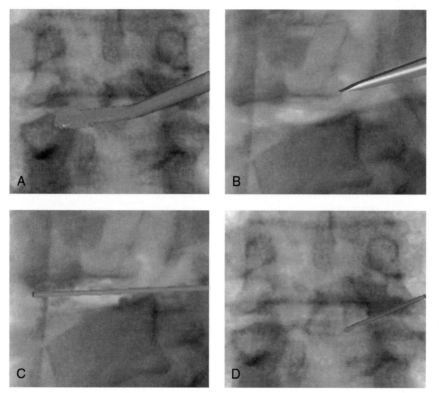

Figure 4 Computer navigation images demonstrate the use of CAS in MIS diskectomy and decompression. The surgical target site is the disk space within the Kambin triangle. Subtotal diskectomy is performed using various navigation instruments such as angled curets (**A**) and osteotomes (**B**). The navigation pointer is used to determine the extent of the diskectomy anteriorly (**C**) and the location of the interbody spacer relative to the midline (**D**).

unilateral approach (**Figure 4**, *A*). If necessary, a navigated osteotome is used to remove the overhanging rim of the posterior vertebral end plate during diskectomy (**Figure 4**, *B*). The navigation pointer can be used to de-

termine the extent of the diskectomy anteriorly (**Figure 4**, *C* and *D*). Fusion is performed using interbody spacers that can be placed anteriorly for maximum correction of lordosis (**Figure 5**). Final C-arm images are ob-

tained to confirm satisfactory implant position and spinal alignment. The surgical team may step away from the surgical field during image acquisition.

Surgical Technique for Percutaneous Pedicle Screw Insertion

CAS is particularly useful for MIS percutaneous pedicle screw insertion. Using a split-screen monitor, four separate images can be viewed simultaneously (**Figure 6**). The pedicle is entered using a navigation awl or Jamshidi-type needle. The availability of simultaneous AP and lateral images provides real-time multidimensional visualization. Navigated blunt pedicle probes and taps can be used to prepare the pedicle for screw insertion. The pedicle screw of the appropriate size is inserted with the navigation screwdriver (**Figure 7**, *A* and *B*). Rods are inserted percutaneously to minimize soft-tissue trauma (**Figure 7**, *C* and *D*).

Tomographic Three-Dimensional Navigation

Emerging technology such as isocentric C-arms and the O-arm can provide CT-like images intraoperatively (**Figure 8**). The use of axial images in particular aids in optimum screw insertion. Using the author's (C.W.K.'s)

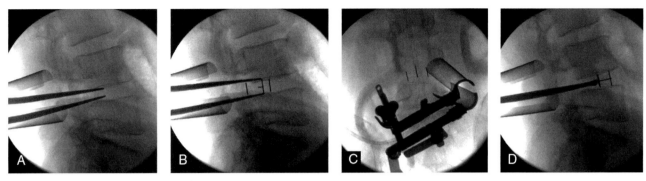

Figure 5 Intraoperative fluoroscopic views show, after a thorough diskectomy, special instruments opening the disk space and protecting the traversing and exiting nerve roots (**A**) as the graft is inserted (**B**). AP (**C**) and lateral (**D**) fluoroscopic views show the graft being pushed to the anterior rim at the midline of the disk space.

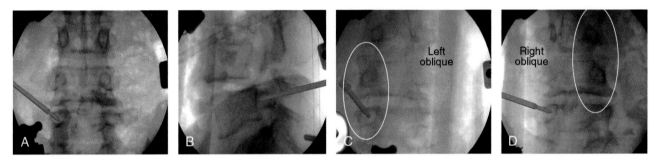

Figure 6 CAS in MIS percutaneous pedicle screw insertion. Using a four-panel split-screen format, AP, lateral, and oblique views of the spine can be visualized simultaneously. Trajectories in the AP (**A**) and lateral (**B**) plane can ensure optimum screw position. Oblique views (**C** and **D**) provide additional information to prevent pedicle breaches. The contralateral oblique is not necessary for screw insertion and thus alternate images can be used, such as another lateral image at a distant surgical level.

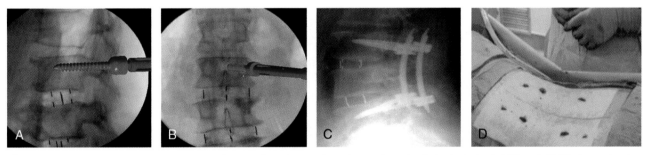

Figure 7 MIS pedicle screw insertion using CAS. CAS allows monitoring of screw insertion in both the lateral (**A**) and AP (**B**) planes simultaneously. Postoperative lateral radiograph (**C**) shows the percutaneous rod systems that allow fixation through small stab incisions. Intraoperative photograph (**D**) demonstrates the small incisions that minimize soft-tissue trauma.

10-point scoring system that grades six parameters of screw position, the accuracy of screw insertion can be assessed readily (**Figure 9**). Use of the O-arm during image-guided MIS pedicle screw insertion may improve the accuracy of pedicle screw insertion compared with image-guided fluoroscopy and standard fluoroscopy.

━━━━━━ ■

■ Avoiding Pitfalls and Complications

The reasons for the poor utilization of spinal navigation include increased surgical time, unreliable accuracy, and intraoperative glitches. Although numerous studies show that navigation reduces surgical times and increases the accuracy of pedicle screw inser-

tion, it is likely that a significant learning curve contributes to the poor utilization. The novice user will experience longer surgical times, greater deviations in accuracy, and an increase in the number of intraoperative software glitches that disrupt the tempo and pace of surgery. A vital step in avoiding pitfalls and complications is proper training not only of the sur-

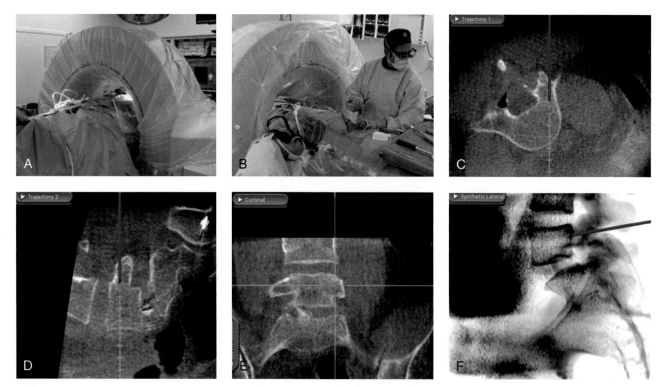

Figure 8 Computer navigation using three-dimensional imaging. Intraoperative CT-like images can be generated using isocentric fluoro-scopic tomography machines. **A,** Initial images are obtained with the surgical team away from the radiation field. **B,** Once images are uploaded onto the navigation computer, the fluoroscopic tomography machine is rolled out of the surgical field to allow the surgical team to operate in an unimpeded environment. Real-time axial (**C**), sagittal (**D**), coronal (**E**) and lateral (**F**) fluoroscopic images can be viewed simultaneously.

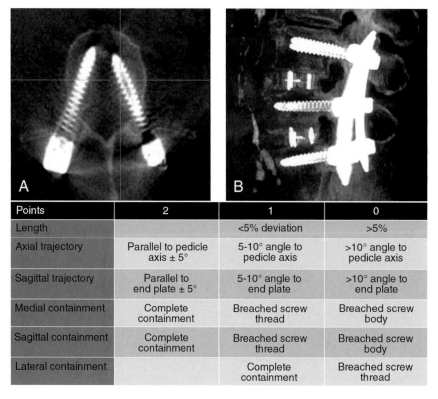

Points	2	1	0
Length		<5% deviation	>5%
Axial trajectory	Parallel to pedicle axis ± 5°	5-10° angle to pedicle axis	>10° angle to pedicle axis
Sagittal trajectory	Parallel to end plate ± 5°	5-10° angle to end plate	>10° angle to end plate
Medial containment	Complete containment	Breached screw thread	Breached screw body
Sagittal containment	Complete containment	Breached screw thread	Breached screw body
Lateral containment		Complete containment	Breached screw thread

Figure 9 The accuracy of screw insertion can be analyzed intraoperatively using axial (**A**) and sagittal (**B**) images. Screw accuracy can be assessed with a scoring system that uses a theoretically optimal screw as a reference standard. Screw placement is scored on six graded parameters: length; axial and sagittal trajectory; and medial, sagittal, and lateral breaches. A total score out of 10 possible points is calculated for each pedicle screw. The accuracy of screw length is assessed using axial images. The goal of screw placement is 75% of the length of the vertebral body. The goal of screw trajectory is placement within 5° of parallel of the pedicle axis for axial trajectory and the end plate for sagittal trajectory. Inferior-superior breaches are detected using sagittal cuts, and medial-lateral breaches are detected using axial cuts.

geon but also of the entire surgical team, including the radiology technician, scrub nurse, circulator, and surgical assistant. This remains a significant investment of time and effort.

Loss of accuracy appears to result from the bending of the navigated instrument or the shifting of the patient reference frame. The most vulnerable instrument is the navigation Jamshidi needle. Because of its thin shaft, the instrument may flex during insertion into hard bone. At L5 and S1 in particular, efforts to redirect the needle trajectory may lead to shifting of the navigation spheres out of plane to the axis of the shaft. Because the tip of the needle and the navigation spheres are on opposite ends of the instrument, bending of the shaft will lead to a discrepancy between the true position of the needle tip and the position seen on the navigation monitor. Great care must be exercised to allow the virtual image to display the instrument "as it lies," without any bending forces acting upon it.

Operating room personnel bumping into the patient reference frame is another common cause of accuracy problems. Unless the patient reference frame is positioned purposefully out of the surgical field, inadvertent jarring of the navigation frame is difficult to avoid. For navigated pedicle screw insertion, it is best to lean the reference frame medially and distally as it is inserted into the posterior superior iliac spine. This facilitates the trajectory of screw insertion, which is from lateral to medial and cranial to caudal at L5 and S1. A secondary reference point serves as a convenient verification method for navigation accuracy. If a readily recognizable bony landmark is available, then frequent matching of this position with the corresponding location on the navigation image serves to confirm that no egregious deviations were sustained. Awareness, combined with adequate training and education, offers the best means of avoiding this potential pitfall.

———————————■

■ Bibliography

Choo AD, Regev G, Garfin SR, Kim CW: Surgeon's perceptions of spinal navigation: Analysis of key factors affecting the lack of adoption of spinal navigation technology. *SAS Journal* 2008;2(4):189-194.

Foley KT, Simon DA, Rampersaud YR: Virtual fluoroscopy: Computer-assisted fluoroscopic navigation. *Spine (Phila Pa 1976)* 2001;26(4):347-351.

Kalfas IH, Kormos DW, Murphy MA, et al: Application of frameless stereotaxy to pedicle screw fixation of the spine. *J Neurosurg* 1995;83(4):641-647.

Kim CW, Lee YP, Taylor W, Oygar A, Kim WK: Use of navigation-assisted fluoroscopy to decrease radiation exposure during minimally invasive spine surgery. *Spine J* 2008;8(4):584-590.

Kosmopoulos V, Schizas C: Pedicle screw placement accuracy: A meta-analysis. *Spine (Phila Pa 1976)* 2007;32(3):E111-E120.

Laine T, Lund T, Ylikoski M, Lohikoski J, Schlenzka D: Accuracy of pedicle screw insertion with and without computer assistance: A randomised controlled clinical study in 100 consecutive patients. *Eur Spine J* 2000;9(3):235-240.

Papadopoulos EC, Girardi FP, Sama A, Sandhu HS, Cammisa FP Jr : Accuracy of single-time, multilevel registration in image-guided spinal surgery. *Spine J* 2005;5(3):263-268.

Quiñones-Hinojosa A, Kolen ER, Jun P, Rosenberg WS, Weinstein PR: Accuracy over space and time of computer-assisted fluoroscopic navigation in the lumbar spine in vivo. *J Spinal Disord Tech* 2006;19(2):109-113.

Rampersaud YR, Foley KT, Shen AC, Williams S, Solomito M: Radiation exposure to the spine surgeon during fluoroscopically assisted pedicle screw insertion. *Spine (Phila Pa 1976)* 2000;25(20):2637-2645.

Rampersaud YR, Pik JH, Salonen D, Farooq S: Clinical accuracy of fluoroscopic computer-assisted pedicle screw fixation: A CT analysis. *Spine (Phila Pa 1976)* 2005;30(7):E183-E190.

Resnick DK: Prospective comparison of virtual fluoroscopy to fluoroscopy and plain radiographs for placement of lumbar pedicle screws. *J Spinal Disord Tech* 2003;16(3):254-260.

Sasso RC, Garrido BJ: Computer-assisted spinal navigation versus serial radiography and operative time for posterior spinal fusion at L5-S1. *J Spinal Disord Tech* 2007;20(2):118-122.

Coding

CPT Codes		Corresponding ICD-9 Codes	
22630	Arthrodesis, posterior interbody technique, including laminectomy and/or discectomy to prepare interspace (other than for decompression), single interspace; lumbar	722.10 738.4 756.12	722.52 756.11 905.1
20660	Arthrodesis, posterior interbody technique, including laminectomy and/or discectomy to prepare interspace (other than for decompression), single interspace; lumbar	805.11 805.13	805.12 839.30
22840	Posterior non-segmental instrumentation (eg, Harrington rod technique, pedicle fixation across one interspace, atlantoaxial transarticular screw fixation, sublaminar wiring at C1, facet screw fixation) (List separately in addition to code for primary procedure)	170.2 342.9 343	342.1 342.90 343.0
22842	Posterior segmental instrumentation (eg, pedicle fixation, dual rods with multiple hooks and sublaminar wires); 3 to 6 vertebral segments (List separately in addition to code for primary procedure)	342.1 342.90 343.0	342.9 343

CPT copyright © 2011 by the American Medical Association. All rights reserved.

Chapter 70

Kyphoplasty and Vertebroplasty

Richard Todd Allen, MD, PhD
Frank M. Phillips, MD

■ Indications

Kyphoplasty and vertebroplasty are minimally invasive surgical procedures used for the treatment of painful vertebral compression fractures (VCFs). Both techniques use a percutaneous transpedicular or extrapedicular approach to access the vertebral body. Vertebroplasty involves the direct injection of bone filler, most commonly polymethyl methacrylate (PMMA), into the fractured vertebral body. Kyphoplasty involves the insertion of an inflatable bone tamp into the fractured vertebral body. The bone tamp is expanded to elevate the fractured vertebral end plates, thereby "reducing" the fracture. Subsequently, a viscous PMMA filler is injected into the cavity created by the bone tamp to reinforce the fractured vertebral body.

General indications for kyphoplasty include acute, painful pathologic VCFs resulting from osteoporosis, multiple myeloma, and other lytic vertebral lesions. It should be noted that according to a recent clinical practice guideline from the American Academy of Orthopaedic Surgeons

(AAOS), vertebroplasty is strongly *not* recommended "for patients who present with an osteoporotic spinal compression fracture on imaging with correlating clinical signs and symptoms and who are neurologically intact." Most pathologic VCFs are due to osteoporosis, a disease of decreased bone mass and microstructural collapse that affects more than 10 million Americans and is the underlying etiology of up to 700,000 VCFs in the U.S. each year. VCFs are the most common type of osteoporotic fracture and the most common skeletal complication of metastatic cancer. In patients with an acute vertebral compression fracture, vertebral augmentation may be indicated for pain that is refractory to nonsurgical management. The ideal timing of vertebral augmentation has not been well defined. There is evidence that painful subacute and chronic pathologic VCFs that have not healed can be treated successfully with kyphoplasty or, in certain patients, with vertebroplasty. Some evidence suggests that acute VCFs may respond to vertebral augmentation more predictably, in terms of de-

creased pain and improvement in kyphosis, than chronic (or subacute) fractures.

The reported advantages of vertebroplasty include a shorter procedural time and lower costs than those incurred with kyphoplasty. Rates of extravertebral cement leakage of up to 60% have been associated with vertebroplasty. Although in most cases the cement leak has no apparent clinical consequence, neurologic compromise and an increased risk of adjacent-level VCF have been reported. Kyphoplasty has been associated with lower rates of cement leakage (generally <10%) and generally modest improvements in vertebral height and local kyphosis correction.

────────■

■ Contraindications

Kyphoplasty and vertebroplasty are contraindicated in patients with spinal infections, coagulopathies, burst fractures with significant bony retropulsion into the spinal canal, VCFs with neurologic deficit, and allergies to bone filler or contrast media. Additionally, advanced vertebral collapse ("vertebra plana") may limit safe access to the vertebral body and make the procedure inadvisable.

────────■

Dr. Allen or an immediate family member has received research or institutional support from DePuy and Medtronic Sofamor Danek. Dr. Phillips or an immediate family member has received royalties from DePuy and Nuvasive; serves as a paid consultant to DePuy, Kyphon, AxioMed, and Flexuspine; has received research or institutional support from Cervitech, Nuvasive, and Stryker; and owns stock or stock options in AxioMed, Nuvasive, Arcus, SpinalMotion, Spinal Kinetics, Salient Surgical Technologies, and Flexuspine.

Alternative Treatments

Nonsurgical Treatments of VCFs

Nonsurgical treatments of symptomatic VCFs related to osteoporosis have variable effectiveness. Treatments include activity modification after a short period of bed rest, braces/orthoses, functional rehabilitation, and medications such as analgesics and anti-inflammatory drugs. Many of these nonsurgical treatments, such as anti-inflammatory drugs, narcotics, and braces/orthoses, are not well tolerated in the elderly. Some evidence suggests that an L2 nerve root block may be beneficial for mid-lumbar VCFs. Even when acute fracture pain resolves, a considerable number of patients with VCFs develop chronic symptoms related to kyphotic deformity, including chronic pain, impaired functional and ambulatory ability, compromised pulmonary function, and increased risk of further fractures. Recent AAOS guidelines, based on a systematic literature review, suggest that the following nonsurgical treatments may be beneficial in select cases. In cases of osteoporotic VCFs seen within 5 days of fracture symptoms, a 4-week course of calcitonin may be beneficial. Additionally, the use of ibandronate and strontium ranelate have been reported to help prevent additional symptomatic VCFs in patients with existing osteoporotic VCFs.

The adverse consequences of osteoporotic VCFs are well described in the literature. Nonsurgical care or natural history does not predictably restore function, improve quality of life, or prevent deformity. In matched cohorts of patients with osteoporotic vertebral and hip fractures, VCFs produced more severe impairments than hip fracture at up to 30-month follow-up. Several studies have documented that VCF-related deformity, independent of acute fracture pain, profoundly impairs physical function, health, quality of life, and survival. When compared with patients without vertebral deformities, those with deformity resulting from VCFs spend more days in bed; have a lower peak expiratory flow; have lower performance scores for walking, standing, and self-care; and have worse scores on health-related quality of life questionnaires. Several studies confirm reductions in health-related quality of life with increased number and severity of VCF-related deformities.

Surgical Alternatives for the Treatment of VCFs

Conventional reconstructive surgery is usually reserved for patients with neurologic deficit and/or severe deformity as a result of osteoporotic VCFs. Surgery in this setting typically involves instrumented stabilization and neural decompression. Poor bone quality places these patients at risk for instrumentation failure and adjacent-segment fracture. Although this form of surgical management may be necessary in some patients, such procedures have high morbidity and complication rates and are typically poorly tolerated by elderly patients.

Results

Vertebral Augmentation

Clinical case series, prospective studies, and systematic meta-analyses have reported on the efficacy of kyphoplasty and vertebroplasty in treating symptomatic VCFs (**Table 1**). Both procedures are reported to provide good short- and long-term pain relief and improve function and have good safety profiles. Two recent randomized controlled trials comparing vertebroplasty with a sham procedure have created contention about the efficacy of the procedure. Potential flaws confounding the outcomes of these studies such as low patient accrual rates at busy centers, inclusion of patients with chronic fractures, sham design, and radiographic evaluation of fractures without clinical correlation significantly limit conclusions that may be drawn.

One recent multicenter, prospective, randomized study in Europe reported that patients treated with kyphoplasty demonstrated statistically significant improvements in quality of life (according to results of the Short Form Health Survey-36 and the EuroQol EQ-5D questionnaire) and reduced back pain and disability, compared with the nonsurgical control. One access device–related adverse event (a soft-tissue hematoma at the surgical site) and one procedure-related adverse event (a postoperative urinary tract infection) were reported. After vertebral augmentation of symptomatic osteoporosis-related VCFs, 80% to 90% of patients experienced rapid and lasting pain relief. In addition, kyphoplasty may improve vertebral body height and decrease local kyphosis. Global sagittal balance may not be affected, however, particularly if fewer than three levels are treated.

Overall, serious adverse events are rare with both vertebroplasty and kyphoplasty. A comparative, comprehensive literature review of safety and efficacy outcomes showed that cement leakage is the most common complication, occurring in 8% of kyphoplasty procedures and in 40% of vertebroplasty procedures. Other reported complications that are rare but are notably more common with vertebroplasty than with kyphoplasty include pulmonary embolism (1.8% versus 0.3%, respectively), spinal cord compression (0.5% versus 0%), and radiculopathy (2.5% versus 0.3%).

Adjacent-Level Fracture Risk

Patients with osteoporotic vertebral fractures have an increased risk of future vertebral fracture, and the risk increases with each additional fracture. Lunt and colleagues found that among

Table 1 Results of Kyphoplasty or Vertebroplasty for Symptomatic Osteoporotic VCFs

Authors (Year)	Number of Patients	Mean Follow-up (Range)	Study Design	Mean Patient Age in Years (Range)	Outcome Measures	Results
Grohs et al (2005)	KP = 28 V = 23	24 months	Prospective, non-randomized comparison	KP: 70 (65-74) V: 70 (64-77)	Pain scores Kyphotic wedging of vertebrae ODI scores	No significant difference in V versus KP postop (pain decreased by half postop) KP (not V) decreased kyphotic wedging by 6° Significantly decreased ODI scores at 1 year with KP only Benefits sustained only by KP at 2 months and 2 years
Alvarez et al (2006)	V = 101 NS = 27	12 months	Prospective, double-cohort	V: 73.3 (52-90) NS: 69.7 (46-80)	VAS pain scores	V group: higher baseline VAS scores V group had significantly better pain and function scores at 3 months No significant differences at 6 or 12 months
Köse et al (2006)	V = 16 (28 levels) KP = 18 (22 levels)	12 months	Retrospective comparison	V: 62.2 (45-80) KP: 63.7 (48-82)	50-point VAS pain score	Both V and KP significantly reduced pain, but KP had significantly greater pain relief at 6 and 12 months KP decreased pain from 36 preop to 12.13, 8.63, and 9.72 at 6 weeks, 6 months, and 12 months, respectively
Voormolen et al (2007)	V = 18 NS ("optimal pain medication") = 16	2 weeks 12 months	Prospective, randomized controlled trial	V: 72 (59-84) NS: 74 (55-88)	VAS pain scores Analgesic use QUALEFFO RMD scores	High crossover: 14 patients in NS group requested V within 2 weeks, severely limiting study results VAS 4.9 (V) versus 6.4 (NS) at 2 weeks Significantly better pain relief, less analgesic use, and improvement in mobility, function, and stature (all short-term) in V versus NS treatment (VAS scores significantly better without the 2 patients with a new VCF)
Wardlaw et al (2009) (FREE trial)	KP = 149 NS = 151	12 months	Prospective, randomized controlled trial	KP: 72.2 ± 9.3 NS: 74.1 ± 9.4	Primary outcome: SF-36 PCS different at 1 month Secondary outcomes: quality of life, efficacy, and safety	SF-36 PCS improved by 7.2 pts in KP versus 2.0 pts in NS group ($P < 0.0001$)

VCF = vertebral compression fracture; KP = kyphoplasty; V = vertebroplasty; ODI = Oswestry Disability Index; NS = nonsurgical; VAS = visual analog scale; QUALEFFO = Quality of Life Questionnaire of European Foundation for Osteoporosis; RMD = Roland-Morris Disability Questionnaire; FREE = fracture reduction evaluation; SF-36 = Short Form Health Survey-36; PCS = Physical Component Score.

patients medically managed for osteoporosis, those with one, two, or three compression fractures had a threefold, ninefold, or twenty-threefold increased risk, respectively, of additional fracture compared with patients with no compression fractures matched for age and bone mineral density. Spinal biomechanics may explain the increased risk of future fracture, at least in part. In spinal kyphosis resulting from vertebral fractures, forces on the

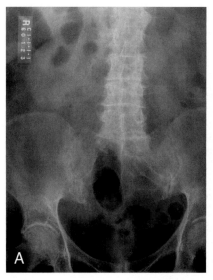
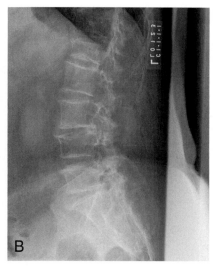
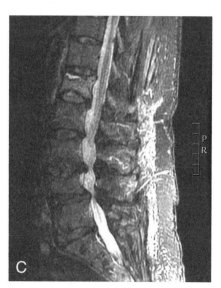

Figure 1 AP (**A**) and lateral (**B**) radiographs demonstrate osteoporotic VCFs at L1 and L4. **C,** Sagittal STIR MRI shows compression fractures at L1 and L4, with associated bony edema primarily at L1.

anterior spine are increased, thereby increasing loads on the vertebral bodies, resulting in an increased risk of fracture. Controversy exists as to whether the risk of additional VCFs is higher following vertebral augmentation than for natural history alone. Cement leakage into the disk during vertebral augmentation has been reported to increase adjacent-level VCF risk, and patients with severe osteoporosis have a higher incidence of adjacent level fracture, possibly because of the severity of their disease (**Table 1**).

■ Technique

Preoperative Workup
Preoperative clinical history and examination are important to determine the acuity of any VCF and to determine whether the fracture is indeed the source of pain. Radiographs are useful for defining the bony vertebral anatomy and help in planning an appropriate trajectory for the procedure (**Figure 1**, *A* and *B*). MRI is ideal for determining the acuity of the fracture

and helps to exclude a metastatic lesion (**Figure 1**, *C*). When MRI is contraindicated, bone scan may help evaluate for fracture acuity.

Positioning and Setup
Kyphoplasty and vertebroplasty can be performed under general or local anesthesia with intravenous sedation. The patient is positioned prone (**Figure 2**), often using a Jackson table or a Wilson frame. Biplanar fluoroscopy is preferred for this procedure. It is critical to obtain good AP and lateral fluoroscopic images before beginning the procedure. AP images should show the spinous process centered between the pedicles (**Figure 3**). The lateral image should display the end plates overlapped, and a single pedicle outline should be seen. A 10° to 15° oblique or *en face* view also may be helpful, particularly in cases of severe osteoporosis or rotational deformities.

Instruments and Equipment
The following equipment is needed for kyphoplasty and vertebroplasty:
- 0.25% bupivacaine hydrochloride with epinephrine (a 1:1 ratio mixed with 1% lidocaine also

can be used) injected via a small-gauge needle, such as a 25-gauge needle
- Scalpel
- 11-gauge soft-tissue biopsy needle (alternatively, a one-step device can be used)
- Mallet and guide pin
- 4.3-mm diameter working cannula
- Hollow-core 3.5-mm diameter biopsy tool
- Inflatable bone tamp (balloon lengths include 10-mm, 15-mm, 20-mm)
- Hand-held drill and bit
- PMMA, radiopaque contrast, liquid monomer
- (5) 5-mL syringes with threaded, locking connections
- Bone filling device (carries ~1.5 mL cement)
- PMMA mixer
- Suture (either 3-0 or 4-0), dermal sealant, and adhesive skin-closure strips

Approach Tips
In the mid- and upper thoracic spine, the smaller, medially angled pedicles may make an extrapedicular approach

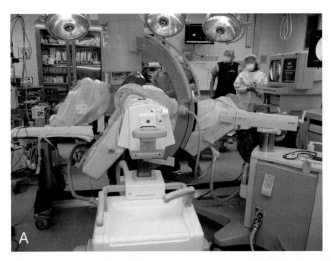

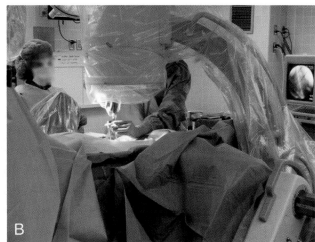

Figure 2 Photographs of the operating room setup for kyphoplasty. **A,** Patient positioning and C-arm placement. **B,** C-arm positioning allows for biplanar fluoroscopy during the procedure.

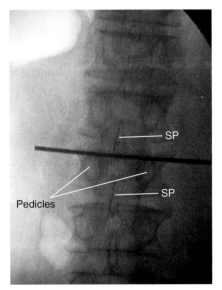

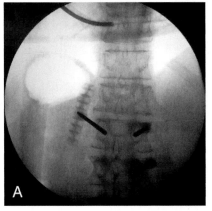

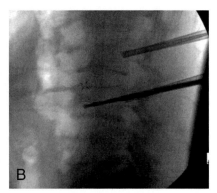

Figure 4 A, AP fluoroscopic image demonstrates cannula entry into the pedicles and advancement into the vertebral body. As the needle and cannula reach the midpoint of the pedicle on the AP view, the tip of the needle should be about halfway down the pedicle on the lateral view. Subsequently, entry into the posterior vertebral body is safe if one maintains the entry point lateral to the medial pedicle wall when entering the VCF. **B,** On this lateral fluoroscopic image, the working cannula has advanced into the posterior vertebral body. Note that the lateral image clearly shows the vertebral end plate overlap and a single pedicle outline.

Figure 3 Intraoperative AP fluoroscopic image demonstrates the use of a metal wire (held above the surgical field during imaging) to assist in localization, as the spinous process (SP) of the vertebral body, best seen at the caudal vertebral body, is centered between the pedicles.

preferable. The initial entry point is superolateral to the pedicle just medial to (or sometimes through) the rib head. The vertebral body is then entered at the base of the pedicle, near the vertebral body/pedicle junction. Care must be taken to avoid entering

the pulmonary cavity. A transpedicular approach also may be a safe alternative.

A transpedicular approach is most often preferred for VCFs below T8 or T9. Initially, the 11-gauge soft-tissue biopsy needle or working cannula should enter the pedicle superolaterally on the AP image, aiming toward the anteroinferior body. With significant superior end plate fractures, a tra-

jectory that enters the pedicle more inferiorly permits optimal elevation of the superior vertebral body (**Figure 4**). Conversely, inferior end plate fractures may require a starting point placed more superiorly. Before the needle is advanced, a lateral view should be obtained to confirm the trajectory. On the AP view, the needle should be advanced down the pedicle until it approximates the midpoint of

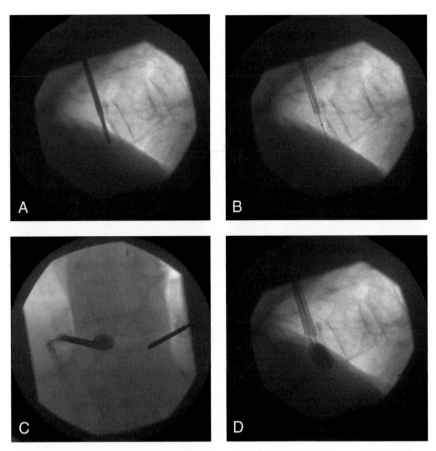

Figure 5 Fluoroscopic images demonstrate drilling, balloon tamp placement, and balloon filling/fracture reduction during kyphoplasty. **A,** Lateral view shows the drilling of the VCF via the working cannula. **B,** Placement of the inflatable balloon before inflation next to the superior end plate fracture. **C,** AP image shows balloon tamp at approximately 75% inflation. Some fracture reduction has begun. **D,** Lateral image shows balloon tamp inflation and fracture reduction. Following maximal inflation and fracture reduction, the inflated balloon tamps should optimally meet at the midline on the AP image.

the pedicle. The tip of the needle should be about halfway down the pedicle on the lateral view. The needle tip should be advanced to approximately 2 to 3 mm beyond the posterior cortex of the vertebral body. The risk of entering the spinal canal can be minimized by ensuring that the needle tip remains lateral to the medial pedicle wall (on the AP image) until the vertebral body is reached (on the lateral image). When performing kyphoplasty, once the working cannula is positioned, the hand drill should be advanced down the cannula toward the anterior vertebral cortex to create a path for the placement of the inflat-able bone tamp (**Figure 5,** A and B). The working cannula should be positioned beyond the pedicle into the vertebral body by a few millimeters. The drill tip should approximate the midline on the AP view and be posterior to the anterior vertebral body cortex on the lateral view. The drill is removed, and the inflatable bone tamp is placed through the cannula (**Figure 5,** C). This procedure is repeated on the contralateral side. As a general rule, in the thoracic spine, 15-mm balloons that can hold volumes of 4 mL can be used, whereas in the lumbar spine, 20-mm balloons that can hold 6 mL may be preferable.

Bone Tamp Inflation and Fracture Cementation

AP and lateral views should show that the inflatable bone tamp is in the correct final position (3 to 4 mm posterior to the anterior vertebral cortex). The tamp should be inflated slowly while obtaining repeat fluoroscopic images (**Figure 6**). If pressure increases and remains high as the bone tamp is inflated, a sclerotic region of fractured vertebral body could be present or a vertebral cortex could be contacted. The bone tamps are inflated until fracture reduction occurs, the bone tamp contacts a vertebral body cortex, or the maximal pressure rating is reached.

Once the desired height has been restored, the bone tamp pressure is slowly released and the device is removed. If vertebral height is lost with bone tamp deflation, it may be helpful to keep one balloon elevated to hold up the end plate while filling the other side with PMMA. Cement is then placed in the bone-filling devices. Once the PMMA has attained a doughy consistency, it is ready to be injected into the vertebral body. The bone-filling device containing the cement should be placed anteriorly into the vertebral body. With the aid of intraoperative fluoroscopy, the plunger of the device is then advanced, injecting cement into the vertebral body while slowly withdrawing the device as cement fills the cavity. At the completion of the cement injection, the PMMA should fill the cavity and interdigitate within the bony trabeculae of the fractured vertebral body (**Figure 7**). We prefer to inject the PMMA with the aid of live fluoroscopy, which permits immediate identification of any extravertebral leaks so that injection can be stopped immediately if necessary. Generally, when cement approaches within approximately 5 mm of the posterior cortex of the vertebral body, injection should stop.

Wound Closure

The irrigated wound can be closed by several methods. Typically, we use nonbraided sutures, such as 3-0 poliglecaprone 25 sutures in the dermal layer, depending on the size of the incision. This step can be followed by a dermal sealant or adhesive skin-closure strips, depending on wound size. Closure also can be performed with a simple nylon suture or staples. Smaller incisions may require only a dermal sealant. The surgeon must ensure excellent hemostasis before closure, as this may guide the choice for closure, especially if the patient is on warfarin sodium or another anti-thrombotic agent. A sterile dressing is then placed.

Postoperative Regimen

The postoperative regimen consists of early mobilization and ambulation on the day of surgery or the following day. Patients should resume their daily activities as tolerated. Formal physical therapy is prescribed if ambulation and function have been significantly limited by the fracture or if deconditioning could limit rehabilitation. Patients with osteoporosis should undergo a medical workup and be placed on anti-osteoporosis medications. Typically, no bracing is required.

Avoiding Pitfalls and Complications

To avoid postoperative complications, the integrity of the posterior cortex of the fractured vertebra should be evaluated carefully. If a burst fracture is suspected, a CT scan should be performed. When bony retropulsion or deficiencies of the posterior vertebral

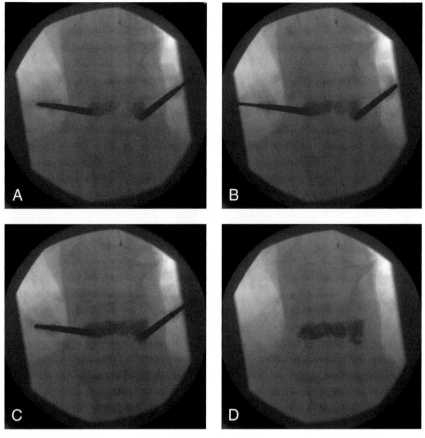

Figure 6 Serial AP fluoroscopic images of vertebral body cementation. **A,** The initial stages of filling of the bilateral balloon tamp voids and early crossing of the cement between cavities. Interconnecting cement migration between voids (**B** and **C**). **D,** final cemented VCF following kyphoplasty after cannula removal.

wall are identified, vertebral augmentation may be contraindicated. Ensure that no fissures are present that extend into the posterior wall.

When accessing the vertebral body, the needle tip should be lateral to the medial pedicle wall on the AP fluoroscopic image until the posterior vertebral body is reached on the lateral image to prevent entry into the spinal canal.

The inflatable bone tamp should not violate the vertebral body cortex or vertebral end plates. If partial healing of a VCF prevents the inflatable bone tamp from being fully expanded, an articulated curet can be used to break up sclerotic regions to facilitate

full bone tamp expansion and fracture reduction.

The vertebral body is slowly filled with cement while being monitored under live fluoroscopy for an extravertebral cement leak. If posterior leakage of cement into the spinal canal or neural foramen occurs, injection of the cement should be stopped immediately.

During cement injection, extravertebral spread can occur via the venous system or through deficiencies in the vertebral body cortex. If extravertebral cement extravasation occurs, the tip of the cement injection tool should be repositioned and the cement allowed to begin hardening before com-

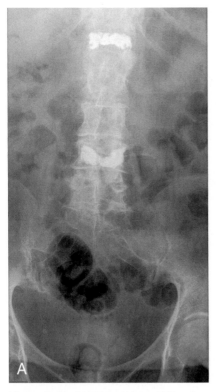
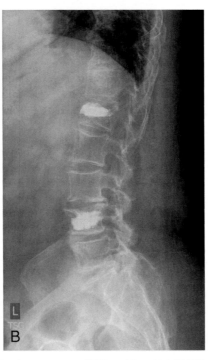

pleting the injection. The bone tamp is reinserted and reinflated within the cement bolus in the vertebral body, creating a cement "shell" around the balloon and at the periphery of the cavity. Once the cement shell is cured, additional cement can be injected.

In most cases, cement leakage is asymptomatic, and no specific treatment is warranted. If cement leaks into the spinal canal or neural foramen and the patient develops a neurologic deficit, urgent surgical decompression is required. When a patient develops a postoperative neurologic deficit and no cement leakage is present, an epidural hematoma should be considered, especially when history of a bleeding diathesis or recent anticoagulation use exists. An MRI should be performed immediately, and if hematoma is confirmed, urgent surgical decompression is indicated.

Figure 7 Final AP (**A**) and lateral (**B**) radiographs show cemented VCFs at L1 and L4. PMMA should fill the cavity and interdigitate within the bony trabeculae of the fractured vertebral body.

Bibliography

Alvarez L, Alcaraz M, Pérez-Higueras A, et al: Percutaneous vertebroplasty: Functional improvement in patients with osteoporotic compression fractures. *Spine (Phila Pa 1976)* 2006;31(10):1113-1118.

American Academy of Orthopaedic Surgeons: *Clinical Practice Guideline on the Treatment of Osteoporotic Spinal Compression Fractures.* Rosemont, IL, American Academy of Orthopaedic Surgeons, September 2010. http://www.aaos.org/research/guidelines/SCFguideline.pdf. Accessed April 11, 2011.

Bouza C, López T, Magro A, Navalpotro L, Amate JM: Efficacy and safety of balloon kyphoplasty in the treatment of vertebral compression fractures: A systematic review. *Eur Spine J* 2006;15(7):1050-1067.

Buchbinder R, Osborne RH, Ebeling PR, et al: A randomized trial of vertebroplasty for painful osteoporotic vertebral fractures. *N Engl J Med* 2009;361(6):557-568.

Garfin SR, Buckley RA, Ledlie J, Balloon Kyphoplasty Outcomes Group: Balloon kyphoplasty for symptomatic vertebral body compression fractures results in rapid, significant, and sustained improvements in back pain, function, and quality of life for elderly patients. *Spine (Phila Pa 1976)* 2006;31(19):2213-2220.

Glassman SD, Alegre GM: Adult spinal deformity in the osteoporotic spine: Options and pitfalls. *Instr Course Lect* 2003; 52:579-588.

Grohs JG, Matzner M, Trieb K, Krepler P: Minimal invasive stabilization of osteoporotic vertebral fractures: A prospective nonrandomized comparison of vertebroplasty and balloon kyphoplasty. *J Spinal Disord Tech* 2005;18(3):238-242.

Hadjipavlou AG, Tzermiadianos MN, Katonis PG, Szpalski M: Percutaneous vertebroplasty and balloon kyphoplasty for the treatment of osteoporotic vertebral compression fractures and osteolytic tumours. *J Bone Joint Surg Br* 2005;87(12): 1595-1604.

Hallberg I, Rosenqvist AM, Kartous L, Löfman O, Wahlström O, Toss G: Health-related quality of life after osteoporotic fractures. *Osteoporos Int* 2004;15(10):834-841.

Kallmes DF, Comstock BA, Heagerty PJ, et al: A randomized trial of vertebroplasty for osteoporotic spinal fractures. *N Engl J Med* 2009;361(6):569-579.

Kasperk C, Hillmeier J, Nöldge G, et al: Treatment of painful vertebral fractures by kyphoplasty in patients with primary osteoporosis: A prospective nonrandomized controlled study. *J Bone Miner Res* 2005;20(4):604-612.

Köse KC, Cebesoy O, Akan B, Altinel L, Dinçer D, Yazar T: Functional results of vertebral augmentation techniques in pathological vertebral fractures of myelomatous patients. *J Natl Med Assoc* 2006;98(10):1654-1658.

Lunt M, O'Neill TW, Felsenberg D, et al: Characteristics of a prevalent vertebral deformity predict subsequent vertebral fracture: Results from the European Prospective Osteoporosis Study (EPOS). *Bone* 2003;33(4):505-513.

Mudano AS, Bian J, Cope JU, et al: Vertebroplasty and kyphoplasty are associated with an increased risk of secondary vertebral compression fractures: A population-based cohort study. *Osteoporos Int* 2009;20(5):819-826.

Ohtori S, Yamashita M, Inoue G, et al: L2 spinal nerve-block effects on acute low back pain from osteoporotic vertebral fracture. *J Pain* 2009;10(8):870-875.

Pflugmacher R, Taylor R, Agarwal A, et al: Balloon kyphoplasty in the treatment of metastatic disease of the spine: A 2-year prospective evaluation. *Eur Spine J* 2008;17(8):1042-1048.

Phillips FM: Minimally invasive treatments of osteoporotic vertebral compression fractures. *Spine (Phila Pa 1976)* 2003;28(15 suppl)S45-S53.

Pluijm SM, Koes B, de Laet C, et al: A simple risk score for the assessment of absolute fracture risk in general practice based on two longitudinal studies. *J Bone Miner Res* 2009;24(5):768-774.

Resnick DK, Garfin SR: *Vertebroplasty and Kyphoplasty*. New York, NY, Thieme Medical Publishers, 2005, pp 62-75.

Riggs BL, Melton LJ III: The worldwide problem of osteoporosis: Insights afforded by epidemiology. *Bone* 1995;17 (5 suppl):505S-511S.

Taylor RS, Fritzell P, Taylor RJ: Balloon kyphoplasty in the management of vertebral compression fractures: An updated systematic review and meta-analysis. *Eur Spine J* 2007;16(8):1085-1100.

Taylor RS, Taylor RJ, Fritzell P: Balloon kyphoplasty and vertebroplasty for vertebral compression fractures: A comparative systematic review of efficacy and safety. *Spine (Phila Pa 1976)* 2006;31(23):2747-275.

Voormolen MH, Mali WP, Lohle PN, et al: Percutaneous vertebroplasty compared with optimal pain medication treatment: Short-term clinical outcome of patients with subacute or chronic painful osteoporotic vertebral compression fractures. The VERTOS study. *AJNR Am J Neuroradiol* 2007;28(3):555-560.

Wardlaw D, Cummings SR, Van Meirhaeghe J, et al: Efficacy and safety of balloon kyphoplasty compared with non-surgical care for vertebral compression fracture (FREE): A randomised controlled trial. *Lancet* 2009;373(9668):1016-1024.

Coding

CPT Codes		Corresponding ICD-9 Codes		
22520	Percutaneous vertebroplasty, one vertebral body, unilateral or bilateral injection; thoracic	733.0 733.01 733.09	733.00 733.02 733.13	
22521	Percutaneous vertebroplasty, one vertebral body, unilateral or bilateral injection; lumbar	733.0 733.01 733.09	733.00 733.02 733.13	
22522	Percutaneous vertebroplasty, one vertebral body, unilateral or bilateral injection; each additional thoracic or lumbar vertebral body (List separately in addition to code for primary procedure)	733.0 733.01 733.09	733.00 733.02 733.13	
22523	Percutaneous vertebral augmentation, including cavity creation (fracture reduction and bone biopsy included when performed) using mechanical device, one vertebral body, unilateral or bilateral cannulation (eg, kyphoplasty); thoracic	733.13	805.2	
22524	Percutaneous vertebral augmentation, including cavity creation (fracture reduction and bone biopsy included when performed) using mechanical device, one vertebral body, unilateral or bilateral cannulation (eg, kyphoplasty); lumbar	733.13	805.4	
22525	Percutaneous vertebral augmentation, including cavity creation (fracture reduction and bone biopsy included when performed) using mechanical device, one vertebral body, unilateral or bilateral cannulation (eg, kyphoplasty); each additional thoracic or lumbar vertebral body (List separately in addition to code for primary procedure)	733.13 805.4	805.2	
72291	Radiological supervision and interpretation, percutaneous vertebroplasty, vertebral augmentation, or sacral augmentation (sacroplasty), including cavity creation, per vertebral body or sacrum; under fluoroscopic guidance	733.0 733.01 733.09 805.2	733.00 733.02 733.13 805.4	
72292	Radiological supervision and interpretation, percutaneous vertebroplasty, vertebral augmentation, or sacral augmentation (sacroplasty), including cavity creation, per vertebral body or sacrum; under CT guidance	733.0 733.01 733.09 805.2	733.00 733.02 733.13 805.4	

Chapter 71

Spinal Epidural Injections
for Lumbar Spinal Radiculopathy Pain

David E. Fish, MD, MPH

Indications

Epidural corticosteroid injection represents the most common interventional pain procedure performed in the United States. The available literature demonstrates moderate evidence that lumbar epidural corticosteroid injections are effective in reducing pain in the short term and in improving functional outcomes. Furthermore, convincing evidence shows that all commonly used approaches for lumbar epidural corticosteroid injections, including transforaminal, caudal, and interlaminar approaches, are relatively safe, with low reported rates of complications. This combination of documented efficacy and a high safety margin makes these procedures well accepted and justifies their common use.

The rationale for spinal epidural injection using either the interlaminar approach or the transforaminal approach is to block lumbar radicular pain in a patient with symptoms that interfere with daily functioning. In performing an epidural injection, the goal is to provide a window of opportunity in which the patient can perform functional activities and experience improved pain symptoms. Other goals of an epidural injection are to locate the source of pain and to help the surgeon determine the level of the spinal pathology that should be targeted for potential surgical treatment. Individuals with symptoms that fail to respond to nonsurgical treatment may be considered for an epidural injection because of their limited ability to participate in physical therapy. A series of injections are given if the initial goals of reduced pain and increased function are achieved. These injections usually are spaced 21 to 28 days apart.

Epidural injections may provide good sensitivity and specificity in identifying the nerve root involved. The literature is unclear as to the value of epidural injections in predicting surgical outcome. Derby and associates reported that patients who responded well to epidural injections tended to have more favorable surgical outcomes compared with those who had poor responses to injections. It has been shown, however, that epidurals may not be specific enough for identifying the nerve root level involved in radicular pain to assist with the surgical planning of sensory rhizotomies.

———————■

Contraindications

One absolute contraindication to spinal epidural injection is the presence of a bacterial infection, either systemic or in the epidural space. Another is a bleeding diathesis, which can lead to an epidural hematoma. Relative contraindications include allergy to corticosteroids or local anesthetics, pregnancy, and the use of nonsteroidal anti-inflammatory drugs (NSAIDs), aspirin, or antiplatelet agents such as clopidogrel or warfarin. Further relative contraindications include hyperglycemia, adrenal suppression, immunocompromise, high blood pressure, and congestive heart failure.

The community standard of care is to use fluoroscopic guidance for both the interlaminar and transforaminal approaches. The goal is to target a level of spinal pathology and determine the source of isolated nerve pain. In a person with a prior laminectomy, the interlaminar approach is not indicated because the loss-of-resistance

---

Dr. Fish or an immediate family member is a member of a speakers' bureau or has made paid presentations on behalf of Allergan and Sanofi-aventis.

© 2011 American Academy of Orthopaedic Surgeons

Table 1 Results of Lumbar Epidural Injections

Authors (Year)	Number of Patients	Procedure or Approach	Mean Patient Age in Years (Range)
Cuckler et al (1985)	73	Interlaminar epidural injection with either methylprednisolone and procaine or saline solution and procaine	48.5
Carette et al (1997)	158	3 interlaminar epidural injections of methylprednisolone vs epidurals with isotonic saline	> 18
Lutz et al (1998)	69	Transforaminal epidural injection with corticosteroid and anesthetic directly at the level and side of documented pathology	43.5 (22-77)
Riew et al (2000)	55	Bupivacaine vs bupivacaine and betamethasone Up to 4 injections allowed	> 21
Karppinen et al (2001)	160	Transforaminal lumbar epidural injections using either corticosteroid or normal saline	44.3
Wilson-MacDonald et al (2005)	93	Interlaminar epidural injection of bupivacaine/methylprednisolone vs intramuscular injection of bupivacaine/methylprednisolone	49.1 (26-76)

technique is impossible to perform given the lack of an intact ligamentum flavum.

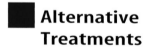

Alternative Treatments

Epidural injections are not used as a mandatory primary treatment option in the paradigm of lumbar radiculopathy therapy. The role of the epidural is to give options to the patient and help promote functional improvements. According to the Cochrane Database for Systematic Reviews, physical therapy with aerobic exercise has been determined to be the best long-term treatment option for lumbar radiculopathy. Oral medications, epidural injections, and superficial modalities

such as ice or heat are used to help a patient with radiculopathy pain progress with aerobic exercises and functional therapies. Epidural injections are not always needed as part of the treatment strategy. An individual who can tolerate the pain symptoms and progress with therapy does not need a spinal injection.

Many variables can limit the success of epidural corticosteroid injection, including the number of spinal pathology levels, the type of corticosteroid used, the volume of injected material, and the type of needle used. Other factors that should be noted and evaluated by the injectionist are patient body habitus and weight, secondary gain issues, and presenting psychologic factors.

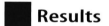 # Results

Based on the studies summarized in **Table 1**, transforaminal epidural injections provide both short-term and long-term benefit. Therefore, in the treatment of patients with lumbar radiculopathy, using a transforaminal approach when performing an epidural injection is potentially more beneficial than using the interlaminar approach. Few studies in the literature compare transforaminal injections with interlaminar injections. Prospective randomized clinical trials will be necessary to properly compare the two types of injection and definitively determine whether the transforaminal approach is superior to the interlaminar approach.

Table 1 *(continued)*

Follow-up	Success Rate	Results
24 hours and 20 months	No difference with outcome vs control	No significant improvement in pain levels between the two groups
12 months	No difference with outcome vs control	At 3 months, no significant difference between the two groups At 12 months, no difference in the rate of back surgery
Mean 80 weeks (range, 28-144)	52 patients (75.4%) had a successful outcome	52 patients (75.4%) Patients reported >50% reduction in pain scores and an ability to return to or near previous level of function Overall, 78.3% satisfied with final outcome
13-28 months	52% did not have surgery based on epidural results	Failed if patient had surgery, which patient could opt to do at any point in the study Rates of surgery significantly lower in those who had betamethasone injections compared with bupivacaine alone
Baseline, 2 and 4 weeks, 3 and 6 months, 1 year	Corticosteroid treatment prevented surgery for contained herniations Corticosteroid not effective for extrusions	Corticosteroid group showed a statistically significant improvement in short-term leg pain, straight-leg raising, lumbar flexion, and patient satisfaction Follow-up at 3 and 6 months failed to show any difference between experimental group receiving corticosteroids and control group receiving normal saline
6 weeks and 24 months	No difference with outcome vs control	Rate of subsequent surgery in the groups was similar Study did not analyze at surgical outcome between the groups

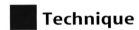

Technique

Instruments/Equipment Required

The materials and equipment to be used with the fluoroscope will depend on the approach. When performing an interlaminar injection, most injectionists use a 16- to 18-gauge, 3.5- to 6.0-inch Tuohy spinal needle. For a transforaminal approach, a 20- to 22-gauge, 3.5- to 6.0-inch needle is used. The volume of injected material used also depends on the approach. The interlaminar epidural space is considered large and can accommodate 3 to 5 mL of injectate, whereas with the transforaminal approach, 2 mL of injectate is typically used. Steroid preparations also are frequently debated with epidural injections based on particle size, diffusion, and

Table 2 Medication Used in Epidural Lumbar Injections

Type	Name	Typical Dose
Contrast	Iohexol or iopamidol	2 mL
Local anesthetic	Lidocaine 1.0%, bupivacaine 0.25%	3 to 5 mL
Corticosteroid	Methylprednisolone Betamethasone	40 to 80 mg 6 to 12 mg

effectiveness. Typical doses are provided in **Table 2**.

Procedure

After standard sterile preparation with the patient prone (**Figure 1**), fluoroscopic views are taken: an AP view for the interlaminar approach and an oblique view (**Figure 2**) for the transforaminal approach. Once the target level is identified, the needle(s) are advanced (**Figure 3**) using intermittent

fluoroscopic images until lamina is struck, indicating the proper depth. With an interlaminar approach, the loss-of-resistance technique is used to advance the needle through the ligamentum flavum (**Figure 4**, *A* and *B*). With the transforaminal approach, the anatomic superior aspect of the foramen seen on the "Scotty dog" view (**Figure 2**) is used to confirm the location of the epidural space. Confirmation with a lateral view of the spine

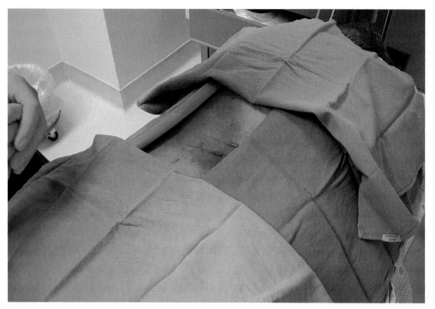

Figure 1 Photograph demonstrates patient position and sterile preparation and draping for epidural injection procedures.

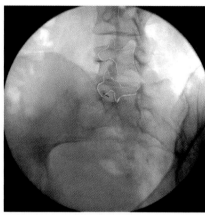

Figure 2 Oblique fluoroscopic view demonstrates the characteristic "Scotty dog" view of L5-S1 and S1-S2 seen when using the transforaminal approach.

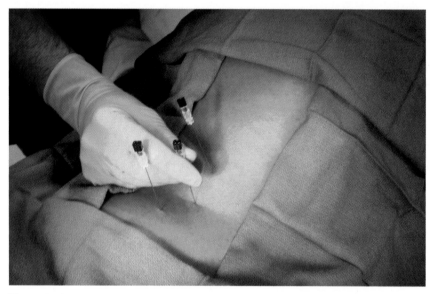

Figure 3 The injectionist maneuvers the 22-gauge, 3.5-inch spinal needles used in the transforaminal approach.

(Figure 5) using a contrast medium can help confirm the location of the epidural space and nerve root. Aspiration is performed to ensure that intravascular injection has not taken place. Contrast medium is used for all epidural injections to ensure that no vascular uptake is present (**Figure 6**).

Postoperative Regimen

Most patients do not require moderate conscious sedation for the procedure; however, for patient comfort and anxiety reduction, sedation using midazolam and fentanyl typically are given by the anesthesia staff and are used in conjunction with surgical monitoring of pulse oximetry, blood pressure, and oxygen saturation. Individuals who have moderate conscious sedation require postoperative monitoring until they are stable enough for discharge in 20 to 30 minutes. Individuals who do not receive sedation usually can be discharged once stable if no neurologic sequelae, such as weakness or numbness in the affected extremity, are present.

Avoiding Pitfalls and Complications

Epidural injections do not always improve function and reduce pain; thus, the patient should be warned that worsening of pain could occur. Any time a needle is placed into the epidural space, the risk of infection (abscess) or hematoma can occur. Because triamcinolone is a neurotoxic agent, betamethasone may be the preferred choice, but studies have shown that triamcinolone can be used safely and effectively.

In 2000, Botwin and associates reviewed the charts of 157 patients who

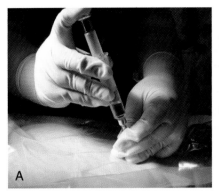
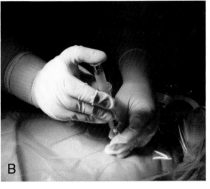
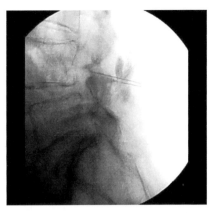

Figure 4 Photographs depict the loss-of-resistance technique for the interlaminar approach. **A,** Constant pressure is applied to a glass syringe with guidance from the opposite hand. **B,** Loss of resistance is accomplished with the needle passing through the ligamentum flavum. The glass syringe has less saline than the one in the previous photo because the loss of resistance allows for easy injection into the epidural space.

Figure 5 Lateral fluoroscopic view of the spine shows a bilateral L4-5 transforaminal approach with the needles in proper position at the upper portion of the foramen.

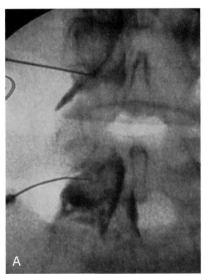
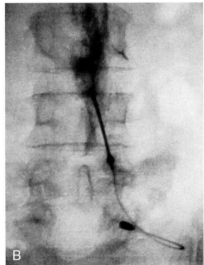
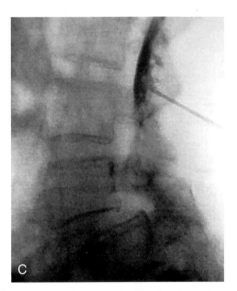

Figure 6 Fluoroscopic views of the spine demonstrate aspiration and use of contrast medium to prevent intravascular injection. **A,** AP view with proper contrast spread shows transforaminal epidural injections at L4-5 and L5-S1. The contrast is seen in the epidural space and along the corresponding nerve root with no vascular uptake. **B,** AP view demonstrates contrast spread in the epidural space at L2-3 using an interlaminar approach. **C,** Lateral view shows contrast in the posterior epidural space using an interlaminar approach at L2-3.

received a total of 345 interlaminar epidural corticosteroid injections. They noted a 16.8% incidence of complications, all of which resolved without significant morbidity or mortality. The authors reported 23 patients (6.7%) with increased pain, 6 patients (1.7%) with vasovagal reactions, 5 patients (1.5%) with facial flushing, 1 patient (0.3%) with fever on the night of the procedure, and 1 patient

(0.3%) with a dural puncture. These side effects and complications were all self-limited.

The common practice of aspiration before injection likely is inadequate to prevent intravascular injection. Furman and associates demonstrated in 2000 that 19.4% of fluoroscopically guided spinal injections resulted in vascular spread despite negative aspiration.

Some interventional pain practitioners have noted that the likely etiology for many of these devastating complications is the injection of particulate corticosteroids into the vascular structures with the transforaminal approach. With this in mind, some practitioners have advocated methods of improving the safety profile of these procedures. Many practitioners have attempted to improve the safety of the transforaminal approach by using digital subtraction angiography and injecting nonparticulate corticosteroids. Although these measures may seem likely in theory to improve the relative safety of epidural corticosteroid injections, to date not a single well-designed published study has demonstrated that using particulate corticosteroid leads to a higher complication rate. Neither has improved safety been demonstrated for digital subtraction angiography or nonparticulate corticosteroid. In fact, limited evidence shows that, in the lumbar spine, interlaminar epidural corticosteroid injections likely are less efficacious than transforaminal epidural corticosteroid injections. Finally, limited evidence also shows that nonparticulate corticosteroids likely are less effective than particulate corticosteroids.

Bibliography

Abdi S, Datta S, Lucas LF: Role of epidural steroids in the management of chronic spinal pain: A systemic review of effectiveness and complications. *Pain Physician* 2005;8:127-143.

Arden NK, Price C, Reading I, et al: A multicentre randomized controlled trial of epidural corticosteroid injections for sciatica: The WEST study. *Rheumatology (Oxford)* 2005;44:1399-1406.

Atlas SJ, Keller RB, Wu YA, Deyo RA, Singer DE: Long-term outcomes of surgical and nonsurgical management of sciatica secondary to a lumbar disc herniation: 10 year results from the Maine Lumbar Spine Study. *Spine (Phila Pa 1976)* 2005;30:927-935.

Boswell MV, Shaw RV, Everett CR, et al: Interventional techniques in the management of chronic spinal pain: Evidence-based practice guidelines. *Pain Physician* 2005;8:1-47.

Botwin KP, Gruber RD, Bouchlas CG, Torres-Ramos FM, Freeman TL, Slaten WK: Complications of fluoroscopically guided transforaminal lumbar epidural injections. *Arch Phys Med Rehabil* 2000;81:1045-1050.

Buchner M, Neubauer E, Zahlten-Hinguranage A, Schiltenwolf M: The influence of the grade of chronicity on the outcome of multidisciplinary therapy for chronic low back pain. *Spine (Phila Pa 1976)* 2007;32:3060-3066.

Bush K, Cowan N, Katz DE, Gishen P: The natural history of sciatica associated with disc pathology: A prospective study with clinical and independent radiologic follow-up. *Spine (Phila Pa 1976)* 1992;17:1205-1212.

Carette S, Leclaire R, Marcoux S, et al: Epidural corticosteroid injections for sciatica due to herniated nucleus pulposus. *N Engl J Med* 1997;336:1634-1640.

Cuckler JM, Bernini PA, Wiesel SW, Booth RE Jr, Rothman RH, Pickens GT: The use of epidural steroids in the treatment of radicular pain: A prospective, randomized, double-blind study. *J Bone Joint Surg Am* 1985;67:63-66.

Derby R, Kine G, Saal JA, et al: Response to steroid and duration of radicular pain as predictors of surgical outcome. *Spine (Phila Pa 1976)* 1992;17:S176-S183.

Deyo RA, Weinstein JN: Low back pain. *N Engl J Med* 2001;344:363-370.

Furman MB, O'Brien EM, Zgleszewski TM: Incidence of intravascular penetration in transforaminal lumbosacral epidural steroid injections. *Spine (Phila Pa 1976)* 2000;25:2628-2632.

Hayden J, van Tulder MW, Malmivaara A, Koes BW: Exercise therapy for treatment of non-specific low back pain. *Cochrane Database Syst Rev* 2005;3:CD000335.

Karppinen J, Ohinmaa A, Malmivaara A, et al: Cost effectiveness of periradicular infiltration for sciatica: Subgroup analysis of a randomized controlled trial. *Spine (Phila Pa 1976)* 2001;26:2587-2595.

Lee HM, Weinstein JN, Meller ST, Hayashi N, Spratt KF, Gebhardt GF: The role of steroids and their effects on phospholipase A2: An animal model of radiculopathy. *Spine (Phila Pa 1976)* 1998;23:1191-1196.

Loyd R, Fanciullo GJ, Hanscom B, Baird JC: Cluster analysis of SF-36 scales as a predictor of spinal pain patients response to a multidisciplinary pain management approach beginning with epidural steroid injection. *Pain Med* 2006;7:229-236.

Lutz GE, Vad VB, Wisneski RJ: Fluoroscopic transforaminal lumbar epidural steroids: An outcome study. *Arch Phys Med Rehabil* 1998;79:1362-1366.

Manchikanti L, Bakhit CE, Pakanati RR, Fellows B: Fluoroscopy is medically necessary for the performance of epidural steroids. *Anesth Analg* 1999;89:1330-1331.

Okubadejo GO, Talcott MR, Schmidt RE, et al: Perils of intravascular methylprednisolone injection into the vertebral artery: An animal study. *J Bone Joint Surg Am* 2008;90:1932-1938.

Riew KD, Yin Y, Gilula L, et al: The effect of nerve-root injections on the need for operative treatment of lumbar radicular pain: A prospective, randomized, controlled, double-blind study. *J Bone Joint Surg Am* 2000;82:1589-1593.

Schaufele MK, Hatch L, Jones W: Interlaminar versus transforaminal epidural injections for the treatment of symptomatic lumbar intervertebral disc herniations. *Pain Physician* 2006;9:361-366.

Smuck M, Abbott Z, Zemper E: Interpretation of contrast dispersal patterns by experienced and inexperienced interventionalists. *PM R* 2009;1:55-59.

Smuck M, Fuller BJ, Chiodo A, et al: Accuracy of intermittent fluoroscopy to detect intravascular injection during transforaminal epidural injections. *Spine (Phila Pa 1976)* 2008;33:E205-E210.

Staal JB, de Bie R, de Vet HC, Hildebrandt J, Nelemans P: Injection therapy for subacute and chronic low-back pain. *Cochrane Database Syst Rev* 2008;3:CD001824.

Stanczak J, Blankenbaker DG, De Smet AA, Fine J: Efficacy of epidural injections of Kenalog and Celestone in the treatment of lower back pain. *AJR Am J Roentgenol* 2003;181:1255-1258.

Thomas E, Cyteval C, Abiad L, Picot MC, Taourel P, Blotman F: Efficacy of transforaminal versus interspinous corticosteroid injection in discal radiculalgia: A prospective, randomized, double-blind study. *Clin Rheumatol* 2003;22:299-304.

Tiso RL, Cutler T, Catania JA, Whalen K: Adverse central nervous system sequelae after selective transforaminal block: The role of corticosteroids. *Spine (Phila Pa 1976)* 2004;4:468-474.

van der Windt DA, Simons E, Riphagen II, et al: Physical examination for lumbar radiculopathy due to disc herniation in patients with low-back pain. *Cochrane Database Syst Rev* 2010;2:CD007431.

Wilson-MacDonald J, Burt G, Griffin D, Glynn C: Epidural steroid injection for nerve root compression: A randomized, controlled trial. *J Bone Joint Surg Br* 2005;87:352-355.

Coding

CPT Codes		Corresponding ICD-9 Codes	
62311	Injection, single (not via indwelling catheter), not including neurolytic substances, with or without contrast (for either localization or epidurography), of diagnostic or therapeutic substance(s) (including anesthetic, antispasmodic, opioid, steroid, other solution), epidural or subarachnoid; lumbar, sacral (caudal)	722.1 722.52 724.02	722.2 722.83 724.3
64483	Injection, anesthetic agent and/or steroid, transforaminal epidural; lumbar or sacral, single level	722.10	722.83
64484	Injection, anesthetic agent and/or steroid, transforaminal epidural; lumbar or sacral, each additional level (List separately in addition to code for primary procedure)	722.10	722.83

CPT copyright © 2010 by the American Medical Association. All Rights Reserved.

Index

Page numbers with *f* indicate figures.
Page numbers with *t* indicate tables.

A

ACCF. *See* Anterior cervical corpectomy and fusion
ACDF. *See* Anterior cervical diskectomy and fusion
Adolescent idiopathic scoliosis (AIS), 339
AIDSF (anterior instrumentation, deformity correction, and spinal fusion), 339
AIS (adolescent idiopathic scoliosis), 339
ALIF. *See* Anterior lumbar interbody fusion
ALPA (anterolateral transpsoatic approach), 396
Anatomic zones of sacropelvic region, 583–584, 583*f*
    fixation, 584–585, 584*f*, 585*f*
Annular tears, symptomatic, 611–612, 612*f*
Annular tissue, anomalous nerve fibers, 622
Anterior approach
    costotransversectomy approach compared with, 243
    for lumbar arthroplasty, 415–424
        alternative treatments, 415–418
        contraindications, 415, 415*t*
        disk-space preparation and remobilization, 421, 421*f*
        exposure/approach, 419–420, 419*f*, 420*f*
        implant insertion, 421–422, 422*f*
        indications, 415
        instruments/equipment/implants required, 420–421
        pitfalls and complications, avoiding, 423
        postoperative regimen, 422–423
        procedure, 421–422
        results, 416*t*, 418
        setup/patient positioning, 418–419, 418*f*
        technique, 418–422
        wound closure, 421–422, 422*f*
    to lumbar spine, 395-404
        alternative treatments, 396
        contraindications, 395–396
        indications, 395
        instruments/equipment/implants required, 397
        pitfalls and complications, avoiding, 402–403
        postoperative regimen, 402
        procedure, 397–402, 397*f*, 398*f*, 399*f*, 400*f*, 401*f*, 402*f*
        results, 396
        setup/exposure, 396
        technique, 396–402
        wound closure, 402
    for transthoracic diskectomy
        alternative treatments, 303–304
        contraindications, 303
        indications, 303
        instruments/equipment required, 305–306
        pitfalls and complications, avoiding, 307

        postoperative regimen, 307
        procedure, 306
        results, 304, 305*t*
        role of fusion, 306
        setup/exposure/patient positioning, 304–305, 306*f*
        technique, 304–306
        wound closure, 306
Anterior cervical corpectomy and fusion (ACCF), 21–29
    alternative treatments, 21
    contraindications, 21
    indications, 21, 22*f*
    pitfalls and complications, avoiding, 27
    postoperative regimen, 26
    results, 21–22, 22*f*, 23*t*
    technique
        instruments/equipment/implants required for, 23, 24*f*
        procedure for, 23–26, 24*f*, 25*f*, 26*f*
        setup/exposure for, 22–23, 23*f*
    wound closure, 26, 26*f*
Anterior cervical diskectomy and fusion (ACDF), 1–12
    alternative treatments, 3–4
    contraindications, 3
    decompression/diskectomy, 8
    diskectomy in, 3
    fusion in, 3
    graft options, 6–7
    indications, 3
    pitfalls and complications, avoiding, 9–10, 9*f*, 10*f*
        harvest site, 9
        neurologic, 9–10
    postoperative regimen, 9
    results, 4, 5*t*
    techniques
        instruments/equipment/implants required, 6–7
        procedure, 7–8, 8*f*
        setup/exposure, 4–6, 5*f*, 6*f*, 7*f*
    wound closure, 8
Anterior cervicothoracic fusion, 63–70
    alternative treatments, 63
    contraindications, 63
    indications, 63
    pitfalls and complications, avoiding, 68–69
    postoperative regimen, 68
    results, 63, 64*t*
    techniques
        instruments/equipment/implants required, 64
        procedure, 64–68
        setup/exposure, 64
        wound closure, 68
Anterior instrumentation, deformity correction, and spinal fusion (AIDSF), 339
Anterior lumbar corpectomy, 425–433
    alternative treatments, 425
    contraindications, 425

indications, 425, 426*f*, 427*f*
  pitfalls and complications, avoiding, 432–433
  postoperative regimen, 432
  results, 425–427, 428*t*
  technique
    anterior corpectomy, 431
    anterolateral corpectomy, 430–431, 431*f*
    deep exposure, T12 through L5, 429–430, 430*f*
    deep exposure of L4 and L5, 429–430, 430*f*
    exposure, 427–430
    instruments/equipment/implants required, 430
    procedure, 430–432
    reconstruction, 431–432, 432*f*
    setup/patient positioning, 427, 429*f*
    superficial exposure, L2 through L4, 429
    superficial exposure, L4 and L5, 429
    superficial exposure, T12 through L2, 428–429
    wound closure, 432
Anterior lumbar interbody fusion (ALIF), 395, 525, 535, 582
  indications, 415
  with plating, 405–414
    alternative treatments, 406–407
    contraindications, 406
    equipment, 409–410, 409*f*
    indications, 405, 406*f*
    interbody implants, 409, 409*f*
    pitfalls and complications, avoiding, 412
    plating systems, 410, 410*f*
    postoperative regimen, 412
    procedure, 410–411, 411*f*, 412*f*
    results, 407, 408*t*
    setup/exposure, 407–408, 409*f*
    technique, 407–411
    wound closure, 411
Anterior mini-open approach for scoliosis correction, 339–350
  alternative treatments, 339–340
  contraindications, 339, 340*f*
  indications, 339
  pitfalls and complications, avoiding, 346
  postoperative regimen, 345–346
  results, 340, 341*t*
  technique
    deformity correction, 345, 346*f*
    instrumentation, 345
    setup, 340–343, 343*f*
    surgical exposure, 343–345, 343*f*, 344*f*
    wound closure, 345, 348*f*
Anterior odontoid screw placement, 55–62
  alternative treatments, 56–57
  contraindications, 55–56, 56*f*, 57*f*
  indications, 55, 56*f*
  pitfalls and complications, avoiding, 61
  postoperative regimen, 60–61
  results, 57, 58*t*

  technique
    complications, 60
    instruments/equipment/implants required, 58
    procedure, 59–60, 60*f*, 61*f*
    setup/exposure, 57–58, 58*f*, 59*f*
  wound closure, 60
Anterior thoracoscopic diskectomy and release, 309–317
  alternative treatments, 309–310
  contraindications, 309, 311*f*
  indications, 309, 310*f*
  instruments/equipment/implants required, 311–313
  pitfalls and complications, avoiding, 315
  postoperative regimen, 314–315
  procedure, 313–314, 313*f*, 314*f*
  results, 310–311, 312
  setup/exposure, 311, 312*f*
  technique, 311–314
  wound closure, 314, 315*f*
Anterolateral corpectomy, 430–431, 431*f*
Anterolateral retroperitoneal approach (ARPA), 396
Anterolateral transpsoatic approach (ALPA), 396
ARPA (anterolateral retroperitoneal approach), 396
Arthrodesis
  C1-C2, 149
  lumbar, 571
  posterior cervical, 157
Arthroplasty, 13-20
  cervical
    alternative treatments to, 13
    contraindications, 13, 14*t*
    indications, 13
    pitfalls and complications, avoiding, 18
    postoperative regimen, 18
    results, 13, 14*t*
    technique, 13–18
    wound closure, 18
  lumbar, anterior approach, 415-424
    alternative treatments, 415–418
    contraindications, 415, 415*t*
    disk-space preparation and remobilization, 421, 421*f*
    exposure/approach, 419–420, 419*f*, 420*f*
    implant insertion, 421–422, 422*f*
    indications, 415
    instruments/equipment/implants required, 420–421
    pitfalls and complications, avoiding, 423
    postoperative regimen, 422–423
    procedure, 421–422
    results, 416*t*, 418
    setup/patient positioning, 418–419, 418*f*
    technique, 418–422
    wound closure, 421–422, 422*f*
  total disk, 407
Atlantoaxial dislocation, congenital, 125
Atlantoaxial instability, 149
  C1-C2 fixation and, 159
Atrophic lumbar pseudarthrosis, 571, 573–574

B

Balloon kyphoplasty, 629

BMD (bone mineral density), 478, 627

Bohlman fibular technique for interbody fusion in lumbosacral spine, 517–523
   alternative treatments, 517–519
   contraindications, 517
   indications, 517, 517*f*
   pitfalls and complications, avoiding, 521
   postoperative regimen, 521
   results, 518*t*, 519
   technique
      instruments/equipment/implants required, 519
      procedure, 519–520, 520*f*, 521*f*
      setup/exposure, 519, 519*f*
      wound closure, 520, 520*f*, 521*f*

Bone grafting
   in decompression/fusion for spondylolisthesis, 512–513, 512*f*, 513*f*
   in thoracoscopic corpectomy and fusion, 325

Bone mineral density (BMD), 478, 627

Burst fractures, posterior fixation of thoracolumbar, 371–377

C

C1-C2 arthrodesis, 149

C1-C2 fixation, 159–165
   alternative treatments, 159
   contraindications, 159
   indications, 159, 160*f*
   pitfalls and complications, avoiding, 164–165
   postoperative regimen, 164
   results, 159–162, 160*t*, 161*f*
   technique
      instruments/equipment/implants required, 162–163
      procedure, 163, 163*f*, 164*f*
      setup/exposure, 162, 162*f*, 163*f*
      wound closure, 163

C1-C2 fusion, 155

C1-C2 segmental screws, in occipitocervical fusion and fixation, 179

C1-C2 transarticular fixation, 149-157
   alternative treatments, 149–150
   contraindications, 149
   indications, 149
   pitfalls and complications, avoiding, 155
   postoperative regimen, 154–155
   results, 150, 150*t*
   technique
      instruments/equipment/implants required, 151
      procedure, 151–154, 152*f*, 153*f*, 154*f*, 155*f*
      setup/exposure, 150–151, 151*f*
      wound closure, 154

C1-C2 transarticular screws, in occipitocervical fusion and fixation, 179

C2 fixation, posterior, 139-147
   alternative treatments, 140
   contraindications, 139–140
   indications, 139
   pitfalls and complications of, avoiding, 145–146
   postoperative regimen for, 145
   results, 140, 141*t*
   technique, 140–145

Carotid tubercle, 6

CAS. *See* Computer-assisted surgery

Central stenosis, minimally invasive decompression for, 505–506

Cervical approach
   for anterior cervicothoracic fusion, 64–65
   thoracic approach combined with, for anterior cervicothoracic fusion, 67–68

Cervical arthrodesis, posterior, 157

Cervical arthroplasty, 13-20
   alternative treatments, 13
   contraindications, 13, 14*t*
   indications, 13
   pitfalls and complications, avoiding, 18
   postoperative regimen, 18
   results, 13, 14*t*
   technique
      preoperative planning, 13–16, 15*t*
      procedure, 15*f*, 16–17, 16*f*, 17*f*
      setup/patient positioning, 16
   wound closure, 18

Cervical deformities, 196

Cervical fusion, 97–105
   cervical laminectomy and, 97–105
      alternative treatments, 97–98
      contraindications, 97
      indications, 97
      pitfalls and complications, avoiding, 103
      postoperative regimen, 103
      results, 98–99, 98*t*
      techniques, 99–103, 99*f*, 101*f*, 102*f*
   posterior subaxial, 89-96
      alternative treatments, 90
      contraindications, 89–90
      indications, 89
      pitfalls and complications, avoiding, 95, 95*f*
      postoperative regimen, 94
      results, 90, 90*t*
      techniques, 90–94
   procedure, 100–101, 102*f*

Cervical laminaplasty
   French door, 115–123
      alternative treatments, 115
      contraindications, 115
      indications, 115, 116*f*
      pitfalls and complications, avoiding, 121
      postoperative regimen, 120–121
      results, 115–116, 117*f*

technique, 116–120
    open-door, 107–113
        alternative treatments, 107–108
        contraindications, 107
        indications, 107, 108*f*
        pitfalls and complications, avoiding, 111–112
        postoperative regimen, 111, 112*f*
        results, 108, 109*t*
        techniques, 108–111
Cervical laminectomy
    cervical fusion and, 97–105
        alternative treatments, 97–98
        contraindications, 97
        indications, 97
        pitfalls and complications, avoiding, 103
        postoperative regimen, 103
        procedure, 100, 101*f*
        results, 98–99, 98*t*
        techniques, 99–103, 99*f*, 101*f*, 102*f*
Cervical osteotomy, 203–211
    alternative treatments, 203–204
    contraindications, 203
    indications, 203
    pitfalls and complications, avoiding, 208
    postoperative regimen, 208
    results, 204–205
    risks, 203
    technique
        instruments/equipment required, 206
        procedure, 206–207
        setup/exposure, 205–206
        wound closure, 207–208
Cervical pedicle screw fixation, 191-201
    alternative treatments, 191–192
    contraindications, 191
    indications, 191
    pitfalls and complications, avoiding, 199
    postoperative regimen, 199
    preoperative radiologic examination, 192–194
    results, 192, 192*t*
    screw placement, 195–197
    technique
        instruments/equipment/implants required, 195
        procedure, 195–197
        setup/exposure, 194–195, 194*f*, 195*f*
        wound closure, 197
Cervical radiculopathy, 81
Cervicothoracic fusion
    anterior, 63–70
        alternative treatments, 63
        contraindications, 63
        indications, 63
        pitfalls and complications, avoiding, 68–69
        postoperative regimen, 68
        results, 63, 64*t*
        techniques, 64–68

posterior, 183–189
        alternative treatments, 184
        contraindications, 183–184, 184*f*
        indications, 183–184, 184*f*
        pedicle screw placement, 186
        pitfalls and complications, avoiding, 187
        postoperative regimen, 187
        results, 184–185, 185*t*
        technique, 185–187, 186*f*, 187*f*
        wound closure, 187
Chromodiskography, 618, 619*f*
Clavicle-splitting approach for anterior cervicothoracic
    fusion, 65–66, 67*f*
Cobb angle, 288, 339
Complex lumbar pseudarthrosis, 571, 575
Computer-assisted surgery (CAS), 643–650
    contraindications, 643–644
    image acquisition, 645, 645*f*
    indications, 643
    instruments/equipment required, 645
    pitfalls and complications, avoiding, 647–649
    results, 644–645, 644*t*
    techniques, 645–647
        for navigation-assisted minimally invasive TLIF,
            645–646, 646*f*, 647*f*
        for percutaneous pedicle screw insertion, 646, 647*f*
        tomographic three-dimensional navigation, 646–647, 648*f*
Congenital atlantoaxial dislocation, 125
Corpectomy
    anterior lumbar, 425–433
        alternative treatments, 425
        contraindications, 425
        indications, 425, 426*f*, 427*f*
        pitfalls and complications, avoiding, 432–433
        postoperative regimen, 432
        results, 425–427, 428*t*
        technique, 427–432
    anterolateral, 430–431, 431*f*
    thoracoscopic, 319–329
        alternative treatments, 319
        contraindications, 319
        indications, 319, 320*f*
        partial, 325, 325*f*
        pitfalls and complications, avoiding, 327
        postoperative regimen, 327, 327*f*
        results, 319–320, 321*t*
        technique, 320–326
    transthoracic, open, 331–338
        alternative treatments, 331–332
        contraindications, 331
        indications, 331
        pitfalls and complications, avoiding, 336–337
        postoperative regimen, 336
        results, 332, 332*t*
        technique, 332–335

Costotransversectomy approach
  for thoracic diskectomy, 235, 237*f*, 239*f*
  for vertebrectomy, 243–251
    alternative treatments, 243
    contraindications, 243
    indications, 243
    pitfalls and complications, avoiding, 248–249
    postoperative regimen, 248
    results, 243–245, 244*f*, 244*t*
    technique, 245–248

D

DDD. *See* Degenerative disk disease
Decompression
  ACDF, 8
  bilateral, unilateral partial laminotomy for, 455–461
    alternative treatments, 455
    contraindications, 455
    indications, 455
    pitfalls and complications, avoiding, 459–460
    postoperative regimen, 459
    results, 455, 456*t*
    technique, 455–459
  minimally invasive, for central and subarticular stenosis, 505–506
Decompression and fusion
  minimally invasive lumbar, 493–499
    alternative treatments, 493
    contraindications, 493
    indications, 493, 494*f*
    pitfalls and complications, avoiding, 498
    postoperative regimen, 497–498
    procedure, 496
    results, 493–495, 494*t*
    technique, 495–497
  mini-open (Wiltse approach), 501–508
    alternative treatments, 501
    contraindications, 501
    indications, 501
    pitfalls and complications, avoiding, 507
    postoperative regimen, 506–507
    results, 501–504, 502*t*
    technique, 505–506
  for spondylolisthesis, 509–510
    alternative treatments, 510
    contraindications, 510
    indications, 509
    instruments/equipment/implants required, 511
    pitfalls and complications, avoiding, 513–514
    positioning/setup/exposure, 511, 511*f*
    procedure, 511–513
    results, 510–511, 510*t*
    technique, 511–513
    wound closure, 513

Deformities
  cervical, 196
  congenital, 309
  fixed flexion, 191, 197*f*
  sagittal, 277, 563, 564*f*
Deformity correction
  AIDSF, 339
  anterior mini-open approach for scoliosis, 345, 346*f*
  fusionless scoliosis surgery, 357
  principles of, 277–278
  revision, 265
Degenerative disk disease (DDD), 582, 627
  ALIF for, 405
Denis classification system, 380, 380*f*
DEXA scan, 627
Direct facet screw placement. *See* Facet screw placement
Diskectomy. *See also specific procedures*
  ACDF, 1–12
  anterior thoracoscopic, 309–317
    alternative treatments, 309–310
    contraindications, 309, 311*f*
    indications, 309, 310*f*
    instruments/equipment/implants required, 311–313
    pitfalls and complications, avoiding, 315
    postoperative regimen, 314–315
    procedure, 313–314, 313*f*, 314*f*
    results, 310–311, 312
    setup/exposure, 311, 312*f*
    technique, 311–314
    wound closure, 314, 315*f*
  PLF with/without, minimally invasive, 81–87
  posterior cervical, 71–79
    alternative treatments, 72
    contraindications, 72, 73*f*
    indications, 71, 71*f*, 72*f*
    results, 72–73, 74*t*
    surgical technique, 73–75
  posterior thoracic VCR, 269
  posterolateral endoscopic lumbar, 611–624
    alternative treatments, 612–613
    contraindications, 612
    indications, 611–612
    pitfalls and complications, avoiding, 622
    postoperative regimen, 620
    results, 613, 613*t*, 614*t*, 615*f*
    technique, 613–620
  retropharyngeal approaches to upper cervical spine, 47
  technique, 619–620, 620*f*, 621*f*, 622*f*
Disk herniations
  acute, 441
  imaging of, 441–442
  lumbar,.611
  thoracic, 303–304, 304*f*, 443*t*
Diskitis, 612
Diskography, provocative, in spinal surgery, 635–642
  alternative diagnostic methods, 637

anesthesia and positioning, 638
antibiotics, 638
assessment, 639
contraindications, 635–636
disk morphologic characteristics, 639, 640*f*
indications, 635, 635*t*, 636*t*
injection pressure, 639
instruments/equipment required, 638
pain response, 639
pitfalls and complications, avoiding, 640–641
positive test, criteria for, 639–640
postoperative regimen, 640
procedure, 638–640, 638*f*
results, 637–638, 637*t*
setup/exposure, 638
technique, 638–640
Dislocation(s)
congenital atlantoaxial, 125
spinopelvic junction fractures and, treatment of, 379–392
alternative treatments, 381
contraindications, 381
external fixation, 384–385
iliosacral screw fixation, percutaneous, 384, 384*f*
indications, 379
neural element decompression, 385
open reduction and fixation with plates and screws, 385
pitfalls and complications, avoiding, 388–389
procedure, 386–387, 386*f*, 387*f*, 388*f*
results, 382–383, 382*t*
segmental lumbopelvic fixation, 385
setup/exposure, 386
techniques, 383–388, 383*f*
wound closure, 387–388
Distraction-based growing spine implants, rib anchors in, 359-369
alternative treatments, 360–361, 360*f*
contraindications, 359
indications, 359
pitfalls and complications, avoiding, 367–368, 367*f*
postoperative regimen, 367
results, 361–362, 361*f*
technique
instruments/equipment/implants required, 363
procedure, 363–366, 363*f*, 364*f*, 365*f*, 366*f*, 367*f*
setup/exposure, 362–363
wound closure, 366–367
Dorsal root ganglion, 245
Double screws, pedicle screw fixation in osteoporotic bone, 628
Double thoracic curve, 287
Dual-energy x-ray absorptiometry (DEXA) scan, 627
Dynesys Dynamic Stabilization System, 599, 600*f*, 600*t*, 604
Dysesthesia, 622
Dysphagia, 10, 97

E

Electromyography (EMG), 282
Epidural injections. *See* Spinal epidural injections for spinal radiculopathy pain
Extreme lateral interbody fusion (XLIF), 407

F

Facetectomy, partial medial, 449, 450*f*
Facet screw placement, 549–555
direct, 549–555
alternative treatments, 550
contraindications, 549–550
indications, 549
pitfalls and complications, avoiding, 554
postoperative regimen, 554
results, 550, 550*t*, 551*t*
technique, 550–553
translaminar, 549–555
alternative treatments, 550
contraindications, 549–550
indications, 549
pitfalls and complications, avoiding, 554
postoperative regimen, 554
results, 550, 550*t*, 551*t*
technique, 550–553
Fixation. *See also specific fixation methods*
C1-C2, 159–166
alternative treatments, 159
coding, 166
contraindications, 159
indications, 159, 160*f*
pitfalls and complications, avoiding, 164–165
postoperative regimen, 164
results, 159–162, 160*t*, 161*f*
technique, 162–163
transarticular, 149–155
C2, posterior, 139–147
alternative treatments, 140
contraindications, 139–140
indications, 139
pitfalls and complications, avoiding, 145–146
postoperative regimen, 145
results, 117*t*, 140
technique, 140–145
rigid, techniques for posterior occipitocervical fusion, 132–133
sacroiliac, 581–588
alternative treatments, 582
anatomic zones, 583–586, 583*f*, 584*f*, 585*f*
contraindications, 582
indications, 581–582, 582*t*
instrumentation prominence and, 582
pitfalls and complications, avoiding, 586
postoperative regimen, 586

results, 582–583, 583*t*
technique, 583–586
segmental lumbopelvic, spinopelvic junction, 385
Fixed flexion deformity, 191, 197*f*
Fixed sagittal imbalance, 563, 564*f*
Foraminal stenosis, 441–442
Foraminotomy, 449–450, 451*f*. *See also*
Microforaminotomy, minimally invasive
lumbar, 435–439
alternative treatments, 435
contraindications, 435
indications, 435
pitfalls and complications, avoiding, 438
postoperative regimen, 438
results, 435, 436*f*
technique, 435–438
posterior cervical, 71–79
alternative treatments, 72
contraindications, 72, 73*f*
indications, 71, 71*f*, 72*f*
results, 72–73, 74*t*
surgical technique, 73–75
Fracture(s)
cementation, 656–658, 657*f*, 658*f*
posterior fixation of thoracolumbar burst, 371–377
alternative treatments, 372
contraindications, 372
indications, 371–372, 371*f*
pitfalls and complications, avoiding, 376, 376*f*
postoperative regimen, 376
results, 372, 373*t*
technique, 372–375
sacral, 380
spinopelvic junction dislocations and, treatment of, 379–392
alternative treatments, 381
contraindications, 381
external fixation, 384–385
iliosacral screw fixation, percutaneous, 384, 384*f*
indications, 379
neural element decompression, 385
open reduction and fixation with plates and screws, 385
pitfalls and complications, avoiding, 388–389
procedure, 386–387, 386*f*, 387*f*, 388*f*
results, 382–383, 382*t*
segmental lumbopelvic fixation, 385
setup/exposure, 386
techniques, 383–388, 383*f*
wound closure, 387–388
French door cervical laminaplasty, 115–123
alternative treatments, 115
contraindications, 115
indications, 115, 116*f*
pitfalls and complications, avoiding, 121
postoperative regimen, 120–121

results, 115–116, 117*f*
technique
exposure for, 118, 118*f*
instruments/equipment/implants required for, 118
procedure for, 119–120, 119*f*, 120*f*
setup/patient positioning for, 116–118
wound closure and, 120
Fusion. *See also specific fusion techniques*
anterior cervicothoracic, 63–70
alternative treatments, 63
contraindications, 63
indications, 63
pitfalls and complications, avoiding, 68–69
postoperative regimen, 68
results, 63, 64*t*
techniques, 64–68
C1-C2, 155
intervertebral, for lumbar pseudarthrosis, 575–576
lateral transpsoas approach for, 525-533
contraindications, 526
indications, 525–526, 526*f*
pitfalls and complications, avoiding, 531–532
postoperative regimen, 531
results, 526–527, 527*t*, 528*f*
technique, 527–531
mini-open (Wiltse approach) decompression and, 501–508
alternative treatments, 501
contraindications, 501
indications, 501
pitfalls and complications, avoiding, 507
postoperative regimen, 506–507
results, 501–504, 502*t*
technique, 505–506
open transthoracic, 331–337
posterior cervical, 105
posterolateral, for lumbar pseudarthrosis, 575–576
posterolateral, posterior pedicle screw fixation with, 463–470
sacropelvic, degenerative disorders that require, 582*t*
for spondylolisthesis, 509–516
alternative treatments, 510
contraindications, 510
indications, 509
instruments/equipment/implants required, 511
pitfalls and complications, avoiding, 513–514
positioning/setup/exposure, 511, 511*f*
procedure, 511–513
results, 510–511, 510*t*
technique, 511–513
wound closure, 513
thoracoscopic, 319–329
alternative treatments, 319
contraindications, 319
indications, 319, 320*f*
partial, 325, 325*f*

pitfalls and complications, avoiding, 327
postoperative regimen, 327, 327*f*
results, 319–320, 321*t*
surgical technique, 323–326
technique, 320–326
Fusionless scoliosis surgery, 351–358
alternative treatments, 353
contraindications, 353
criteria for, 352–353
indications, 351–352, 352*f*
pitfalls and complications, avoiding, 357
postoperative regimen, 357
progression and, 353
results, 353–354, 354*t*, 355*f*
risk-benefit ratio, 351–352
skeletal maturity and, 353
technique
deformity correction, 357
implantation, 356, 356*f*
instruments/equipment/implants required, 355–356
setup/exposure, 354–355, 355*f*
wound closure, 357

G

Graf Artificial Ligament System, 599, 599*f*, 600*t*, 604
Graft(s)
ACDF, 6–7
harvest-site complications, 9
bone
for spondylolisthesis, 512–513, 512*f*, 513*f*
for vertebral body replacement, 325
options
ACDF, 6–7
keystone, 8
Smith-Robinson, 8
selection, for posterior occipitocervical fusion, 133

H

Hydroxyapatite (HA)-coated screws, 629

I

IAR, 581
Idiopathic scoliosis, 351–352, 352*f*
Iliosacral screw fixation, 383
percutaneous, 384, 384*f*
Infection, PSO and, 285
Injection pressure, in provocative diskography, 641
Instability, following thoracic diskectomy, 240–241
Instantaneous axis of rotation (IAR), 581
Interbody fusion
ALIF with plating, 409, 409*f*
lumbar
minimally invasive, 493–499

posterior transsacral, 535–541
lumbosacral spine, Bohlman fibular technique for, 517–523
alternative treatments, 517–519
contraindications, 517
indications, 517, 517*f*
pitfalls and complications, avoiding, 521
postoperative regimen, 521
results, 518*t*, 519
technique, 519–520
for spondylolisthesis, 512, 513, 513*f*
Intercostal neuralgia, as complication of posterolateral approach for thoracic diskectomy, 240
Interspinous spacers in lumbar spine, 557–562
alternative treatments, 558
contraindications, 557–558
indications, 557, 558*f*
instruments/equipment/implants required, 559
pitfalls and complications, avoiding, 560, 561*f*
postoperative regimen, 560
procedure, 559, 559*f*, 560*f*, 561*f*
results, 558, 558*t*
setup/exposure, 558, 559*f*
technique, 558–559
wound closure, 559
Intervertebral fusion, 575–576

J

Jefferson fracture, 139, 159

K

King classification of thoracic curves, 287–288
type II, 287, 292*f*
type III, 290
type IV, 287
Kyphoplasty
advantages and disadvantages, 651
alternative treatments, 652
balloon, 629
contraindications, 651
indications, 651
pitfalls and complications, avoiding, 657–658
postoperative regimen, 657
results
adjacent-level fracture risk, 652–654
vertebral augmentation, 652
technique
approach tips, 654–656, 655*f*, 656*f*
bone tamp inflation, 656, 656*f*
fracture cementation, 656, 657*f*
instruments and equipment, 656
positioning and setup, 654, 655*f*
preoperative workup, 654, 654*f*

lumbar, 563–570
    alternative treatments, 563
    contraindications, 563
    indications, 563, 564*f*
    pitfalls and complications, avoiding, 568
    postoperative regimen, 568
    results, 563, 564*t*
    technique, 565–568
posterior thoracic, Smith-Petersen approach, 253–263
    alternative treatments, 254
    coding, 262–263
    complications, 256
    contraindications, 254
    indications, 253, 254*f*
    pitfalls and complications, avoiding, 259
    postoperative regimen, 259, 260*f*
    results, 255–256, 255*t*
    technique, 256–259, 257*f*
posterior thoracic VCR, 267
PSO, 277
    pitfalls and complications, avoiding, 284
Smith-Petersen, 253–568

P

Pain
    response, in provocative diskography, 639
    spinal radiculopathy, spinal epidural injections for,
        661–667
        alternative treatments, 662
        contraindications, 661
        indications, 661
        pitfalls and complications, avoiding, 664–666
        postoperative regimen, 664
        results, 662, 662*t*–663*t*
        technique, 663–664, 662*t*–663*t*, 664*f*, 665*f*
Pars repair, 543–548
    alternative treatments, 543
    contraindications, 543
    indications, 543, 544*f*
    pitfalls and complications, avoiding, 547
    postoperative regimen, 546
    results, 544, 544*t*
    technique
        exposure, 544–545, 545*f*
        procedure, 545, 545*f*, 546*f*
        wound closure, 545–546
Pars screws, posterior C2 fixation and placement of, 142–
    144, 143*f*, 144*f*
PCD. *See* Posterior cervical diskectomy
Pedicle, morphology of, 192–193, 193*f*
Pedicle-based posterior dynamic stabilization, 599–610
    alternative treatments, 601
    contraindications, 601
    indications, 599, 599*f*, 600*f*
    pitfalls and complications, avoiding, 608

postoperative regimen, 607
results, 600*t*, 604
technique
    decompression, 604, 604*f*
    implants and implant insertion, 604–607, 605*f*,
        606*f*, 607*f*, 608*f*
    setup/exposure, 604, 604*f*, 605*f*
    wound closure, 607
Pedicle screw(s)
    C2 fixation and placement of, 142–144, 143*f*, 144*f*
    for cervical laminectomy and fusion, 102
    expandable, 628
    insertion of in occipitocervical fusion, 178–179
    placement of in posterior cervicothoracic fusion, 186
    posterior thoracic VCR correction with, 269–270
Pedicle screw fixation
    cervical, 191–201
        alternative treatments, 191–192
        computer-assisted screw insertion, 197
        contraindications, 191
        indications, 191
        longitudinal connection using plate/rod, 197, 197*f*,
            198*f*
        manual screw insertion, 195–197, 195*f*, 196*f*, 197*f*
        pitfalls and complications, avoiding, 199
        postoperative regimen, 199
        preoperative radiologic examination, 192–194
        results, 192, 192*t*
        screw placement, 195–197
        technique, 194–197
    in osteoporotic bone, 627–634
        alternative treatments, 627–629
        concurrent vertebroplasty, 629
        contraindications, 627, 628*f*
        coupler connections for, 629
        CPC for, 628
        double screws for, 629
        HA-coated screws for, 629
        indications, 627
        instruments/implants/equipment required, 629
        kyphoplasty, 629
        laminar hooks for, 628
        novel screws for, 629
        pitfalls and complications, avoiding, 632
        postoperative regimen, 631–632
        procedure, 631–632, 632*f*
        results, 629, 630*t*
        setup and exposure, 631
        sublaminar wires for, 628
        techniques, 629, 631
        wound closure, 631
    percutaneous, in lumbar spine, 471–476
        alternative treatments, 471
        contraindications, 471
        indications, 471
        pitfalls and complications, avoiding, 475

postoperative regimen, 475
results, 472, 472*t*
technique, 472–475
  posterior, with posterolateral fusion, 463–470
    alternative treatments, 464
    contraindications, 463, 463*f*
    indications, 463
    pitfalls and complications, avoiding, 468–469, 469*f*
    postoperative regimen, 468
    results, 464, 465*t*
    technique, 464–468
  thoracic, 221–229
    alternative treatments, 221
    contraindications, 221
    examples of, 222*f*
    indications, 221
    pitfalls and complications, avoiding, 227, 227*f*
    postoperative regimen, 226–227
    results, 221–223
    technique, 223–226
Pedicle screw placement in spondylolisthesis, 512–513, 514*f*
Pedicle subtraction osteotomy (PSO)
  lumbar, 563–570
    alternative treatments, 563
    complications, 563
    contraindications, 563
    indications, 563
    pitfalls and complications, avoiding, 568
    postoperative regimen, 568
    procedure, 565–568, 566*f*, 567*f*
    results, 563, 564*t*
    technique, 565–568
  thoracic, 277–281
    alternative treatments, 279
    complications, 279, 280*t*
    contraindications, 278
    indications, 277–278, 277*f*, 279*f*
    osteotomy level and, 277, 284
    pitfalls and complications, avoiding
      blood loss, 285
      infection, 285
      neurologic injury, 284–285
      osteotomy level, 284
      pseudarthrosis, 285
    postoperative regimen, 284, 284*f*
    results, 279, 280*t*
    techniques
      instruments/equipment/implants required, 282
      procedure, 282–283, 282*f*
      setup and patient positioning, 282
      wound closure, 283–284
PEEK (polyetheretherketone) cages, 4, 267
Percutaneous pedicle screw fixation in lumbar spine, 471–476
  alternative treatments, 471

contraindications, 471
indications, 471
pitfalls and complications, avoiding, 475
postoperative regimen, 475
results, 472, 472*t*
technique
  instruments/equipment/implants required, 472
  procedure, 473–474, 474*f*, 475*f*
  setup/exposure, 472, 473*f*
  wound closure, 474–475
using CAS, 645–647
Pleural defects, as complication in posterolateral approaches, 240
Pleural dissection, in anterior thoracoscopy for diskectomy, 313, 313*f*
PLF. *See* Posterior laminoforaminotomy
PLIF. *See* Posterior lumbar interbody fusion
PMMA (polymethyl methacrylate), 426, 651
Polyetheretherketone (PEEK) cages, 4, 267
Polymethyl methacrylate (PMMA), 426, 651
Posterior C2 fixation, 139–147
  alternative treatments, 140
  contraindications, 139–140
  indications, 139
  pitfalls and complications of, avoiding, 145–146
  postoperative regimen, 145
  results, 140, 141*t*
  technique
    instruments/equipment/implements for, 142
    placement of C2 laminar screws, 144–145, 145*f*
    placement of C2 pedicle, pars screws, 142–144, 143*f*, 144*f*
    procedure, 142–145, 143*f*, 144*f*, 145*f*
    setup/exposure, 140–142, 141*f*
    wound closure, 145
Posterior cervical arthrodesis, 157
Posterior cervical diskectomy (PCD), minimally invasive, 81–88
  access, 83–84, 83*f*
  access complications, 86
  alternative treatments, 81
  contraindications, 81
  decompression complications, 86–87
  indications, 81
  instruments/equipment required, 82–83, 83*f*
  open PLF compared with, 82–83
  PCD procedure and, 84–86, 86*f*
  pitfalls and complications, avoiding, 86–87
  postoperative regimen, 86
  procedure, 83–86, 83*f*, 85*f*, 86*f*
  results, 81–82, 82*t*
  setup/patient positioning, 83
  techniques, 82–86
  wound closure, 86
Posterior cervical foraminotomy and diskectomy, 71–79
  alternative treatments, 72

contraindications, 72, 73*f*

indications, 71, 71*f*, 72*f*

results, 72–73, 74*t*

surgical technique

    instruments/equipment/implants required, 73–74

    pitfalls and complications, avoiding, 77

    postoperative regimen, 77

    procedure, 74–75, 75*f*, 76*f*, 77*f*

    setup/exposure, 73, 75*f*

    wound closure, 75

Posterior cervical lateral mass fusion, minimally invasive, 213–218

alternative treatments, 213

contraindications, 213

indications, 213

instruments/equipment/implants required, 214–215

pitfalls and complications of, avoiding, 217

postoperative regimen, 216–217

procedure, 215–216, 215*f*, 216*f*

results, 213–214, 214*t*

setup/exposure, 214

techniques, 214–216

wound closure, 216, 216*f*

Posterior cervical wiring, 167–172

alternative treatments, 167–168, 167*f*, 168*f*

contraindications, 167

indications, 167

pitfalls and complications, avoiding, 172

postoperative regimen, 170

results, 168, 168*t*

techniques

    instruments/equipment/implants required, 169

    procedure, 169–170, 169*f*, 170*f*, 171*f*

    setup/exposure, 168–169

    wound closure, 170

Posterior cervicothoracic fusion, 183–189

alternative treatments, 184

contraindications, 184

indications, 183

pedicle screw placement, 186

pitfalls and complications, avoiding, 187

postoperative regimen, 187

results, 184–185, 185*t*

technique, 185–187, 186*f*, 187*f*

wound closure, 187

Posterior fixation of thoracolumbar burst fractures. *See* Thoracolumbar burst fractures, posterior fixation of

Posterior laminoforaminotomy (PLF)

with/without diskectomy, minimally invasive, 81–88

    access, 83–84, 83*f*

    access complications, 86

    alternative treatments, 81

    contraindications, 81

    decompression complications, 86–87

    indications, 81

    instruments/equipment required, 82–83, 83*f*

    open PLF compared with, 82–83

    PCD procedure and, 84–86, 86*f*

    pitfalls and complications, avoiding, 86–87

    postoperative regimen, 86

    procedure, 83–86, 83*f*, 85*f*, 86*f*

    results, 81–82, 82*t*

    setup/patient positioning, 83

    techniques, 82–86

    wound closure, 86

open, minimally invasive PLF compared with, 82–83

Posterior lumbar interbody fusion (PLIF), 477–484

as alternative to ALIF, 406

alternative treatments, 478

contraindications, 478

indications, 477–478, 477*f*

pitfalls and complications, avoiding, 482

postoperative regimen, 481–482

results, 479, 479*t*

technique

    procedure, 479–480, 480*f*, 481*f*, 482*f*

    setup/exposure, 479

    wound closure, 481

Posterior occipitocervical fusion, 125–138

alternative treatments, 127, 128*t*

contraindications, 126–127

indications, 125–126, 126*f*

pitfalls and complications, avoiding, 135–136, 136*f*

postoperative regimen, 135

results, 127, 128*f*

techniques

    equipment/instruments/implants required, 130

    exposure, 131

    procedure, 131

    setup, 130–131

    surgical options, 127–130

    wound closure, 134

Posterior pedicle screw fixation with posterolateral fusion, 463–470

alternative treatments, 464

contraindications, 463, 463*f*

indications, 463

pitfalls and complications, avoiding, 468–469, 469*f*

postoperative regimen, 468

results, 464, 465*t*

technique

    instruments/equipment/implants required, 464–466, 466*f*

    procedure, 466–467, 467*f*

    setup/exposure, 464, 466*f*

    wound closure, 467–468

Posterior subaxial cervical fusion, 89–96

alternative treatments, 90

contraindications, 89–90

indications, 89

pitfalls and complications, avoiding, 95, 95*f*

postoperative regimen, 94

results, 90, 90*t*

techniques
    procedure, 91–94, 92*f*, 93*f*, 94*f*
    setup/exposure, 90–91, 91*f*, 92*f*
    wound closure, 94
Posterior thoracic osteotomy: Smith-Petersen approach, 253–263
    alternative treatments, 254
    complications, 256
    contraindications, 254
    indications, 253, 254*f*
    pitfalls and complications, avoiding, 259
    postoperative regimen, 259, 260*f*
    results, 255–256, 255*t*
    technique
        angular correction, 258–259, 258*f*
        exposure, 256
        fusion, 259
        osteotomies, 256, 257*f*
        positioning/setup, 256
        posterior instrumentation, 256
        wound closure, 259
Posterior thoracic VCR, 265–275
    alternative treatments, 265
    contraindications, 265
    correction, 269–270
    diskectomy, 269
    indications, 265
    pitfalls and complications, avoiding, 271, 272*f*, 273*f*
    posterior osteotomy, 267
    postoperative regimen, 271
    results, 265–266, 266*t*
    technique
        instruments/equipment/implants required, 266–267
        procedure, 267–271, 268*f*, 269*f*, 270*f*, 272*f*
        setup/exposure, 266
        wound closure, 271
Posterior transsacral lumbar interbody fusion, 535–541
    alternative treatments, 535–536
    contraindications, 535
    indications, 535
    pitfalls and complications, avoiding, 540
    postoperative regimen, 540
    results, 536–537, 536*t*
    technique
        instruments/equipment/implants required, 537
        procedure, 537–539, 537*f*, 538*f*, 539*f*
        setup/exposure, 537
        wound closure, 539
Posterolateral approaches for thoracic diskectomy. *See* Thoracic diskectomy, posterolateral approaches for
Posterolateral endoscopic lumbar diskectomy. *See* Lumbar diskectomy, posterolateral endoscopic
Posterolateral fusion, lumbar pseudarthrosis and, 575–576
Posterolateral fusion, posterior pedicle screw fixation with. *See* Posterior pedicle screw fixation with posterolateral fusion

Provocative diskography in spinal surgery. *See* Diskography, provocative, in spinal surgery
Pseudarthrosis, lumbar, 571–579
    alternative treatments, 573
    atrophic, 571
    complex, 571
    contraindications, 571–573
    imaging, 571, 572*f*
    indications, 571
    intervertebral fusion, 575–576
    patterns, 571
    pitfalls and complications, avoiding, 576–577
    posterolateral fusion, 575–576
    postoperative regimen, 576
    results, 573, 574*t*
    shingle, 571
    technique, 573–576
    transverse, 571
Pseudarthrosis, thoracic, PSO and, 285
PSO. *See* Pedicle subtraction osteotomy

R

RA (rheumatoid arthritis), 125, 159
Radiculopathy
    cervical, 13, 81
    epidural injections for, 663–669
Radiologic examination, preoperative, for cervical pedicle screw fixation
    morphology of pedicle, 192–193, 193*f*
    neural foramina, preoperative morphology of, 194
Recombinant human bone morphogenetic protein 2 (rhBMP-2), 4
Reduction, of spondylolisthesis, 509–516
    alternative treatments, 510
    contraindications, 510
    indications, 509
    instruments/equipment/implants required, 511
    pitfalls and complications, avoiding, 513–514
    positioning/setup/exposure, 511, 511*f*
    procedure, 511–512, 511–513, 512*f*
    results, 510–511, 510*t*
    technique, 511–513
    wound closure, 513
Retropharyngeal approaches to upper cervical spine, 43–53
    alternative treatments, 43
    anterior approach, 45–47, 46*f*, 47*f*, 48*f*
    contraindications, 43
    diskectomy, 47
    dissection, 46–47
    indications, 43
    instruments/equipment/implants required, 44–45
    lateral approach, 47–48, 49*f*
    pitfalls and complications, avoiding, 49–50
    postoperative regimen, 49

procedure, 45, 45*f*
results, 43, 44*t*
setup/exposure, 43–44, 44*f*
technique, 43–48
wound closure, 48
rhBMP-2 (recombinant human bone morphogenetic
protein 2), 4
Rheumatoid arthritis (RA), 125, 159
Rib(s), spine hooks on, 360
Rib anchors, in distraction-based growing spine implants,
359–369
alternative treatments, 360–361, 360*f*
contraindications, 359
indications, 359
pitfalls and complications, avoiding, 367–368, 367*f*
postoperative regimen, 367
results, 361–362, 361*f*
technique, 362–367
Risser grade, 288
Roy-Camille subclassification, 380, 380*f*

S

Sacral fractures, 380
Sacroiliac fixation, 581-588
alternative treatments, 582
contraindications, 582
indications, 581–582, 582*t*
instrumentation prominence and, 582
pitfalls and complications, avoiding, 586
postoperative regimen, 586
results, 582–583, 583*t*
technique
anatomic zones, 583–584, 583*f*
instruments/equipment/implants required, 584
procedure, 584–586
setup/exposure, 584
wound closure, 586
Sacropelvis, degenerative disorders requiring fusion to,
582*t*
Sagittal deformity, 277, 563, 564*f*
Sagittal imbalance, fixed, 563, 564*f*
Scoliosis
anterior mini-open approach for, 339–350
alternative treatments, 339–340
contraindications, 339, 340*f*
indications, 339
pitfalls and complications, avoiding, 346
postoperative regimen, 345–346
results, 340, 341*t*
technique, 340–345
fusionless, 351–358
alternative treatments, 353
contraindications, 353
curves and, 352–353
indications, 351–352, 352*f*

pitfalls and complications, avoiding, 357
postoperative regimen, 357
progression and, 353
results, 353–354, 354*t*, 355*f*
risk-benefit ratio, 351–352
skeletal maturity and, 353
technique, 354–357
idiopathic, 351–352, 352*f*
lumbar, 589–597
alternative treatments, 589–590
clinical presentation, 589
contraindications, 589
indications, 589, 590*f*
pitfalls and complications, avoiding, 594–595, 595*f*
postoperative regimen, 593–594
results, 590–591, 592*t*
technique, 591–593
thoracic, surgical treatment of, 287–301
alternative treatments, 288
contraindications, 288
indications, 287–288
pitfalls and complications, avoiding, 301
postoperative regimen, 300–301
results, 288
technique, 288–300
Segmental lumbopelvic fixation, 385
Segmental screws, occipitocervical fusion fixation of
C1-C2, 179
Shingle pseudarthrosis, 571
lumbar, 575
Single thoracic curve, 287
Skeletal maturity
fusionless scoliosis surgery and, 353
thoracic curves and, 287–288
surgical treatment of, 293, 296*f*, 297*f*
Smith-Petersen approach for posterior thoracic osteotomy.
See Posterior thoracic osteotomy: Smith-Petersen
approach
Smith-Petersen osteotomies (SPOs), 253, 568
Smith-Robinson graft, 5*t*, 8
Somatosensory-evoked potentials (SSEPs), 266, 282
Spinal cord ischemia, as complication in thoracic
diskectomy, 241
Spinal epidural injections for lumbar spinal radiculopathy
pain, 661-667
alternative treatments, 662
contraindications, 661
indications, 661
pitfalls and complications, avoiding, 664–666
postoperative regimen, 664
results, 662–663, 662*t*
technique
instruments/equipment/required, 663, 665*t*
procedure, 663–664, 664*f*, 665*f*

Spinal radiculopathy pain, lumbar, spinal epidural
injections for. *See* Spinal epidural injections for lumbar
spinal radiculopathy pain
Spine hooks, 360
Spinopelvic junction fractures and dislocations, treatment
of, 379–392
alternative treatments, 381
contraindications, 381
external fixation, 384–385
iliosacral screw fixation, percutaneous, 384, 384*f*
indications, 379
neural element decompression, 385
open fixation with plates and screws, 385
open reduction with plates and screws, 385
pitfalls and complications, avoiding, 388–389
procedure, 386–387, 386*f*, 387*f*, 388*f*
results, 382–383, 382*t*
segmental lumbopelvic fixation, 385
setup/exposure, 386
techniques, 383–388, 383*f*
wound closure, 387–388
Spondylolisthesis, decompression/fusion and possible
reduction, 509-516
alternative treatments, 510
bone grafting, disk-space preparation for, 512, 512*f*,
513*f*
contraindications, 510
decompression, 509–514
indications, 509
instruments/equipment/implants required, 511
interbody implant/grafting material insertion for, 513,
513*f*
lumbosacral, 517
pedicle screw placement, 512-514, 514*f*
pitfalls and complications, avoiding, 513–514
positioning/setup/exposure, 511, 511*f*
procedure, 511–513, 512*f*
results, 510–511, 510*t*
technique, 511–513
wound closure, 513
Spondylosis, cervical, 125–126
SPOs (Smith-Petersen osteotomies), 253, 568
SSEPs (somatosensory-evoked potentials), 266, 282
Stenosis
central, minimally invasive decompression for, 505–506
foraminal, 441–442
lumbar spine, 447
subarticular, minimally invasive decompression for,
505–506
Sternocleidomastoid muscle (SCM), 5
Sternum-splitting approach, for anterior cervicothoracic
fusion, 63, 65, 66*f*, 67*f*
Strange-Vognsen subclassification, 380, 380*f*
Supraclavicular approach, for anterior cervicothoracic
fusion, 65

T
TDR (total disk replacement), 415
Thoracic curve
adult *v.* teenage, 293, 296*f*, 297*f*
double, 287, 290–293
false double major, surgical treatment of, 290, 292*f*
King type II, 287, 290, 292*f*
King type IV, 287, 293
single, 287, 288–290, 291*f*
stiff, 293–299
Thoracic diskectomy, posterolateral approaches for,
231–242
alternative treatments, 231
complications associated with, 234*t*
contraindications for, 231, 232*t*
costotransversectomy approach to, 235, 237*f*, 239*f*
CSF leakage during, 240
inadequate decompression during, 240
indications for, 231, 232*f*
intercostal neuralgia and, 240
lateral extracavitary approach to, 239
misidentification of surgical level and, 240
modified transfacet (pedicle-sparing) approach to,
234–235
mortality and neurologic deterioration by, 232*t*
pitfalls and complications, avoiding, 240–241
pleural defects and, 240
postoperative instability, 240–241
postoperative regimen, 240
results, 231–233, 233*t*, 234*t*
spinal cord ischemia, 241
techniques, 234–239
transpedicular approach to, 235
Thoracic disk excision, 313, 314*f*
Thoracic disk herniations, 303, 304*f*
natural history, 303–304
treatment, anterior approach to, 304, 305*t*
Thoracic pedicle screw fixation, 221–229
alternative treatments, 221
contraindications, 221
examples of, 222*f*
indications, 221
pitfalls and complications, avoiding, 227, 227*f*
postoperative regimen, 226–227
results, 221–223
biomechanical data and, 223, 223*t*
clinical outcomes in, 223
radiographic data and, 223, 224*t*
technique
correction and, 226
instruments/equipment required, 224–225
palpation and, 225*f*, 226
pedicle probing and, 225–226, 225*f*
procedure, 225–226
screw placement confirmation and, 226
setup/exposure, 223–224, 225*f*

starting point creation/identification and, 225–226, 225*f*

   tapping and, 225*f*, 226

   wound closure, 226

Thoracic scoliosis, surgical treatment of, 287-302

   alternative treatments, 288

   anterior surgery, 293, 294*f*, 295*f*

   contraindications, 288

   general concepts, 288

   indications, 287

   instrumentation, 299

   large magnitude curves, 293–299, 298*f*

   pitfalls and complications, avoiding, 301

   postoperative regimen, 300–301

   procedure, 299–300, 300*f*

   results, 288

   setup, 299

   skeletal maturity and, 293, 296*f*, 297*f*

   stiff curves, 293–299, 298*f*

   technique, 288–300

   thoracoplasty, 293

   wound closure, 300

Thoracolumbar burst fractures, posterior fixation of, 371–377

   alternative treatments, 372

   contraindications, 372

   fusion and wound closure, 374–375

   indications, 371–372, 371*f*

   instruments/equipment/implants required, 373, 374*f*

   pitfalls and complications, avoiding, 376, 376*f*

   postoperative regimen, 376

   procedure, 373–374, 374*f*, 375*f*

   results, 372, 373*t*

   setup/exposure, 372

   technique, 372–375

Thoracolumbosacral orthosis (TLSO), 371

Thoracoplasty, 293

Thoracoscopic corpectomy and fusion, 319–329

   alternative treatments, 319

   contraindications, 319

   indications, 319, 320*f*

   partial, 325, 325*f*

   pitfalls and complications, avoiding, 327

   postoperative regimen, 327, 327*f*

   results, 319–320, 321*t*

   technique

      anterior instrumentation, 326, 326*f*

      bone grafting, 325

      decompression, 325, 325*f*

      general principles, 322–323

      instruments/equipment/implants required, 320–321

      landmarks, 323–325, 324*f*

      patient positioning, 321–322, 322*f*

      portal placement and approach, 323, 323*f*, 324*f*

      vertebral body replacement, 325–326, 326*f*

      wound closure, 326, 327*f*

Thoracoscopic diskectomy, anterior. *See* Anterior thoracoscopic diskectomy and release

TLIF. *See* Transforaminal lumbar interbody fusion

TLSO (thoracolumbosacral orthosis), 371

Total disk arthroplasty, 407

Total disk replacement (TDR), 415

Transarticular fixation, C1-C2, 149–155

   alternative treatments, 149–150

   contraindications, 149

   indications, 149

   pitfalls and complications, avoiding, 155

   postoperative regimen, 154–155

   results, 150, 150*t*

   technique, 150–154

Transarticular screws, 149, 153–154

   occipitocervical fusion fixation of C1-C2, 179

Transcranial motor-evoked potentials, 266

Transforaminal lumbar interbody fusion (TLIF), 406, 478, 485–491, 501, 525, 535, 581, 582, 645

   alternative treatments, 485

   contraindications, 485

   indications, 485

   minimally invasive, 501

      exposure, 504

      instruments/equipment/implants required, 504

      patient positioning, 504

      procedure, 504–505, 505*f*, 506*f*

      surgical technique for navigation-assisted, 645–646, 646*f*, 647*f*

      technique, 504–505

      wound closure, 505

   pitfalls and complications, avoiding, 490

   postoperative regimen, 489–490

   results, 485, 486*f*

   techniques

      instruments/equipment/implants required, 486–487

      procedure, 487, 487*f*, 488*f*, 489*f*

      setup/patient positioning, 485–486

      wound closure, 487–489

Translaminar facet screw placement. *See* Facet screw placement

Transoral odontoid excision. *See* Odontoid excision, transoral

Transpedicular approach, posterolateral approaches for thoracic diskectomy, 235

Transsacral lumbar interbody fusion, posterior. *See* Posterior trassacral lumbar interbody fusion

Transthoracic corpectomy, open. *See* Open transthoracic corpectomy

Transthoracic diskectomy, anterior approach, 303–308

   alternative treatments, 303–304

   contraindications, 303

   indications, 303

   instrument/equipment required, 305–306

   pitfalls and complications, avoiding, 307

   postoperative regimen, 307

procedure, 306
results, 304, 305*t*
role of fusion, 306
setup/exposure/patient positioning, 304–305, 306*f*
technique, 304–306
wound closure, 306
Transthoracic fusion, open. *See* Open transthoracic fusion
Transverse pseudarthrosis, 571
lumbar, 574–575, 575*f*

U

Unilateral partial laminotomy (laminaplasty) for bilateral decompression, 455–461
alternative treatments, 455
contraindications, 455
indications, 455
pitfalls and complications, avoiding, 459–460
postoperative regimen, 459
procedure, 456–458
results, 455, 456*t*
setup/exposure, 455–456, 456*f*
technique, 455–459
wound closure, 459, 460*f*
Upper cervical spine
anatomy, 31
retropharyngeal approaches to, 43–53

V

VCFs. *See* Vertebral compression fractures
VCR. *See* Vertebral column resection
VEPTR (Vertical Expandable Prosthetic Titanium Rib), 351, 360
Vertebral artery
cervical pedicle screw fixation and, 193–194, 194*f*
injury to, 10
MRA and, 193–194, 194*f*
Vertebral augmentation, 652, 653*t*
Vertebral body replacement
thoracoscopic corpectomy, 325–326, 326*f*
thoracoscopic fusion, 325–326, 326*f*
Vertebral column resection (VCR), posterior thoracic, 265–275
alternative treatments, 265
contraindications, 265
correction, 269–270
diskectomy, 269
indications, 265
pitfalls and complications, avoiding, 271, 272*f*, 273*f*
posterior osteotomy, 267
postoperative regimen, 271
results, 265–266, 266*t*
technique, 266–271
Vertebral compression fractures (VCFs), 651
adjacent-level, 654

nonsurgical treatments for, 652
surgical alternatives for treatment of, 652
Vertebrectomy, costotransversectomy approach for, 243–251
alternative treatments, 243
contraindications, 243
indications, 243
pitfalls and complications, avoiding, 248–249
postoperative regimen, 248
results, 243–245, 244*f*, 244*t*
technique, 245–248
instruments/equipment/implants required, 245
procedure, 245–247, 245*f*, 246*f*, 247*f*, 248*f*, 249*f*
setup/exposure, 245
wound closure, 247–248
Vertebroplasty, 629, 651–660
alternative treatments, 652
contraindications, 651
indications, 651
pitfalls and complications, avoiding, 657–658
postoperative regimen, 657
results
adjacent-level fracture risk, 652–654
vertebral augmentation, 653*t*, 654
technique
approach tips, 654–656, 655*f*, 656*f*
bone tamp inflation, 656-657, 657*f*
fracture cementation, 656, 657*f*
instruments and equipment, 654
positioning and setup, 654, 655*f*
preoperative workup, 654, 654*f*
Vertical Expandable Prosthetic Titanium Rib (VEPTR), 351, 360

W

Wiltse approach. *See* Mini-open decompression/fusion
Wiring, 167–172
posterior cervical
alternative treatments to, 167–168, 167*f*, 168*f*
contraindications, 167
indications, 167
pitfalls and complications, avoiding, 172
postoperative regimen, 170
results, 168, 168*t*
techniques, 168–170
for posterior occipitocervical fusion, 131–132, 132*f*
for posterior subaxial cervical fusion, 92–93, 93*f*

X

XLIF (Extreme lateral interbody fusion), 407

Z

Zones, anatomic, of the pelvic region, 583–584, 583*f*, fixation of, 584–586